Brain Tumor Imaging

Rajan Jain, MD
Associate Professor, Radiology
Division of Neuroradiology
NYU Langone Medical Center
Clinical Co-Director
Center for Advanced Imaging Innovation and Research
New York University School of Medicine
New York, New York

Marco Essig, MD, PhD, FRCPC
Professor and Chairman
Department of Radiology
University of Manitoba
Medical Director
Winnipeg Regional Health Authority
Winnipeg, Manitoba, Canada

Thieme
New York • Stuttgart • Delhi • Rio de Janeiro

Executive Editor: William Lamsback
Managing Editor: J. Owen Zurhellen IV
Director, Editorial Services: Mary Jo Casey
Production Editor: Sean Woznicki
International Production Director: Andreas Schabert
Vice President, Editorial and E-Product
    Development: Vera Spillner
International Marketing Director: Fiona Henderson
International Sales Director: Louisa Turrell
Director of Sales, North America: Mike Roseman
Senior Vice President and Chief Operating
    Officer: Sarah Vanderbilt
President: Brian D. Scanlan
Printer: Asia Pacific Offset

Library of Congress Cataloging-in-Publication Data

Brain tumor imaging / [edited by] Rajan Jain, Marco Essig.
    p. ; cm.
    ISBN 978-1-60406-806-1 (hardcover) –
ISBN 978-1-60406-830-6 (e-book)
    I. Jain, Rajan, editor. II. Essig, Marco, editor.
    [DNLM: 1. Brain Neoplasms–diagnosis. 2. Brain Neoplasms–
genetics. 3. Diagnostic Imaging–methods. 4. Molecular Imaging–
trends. 5. Neuroimaging. WL 358]
    RC280.B7
616.99'481–dc23   2014026267

© 2016 Thieme Medical Publishers, Inc.

Thieme Publishers New York
333 Seventh Avenue, New York, NY 10001 USA, 1-800-782-3488
customerservice@thieme.com

Thieme Publishers Stuttgart
Rüdigerstrasse 14, 70469 Stuttgart, Germany, +49 [0]711 8931 421
customerservice@thieme.de

Thieme Publishers Delhi
A-12, Second Floor, Sector -2, Noida -201301, Uttar Pradesh, India,
+91 120 45 566 00
customerservice@thieme.in

Thieme Publishers Rio de Janeiro, Thieme Publicações Ltda.
Argentina Building 16th floor, Ala A, 228 Praia do Botafogo
Rio de Janeiro 22250-040 Brazil, +55 21 3736-3631

Printed in China   5 4 3 2 1

ISBN 978-1-60406-806-1

Also available as an e-book:
eISBN 978-1-60406-830-6

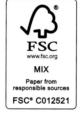

We dedicate this book to our patients, with gratitude.

I would like to dedicate this book also to my parents and the rest of my family, especially my wife Ruchika for helping me balance a prosperous and fulfilling professional life with a happy and healthy family life.

– RJ

I would like to dedicate this book also to my family: my children Nicolai, Alicia, and Luca; and especially my wife Jutta; for their love and their continuous support in both my professional and personal life.

– ME

Contents

Foreword

Rajan Jain and Marco Essig are to be complimented for putting together a superb text on brain tumor imaging. I was particularly impressed with the international list of authors since practice patterns tend to vary somewhat by region. So this text really gives a worldwide perspective. Of course this would be expected of Professor Essig as he has spent time in Germany, Iowa, and is now Chair at the University of Manitoba which I understand is somewhat north and colder than where I reside in San Diego (sorry Marco).

As would be expected, most of the 19 chapters in this book deal with MRI and its major applications: morphology, diffusion imaging, diffusion tensor imaging, dynamic contrast enhanced (T1 weighted DCE) perfusion imaging, dynamic susceptibility contrast (T2*-weighted DSC) perfusion imaging, arterial spin labeling perfusion imaging (without contrast agents), functional imaging, functional imaging with DTI, spectroscopy (including CEST), intraoperative MRI, and ultra-high-field MRI. By comparison, the first edition of Magnetic Resonance Imaging (Stark and Bradley, 1987) had two chapters out of 47 on brain tumors. Clearly the field has come a long way. While CT, PET, and SPECT are all included as well, the "workhorse" (borrowing from the title of Chapter 1) is MRI.

So these MRI topics alone would have warranted a textbook, however, clearly Professors Jain and Essig have been in the trenches, practicing real neuroradiology. So there are also chapters on RANO criteria, paraneoplastic syndromes, and treatment effects (e.g., radiation necrosis).

I also particularly enjoyed reading the On the Horizon chapters: ultra-high-field MRI, tumor genomics, new contrast agents, and molecular imaging. This takes a book that would have useful for a year or two and extends its lifespan several years. While the obvious primary beneficiaries of this book will be neuroradiololists (at all levels of training), I am certain that neurologists, neurosurgeons, and the new breed of "molecular imagers" will find it useful as well.

William G. Bradley, Jr., MD, PhD, FACR
Professor and Chair
Department of Radiology
University of California, San Diego
San Diego, California

Preface

Brain tumors are among the top causes of cancer-related deaths in both Europe and North America. They are categorized as primary or secondary tumors based on the tissue origin and as intra-axial or extra-axial tumors based on the origin of growth. The most common primary intra-axial tumors are of neuroepithelial origin, including astrocytomas, oligodendrogliomas, mixed gliomas, and other, rarer neuronal–glial tumors, with glioblastoma multiforme as the most common of all primary intra-axial lesions. Meningiomas are the most common primary extra-axial tumors and account for about 20% of all brain tumors. Secondary, metastatic brain lesions far outnumber the primary tumors, with a high incidence in systemic cancers such as lung and breast cancer.

The goals and requirements for neuroimaging in brain tumors are multiplex and involve making a diagnosis and a differential diagnosis, whereas accurate lesion grading is needed for overall patient management. Imaging is also involved in the decision-making process for therapy and later for precise planning of surgical or radiotherapeutic interventions. After therapy neuroimaging techniques have shown to be mandatory for monitoring disease and detection as well as management of possible therapy-related side effects.

Aside from lesion pathology, neuroimaging is an essential part of the decision-making process for therapy and later for precise planning of surgical or nonsurgical interventions. In the case of neurosurgery, neuroimaging can precisely define the location and accurately delineate the lesion. In the case of radiotherapy, neuroimaging assists in defining the treatment volume and enables demarcation of margins for targeted interventions.

Of all diagnostic imaging methods, computed tomography (CT) and magnetic resonance imaging (MRI) are accepted as the most sensitive methods for diagnosing brain tumors.

CT is often used as the primary diagnostic step for patients with unknown or acute-onset neurological symptoms. Because of its geometric accuracy, CT is mandatory for treatment planning in radiotherapy.

MRI, with its high tissue contrast and noninvasiveness, makes it possible to recognize and determine with accuracy the dimensions of a tumor and its surrounding affected or nonaffected tissue. This requires a high central nervous system (CNS) to lesion contrast, which depends on the signal intensity of the lesion relative to that of the surrounding normal tissue. Furthermore, detailed information on the internal morphology of the lesion is essential for differential diagnosis, grading, and selection and planning of therapy. For most diseases and for many of the currently available functional MRI methods, the use of magnetic resonance (MR) contrast media is mandatory. The standard dose employed for MRI of the CNS is 0.1 mmol/kg body weight, although numerous studies have shown that lesion detection may be improved with the use of higher doses and dedicated sequences. Contrast-enhanced MRI also helps to distinguish tumors from other pathological processes and to depict basic signs of tumor response to therapy, such as change in size, morphology, and degree of contrast material enhancement.

Neuroimaging initially focused on the superb contrast and spatial resolution of neuronal tissue to enable a detailed morphological analysis. Recent developments, however, have focused on evaluating these in conjunction with additional functional assessments. The characterization of neoplasm using physiological or pathophysiological characteristics has long been the domain of positron-emission tomography (PET).

Although PET has significantly improved our pathophysiological understanding of the CNS, the availability of contrast agents and improved rapid imaging methodologies in CT and MRI are now enabling further noninvasive characterization of physiological tissue and diseases. Functional information can reflect macrovasculature, the breakdown of the blood–brain barrier (BBB) with resulting permeability for the contrast agent, and tissue perfusion. Neurofunctional magnetic resonance imaging (nfMRI) is a recently established technique that increases our diagnostic potential in the neurosciences, whereas MR spectroscopic techniques such as chemical shift imaging (CSI) allow a detailed metabolic analysis of the neuronal or pathological tissue.

The overall diagnostic aim of functional neuroimaging of CNS neoplasm is to optimize tumor characterization, with an emphasis on improved specificity with which to separate benign from malignant features. Specific characterization facilitates planning of the most appropriate treatment. Furthermore, functional neuroimaging of CNS neoplasms can be expanded to monitoring ongoing therapy and early detection of therapeutic side effects. Predictive assessment of therapy response and monitoring ongoing therapy to guide therapeutic intervention are major challenges in the current treatment of CNS neoplasms.

This book provides a broad overview of the currently available diagnostic methods for the complex management of patients with brain tumors. Introductory chapters discuss clinical needs regarding patient management and response assessment and provide overviews of current trends in conventional and advanced brain tumor imaging. The reader learns about the imaging features of brain neoplasms and the most significant differentials.

There is detailed focus on the current use of functional imaging techniques, including CT, PET, and MRI. The reader learns about the indications of functional imaging techniques, the technical requirements and challenges, and how they impact the management of patients with brain tumor. The "on the horizon" chapters discuss methods that are under preclinical and clinical investigations, and that have the potential to significantly impact our evaluations of brain tumor cases.

Overall, the book presents exciting developments in brain tumor imaging that substantially impact our future brain tumor patient management.

Acknowledgments

We wish to thank all our contributors, without whose help this project would not have been possible.

Contributors

Meser M. Ali, PhD
Assistant Scientist
Department of Neurology
Henry Ford Hospital
Detroit, Michigan

Samuel E. Almodóvar, MD
Assistant Professor of Radiology
Division of Molecular Imaging and Therapeutics
Chief of Clinical PET
University of Alabama at Birmingham
Birmingham, Alabama

Ali S. Arbab, MD, PhD
Professor
Department of Biochemistry and Molecular Biology
Leader of Tumor Angiogenesis Initiative, Cancer Center
Georgia Regents University
Augusta, Georgia

Asim K. Bag, MD
Assistant Professor, Department of Radiology
Section of Neuroradiology
University of Alabama at Birmingham School of Medicine
Birmingham, Alabama

Isabella M Björkman-Burtscher, MD, PhD
Associate Professor, Radiology
Clinical Sciences Lund, Lund University, Sweden
Staff Neuroradiologist
Department of Medical Imaging and Physiology
Skane University Hospital
Lund, Sweden

Cem Calli, MD
Ege University Medical Faculty
Department of Radiology
Chief of Neuroradiology Section
Bornova, Izmir, Turkey

Victor Chang, MD
Department of Neurosurgery, Henry Ford Hospital
Director of Spine Research
Co-Director of Minimally Invasive and Deformity
  Spine Surgery
Detroit, Michigan

Wilson Chwang, MD, PhD
Fellow, Neuroradiology
Stanford University School of Medicine
Stanford, California

Rivka R. Colen, MD
Assistant Professor (tenure-track), Radiology
Section of Neuroradiology, Department of Diagnostic
  Radiology
Co-Director, Quantitative Imaging Analysis Core
UT MD Anderson Cancer Center
Houston, Texas

Benjamin M. Ellingson, PhD, MS
Assistant Professor of Radiology, Biomedical Physics,
  Psychiatry and Bioengineering
Director, UCLA Brain Tumor Imaging Laboratory (BTIL)
David Geffen School of Medicine at UCLA
Los Angeles, California

Marco Essig, MD, PhD, FRCPC
Professor and Chairman
Department of Radiology
University of Manitoba
Medical Director
Winnipeg Regional Health Authority
Winnipeg, Manitoba, Canada

Girish M. Fatterpekar, MBBS
Associate Professor, Radiology
Division of Neuroradiology
NYU School of Medicine
New York, New York

David Fussell, MD
Division of Neuroradiology
Medical Director, Los Gatos Imaging Center
Valley Radiology Medical Associates
Los Gatos, California

Brent Griffith, MD
Senior Staff Neuroradiologist
Henry Ford Health System
Detroit, Michigan

Rajan Jain, MD
Associate Professor, Radiology
Division of Neuroradiology, NYU Langone
  Medical Center
Clinical Co-Director, Center for Advanced Imaging
  Innovation and Research
NYU School of Medicine
New York, New York

Anna Knobel, MD
Radiology Resident at Lenox Hill Hospital, North Shore-LIJ
    Health System
Clinical Research Assistant at Memorial Sloan Kettering
    Cancer Center
New York, New York

Sanath Kumar, MD
Department of Radiation Oncology
Henry Ford Hospital
Detroit, Michigan

Ian Lee, MD
Staff Neurosurgeon
Department of Neurosurgery
Hermelin Brain Tumor Center
Henry Ford Health System
Detroit, Michigan

Tom Mikkelsen, MD, FRCP(C)
Professor of Neurology, Wayne State University
Co-Director, Hermelin Brain Tumor Center
Departments of Neurology & Neurosurgery
Henry Ford Hospital
Detroit, Michigan

Suyash Mohan, MD, PDCC
Assistant Professor of Radiology
Department of Radiology, Division of Neuroradiology
University of Pennsylvania School of Medicine
Philadelphia, Pennsylvania

S. Ali Nabavizadeh, MD
Clinical Instructor
Division of Neuroradiology,
Hospital of University of Pennsylvania
Philadelphia, Pennsylvania

Prashant Nagpal, MBBS, MD
Department of Radiology
Brigham and Women's Hospital
Harvard Medical School
Boston, Massachusetts
Department of Medicine
Westchester Medical Center
New York Medical College
Valhalla, New York

Peter Neher, PhD
German Cancer Research Center (DKFZ)
Division Medical and Biological Informatics
Juniorgroup Medical Image Computing
Heidelberg, Germany

Inna Nutanson, MD
Clinical Fellow, Neuroradiology
Division of Neuroradiology, NYU Langone Medical Center
New York, New York

Jeffrey M. Pollock, MD
Associate Professor, Radiology
Division of Neuroradiology, Oregon Health and
    Science University
Director of MRI and Functional MRI
Portland, Oregon

Whitney Pope, MD, PhD
Associate Professor, Radiology
David Geffen School of Medicine at UCLA
Los Angeles, California

Josep Puig, MD, PhD
Associated Professor, Radiology
Faculty of Medicine, University of Girona
Staff Researcher, Girona Biomedical Research
    Institute, IDIBGI
Department of Radiology and Diagnostic
    Imaging Institute
Dr Josep Trueta University Hospital
Girona, Spain

Alexander Radbruch, MD, JD
Dr. med. Assessor juris
Groupleader Neurooncologic Imaging
Department of Neuroradiology,
University of Heidelberg
German Cancer Research Center (DKFZ)
Heidelberg, Germany

Steffen Sammet, MD, PhD, DABR, FAMP
Associate Professor
Director of Clinical MR Physics
Physician and Medical Physicist
University of Chicago Medical Center
Department of Radiology
Chicago, Illinois

Bram Stieltjes, MD, PhD
Research Coordinator
Department of Radiology and Nuclear Medicine
University Hospital Basel
Basel, Switzerland

Pia C. Sundgren, MD, PhD
Professor of Radiology
Clinical Sciences Lund, Lund University, Sweden
Staff Neuroradiologist
Department of Medical Imaging and Physiology
Skane University Hospital
Lund, Sweden

Faisal Tai, MD
Resident, Psychiatry
University of Iowa Hospitals and Clinics
Iowa City, Iowa

Tobias Walbert, MD, PhD, MPH
Neuro-Oncologist
Medical Co-Director Hermelin Brain Tumor Center
Henry Ford Health System Detroit
Detroit, Michigan

Bryan Yoo, MD
Assistant Professor, Radiology
David Geffen School of Medicine at UCLA
Los Angeles, California

Robert J. Young, MD
Assistant Professor, Radiology
New York Presbyterian Hospital/Weill Cornell
   Medical College
Director, 3T MRI Neuroradiology
Assistant Attending, Neuroradiology Service, Radiology
Memorial Sloan Kettering Cancer Center
New York, New York

Pascal O. Zinn, MD, PhD
Department of Neurosurgery
Baylor College of Medicine
Houston, Texas

1 Conventional Morphological Imaging: MRI Remains the Workhorse

Benjamin Cohen, Inna Nutanson, and Girish M. Fatterpekar

1.1 Introduction

The term *brain tumor* refers to a collection of neoplasms, each with its own biology, imaging appearance, treatment, and prognosis.[1] This chapter provides an overview of the magnetic resonance imaging (MRI) appearance of common intracranial neoplasms, primarily focusing on intra-axial neoplasms.

For the purpose of discussion and based on the cell of origin, the intracranial tumors discussed herein have been classified as follows:
- Tumors of the neuroepithelial tissue
  - Astrocytic tumors
  - Oligodendroglial/oligoastrocytic tumors
  - Neuronal and mixed neuronal–glial tumors
  - Embryonal tumors
- Lymphoma
- Metastasis

1.2 Tumors of the Neuroepithelial Tissue

1.2.1 Astrocytic Tumors

These can be categorized into eight types based on their histopathological appearance:
- Pilocytic astrocytoma
- Subependymal giant cell astrocytoma (SEGA)
- Pleomorphic xanthoastrocytoma (PXA)
- Diffuse astrocytoma
- Anaplastic astrocytoma
- Glioblastoma
- Gliosarcoma
- Gliomatosis cerebri

Pilocytic Astrocytoma

Pilocytic astrocytoma is the most common pediatric central nervous system (CNS) glial neoplasm.[2] The tumor has a benign biological behavior, categorized as World Health Organization (WHO) grade I, with an extremely high survival rate of 94% at 10 years, the best of any glial tumor. The cerebellum, optic nerve and chiasm, and hypothalamic region are the most common locations, but the tumor can be found anywhere in the brain and spinal cord. Leptomeningeal metastases are rare. Most patients present in the first 2 decades, and clinical symptoms and signs are usually of several months' duration and are directly related to the specific location of the tumor.

MRI typically demonstrates a slow-growing, relatively well circumscribed tumor, with a predominant cystic component (▶ Fig. 1.1). A variable degree of enhancement is seen following contrast administration. The most common pattern of enhancement is that of an avidly enhancing mural nodule with a nonenhancing cyst (50% of cases). The wall of the cyst occasionally

enhances. Other tumor patterns include a heterogeneously enhancing lesion and a solid homogeneous enhancement.[3] Surrounding vasogenic edema is rarely present. Foci of susceptibility likely related to calcifications can be seen in 20% of cases. Hemorrhage is very rare. These masses often cause obstructive hydrocephalus.

Subependymal Giant Cell Astrocytoma

SEGA is an intraventricular glioneuronal tumor arising from the ventricular wall near the foramen of Monro. It is the most common cerebral neoplasm in tuberous sclerosis. The tumor is characterized by slow growth and a benign biological behavior (WHO grade I).

MRI demonstrates a well-circumscribed, lobulated, heterogeneous mass, with avid enhancement (▶ Fig. 1.2). Associated foci of susceptibility related to calcification can sometimes be seen. There is typically no leptomeningeal spread.[4]

Pleomorphic Xanthoastrocytoma

PXA is a rare, usually benign brain tumor. It is seen almost exclusively as a neoplasm of children and young adults. It is characterized as a WHO grade II tumor. It is supratentorial in approximately 98% of cases. Most often, it involves the superficial cortex of the temporal lobes. The overlying leptomeninges are commonly involved.

MRI demonstrates a round to oval, predominantly cystic, cortical mass with an enhancing mural nodule (▶ Fig. 1.3). The enhancing nodule tends to abut the pial surface.[5] Adjacent leptomeningeal enhancement and an enhancing dural "tail" are commonly seen. Minimal surrounding edema is rarely present. Calcifications, hemorrhage, and skull erosion are rarely seen.

Diffuse Astrocytoma

Diffuse astrocytoma is a well differentiated but diffusely infiltrating primary brain neoplasm of astrocytic origin (WHO grade II). It represents approximately 10 to 15% of all astrocytomas, and it typically affects young adults in the third to fourth decade of life. It has an intrinsic tendency for malignant progression to anaplastic astrocytoma, and glioblastoma.[6]

Diffuse astrocytoma is a white matter neoplasm that may extend into the cortex. Frontal and temporal lobes are the sites most commonly involved. About 20% involve the deep gray matter structures, thalamus, and basal ganglia. Involvement of the spinal cord is less common. In children and adolescents, the brainstem (mostly pons and medulla) is the most common site of involvement.

MRI demonstrates an ill-defined mass iso- to hypointense to the gray matter on T1-weighted imaging (T1WI), and hyperintense on T2WI (▶ Fig. 1.4). Minimal surrounding edema is occasionally seen. Cysts, calcification, and hemorrhage are rarely seen. Restricted diffusion is typically absent. There is

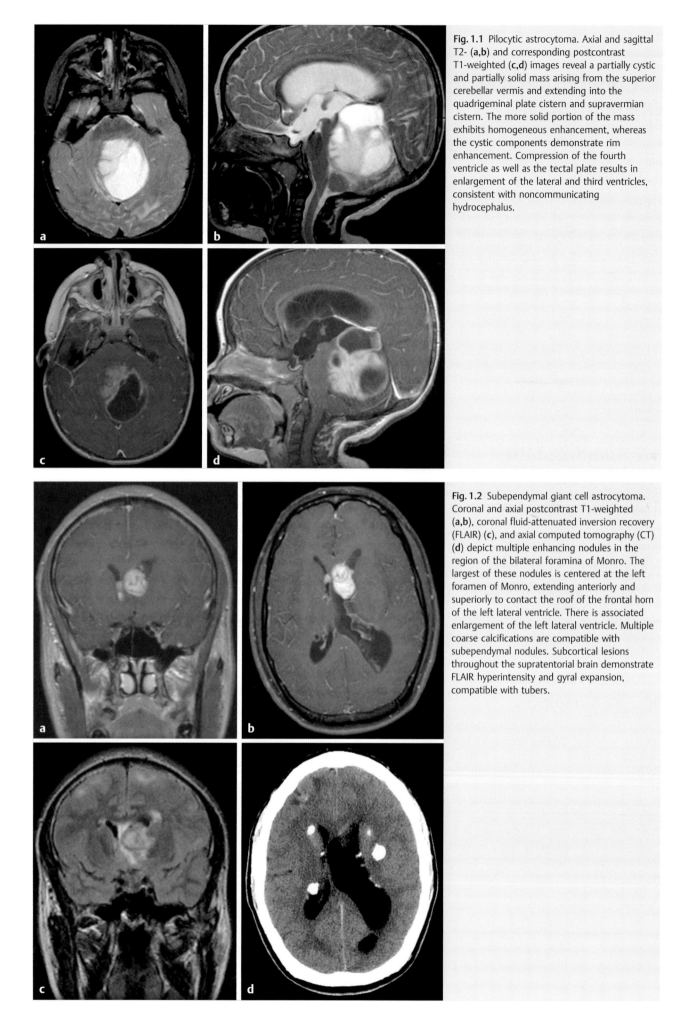

Fig. 1.1 Pilocytic astrocytoma. Axial and sagittal T2- (**a,b**) and corresponding postcontrast T1-weighted (**c,d**) images reveal a partially cystic and partially solid mass arising from the superior cerebellar vermis and extending into the quadrigeminal plate cistern and supravermian cistern. The more solid portion of the mass exhibits homogeneous enhancement, whereas the cystic components demonstrate rim enhancement. Compression of the fourth ventricle as well as the tectal plate results in enlargement of the lateral and third ventricles, consistent with noncommunicating hydrocephalus.

Fig. 1.2 Subependymal giant cell astrocytoma. Coronal and axial postcontrast T1-weighted (**a,b**), coronal fluid-attenuated inversion recovery (FLAIR) (**c**), and axial computed tomography (CT) (**d**) depict multiple enhancing nodules in the region of the bilateral foramina of Monro. The largest of these nodules is centered at the left foramen of Monro, extending anteriorly and superiorly to contact the roof of the frontal horn of the left lateral ventricle. There is associated enlargement of the left lateral ventricle. Multiple coarse calcifications are compatible with subependymal nodules. Subcortical lesions throughout the supratentorial brain demonstrate FLAIR hyperintensity and gyral expansion, compatible with tubers.

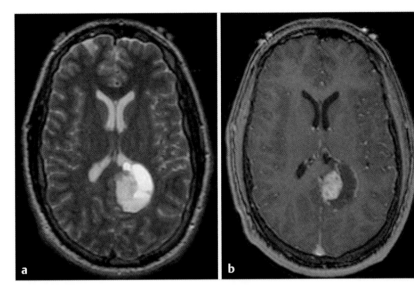

Fig. 1.3 Pleomorphic xanthoastrocytoma. Axial T2- (**a**) and corresponding postcontrast T1-weighted (**b**) images show a mixed solid and cystic mass involving the left parietal lobe cortex and left splenium of the corpus callosum. This mass abuts and deforms the left atrium.

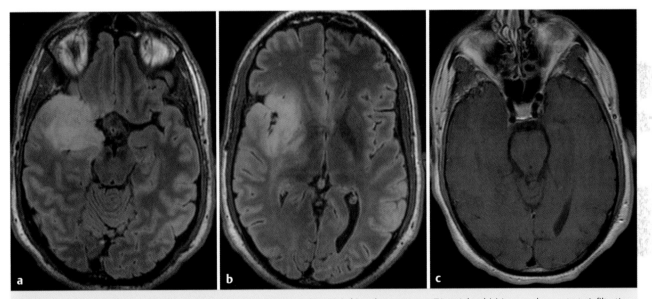

Fig. 1.4 Diffuse astrocytoma. Axial fluid-attenuated inversion recovery (FLAIR) (**a,b**) and postcontrast T1-weighted (**c**) images demonstrate infiltrative masslike nonenhancing abnormal T2 signal hyperintensity involving the right anterior/inferior temporal lobe extending into the inferior frontal gyrus, insular cortex, temporal operculum, and temporal stem, and medially into the hippocampus and lentiform nucleus.

usually no associated enhancement seen. In fact, the presence of enhancement can suggest progression to a higher-grade neoplasm.[7]

Anaplastic Astrocytoma

Anaplastic astrocytoma is a diffusely infiltrating astrocytoma with focal or diffuse anaplasia and marked proliferative potential. It is a WHO grade III neoplasm and represents approximately 25% of all astrocytomas. Anaplastic astrocytoma predominantly involves the hemispheric white matter and is commonly found in the frontal and temporal lobes. Less commonly, it involves the brainstem and spinal cord. In children, it may involve the pons and the thalamus.

MRI demonstrates an ill-defined mass iso- to hypointense to the gray matter on T1WI, and hyperintense on T2WI. Minimal

surrounding edema can sometimes be seen. Enhancement, when seen, is often focal, patchy, and heterogeneous. Cysts, calcification, and hemorrhage are rarely seen. Restricted diffusion is typically absent. Presence of prominent flow voids and ringlike enhancement are features suggestive of progression to glioblastoma.[7]

Glioblastoma

Glioblastoma is the most common primary brain malignancy, accounting for 12 to 15% of all intracranial neoplasms. It is a WHO grade IV tumor and accounts for 60 to 75% of all astrocytic tumors. It occurs most frequently in the cerebral hemispheres of adults between 45 and 70 years of age. Most glioblastomas arise de novo. The mean age of such patients who present with *primary glioblastoma* is 55 years. Glioblastomas may also arise

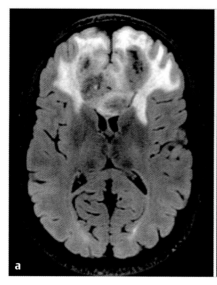 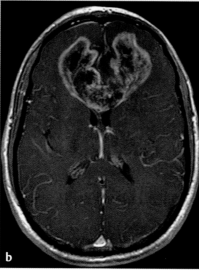

Fig. 1.5 Glioblastoma. Axial fluid-attenuated inversion recovery (FLAIR) (**a**) and postcontrast T1-weighted (**b**) images depict a heterogeneous, irregular, enhancing mass centered within the bifrontal lobes that crosses the midline at the genu of the corpus callosum, extending to the margins of the frontal horns of the lateral ventricles with mass effect. Surrounding associated diffuse, infiltrative FLAIR signal abnormality within the bifrontal white matter is seen.

from an existing astrocytoma that has undergone progression to a higher grade. Such *secondary glioblastomas* are found in a younger patient population (mean age, 40 years) and are characterized by a longer clinical course.[8,9]

Glioblastoma is a rapidly enlarging malignant astrocytic tumor characterized by necrosis and neovascularity. Glioblastomas are more frequently found in the supratentorial white matter, most commonly in the frontal, temporal, and parietal lobes. The occipital lobes are relatively spared. Glioblastomas typically appear as poorly marginated, diffusely infiltrating, necrotic, hemispheric masses. These tumors cross the white matter tracts to involve the contralateral hemisphere. They frequently extend across the corpus callosum ("butterfly glioma") and can also involve the anterior and posterior commissures (▶ Fig. 1.5). These tumors may be multifocal or multicentric.

Most often, imaging shows heterogeneously enhancing, partially necrotic mass lesion with surrounding edema and mass effect.[9] Based on the underlying genetic profile, this appearance can vary. Diffusion restriction from some of the solid components suggestive of hypercellularity is commonly seen. Foci of susceptibility suggestive of hemorrhage are commonly seen. Calcifications are rare because these tend to be related to low-grade tumor degeneration. Surrounding fluid-attenuated inversion recovery (FLAIR) signal abnormality suggests edema and tumor infiltration, which in fact extends far beyond the signal abnormality changes.[9]

Gliosarcoma

Gliosarcoma is a rare primary brain tumor that is composed of neoplastic glial cells mixed with a spindle cell sarcomatous element (WHO grade IV). The sarcomatous element is thought to arise from neoplastic transformation of vascular elements within the glioblastoma. Gliosarcomas present in the sixth to seventh decade of life. The temporal lobes are commonly involved. Imaging findings and clinical presentation can be indistinguishable from glioblastoma. The presence of dural involvement can suggest the presence of gliosarcoma.[10]

Gliomatosis Cerebri

According to the current WHO classification system for brain tumors, gliomatosis cerebri is a distinct malignant neuroepithelial neoplasm of uncertain origin.[11] The overall biological behavior corresponds to WHO grade III in a majority of cases. Gliomatosis cerebri typically involves the hemispheric white matter. Associated involvement of the cortex is often seen. There is diffuse white matter infiltration of three or more lobes and also involvement of the basal ganglia, thalami (in 75% of cases), corpus callosum (in 50% of cases), and brainstem and spinal cord (in 10–15% of cases). In 10% of cases there is also cerebellar involvement. This tumor infiltrates and enlarges the involved structures. However, it preserves the underlying brain architecture.[12] Patients usually present between the third and fifth decades of life, but cases have been described in patients of all ages, from neonates to the elderly. There is no gender predilection.

Imaging shows a poorly defined, nonenhancing, infiltrative lesion involving three or more lobes, with blurring of the gray–white differentiation and expansion of the involved parenchyma (▶ Fig. 1.6). Associated mass effect is common but is less when compared with the size of the tumor. Enhancement may indicate malignant progression or a focus of malignant glioma. There is usually no abnormal diffusion restriction on diffusion-weighted imaging (DWI).[13]

1.2.2 Oligodendroglial/Oligoastrocytic Tumors

Oligodendroglioma

Oligodendroglioma is the third most common glial neoplasm. It accounts for 2 to 5% of primary brain tumors and 5 to 18% of all glial neoplasms.[14] Males are affected more frequently, and the peak manifestation is during the fifth and sixth decades.

Currently two main types of tumors are recognized histopathologically: well-differentiated oligodendroglioma (WHO grade II) and its anaplastic variant (WHO grade III). Less

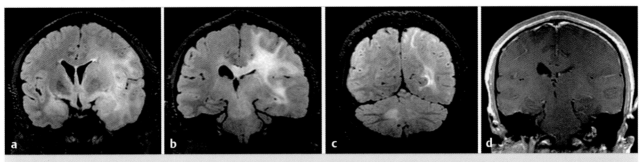

Fig. 1.6 Gliomatosis cerebri. Coronal fluid-attenuated inversion recovery (FLAIR) (**a–c**) and postcontrast T1-weighted (**d**) images illustrate diffuse masslike FLAIR signal consistent with tumor infiltration, primarily involving the left frontal, temporal, and parietal lobes' white matter with extension across the corpus callosum splenium to involve the right parietal corona radiata. Posteriorly, extension along the left optic tracts into the left occipital lobe is also seen. Medially, there is infiltration of the left basal ganglia, thalamus, insula, and subinsular white matter. There is also involvement of the right thalamus and bilateral anterior and medial temporal lobes, greater on the left. Inferiorly, tumor infiltration extends into the midbrain, dorsal pons, middle cerebellar peduncles, and cerebellum. No abnormal enhancement is seen. There is mass effect on the left lateral ventricle and a slight left to right midline shift.

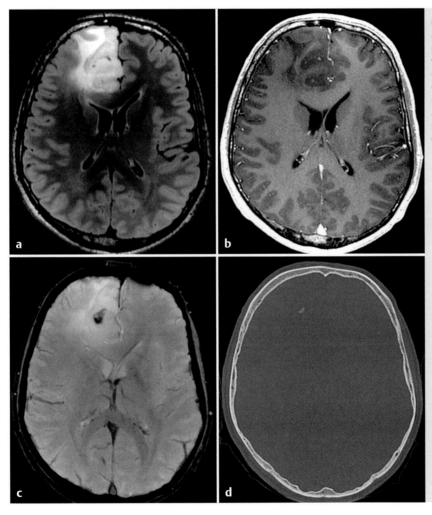

Fig. 1.7 Oligodendroglioma. Axial fluid-attenuated inversion recovery (FLAIR) (**a**), postcontrast T1-weighted (**b**), susceptibility-weighted (**c**), and computed tomographic (CT) (**d**) images reveal cortical and subcortical expansion of the right cingulate gyrus and right paramedian superior frontal gyrus without associated enhancement. Additionally, curvilinear susceptibility-related signal loss correlates with calcification seen on CT.

commonly, neoplastic mixtures of both oligodendroglial and astrocytic components occur. These have both well-differentiated and anaplastic forms and are referred to as oligoastrocytomas.[15]

Although it is most common in the frontal lobes, additional sites of involvement include temporal, parietal, and occipital lobes. Posterior fossa involvement is rare. There is an uncommon intraventricular variant of oligodendroglioma seen in approximately 1 to 10% of cases.[14,15]

Imaging shows a heterogeneous mass lesion within the subcortical white matter with extension to the cortex (▶ Fig. 1.7). Heterogeneity is related to calcifications (70–90%), cystic change (20%), and, uncommonly, blood products. Mild surrounding edema may be seen. The tumor may expand, remodel, or erode the adjacent calvarium. On occasion, frontal lobe tumors may extend through the corpus callosum to produce a "butterfly glioma" pattern. No diffusion restriction is seen. The presence of enhancement is usually associated with a higher-grade tumor. However, such enhancement is uncommonly seen with low-grade oligodendrogliomas as well. In fact, the absence of enhancement does not definitely indicate a low-grade tumor. Histological confirmation is always desired.[15]

Tumors with 1p and 19q deletions have interesting imaging features. They are more likely to demonstrate calcification and demonstrate ill-defined margins on T1WI.[16] They are also more likely to be found in the frontal lobe and extend across the midline than tumors that lack these deletions, which are more common in the temporal lobe, insula, and midbrain.[17]

Mixed Oligoastrocytoma

There are no unique features at cross-sectional neuroimaging that allow distinction of a mixed oligoastrocytoma from an oligodendroglioma.[18,19] However, enhancement is seen more commonly (50%) than in pure oligodendrogliomas. Also, calcification is not as commonly seen (14%).[20,21,22]

1.2.3 Neuronal and Mixed Neuronal–Glial Tumors

Neoplasms of the CNS containing abnormal neuronal elements are termed neuronal tumors. These neoplasms represent approximately 1% of all brain tumors. They have favorable clinical outcomes and are generally cured with surgery alone. Neuronal tumors are usually classified as pure neuronal cell tumors (gangliocytoma, Lhermitte-Duclos disease [dysplastic cerebellar gangliocytoma], central neurocytoma) and mixed neuronal–glial tumors (ganglioglioma, desmoplastic infantile ganglioglioma, dysembryoplastic neuroepithelial tumor).[23]

Gangliocytoma

Gangliocytoma refers to a spectrum of rare tumors that originate from a neuronal cell lineage.[24] In addition to the neuronal population, there is a highly variable network of nonneoplastic glial cells.[25] This distinguishes gangliocytomas from gangliogliomas, which contain anaplastic glial cells. However, such a clear distinction between these two tumors is not always possible on pathology. Hence the term *ganglion cell tumor*, which can refer to either of these two tumors, is occasionally used. Essentially, gangliocytomas and gangliogliomas represent opposite ends of a spectrum of differentiated ganglion cell tumors.

According to the WHO system of grading, gangliocytoma is a grade I tumor. Most lesions become clinically symptomatic in children and young adults. The most common sites are the cerebral hemispheres and the cervicothoracic spinal cord. Within the cerebral hemispheres, the temporal lobe, either alone or in combination with the frontal or parietal lobes, is the favored site of involvement.[24,25] Patients typically present with seizures or focal neurologic signs according to the location of the mass.

On imaging, the tumor presents as a cortically located, cystic mass with a mural enhancing nodule. Occasionally, it appears as a circumscribed solid mass or as a mass containing multiple cysts. Calcification can sometimes be seen. Some cases are

accompanied by an enhancing dura, also known as the dural tail sign.[23]

Lhermitte-Duclos Disease

Lhermitte-Duclos disease is also known as dysplastic cerebellar gangliocytoma. There is considerable controversy regarding the etiology of this disease: It may have a hamartomatous, neoplastic, or congenital malformative origin. Clinical evidence and the close association with multiple hamartoma–neoplasia complex (Cowden disease) favors a hamartomatous origin.[26] Most cases of Lhermitte-Duclos disease occur in young adults. There is no definite gender predilection. This lesion is typically located in the cerebellar hemisphere and occasionally extends to the vermis. Hydrocephalus or syrinx may be present due to mass effect and compression of the fourth ventricle.

The characteristic MRI finding is of a nonenhancing mass in the cerebellar hemisphere with an alternating striated pattern of isointense and hypointense signal on T1WI and alternating isointense and hyperintense signal on T2WI. This alternating striated pattern is also referred to as a laminated, corduroy, lamellar, or folial pattern.[27] The characteristic striations demonstrated on MRI represent the abnormally thickened cerebellar folia. Rarely, calcifications or enhancement may be seen. Hyperintense signal on DWI reflects T2 shine-through.

Central Neurocytoma

Central neurocytoma is a WHO grade II neuroepithelial intraventricular tumor with neuronal differentiation. It accounts for less than 1% (0.25–0.5%) of all *intracranial tumors*. This tumor affects mainly young adults and has a favorable prognosis. There is no gender predilection. It is often located in the lateral ventricles near the foramen of Monro attached to the septum pellucidum. Most patients present with symptoms of increased intracranial pressure secondary to obstructive hydrocephalus.

On imaging, a moderately enhancing, well-demarcated, lobulated, heterogeneous (mixed cystic and solid) mass is seen (▶ Fig. 1.8).[28] Hemorrhage and prominent flow voids can be occasionally seen. Calcification is seen in about half of the cases.

Ganglioglioma

Ganglioglioma is the most common of the mixed neuronal–glial neoplasms arising within the CNS.[23] The main histopathological feature of ganglioglioma is the admixture of both atypical ganglion cells and neoplastic glial cells in varying amounts. Most gangliogliomas are WHO grade I tumors. However, when they exhibit anaplastic features, they correspond to WHO grade III tumors. Most gangliogliomas occur in children and young adults, with the majority of tumors arising within the temporal lobe. Most patients present with medically refractory seizures of the partial complex type.

On imaging, three main patterns of gangliogliomas are recognized, with the most common being that of a well circumscribed cystic-appearing mass with a mural nodule (▶ Fig. 1.9).[29] The mural nodule often demonstrates homogeneous enhancement but sometimes is seen to exhibit sparse or ringlike enhancement. Other patterns include a solid tumor that thickens and expands the overlying cortex, and an uncommon pattern of a poorly

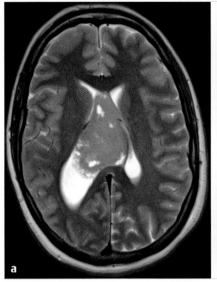
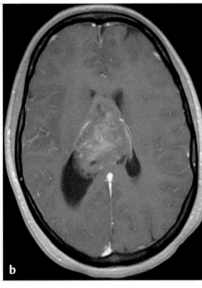

Fig. 1.8 Central neurocytoma. Axial T2- (a) and corresponding postcontrast T1-weighted (b) images show a heterogeneous, partially enhancing, lobular right lateral ventricular mass, which abuts the septum pellucidum. There is predominant T2 isointensity with cystic foci.

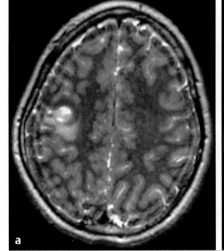
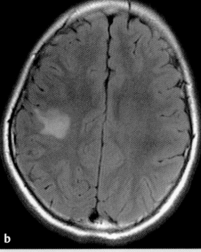
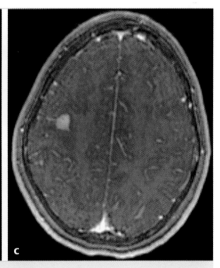

Fig. 1.9 Ganglioglioma. Axial T2-weighted (a), fluid-attenuated inversion recovery (FLAIR) (b), and postcontrast T1-weighted (c) images demonstrate a well-demarcated, T2 hyperintense, homogeneously enhancing, cortically based lesion within the anterior bank of the right postcentral gyrus. There is surrounding T2 prolongation, most consistent with vasogenic edema.

delineated mass. Calcifications are seen in about 30% of cases of ganglioglioma.

Rarely meningeal enhancement may be seen. There is usually little associated mass effect or surrounding vasogenic edema.

Desmoplastic Infantile Ganglioglioma

Desmoplastic infantile ganglioglioma is an uncommon variant of ganglioglioma, often seen in the first year of life. It is a benign tumor corresponding to WHO grade I. It typically demonstrates a large cystic component and a smaller solid component. The smaller solid component is often seen to be associated with a desmoplastic reaction and is typically located adjacent to the meninges and dura.[30]

Imaging shows a cystic mass with a peripheral solid component that enhances intensely following contrast administration. The enhancing portion is seen to extend to the leptomeninges and correlates with the firm dural attachment of the solid component of the mass.[31]

Dysembryoplastic Neuroepithelial Tumor

Dysembryoplastic neuroepithelial tumor (DNET) is a benign (WHO grade I) slow-growing tumor arising from either cortical or deep gray matter. Most such tumors are centered in the cortical gray matter, arising from *secondary germinal layers* and are frequently associated with *cortical dysplasia* (up to 80% of cases). The temporal lobe, amygdala, and hippocampus are the most common sites of origin (seen in 50–60%), followed by the frontal lobes (30%). The tumor characteristically presents with intractable partial seizures.

On imaging, it appears as a well-demarcated, "bubbly" intracortical mass that remodels the inner table of the skull (44–60%) and "points" toward the ventricle (30%).[32,33] The mass

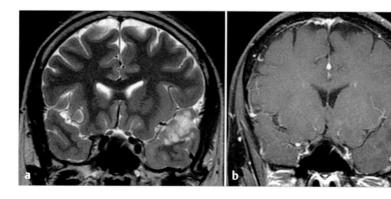

Fig. 1.10 Dysembryoplastic neuroepithelial tumor. Coronal T2- (**a**) and corresponding postcontrast T1-weighted (**b**) images depict abnormal cortical T2 hyperintensity with a cystlike appearance in the left superior temporal gyrus with extension into the middle temporal gyrus. No abnormal contrast enhancement is seen.

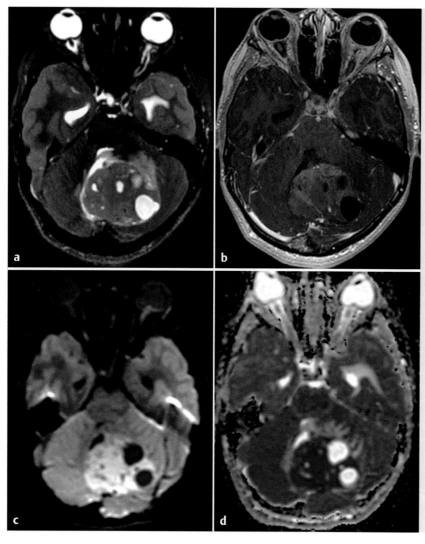

Fig. 1.11 Medulloblastoma. Axial T2- (**a**), postcontrast T1- (**b**), and diffusion-weighted (**c**) images with apparent diffusion coefficient ADC map (**d**) illustrate a large, well-circumscribed, heterogeneously enhancing, predominantly solid mass with multiple cystic components centered just to the left of midline within the cerebellum. The mass has markedly reduced diffusion within its solid enhancing components, suggesting high cellularity. There is a mild amount of surrounding vasogenic edema within the paramedian cerebellar hemispheres. Marked mass effect on the fourth ventricle results in obstructive hydrocephalus. The optic nerve sheaths are markedly dilated with cupping of the optic discs, suggesting papilledema.

appears hypointense to the gray matter on T1WI, and hyperintense on T2WI, and it does not demonstrate any enhancement (▶ Fig. 1.10). It can mimic an infarction on initial computed tomographic (CT) scan. However, there is no temporal evolution to atrophy. On FLAIR pulse sequence, a "bright rim" is seen. There is often minimal or no mass effect. The tumor lacks surrounding edema. Calcifications are seen in 20 to 36% of cases. Hemorrhage into DNET is uncommon but does occur, possibly in association with microvascular abnormalities. The tumor usually lacks abnormal restricted diffusion.

1.2.4 Embryonal Tumors

Embryonal tumors are a unique group of poorly differentiated malignant tumors (WHO grade IV) with a propensity to disseminate throughout the neuraxis and exhibit aggressive clinical behavior.[34] Imaging of the entire craniospinal axis is therefore necessary for complete evaluation of an embryonal tumor. They most commonly occur in young children and represent approximately 25% of all primary CNS neoplasms seen in the pediatric population. These tumors are classified into medulloblastoma (they contribute to an overwhelming majority of all embryonal tumors), CNS primitive neuroectodermal tumor, and atypical teratoid/rhabdoid tumor.[35]

Medulloblastoma

Medulloblastoma is a malignant neuroepithelial tumor of the cerebellum. Medulloblastomas account for approximately 25% of all pediatric CNS tumors, 40% of all pediatric posterior fossa tumors, and 0.4 to 1% of all adult CNS tumors.[36] They are seen more commonly in males, with a M:F ratio of 2 to 4:1. The median age of diagnosis is 9 years. When diagnosed in adults, they typically present in the third to fourth decade and are more likely to arise in atypical locations. Medulloblastomas carry a better prognosis when diagnosed in older children and adults.

The cerebellar vermis is the most common location for medulloblastomas (>75%). More lateral locations within the cerebellar hemisphere are typical when these tumors manifest in older children, adolescents, and adults.[36] This difference in location is thought to be related to the migration of undifferentiated cells from the posterior medullary velum in a lateral and superior direction.

Most patients present with headache and vomiting. Symptom duration is often less than 3 months, reflecting the aggressive biological behavior of the tumor. Truncal ataxia, secondary to destruction of the cerebellar vermis, is the most common objective clinical sign and is frequently accompanied by spasticity. Seizure activity is uncommon and may indicate metastatic spread.

On imaging, medulloblastoma is seen as a well-defined mass iso- to hypointense to the gray matter on T1WI, and iso- to hypointense on T2WI. Diffusion restriction reflecting hypercellularity is characteristic of this tumor.[37] There is homogeneous enhancement seen following contrast administration (► Fig. 1.11). Surrounding vasogenic edema and hydrocephalus are often present. Cyst formation (approximately 40–60% of cases) and calcifications (20%) may also be seen. Up to one third of patients have subarachnoid metastatic disease at the time of initial presentation.

Medulloblastomas in the adult population are often of the desmoplastic histological type. On imaging, a peripherally located mass along the lateral aspect of the cerebellar hemispheres and extending into the cerebellopontine angle cisterns is seen. Heterogeneous signal is noted on both T1WI and T2WI. Patchy diffusion restriction can be seen. Intratumoral cysts are commonly seen. Minimal enhancement is typical of desmoplastic medulloblastoma.[37]

Central Nervous System Primitive Neuroectodermal Tumor

CNS primitive neuroectodermal tumors (PNETs) are a heterogeneous group of tumors that may arise in the cerebral hemispheres (most commonly), brainstem, or spinal cord, and are composed of undifferentiated or poorly differentiated neuroepithelial cells.[38] These tumors are most frequently encountered during the first decade of life, with a recognized male predilection. Clinical presentation is nonspecific, with symptoms of raised intracranial pressure, seizures, and focal neurologic deficits.

Imaging shows a heterogeneous mass demonstrating solid and cystic components.[39] Calcifications (50–70%), hemorrhage, and necrosis are common. The extent of peritumoral vasogenic edema is surprisingly low given the size of the mass and the aggressive tumor characteristics. Abnormal restricted diffusion is commonly seen. Postcontrast imaging demonstrates marked heterogeneous enhancement (► Fig. 1.12). Leptomeningeal and subarachnoid involvement are commonly seen.

Atypical Teratoid/Rhabdoid Tumor

Atypical teratoid/rhabdoid tumors (AT/RTs) are pediatric tumors most often presenting in the first 3 years of life, with a male predominance.[40] They are more often seen in the supratentorial rather than the infratentorial compartment. Clinical presentation is nonspecific, with symptoms of raised intracranial pressure, seizures, and focal neurologic deficits.

Imaging features are similar to those for PNETs.[41]

1.3 Lymphoma

Primary central nervous system lymphoma (PCNSL) is a malignant neoplasm composed of B lymphocytes involving the craniospinal neuraxis without evidence of metastasis outside the CNS at primary diagnosis. It accounts for 1 to 5% of all brain tumors and approximately 1% of all non-Hodgkin lymphomas. PCNSL was more commonly seen in the immunocompromised patient population. However, with the introduction of highly active antiretroviral therapy (HAART) during the past decade, the incidence of PCNSL in the human immunodeficiency virus (HIV) population has declined.[42]

The imaging appearance of PCNSL varies between the immunocompromised and immunocompetent populations.[43,44] In the immunocompromised patients, a centrally necrotic, peripherally enhancing lesion is seen. The periventricular region is a favored location in an HIV-positive patient. Detection of enhancement along the perivascular spaces is strongly suggestive of PCNSL. Multiple such lesions can sometimes be seen. Hemorrhage and calcification are usually absent. In the immunocompetent individuals, a solid mass appearing isointense to the gray matter on T1WI, hypointense on T2WI, is seen. Most lesions demonstrate diffusion restriction reflecting the cellular component of the tumor. Homogeneous enhancement is seen following contrast administration. Most lesions are located in the basal ganglia or the hemispheric white matter, including the corpus callosum (► Fig. 1.13). A superficial location adjacent to the meninges is also common.

1.4 Metastases

Intraparenchymal metastases represent the most common intracranial tumor, exceeding gliomas in prevalence by tenfold, and occur in 20 to 25% of all patients with systemic cancer. Lung cancer accounts for 60% of all such metastases, and 25% of patients with lung cancer will develop metastases.[45] Other common cancers to metastasize to the brain include breast

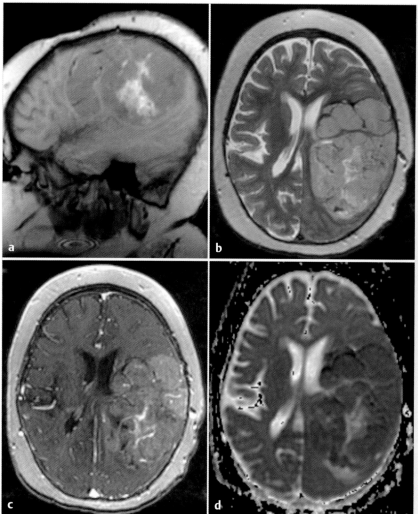

Fig. 1.12 Primitive neuroectodermal tumor. Sagittal T1- (**a**), axial T2- (**b**), and axial postcontrast T1-weighted (**c**) images with axial apparent diffusion coefficient (ADC) map (**d**) reveal a large heterogeneous lobulated mass centered within the left frontal lobe but also involving the left parietal and temporal lobes. The mass demonstrates intrinsic T1-shortening and susceptibility on the T2-weighted image, compatible with hemorrhage. There is irregular enhancement of this mass without significant surrounding vasogenic edema. There is minimal midline shift toward the right. Extensive lipomatous hypertrophy within the scalp is most likely related to exogenous steroid administration.

cancer and melanoma. A favored location for metastasis to occur is at the gray–white matter interface.

Solitary or multiple intraparenchymal lesions can be seen. Imaging appearance can be variable. A nodular enhancing lesion(s), or larger more solid appearing mass(es), or centrally necrotic peripherally enhancing lesion(s) can be seen (▶ Fig. 1.14). Surrounding edema is commonly seen. Certain systemic primary tumors, including thyroid and renal tumors and choriocarcinoma, are commonly associated with hemorrhage when they metastasize to the brain. The presence of intrinsic hyperintense signal on T1WI seen within the mass, having ruled out hemorrhage, should be suggestive of a melanotic melanoma deposit. However, distinction from primary intracranial neoplasm can be difficult based on imaging alone when a solitary lesion is seen. A history of a primary cancer known to metastasize to the brain and the use of advanced imaging techniques such as dynamic susceptibility contrast magnetic resonance perfusion imaging and magnetic resonance spectroscopy can help in differentiating a primary intracranial mass from a metastatic lesion.[46]

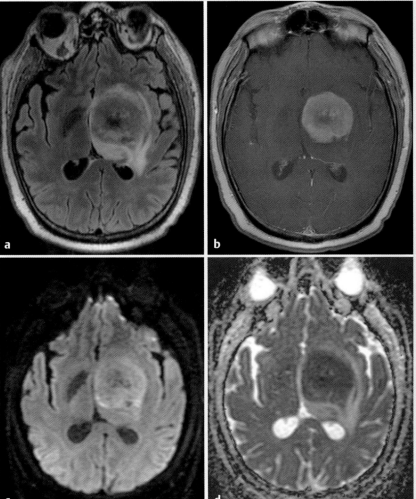

Fig. 1.13 Lymphoma. Axial fluid-attenuated inversion recovery (FLAIR) (**a**), postcontrast T1-weighted (**b**), and diffusion-weighted (**c**) images with apparent diffusion coefficient (ADC) map (**d**) show an avidly enhancing mass centered within the left basal ganglia. Reduced diffusion is in keeping with high cellularity. There is local mass effect, which results in compression of the left lateral and third ventricles and mild left-to-right midline shift.

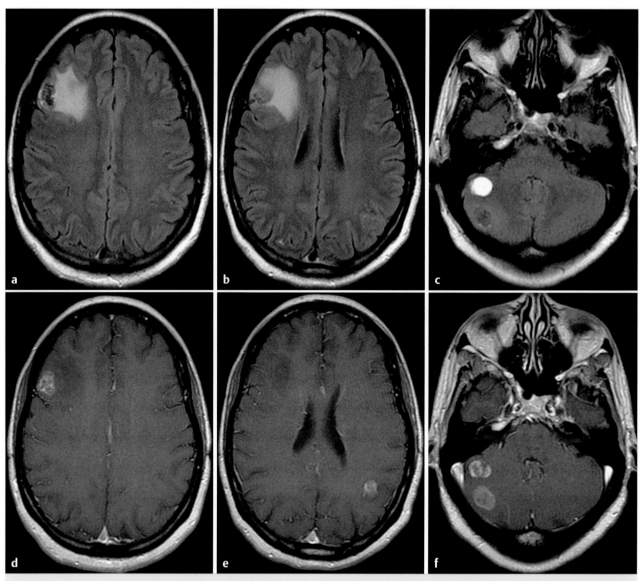

Fig. 1.14 Metastases. Axial postcontrast fluid-attenuated inversion recovery (FLAIR) (**a–c**) and T1-weighted (**d–f**) images demonstrate multiple intraparenchymal enhancing lesions surrounded by varying degrees of FLAIR hyperintensity, compatible with vasogenic edema.

References

[1] DeAngelis LM. Brain tumors. N Engl J Med 2001; 344: 114–123

[2] Ohgaki H, Kleihues P. Population-based studies on incidence, survival rates, and genetic alterations in astrocytic and oligodendroglial gliomas. J Neuropathol Exp Neurol 2005; 64: 479–489

[3] Koeller KK, Rushing EJ. From the archives of the AFIP: pilocytic astrocytoma: radiologic-pathologic correlation. Radiographics 2004; 24: 1693–1708

[4] Koeller KK, Sandberg GD Armed Forces Institute of Pathology. From the archives of the AFIP. Cerebral intraventricular neoplasms: radiologic-pathologic correlation. Radiographics 2002; 22: 1473–1505

[5] Tien RD, Cardenas CA, Rajagopalan S. Pleomorphic xanthoastrocytoma of the brain: MR findings in six patients. AJR Am J Roentgenol 1992; 159: 1287–1290

[6] Brasil Caseiras G, Ciccarelli O, Altmann DR et al. Low-grade gliomas: six-month tumor growth predicts patient outcome better than admission tumor volume, relative cerebral blood volume, and apparent diffusion coefficient. Radiology 2009; 253: 505–512

[7] Pierallini A, Bonamini M, Bozzao A et al. Supratentorial diffuse astrocytic tumours: proposal of an MRI classification. Eur Radiol 1997; 7: 395–399

[8] Kleihues P, Louis DN, Scheithauer BW et al. The WHO classification of tumors of the nervous system. J Neuropathol Exp Neurol 2002; 61: 215–225, discussion 226–229

[9] Altman DA, Atkinson DS, Jr, Brat DJ. Best cases from the AFIP: glioblastoma multiforme. Radiographics 2007; 27: 883–888

[10] Han L, Zhang X, Qiu S et al. Magnetic resonance imaging of primary cerebral gliosarcoma: a report of 15 cases. Acta Radiol 2008; 49: 1058–1067

[11] Kleihues P, Cavenee WK. Pathology and Genetics of Tumors of the Nervous System. Lyon, France: IARC; 2000

[12] McLendon RE, Enterline DS, Tien RD, Thorstad WL, Bruner JM. Pathologic anatomy: tumors of central neuroepithelial origin. In: Bigner DD, Mclendon RE, Bruner JM, eds. Russel and Rubinstein's Pathology of Tumors of the Nervous System. 6th ed. London, England: Arnold; 1998;340–342

[13] Yip M, Fisch C, Lamarche JB. AFIP archives: gliomatosis cerebri affecting the entire neuraxis. Radiographics 2003; 23: 247–253

[14] Reifenberger G, Kros JM, Burger PC, Louis DN, Collins VP. Oligodendroglioma. In: Kleihues P, Cavenee WK, eds. Pathology and Genetics of Tumours of the Nervous System. Lyon, France: IARC Press; 2000:56–61

[15] Koeller KK, Rushing EJ. From the archives of the AFIP: Oligodendroglioma and its variants: radiologic-pathologic correlation. Radiographics 2005; 25: 1669–1688

[16] Megyesi JF, Kachur E, Lee DH et al. Imaging correlates of molecular signatures in oligodendrogliomas. Clin Cancer Res 2004; 10: 4303–4306

[17] Zlatescu MC, TehraniYazdi A, Sasaki H et al. Tumor location and growth pattern correlate with genetic signature in oligodendroglial neoplasms. Cancer Res 2001; 61: 6713–6715

[18] Behin A, Hoang-Xuan K, Carpentier AF, Delattre JY. Primary brain tumours in adults. Lancet 2003; 361: 323–331

[19] Beckmann MJ, Prayson RA. A clinicopathologic study of 30 cases of oligoastrocytoma including p53 immunohistochemistry. Pathology 1997; 29: 159–164

[20] Ricci PE, Dungan DH. Imaging of low- and intermediate-grade gliomas. Semin Radiat Oncol 2001; 11: 103–112

[21] Shaw EG, Scheithauer BW, O'Fallon JR, Davis DH. Mixed oligoastrocytomas: a survival and prognostic factor analysis. Neurosurgery 1994; 34: 577–582, discussion 582

[22] Lee YY, Van Tassel P. Intracranial oligodendrogliomas: imaging findings in 35 untreated cases. AJR Am J Roentgenol 1989; 152: 361–369

[23] Shin JH, Lee HK, Khang SK et al. Neuronal tumors of the central nervous system: radiologic findings and pathologic correlation. Radiographics 2002; 22: 1177–1189

[24] Lantos PL, Vandenberg SR, Kleihues P. Tumours of the nervous system. In: Graham DI, Lantos PL, eds. Greenfield's Neuropathology. 6th ed. London, England: Arnold; 1997:583–879

[25] Russo CP, Katz DS, Corona RJ, Jr, Winfield JA. Gangliocytoma of the cervicothoracic spinal cord. AJNR Am J Neuroradiol 1995; 16 Suppl: 889–891

[26] Padberg GW, Schot JD, Vielvoye GJ, Bots GT, de Beer FC. Lhermitte-Duclos disease and Cowden disease: a single phakomatosis. Ann Neurol 1991; 29: 517–523

[27] Meltzer CC, Smirniotopoulos JG, Jones RV. The striated cerebellum: an MR imaging sign in Lhermitte-Duclos disease (dysplastic gangliocytoma). Radiology 1995; 194: 699–703

[28] Chang KH, Han MH, Kim DG et al. MR appearance of central neurocytoma. Acta Radiol 1993; 34: 520–526

[29] Castillo M, Davis PC, Takei Y, Hoffman JC, Jr. Intracranial ganglioglioma: MR, CT, and clinical findings in 18 patients. AJNR Am J Neuroradiol 1990; 11: 109–114

[30] Paulus W, Schlote W, Perentes E, Jacobi G, Warmuth-Metz M, Roggendorf W. Desmoplastic supratentorial neuroepithelial tumours of infancy. Histopathology 1992; 21: 43–49

[31] Tenreiro-Picon OR, Kamath SV, Knorr JR, Ragland RL, Smith TW, Lau KY. Desmoplastic infantile ganglioglioma: CT and MRI features. Pediatr Radiol 1995; 25: 540–543

[32] Fernandez C, Girard N, Paz Paredes A, Bouvier-Labit C, Lena G, Figarella-Branger D. The usefulness of MR imaging in the diagnosis of dysembryoplastic neuroepithelial tumor in children: a study of 14 cases. AJNR Am J Neuroradiol 2003; 24: 829–834

[33] Ostertun B, Wolf HK, Campos MG et al. Dysembryoplastic neuroepithelial tumors: MR and CT evaluation. AJNR Am J Neuroradiol 1996; 17: 419–430

[34] Louis DN, Ohgaki H, Wiestler OD et al. The 2007 WHO classification of tumours of the central nervous system. Acta Neuropathol 2007; 114: 97–109

[35] Pomeroy SL, Tamayo P, Gaasenbeek M et al. Prediction of central nervous system embryonal tumour outcome based on gene expression. Nature 2002; 415: 436–442

[36] Roberts RO, Lynch CF, Jones MP, Hart MN. Medulloblastoma: a population-based study of 532 cases. J Neuropathol Exp Neurol 1991; 50: 134–144

[37] Koeller KK, Rushing EJ. From the archives of the AFIP: medulloblastoma: a comprehensive review with radiologic-pathologic correlation. Radiographics 2003; 23: 1613–1637

[38] Altman N, Fitz CR, Chuang S, Harwood-Nash D, Cotter C, Armstrong D. Radiologic characteristics of primitive neuroectodermal tumors in children. AJNR Am J Neuroradiol 1985; 6: 15–18

[39] Borja MJ, Plaza MJ, Altman N, Saigal G. Conventional and advanced MRI features of pediatric intracranial tumors: supratentorial tumors. AJR Am J Roentgenol 2013; 200: W483–503

[40] Biegel JA. Molecular genetics of atypical teratoid/rhabdoid tumor. Neurosurg Focus 2006; 20: E11

[41] Meyers SP, Khademian ZP, Biegel JA, Chuang SH, Korones DN, Zimmerman RA. Primary intracranial atypical teratoid/rhabdoid tumors of infancy and childhood. MRI features and patient outcomes. AJNR Am J Neuroradiol 2006; 27: 962–971

[42] Grogg KL, Miller RF, Dogan A. HIV infection and lymphoma. J Clin Pathol 2007; 60: 1365–1372

[43] Erdag N, Bhorade RM, Alberico RA, Yousuf N, Patel MR. Primary lymphoma of the central nervous system: typical and atypical CT and MR imaging appearances. AJR Am J Roentgenol 2001; 176: 1319–1326

[44] Haque S, Law M, Abrey LE, Young RJ. Imaging of lymphoma of the central nervous system, spine, and orbit. Radiol Clin North Am 2008; 46: 339–361, ix

[45] Norden AD, Wen PY, Kesari S. Brain metastases. Curr Opin Neurol 2005; 18: 654–661

[46] Fink KR, Fink JR. Imaging of brain metastases. Surg Neurol Int 2013; 4 Suppl 4: S209–S219

2 Response Assessment in Neuro-oncology

Tom Mikkelsen and Tobias Walbert

2.1 Introduction

The gold standard for outcome in oncology and in the treatment of brain tumors is measured as overall survival. Beyond showing improved survival, clinical trials have relied on surrogate markers such as progression-free survival (PFS) and radiographic response to show improvements with brain tumor treatment. As with other solid tumors, radiographic response has been the most important end point in clinical trials for brain tumors. Reduction in tumor mass has traditionally been seen as an important correlate marker for improved quality of life, longer survival, and overall clinical benefit.[1] The assessment of tumor burden in high-grade glioma (HGG) patients in clinical trials has been based on the contrast extravasation as measured on computed tomography (CT) or, more recently, by magnetic resonance imaging (MRI). This two-dimensional planar measurement has worked reasonably well in the era of cytotoxic chemotherapy, but the development of antiangiogenic agents such as bevacizumab in brain tumors has challenged this paradigm and has triggered the requirement for and development of new imaging end points. In 2010, new response criteria from the Response Assessment in Neuro-Oncology (RANO) Working Group addressed some of these challenges.[2]

2.2 Traditional Assessments of Brain Tumors

Early attempts to use and standardize imaging criteria for evaluating patients undergoing therapy for HGGs go back to the 1970s when CT scans were first used to define tumor progression in brain tumor patients.[3] In 1990, the so-called Macdonald criteria further developed the Levin criteria and established, for the first time, a set of objective radiological and clinical response criteria for the standardized assessment of brain tumor response.[4] They provided a standardized radiological assessment tool for tumor response in clinical trials and were based on the two-dimensional measurement of tumor enhancement with contrast (sum of the products of the maximum perpendicular tumor diameters) (▸ Table 2.1). In addition to the imaging features, the so-called Macdonald criteria also considered the impact of corticosteroids and changes in neurologic status of patients. This new set of criteria enabled response rates to be standardized for clinical trials and has been widely used in clinical trials. Although the Macdonald criteria were originally developed for use in CT scans, they were successfully extrapolated to MRI as well. In either case imaging interpretation is based on the disruption of the blood–brain barrier and the extravasation of contrast material into the peritumoral brain tissue.

During the same time period, one-dimensional assessment of solid tumors became the standard to assess response to treatment. The Response Evaluation Criteria in Solid Tumors (RECIST) were first published in 2000[5] and later revised in 2009.[6] The one-dimensional RECIST have been widely used in systemic cancers. Although they were found to correlate with two-dimensional and volumetric assessment in retrospective HGG studies,[7,8] they were inferior to three-dimensional assessment. To this point the RECIST have not been prospectively validated in brain tumors and the Macdonald criteria remain the most extensively used brain tumor imaging criteria.

2.3 Limitations of Macdonald Criteria

Although there are several limitations to using the Macdonald criteria (reviewed in detail by van den Bent et al[9]) the most prominent is its reliance on contrast-enhancing lesions to define tumor progression.[9] Contrast enhancement in the brain is a reflection of the blood–brain barrier and is nonspecific. Although this is commonly seen in HGGs, it can also be caused by other nontumor processes such as postsurgical changes,[10] ischemia,[11] seizure activity,[12] radiation-induced pseudoprogression, or radiation necrosis.[13] The often irregularly shaped tumors make proper measurement difficult and create another layer of complexity while increasing the chances of interobserver variability. Enhancement itself can be influenced by steroids and antiangiogenic agents.[14] The use of the latter, creating

Table 2.1 Macdonald response criteria for malignant glioma

Response	Definition
Complete response	Requires all of the following:
	Complete disappearance of all enhancing measurable and nonmeasurable disease sustained for at least 4 weeks
	No new lesions
	No corticosteroids
	Clinically stable or improved
Partial response	Requires all of the following:
	50% or more decrease compared with baseline in the sum of products of perpendicular diameters of all measurable enhancing lesions sustained for at least 4 weeks
	No new lesions
	Stable or reduced corticosteroid dose
	Clinically stable or improved
Stable disease	Requires all of the following:
	Does not qualify for complete or partial response, or progression
	Clinically stable
Progression	Defined by any of the following:
	25% or more increase in sum of the products of perpendicular diameters of enhancing lesions
	Any new lesion
	Clinical deterioration

Source: Data from Macdonald DR, Cascino TL, Schold SC Jr, Cairncross JG. Response criteria for phase II studies of supratentorial malignant glioma. J Clin Oncol 1990;8(7):1277–1280.

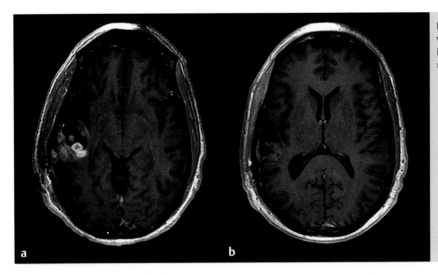

Fig. 2.1 (a) Response to radiation treatment with concurrent temozolomide and additional investigational agent. (b) Shows complete response after 3 months of treatment.

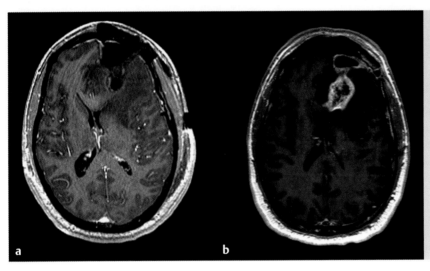

Fig. 2.2 Pseudoprogression. (a) A 54-year-old patient who underwent gross total resection for a glioblastoma. (b) Increased enhancement and edema after completion of radiation therapy with concurrent temozolomide and an investigational agent. The patient underwent repeat surgery, and pathological assessment did not find any active tumor tissue.

the picture of a so-called pseudoresponse, triggered the requirement for the development of new imaging criteria.

2.4 Pseudoprogression and Radiation Effects

The standard of care for patients with glioblastoma (GBM) consists of maximal safe tumor resection followed by radiation with concurrent and adjuvant chemotherapy with temozolomide (▶ Fig. 2.1).[15] On the first MRI scan following radiation therapy up to one third of patients present with contrast enhancement, which eventually subsides without changing the therapeutic regimen.[16,17] These occurrences are thought to be caused by a transient increase of blood vessel permeability due to radiation and are commonly called pseudoprogression. Temozolomide acts as a radiosensitizer when given concurrently with radiation therapy for GBM.[18] The incidence of pseudoprogression appears to be increased with its use during radiation and correlates with the methylation of the *MGMT* gene promoter.[19] This treatment effect has not been formally addressed in the Macdonald criteria while having implications on patient management and treatment evaluation. Despite the

development of new radiographic assessment, such as perfusion imaging,[20,21] there is no reliable imaging to differentiate between true tumor progression and pseudoprogression (▶ Fig. 2.2). In addition, the combination of radiation with chemotherapy appears to result in more frequent and earlier radiation necrosis than treatment with radiation alone.[22] The inability to differentiate between pseudoprogression, radiation necrosis, and tumor progression limits the validity of PFS as the primary end point in clinical trials. Patients with pseudoprogression who participate in clinical trials for recurrent disease would create falsely high response rates and prolonged survival rates. Although most clinical trials use a 90-day minimum interval after radiation therapy to participate in clinical trials, the Macdonald criteria have not formally addressed this issue.

2.5 Enhancement from Local Treatment

Increased enhancement can be seen postsurgically and after the administration of locally administered therapies. Because postsurgical enhancement is often developing in the wall of the surgical cavity 48 to 72 hours after resection, postoperative

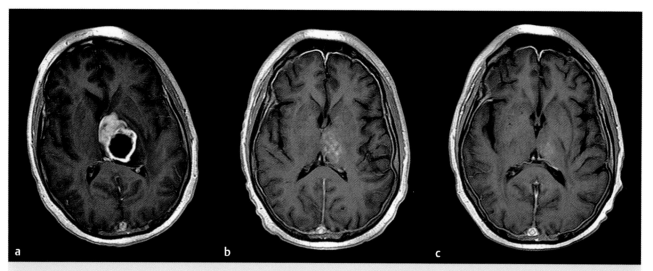

Fig. 2.3 Treatment response to bevacizumab. (a) A 41-year-old man with recurrent glioblastoma. (b) A partial response is seen after 2 months, and (c) there is a complete response after 6 months of treatment with bevacizumab.

MRI should be performed within the first 24 to 48 hours for comparison purposes.[10] This MRI scan should include diffusion-weighted images to assess for postsurgical ischemia. Local therapies such as chemotherapy wafers, immunotherapy, and locally administered gene and viral therapies further complicate the reliance on enhancement only to diagnose tumor progression.[9,23]

2.6 Pseudoresponse with Antiangiogenic Agents

Antiangiogenic agents targeting the vascular endothelial growth factor (VEGF) and its receptor are known to produce dramatic reduction in enhancement (▶ Fig. 2.3). The application of bevacizumab as well as cediranib can produce reduction in swelling and enhancement within 1 or 2 days of starting therapy, and radiological response rates of 25 to 60% have been described in the literature and can be observed in daily clinical practice.[24,25,26] This rapid presumed "response" to therapy is thought to be caused by a stabilization of the blood–brain barrier, based on the specific inhibition of VEGF (previously also known as vascular permeability factor). Based on the original Macdonald criteria, antiangiogenic therapy resulted in outstanding response rates, which, so far, have not been associated with major improvement in overall survival.[24,27]

2.7 Nonenhancing Tumors

Another limitation of the Macdonald criteria is due to the infiltrative nature of HGG that does not always result in a breakdown of the blood–brain barrier and enhancement with gadolinium.[28] The Macdonald criteria do not account for the extent of nonenhancing tumor mass that is routinely observed as hyperintensity on fluid-attenuated inversion recovery (FLAIR) and T2-weighted imaging. Although being highly sensitive to new changes in the brain, FLAIR changes can be difficult to interpret because they are caused not only by tumor

progression but also by peritumoral edema and radiation-induced white matter changes. The application of the Macdonald criteria has been limited in trials for low-grade (World Health Organization [WHO] II) and anaplastic tumors (WHO III), which often present without any enhancement and intact blood–brain barrier. Several studies have shown that a subpopulation of patients that showed initial response to antiangiogenic therapy subsequently presented with increasing areas of nonenhancing infiltrating disease observed on FLAIR sequences (▶ Fig. 2.4). It has been shown that VEGF-targeting agents lead to a decrease of the vascular supply and a reduction of large- and medium-sized blood vessels. At the same time the brain tumor showed increased infiltration into the parenchyma along with increased FLAIR hyperintensity. This phenomenon is thought to be a reflection of the tumor cells' increased usage of existing blood vessels, resulting in more tumor cell invasion and nonenhancing disease on FLAIR sequence.[29,30]

2.8 Development of Updated Response Assessment Criteria in Neuro-oncology

The aforementioned limitations of the Macdonald criteria have led to an international effort in the neuro-oncology community to develop more specific criteria to define response in clinical trials with HGG patients. This international group effort was initiated after it became obvious that the Macdonald criteria were insufficient to assess brain tumors with the validity, objectivity, reproducibility, and comprehensiveness that are required by regulatory agencies. The RANO Working Group consisted of international opinion leaders in the field of neuro-oncology and included neuro-oncologists, neurosurgeons, radiation oncologists, neuroradiologists, and neuropsychologists as well as specialists in the assessment of quality of life.[2] The RANO Working Group includes members with leadership responsibility in major research cooperative groups in the United States and Europe. The members were selected as part of an informal

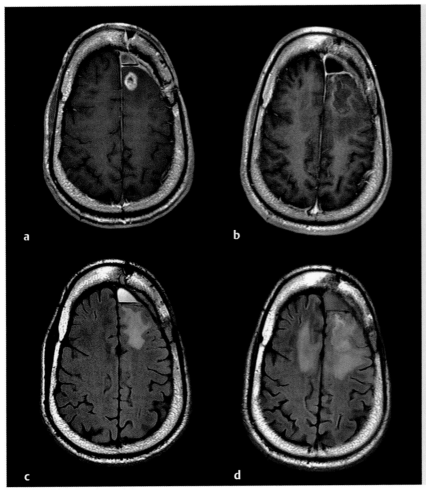

Fig. 2.4 (a–d) Progressive disease based on fluid-attenuated inversion recovery (FLAIR) imaging during therapy with bevacizumab, **(b)** A sustained response based on contrast enhancement after 6 months of treatment. **(c,d)** A patient with recurrent glioblastoma. **(d)** Disease progression at the same time based on FLAIR imaging.

process, and input of patient representative groups is not described. The suggested guidelines on how to assess response in HGG and in low-grade glioma, and the evaluation of surgically based therapies, were published in 2010, 2011, and 2012, respectively.[2,23,31] Rather than being definite, the recommendations of the RANO group should be seen as a work in progress to better define response to therapy in patients with malignant brain tumors not only in the setting of clinical trials but in daily practice as well.

2.9 The RANO Criteria

The updated response criteria for HGG by the RANO group is a further development of the Macdonald criteria and is similarly based on the serial assessment of specific lesions; however, in addition to the enhancing lesions, nonenhancing parts of the tumor are also assessed (▶ Table 2.2). As before, the product of the maximal cross-section diameters is used to measure the contrast-enhancing lesions.[2] Similar to the Macdonald criteria, measurable enhancing lesions must have at least two perpendicular diameters that measure at least 10 mm each and that are visible on two or more slices of an MRI that are at most 5 mm apart. Cystic parts and the surgical cavity are not included in the measurement. Nonmeasurable enhancing disease is defined by lesions that are only unidimensionally measurable (i.e., masses without clear margins or with a

perpendicular diameter < 10 mm). Patients with a gross total resection can achieve only stable disease as the best radiographic outcome, and patients without measurable disease cannot participate in studies intending to measure response rate as the primary outcome. However, patients without measurable disease can participate when the primary end point is duration until disease progression (tumor control).

2.9.1 Assessment of Multiple Lesions

In the setting of more than one enhancing lesion, a minimum of the two largest and a maximum of up to five lesions should be measured. Similarly to the RECIST, the sum of the product of the perpendicular diameters of these lesions should be calculated.[6] The RANO Working Group realizes that sometimes a smaller lesion should be favored over the largest one if it can be measured more precisely. When assessing patients with multiple lesions of which not all are increasing in size, the enlarging lesions should be the ones considered for response evaluation.

2.9.2 Precautions to Avoid Pseudoprogression

As described earlier, approximately 30% of all patients undergoing radiation with concurrent chemotherapy will develop so-called pseudoprogression.[16,17] This transient increase of blood

Table 2.2 Response Assessment in Neuro-Oncology (RANO) Working Group response criteria

Response	Definition
Complete response (CR)	Requires all of the following:
	Complete disappearance of all enhancing measurable and nonmeasurable disease for at least 4 weeks
	No new enhancing lesions
	Stable or improved nonenhancing (T2/FLAIR) lesions
	Off corticosteroids
	Clinically stable or improved
	Patients with nonmeasurable disease only, cannot have CR: best response possible is SD
Partial response (PR)	Requires all of the following:
	50% or more decrease compared with baseline of all measurable enhancing lesions sustained for at least 4 weeks
	No progression of nonmeasurable disease
	No new enhancing lesions
	Stable or improved nonenhancing (T2/FLAIR) lesions
	Same or lower dose of corticosteroids compared with baseline scan
	Clinically stable or improved
Stable disease (SD)	Requires all of the following:
	Does not qualify for CR, PR, PD
	No new lesions
	Stable nonenhancing (T2/FLAIR) lesions
	Same or lower dose of corticosteroids compared with baseline scan
	Clinically stable or improved
Progressive disease (PD)	Defined by any of the following:
	25% or more increase in enhancing lesions compared with the smallest tumor measurement obtained either at baseline (if no decrease) or best response
	Significant increase in T2/FLAIR nonenhancing lesion compared with baseline scan or best response after initiation of therapy
	Any new lesion
	Above imaging changes on stable or increasing doses of corticosteroids
	Clear clinical deterioration not attributable to other causes than tumor or changes in corticosteroid dose
	Failure to return for evaluation as a result of death, deteriorating condition, or clear progression of nonmeasurable disease

Abbreviations: FLAIR, fluid-attenuated inversion recovery.
Source: Adapted from Wen P, Macdonald DR, Reardon DA, et al. Updated response assessment criteria for high-grade gliomas: Response Assessment in Neuro-Oncology Working Group. J Clin Oncol 2010;28(11):1963–1972.

vessel permeability due to radiation is especially prevalent within the first 3 months after finishing radiation therapy. Therefore, the RANO Working Group suggests excluding all patients showing new enhancement within the first 90 days after irradiation, except when the new enhancing lesion is beyond the high-dose radiation field. This recommendation only formalizes current practice because most current clinical trials already exclude patients within this time window.

2.9.3 Radiographic Response

Radiographic response is assessed by comparing sequential MRIs. To obtain best results, all images should be obtained with the same techniques as the baseline MRI. If it is not possible to use the same MRI scanner, at least the same magnet strength should be used to obtain the follow-up MRI scans. When it is not possible to clearly identify disease progression, when the MRI does not clearly indicate disease progression, but shows the questionable disease progression, the RANO criteria allow for continuing with the current treatment for another 4 weeks and to repeat the MRI at that point. If, after a subsequent MRI scan, disease progression is identified, the date of progression should be noted according to when the first MRI signs of progression were identified. Because it is challenging to determine disease progression when one is using antiangiogenic agents, a follow-up MRI scan is recommended 4 weeks after initiating antiangiogenic therapy. Based on comparison with the pretreatment or baseline MRI scan, the RANO criteria differentiate between complete response (CR), partial response (PR), stable disease (SD), and progressive disease (PD) (▶ Table 2.3).

2.9.4 Complete Response

A CR is defined by the complete disappearance of all enhancing measurable and nonmeasurable lesions. This absence of enhancement must be sustained for at least 4 weeks. At the same time no new lesions are permitted, and nonenhancing

Table 2.3 Response Assessment in Neuro-Oncology response criteria schematic summary

Criteria	Complete response	Partial response	Stable disease	Progressive disease
T1 enhancement	No	≥50% ↓	<50% ↓ but <25% ↑	≥25% ↑
T2/FLAIR	↔ or ↓	↔ or ↓	↔ or ↓	↑—sufficient to define PD
New lesions	No	No	No	Yes—sufficient to define PD
Corticosteroids	No	↔ or ↓	↔ or ↓	Not sufficient to define PD
Clinical status	↔ or ↑	↔ or ↑	↔ or ↑	↓—sufficient to define PD
Required change	All	All	All	Any

Abbreviations: FLAIR, fluid-attenuated inversion recovery; PD, progressive disease.
Source: Adapted from Wen PY, Macdonald DR, Reardon DA, et al. Updated response assessment criteria for high-grade gliomas: response assessment in neuro-oncology working group. J Clin Oncol 2010;28(11):1963–1972.

disease on T2/FLAIR must be at least stable or improved as well. Patients must be off corticosteroids or on physiological replacement doses while their clinical status must remain unchanged or improved.

2.9.5 Partial Response

To qualify as a PR according to the RANO criteria, the patient's MRI scan must show at least a 50% decrease of the sum of products of perpendicular diameters of all measurable enhancing lesions for at least 4 weeks. Nonenhancing or nonmeasurable disease must be stable at the same time, and the patient's steroid dosage must be the same or lower than at baseline. A follow-up scan is required in 4 weeks to reach the definition of PR, otherwise the response must be rated as SD.

In the setting of multifocal tumors, PR is defined as the decrease of 50% or more of the sum of products of perpendicular diameters of all measurable disease when compared with the baseline. Similar to singular lesions, this response must be achieved on stable or decreasing doses of corticosteroids and must be sustained for at least 4 weeks.

2.9.6 Progression

PD is defined by a variety of changes. A 25% or greater increase in the sum of the products of perpendicular diameters of the enhancing disease when compared with the baseline defines PD. A recent decrease in corticosteroids disqualifies the finding from PD even if there is an increase in enhancement. A significant increase of nonenhancing lesions observed in T2/FLAIR images with a stable or increasing regimen of corticosteroids when compared to the baseline MRI scan or the best response after the start of therapy is also considered as PD. It is important to understand that *significant* in this context is used in the sense of *relevant* and is dependent on the clinician's interpretation. Clear progression of nonmeasurable lesions or any new enhancing lesions also qualify as PD.

Definite clinical deterioration not attributable to any other causes but tumor is to be considered PD. This specifically excludes clinical decline due to the decrease of corticosteroids.

Multifocal lesions represent PD if there is an increase of 25% or more of the sum of products of perpendicular diameters of all measurable lesions. Similar to singular lesions, the image should be compared with the smallest tumor measurement after the start of therapy. The appearance of a new lesion as part of the multifocal tumor is also to be considered PD. Patients who initially present with enhancing lesions that are considered nonmeasurable are considered to have PD if their lesions expand to or beyond the foregoing definition of measurable disease (≥10 mm in bidirectional diameter and visible on at least two slides that are at most 5 mm apart). If there is any doubt that a patient is presenting with PD, the general recommendation of the RANO criteria is to continue with the current treatment and to repeat MRI in 4 to 8 weeks.

Patients who do not return for follow-up due to clinical deterioration or due to death are considered to have had PD.

2.9.7 Stable Disease

Follow-up MRI findings are considered as SD if the findings are not consistent with CR, PR, or PD and if nonenhancing (FLAIR/T2) lesions are stable as well. Stable disease requires the patient to be clinically stable and to be on a lower or stable dose of corticosteroids when the MRI scan is compared to the baseline imaging.

2.9.8 Corticosteroid Use as Defining Criteria

The role of steroids is rather complex in the RANO criteria. In addition to the radiographic criteria just outlined, the use of steroids must be considered in order to assess radiographic responses according to the RANO criteria. It is important to realize that it is not feasible to interpret imaging changes without having detailed knowledge about possible changes in corticosteroid therapy. A patient cannot be on any therapeutic steroids to qualify for a CR. To qualify as PR or even stable disease, patients must be on stable or decreasing doses of corticosteroids. However, an increase in corticosteroids without neurologic decline is not sufficient to categorize an otherwise stable MRI scan as PD. These patients should be followed closely and their radiographic response should be considered as SD if the corticosteroids can be reduced back to baseline levels. Should it become apparent that they continue to decline due to the tumor, their disease should be categorized as PD. In this situation, the date of progression is the time of steroid increase.

2.9.9 Clinical Assessment

The clinical assessment is not clearly defined in the RANO criteria, but it plays an important role. If a patient with a baseline Karnofsky performance scale (KPS) score from 100 to 90 declines to 70 or less, or a patient with a KPS score of 90 declines by 20, the clinicians should consider this deterioration as significant if it cannot be attributed to any other non-tumor-related events. A decline to 50 or less from any baseline should always be considered significant as well when using the RANO criteria. Similar guidelines apply to the use of Eastern Cooperative Oncology Group or WHO performance scores where a decline from 0 or 1 to 2 or from 2 to 3 should be considered as a clinical deterioration. Therefore, changes in clinical status even without imaging changes can be a defining factor when assessing treatment response according to the RANO criteria.

Although the importance of performance status was strengthened in the new response criteria, the RANO group did not recommend the adoption of neurocognitive measures, quality of life, or symptom assessment to be used to assess disease progression.

2.9.10 Role of New Imaging

The authors of the RANO criteria realize that the two-dimensional assessment of tumors has significant shortcomings. Although there is continuous and growing academic interest in three-dimensional imaging, the lack of standardization and availability outside specialized centers precludes the integration of volumetric measures into daily clinical practice.

A similar approach was taken to other emerging MRI techniques such as dynamic susceptibility MRI (perfusion imaging), dynamic contrast-enhanced MRI (permeability imaging), diffusion imaging, magnetic resonance spectroscopy, and positron-emission tomography. Although some of these advanced techniques might be helpful in daily clinical decision making at experienced sites, more research and standardization is required to recommend them as criteria to base response assessment across multiple clinical sites.

2.9.11 Limitations

The new RANO criteria are an important step to standardize response criteria for HGG (▶ Table 2.4). The introduction of antiangiogenic agents unmasked the deficiencies of relying primarily on contrast enhancement to represent disease burden in order to define treatment response. The integration of FLAIR/T2 imaging has added an important feature to the assessment of disease burden, despite the relative nonspecificity of these MRI features for tumor, being influenced by edema, treatment effects, and other pathology. Despite the value of broadening the criteria by incorporating other MR features, the current RANO criteria have persisting limitations. First, the criteria refer to "significant" changes in FLAIR signal, but without any definition of *significant*, because the working group acknowledges that it is difficult to assess nonenhancing tumors. Second, the lack of a clear definition of clinical symptoms is problematic. The limitations of arbitrary scales for performance status for the evaluation of brain tumor patients are well documented.[32] The validity and reliability of the KPS are questionable in brain tumor patients because the scale does not incorporate neurologic symptoms such as memory loss, speech disturbances, and seizure activity.[33,34] Nevertheless, the assessment of performance status has been given an important role in defining disease progression, especially when the use of corticosteroids to manage symptoms is concerned.

Of course, it must be understood that the RANO criteria have not been subjected to any rigorous testing process that would be required by any new laboratory test before being implemented in clinical practice. Thus the validity of these criteria to predict survival or true clinical deterioration remains unknown. Admittedly a work in progress, the criteria do begin to address the major limitations of the prior Macdonald criteria, limitations which have come to light primarily in the context of antiangiogenic therapies.

The RANO recommendations deal with many issues that apply to the clinical practice of neuro-oncologists but might be challenging for the radiologist. Although it is practical from a clinician's perspective to continue treatment when there is doubt about PD and to review earlier MRI scans when necessary, this retrospective approach will be challenging in a clinical trial setting where the continuation or extension of a trial or cohort is based on the immediate evaluation of disease progression. Furthermore, radiologists seldom have direct knowledge of a patient's clinical status and corticosteroid dosing.

Objectively, there are also a number of clinical situations where the ability to assess both contrast and FLAIR images remains problematic. The issue of multifocality whereby up to two separate zones in a single plane are summed sounds more objective than it may be in practice, where heterogeneity in defining a contrast margin is concerned, or where adjacent contrast-enhancing foci may be considered as part of a single lesion or separate. Mixed responses are also seen, either relating to measurable disease or to changes in nonmeasurable lesions, the inclusion or exclusion of which is often arbitrary.

Similarly, the definition of clinical status has been a long-standing issue, where no good objective neurologic scales exist, relying on the subjective impression of a clinician, an assessment that may differ between observers. The use of symptom assessment scales such as the M.D. Anderson Symptom Inventory Brain Tumor (MDASI-BT) might offer important ways to quantify and qualify clinical impairment in the future.[35]

Additionally, the current RANO criteria, which seek to be applicable by the most routine MRI methods, necessarily exclude the potential value of a number of new MRI sequences, including dynamic susceptibility contrast or dynamic contrast-enhanced perfusion, diffusion-weighted imaging, susceptibility-weighted imaging, magnetic resonance spectroscopy, and others, which may significantly enhance the specificity of changes in routine MRI sequences such as postcontrast T1 and FLAIR.

Finally, once a feature set, such as FLAIR and postcontrast T1, is defined, it would seem to be relatively straightforward to employ semiautomated measurement software, which can at least evaluate the arbitrary features in a more reproducible and observer-independent manner (▶ Fig. 2.5).

Table 2.4 Macdonald versus Response Assessment in Neuro-Oncology (RANO) criteria

	Macdonald criteria	RANO criteria
Complete response (CR)	Requires all of the following:	Requires all of the following:
	Complete disappearance of all enhancing measurable and nonmeasurable disease for at least 4 weeks	Complete disappearance of all enhancing measurable and nonmeasurable disease for at least 4 weeks
	No new enhancing lesions	No new enhancing lesions
		Stable or improved nonenhancing (T2/FLAIR) lesions
	No corticosteroids	No corticosteroids
	Clinically stable or improved	Clinically stable or improved
Partial response (PR)	Requires all of the following:	Requires all of the following:
	50% or more decrease compared with baseline in the sum of products of perpendicular diameters of all measurable enhancing lesions for at least 4 weeks	50% or more decrease compared with baseline of all measurable enhancing lesions sustained for at least 4 weeks
		No progression of nonmeasurable disease
	No new enhancing lesions	No new enhancing lesions
		Stable or improved nonenhancing (T2/FLAIR) lesions
	Same or reduced dose of corticosteroids	Same or reduced dose of corticosteroids compared with baseline scan
	Clinically stable or improved	Clinically stable or improved
Stable disease	Requires all of the following:	Requires all of the following:
	Does not qualify for CR, PR, PD	Does not qualify for CR, PR, PD
		No new lesions
		Stable nonenhancing (T2/FLAIR) lesions
		Same or lower dose of corticosteroids compared with baseline scan
	Clinically stable	Clinically stable or improved
Progressive disease (PD)	Defined by any of the following:	Defined by any of the following:
	25% or more increase in sum of the products of perpendicular diameters of enhancing lesions	25% or more increase in enhancing lesions compared with the smallest tumor measurement obtained either at baseline (if no decrease) or best response
		Significant increase in T2/FLAIR nonenhancing lesion compared with baseline scan or best response after initiation of therapy
	Any new lesion	Any new lesion
		Above imaging changes on stable or increasing doses of corticosteroids
	Clinical deterioration	Clear clinical deterioration not attributable to other causes than tumor or changes in corticosteroid dose
		Failure to return for evaluation as a result of death, deteriorating condition, or clear progression of nonmeasurable disease

Abbreviation: FLAIR, fluid-attenuated inversion recovery.
Source: Adapted from Macdonald DR, Cascino TL, Schold SC Jr, Cairncross JG. Response criteria for phase II studies of supratentorial malignant glioma. J Clin Oncol 1990;8(7):1277–1280; and Wen P, Macdonald DR, Reardon DA, et al. Updated response assessment criteria for high-grade gliomas: Response Assessment in Neuro-Oncology Working Group. J Clin Oncol 2010;28(11):1963–1972.

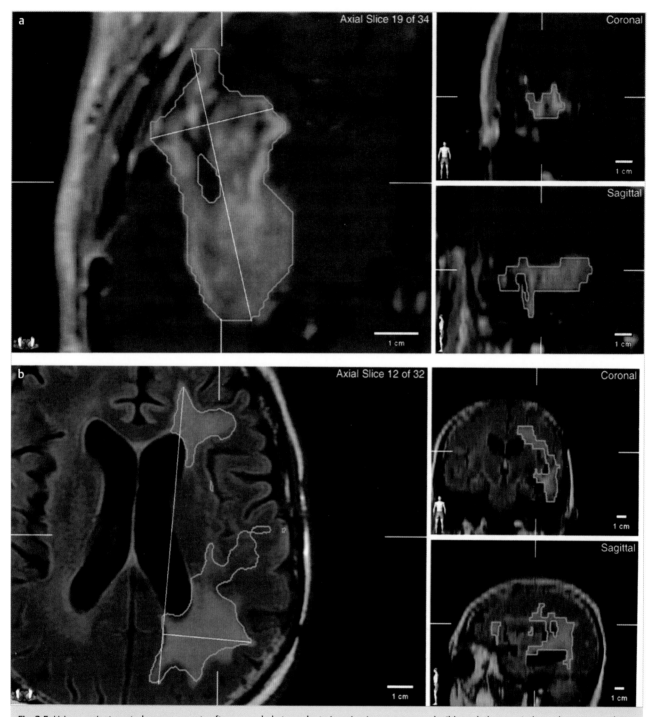

Fig. 2.5 Using semiautomated measurement software can help to evaluate imaging in a more reproducible and observer-independent manner, but it requires further improvement. (**a**) A successful example. (**b**) The pitfall of new automated software.

References

[1] Reardon DA, Galanis E, DeGroot JF et al. Clinical trial end points for high-grade glioma: the evolving landscape. Neuro-oncol 2011; 13: 353–361

[2] Wen PY, Macdonald DR, Reardon DA et al. Updated response assessment criteria for high-grade gliomas: response assessment in neuro-oncology working group. J Clin Oncol 2010; 28: 1963–1972

[3] Levin VA, Crafts DC, Norman DM, Hoffer PB, Spire JP, Wilson CB. Criteria for evaluating patients undergoing chemotherapy for malignant brain tumors. J Neurosurg 1977; 47: 329–335

[4] Macdonald DR, Cascino TL, Schold SC, Jr, Cairncross JG. Response criteria for phase II studies of supratentorial malignant glioma. J Clin Oncol 1990; 8: 1277–1280

[5] Therasse P, Arbuck SG, Eisenhauer EA et al. New guidelines to evaluate the response to treatment in solid tumors. European Organization for Research and Treatment of Cancer, National Cancer Institute of the United States, National Cancer Institute of Canada. J Natl Cancer Inst 2000; 92: 205–216

[6] Eisenhauer EA, Therasse P, Bogaerts J et al. New response evaluation criteria in solid tumours: revised RECIST guideline (version 1.1). Eur J Cancer 2009; 45: 228–247

[7] Shah GD, Kesari S, Xu R et al. Comparison of linear and volumetric criteria in assessing tumor response in adult high-grade gliomas. Neuro-oncol 2006; 8: 38–46

[8] Galanis E, Buckner JC, Maurer MJ et al. Validation of neuroradiologic response assessment in gliomas: measurement by RECIST, two-dimensional, computer-assisted tumor area, and computer-assisted tumor volume methods. Neuro-oncol 2006; 8: 156–165

[9] van den Bent MJ, Vogelbaum MA, Wen PY, Macdonald DR, Chang SM. End point assessment in gliomas: novel treatments limit usefulness of classical Macdonald's Criteria. J Clin Oncol 2009; 27: 2905–2908

[10] Cairncross JG, Pexman JH, Rathbone MP, DelMaestro RF. Postoperative contrast enhancement in patients with brain tumor. Ann Neurol 1985; 17: 570–572

[11] McMillan KM, Rogers BP, Field AS, Laird AR, Fine JP, Meyerand ME. Physiologic characterisation of glioblastoma multiforme using MRI-based hypoxia mapping, chemical shift imaging, perfusion and diffusion maps. J Clin Neurosci 2006; 13: 811–817

[12] Finn MA, Blumenthal DT, Salzman KL, Jensen RL. Transient postictal MRI changes in patients with brain tumors may mimic disease progression. Surg Neurol 2007; 67: 246–250, discussion 250

[13] Kumar AJ, Leeds NE, Fuller GN et al. Malignant gliomas: MR imaging spectrum of radiation therapy- and chemotherapy-induced necrosis of the brain after treatment. Radiology 2000; 217: 377–384

[14] Cairncross JG, Macdonald DR, Pexman JH, Ives FJ. Steroid-induced CT changes in patients with recurrent malignant glioma. Neurology 1988; 38: 724–726

[15] Stupp R, Mason WP, van den Bent MJ et al. European Organisation for Research and Treatment of Cancer Brain Tumor and Radiotherapy Groups, National Cancer Institute of Canada Clinical Trials Group. Radiotherapy plus concomitant and adjuvant temozolomide for glioblastoma. N Engl J Med 2005; 352: 987–996

[16] Brandsma D, Stalpers L, Taal W, Sminia P, van den Bent MJ. Clinical features, mechanisms, and management of pseudoprogression in malignant gliomas. Lancet Oncol 2008; 9: 453–461

[17] Taal W, Brandsma D, de Bruin HG et al. Incidence of early pseudo-progression in a cohort of malignant glioma patients treated with chemoirradiation with temozolomide. Cancer 2008; 113: 405–410

[18] Zhai GG, Malhotra R, Delaney M et al. Radiation enhances the invasive potential of primary glioblastoma cells via activation of the Rho signaling pathway. J Neurooncol 2006; 76: 227–237

[19] Brandes AA, Franceschi E, Tosoni A et al. MGMT promoter methylation status can predict the incidence and outcome of pseudoprogression after concomitant radiochemotherapy in newly diagnosed glioblastoma patients. J Clin Oncol 2008; 26: 2192–2197

[20] Hu LS, Eschbacher JM, Heiserman JE et al. Reevaluating the imaging definition of tumor progression: perfusion MRI quantifies recurrent glioblastoma tumor fraction, pseudoprogression, and radiation necrosis to predict survival. Neuro-oncol 2012; 14: 919–930

[21] Narang J, Jain R, Arbab AS et al. Differentiating treatment-induced necrosis from recurrent/progressive brain tumor using nonmodel-based semiquantitative indices derived from dynamic contrast-enhanced T1-weighted MR perfusion. Neuro-oncol 2011; 13: 1037–1046

[22] Chamberlain MC, Glantz MJ, Chalmers L, Van Horn A, Sloan AE. Early necrosis following concurrent Temodar and radiotherapy in patients with glioblastoma. J Neurooncol 2007; 82: 81–83

[23] Vogelbaum MA, Jost S, Aghi MK et al. Application of novel response/progression measures for surgically delivered therapies for gliomas: Response Assessment in Neuro-Oncology (RANO) Working Group. Neurosurgery 2012; 70: 234–243, discussion 243–244

[24] Vredenburgh JJ, Desjardins A, Herndon JE, II et al. Bevacizumab plus irinotecan in recurrent glioblastoma multiforme. J Clin Oncol 2007; 25: 4722–4729

[25] Batchelor TT, Sorensen AG, di Tomaso E et al. AZD2171, a pan-VEGF receptor tyrosine kinase inhibitor, normalizes tumor vasculature and alleviates edema in glioblastoma patients. Cancer Cell 2007; 11: 83–95

[26] Friedman HS, Prados MD, Wen PY et al. Bevacizumab alone and in combination with irinotecan in recurrent glioblastoma. J Clin Oncol 2009; 27: 4733–4740

[27] Batchelor TT, Duda DG, di Tomaso E et al. Phase II study of cediranib, an oral pan-vascular endothelial growth factor receptor tyrosine kinase inhibitor, in patients with recurrent glioblastoma. J Clin Oncol 2010; 28: 2817–2823

[28] Scott JN, Brasher PM, Sevick RJ, Rewcastle NB, Forsyth PA. How often are non-enhancing supratentorial gliomas malignant? A population study. Neurology 2002; 59: 947–949

[29] Keunen O, Johansson M, Oudin A et al. Anti-VEGF treatment reduces blood supply and increases tumor cell invasion in glioblastoma. Proc Natl Acad Sci U S A 2011; 108: 3749–3754

[30] de Groot JF, Fuller G, Kumar AJ et al. Tumor invasion after treatment of glioblastoma with bevacizumab: radiographic and pathologic correlation in humans and mice. Neuro-oncol 2010; 12: 233–242

[31] van den Bent MJ, Wefel JS, Schiff D et al. Response assessment in neuro-oncology (a report of the RANO group): assessment of outcome in trials of diffuse low-grade gliomas. Lancet Oncol 2011; 12: 583–593

[32] Cheng JX, Liu BL, Zhang X et al. The validation of the standard Chinese version of the European Organization for Research and Treatment of Cancer Quality of Life Core Questionnaire 30 (EORTC QLQ-C30) in pre-operative patients with brain tumor in China. BMC Med Res Methodol 2011; 11: 56

[33] Mackworth N, Fobair P, Prados MD. Quality of life self-reports from 200 brain tumor patients: comparisons with Karnofsky performance scores. J Neurooncol 1992; 14: 243–253

[34] Heimans JJ, Taphoorn MJ. Impact of brain tumour treatment on quality of life. J Neurol 2002; 249: 955–960

[35] Armstrong TS, Mendoza T, Gning I et al. Validation of the M.D. Anderson Symptom Inventory Brain Tumor Module (MDASI-BT) [published correction appears in J Neurooncol 2006;80(1):37. 2006; 80: 27–35

3 Going Beyond the Conventional Morphological Imaging: An Overview of Functional Imaging Techniques

Marco Essig and Cem Calli

3.1 Introduction

The goals and requirements for brain tumor imaging are to make a diagnosis or a differential diagnosis or both, whereas accurate lesion grading and delineation are needed in the case of tumor description and risk assessment. Imaging is also involved in the decision-making process for therapy and later for precise planning of surgical or radiotherapeutic interventions, both of which require an optimal detection and delineation of the lesions. After therapy, neuroimaging techniques are mandatory for monitoring disease and to identify and monitor possible therapy-related side effects.

Magnetic resonance imaging (MRI) is initially focused on the superb contrast and spatial resolution of neuronal tissue to enable a detailed morphological analysis. Recent developments, however, have focused on evaluating contrast and spatial resolution in conjunction with additional functional assessments. The characterization of neoplasm using physiological or pathophysiological characteristics has long been the domain of positron-emission tomography (PET).

Whereas PET has significantly improved our pathophysiological understanding of the central nervous system (CNS), the availability of MRI contrast agents and improved MR rapid imaging sequences are now enabling further noninvasive characterization of physiological tissue and diseases. Functional information can reflect macrovasculature, the breakdown of the blood–brain barrier (BBB) with resulting permeability for the contrast agent, and tissue perfusion. Neurofunctional magnetic resonance imaging (nfMRI) is a recently established technique that increases our diagnostic potential in the neurosciences, whereas MR-spectroscopic techniques such as chemical shift imaging (CSI) allow a detailed metabolic analysis of the neuronal or pathological tissue.

The overall diagnostic aim of functional neuroimaging of CNS neoplasms is to optimize tumor characterization, with an emphasis on improved specificity to separate benign from malignant features. Specific characterization facilitates planning of the most appropriate treatment. Furthermore, functional neuroimaging of CNS neoplasms can be expanded for monitoring ongoing therapy and for early detection of therapeutic side effects. The predictive assessment of therapy response, and monitoring ongoing therapy to guide therapeutic intervention, are major challenges in the current treatment of CNS neoplasms. This chapter provides a broad overview of the available functional neuroimaging methods and their use for detecting and monitoring neoplasms and their therapeutic interventions. Details on the individual techniques and their clinical impact are described separately in this chapter.

3.2 Magnetic Resonance Spectroscopy

Proton magnetic resonance spectroscopy (MRS), or spectroscopic imaging, is one of the first functional imaging techniques that provides detailed tumor information beyond the morphological characteristics. The method has become a common clinical tool, especially in the diagnostic workup of tumors and the differentiation from normal or physiological neuronal tissue changes.

There are different elements that allow a spectroscopic characterization; however, due to its dominant presence that allows the best signal-to-noise ratio, 1 H protons are used most commonly in clinical practice. The spectroscopic characterization of brain abnormalities relies mostly on the calculations of ratios between the main proton spectrum metabolites, notably *N*-acetylaspartate (NAA), a neuronal marker, choline-containing compounds (Cho), a marker of membrane turnover, and creatine (Cr) including the phosphocreatine compound, and on the presence of lipids and lactate.[1–6] Brain tumors typically have loss of NAA and an increase in the Cho content (▶ Fig. 3.1). MRS has also been used to differentiate nontumor lesions, such as hamartomas, from gliomas.[7,8] Several studies have reported that hamartomas did not differ significantly from the normal brain or physiological changes, whereas gliomas had lower NAA:Cr, Cr:Cho, and NAA:Cho ratios (▶ Fig. 3.2). In patients with seizures it is important to identify tumor changes from scar because this has a major impact on the further management of patients. In a study by Vuori et al,[6] patients with seizures and a cortical brain lesion on MRI scan were studied with proton MRS. A metabolite ratio analysis was performed, and the metabolite signals in the lesion core were compared with those in the contralateral centrum semiovale and in the corresponding brain sites of control subjects to separately obtain the changes in NAA, Cho, and Cr. In their study, 10 patients had a low-grade glioma (three, oligodendrogliomas; three, oligoastrocytomas; three, astrocytomas; and one, pilocytic astrocytoma), and eight had focal cortical developmental malformations (FCDM) (five, focal cortical dysplasias, and three, dysembryoplastic neuroepithelial tumors). The authors found that loss of NAA and increase of Cho were more pronounced in low-grade gliomas than in subjects with cortical developmental malformations. MRS was also able to differentiate between subtypes of gliomas.

In a study by Law,[9] which combined MRS with the later-described magnetic resonance perfusion, both methods enabled identification at a high sensitivity and a high positive predictive value for tumor grading when compared with conventional contrast-enhanced MRI. It is well known that a certain percentage of high-grade tumors do not present with a BBB disruption or vice versa. For biopsy planning and for treatment decision and management it is essential to identify the highest tumor grade in those often very morphologically homogeneous-appearing tumors. The author was also able to provide thresholds for the metabolite ratios for the diagnosis of a high-grade tumor. A review of the literature, taking into account differences in MRS technique such as the choice of echo time (TE) and the method used to determine metabolite ratios, demonstrates that the mean maximal values obtained for Cho:Cr and

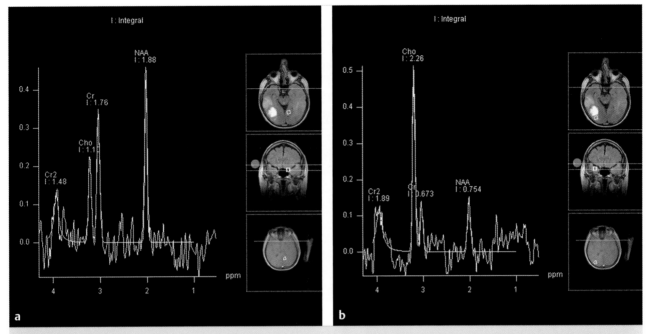

Fig. 3.1 Magnetic resonance spectroscopy of a 36-year-old patient with anaplastic astrocytoma. In normal tissue (**a**) from the contralateral side, N-acetylaspartate (NAA) is the most pronounced metabolite representing normal neuronal tissue, followed by the creatine (Cr) peak for energy metabolism. The choline (Cho) peak is small in normal tissue because there is not a lot of membrane turnover. Lactate or lipids are not present in a normal spectrum. A tumor (**b**) is characterized by an elevated Cho peak representing a high membrane turnover and a reduction or loss of NAA as normal neuronal tissue is replaced by tumor tissue. The higher the grade, the more pronounced is the NAA reduction and the presence of lactate or lipids as a sign of anaerobic glycolysis.

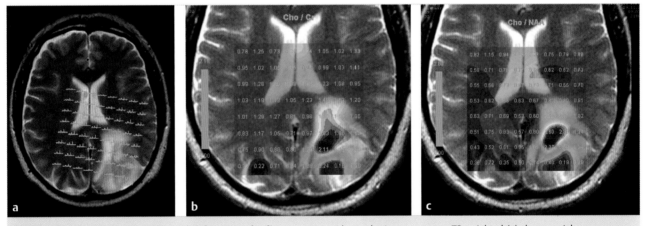

Fig. 3.2 Spectroscopic imaging (chemical shift imaging [CSI]) in a patient with anaplastic astrocytoma. T2-weighted (**a**) shows an inhomogeneous tumor in the left occipito-parietal region. The CSI maps of the ratio of choline (Cho) to creatine (Cr) (**b**) or Cho to N-acetylaspartate (NAA) (**c**) present a hot spot in the anterior aspect of the tumor representing a high proliferation and aggressiveness of the tissue.

Cho:NAA and the mean minimum values for NAA:Cr ratios in the studies[1,7] were comparable to previously published data in differentiating between low- and high-grade gliomas.

As with many functional techniques, one of the challenges is standardized data acquisition and postprocessing. For data acquisition the same TE should be used, and data from the contralateral unaffected white matter should be acquired. Studies comparing long and short TE MRS studies found that a short TE provided a slightly better tumor classification.[10,11] In a study by Majós et al, only meningiomas profited from long TE acquisitions.[12]

The use of modern scanner technology further allows measurement of spectroscopic data from more than a single voxel. Two- or three-dimensional MRS (2D or 3D CSI) enables acquisition from multiple small voxels, which provides more detailed information about lesion heterogeneity (▶ Fig. 3.2). The voxel information can be used to calculate metabolite ratios, which can be color coded and superimposed on the anatomical images to allow better visualization (e.g., hot spots within a tumor).

Follow-up assessment of cerebral tumors is a promising field for MRS. Increases in size and contrast enhancement are typical

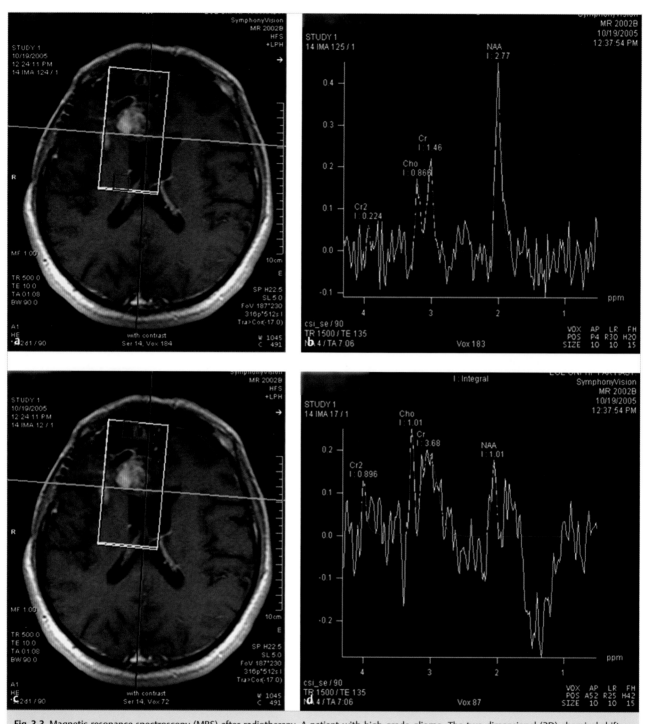

Fig. 3.3 Magnetic resonance spectroscopy (MRS) after radiotherapy. A patient with high-grade glioma. The two-dimensional (2D) chemical shift imaging (CSI) MRS for the follow-up of the patient after surgery and radiotherapy. The magnetic resonance spectra obtained from the normal-appearing area (a) (the voxel represented with blue square in CSI grid) show normal brain MRS findings (b). However, in the anterior part of the grid, the spectra taken from the small ring-enhancing lesion (c) reveal decreased levels of all metabolites and a prominent peak under the baseline at 1.3 ppm at middle echo time (TE) (TE:135 ms) representing the lactate doublet (d). This area represents radiation necrosis.

findings in tumor progression but also reflect therapeutically induced changes. The same is true for postoperative changes. Often microbleeding is seen in the treated tissue. This may cause a local field inhomogeneity, which is a technical challenge for MRS (▶ Fig. 3.3). However, the method allows supplementary information about the possible extent and nature of changes on a routine MRI scan by analyzing the metabolite ratios (▶ Fig. 3.3). The ratio of choline to normal creatine level is usually significantly elevated in those areas consistent with tumor compared with those containing predominantly treatment effect. In fact, treatment effect is generally indicated by a marked depression of all the intracellular metabolite peaks from choline, creatine, and N-acetyl compounds. However, MRS alone may not be helpful in instances where patients have

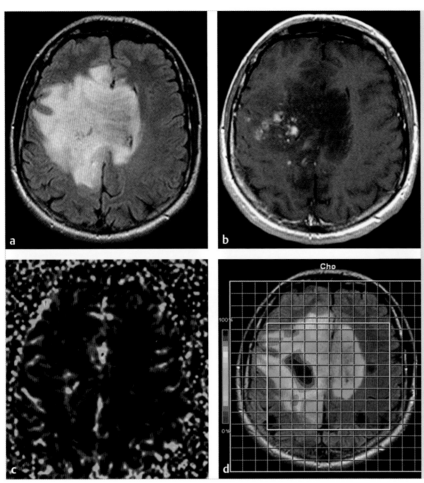

Fig. 3.4 Magnetic resonance imaging (MRI) study including magnetic resonance spectroscopy and dynamic susceptibility contrast (DSC) perfusion MRI in a patient with anaplastic astrocytoma (World Health Organization grade III). Fluid-attenuated inversion recovery (**a**) presents a large infiltrating tumor crossing the midline. After contrast media injection (**b**) multiple inhomogeneous enhancing areas are present in the right part of the tumor presenting areas of blood–brain barrier disruption. The relative cerebral blood volume (rCBV) map of the DSC perfusion study (**c**) depicts an elevated perfusion in good correlation with the enhancing tumor areas. The choline (Cho) map of chemical shift imaging (CSI) (**d**) proved a high proliferation in this area compared with other tumor parts.

mixed histological findings consisting of necrosis and tumor. Because of this heterogeneity and as a result of low spatial resolution, MRS findings of choline and NAA resonances below the normal range may indicate variable histological findings ranging from radiation necrosis, gliosis, and macrophage infiltration to mixed tissues that contain some regions of tumor. The careful choice of voxel placement and interpretation of results in concordance with other imaging and clinical findings is critical in distinguishing between tumor- and treatment-related changes. Furthermore, validation studies using image-guided acquisition of tissue are needed to correlate imaging with biology.

3.3 Contrast-Enhanced Perfusion Magnetic Resonance Imaging in Brain Tumors

Perfusion can be assessed in several ways with MRI which is called the perfusion-weighted imaging (PWI), and has benefits for three major fields: differential diagnosis, biopsy planning, and treatment monitoring.[13] The most common way to assess perfusion in neuro-oncology is the contrast-enhanced first-pass dynamic susceptibility-weighted contrast-enhanced (DSC) magnetic resonance echoplanar imaging approach using the indicator dilution theory model.[14,15] Newer perfusion imaging approaches such as arterial spin labeling (ASL) do not need extrinsic contrast media application and use the blood as an intrinsic contrast medium.[16] Because the contrast media is injected routinely for brain neoplasm imaging, majority of centers prefer to perform DSC-MRI (using the same contrast media) for perfusion imaging.

Because tumor specification is limited, and sometimes conventional MRI cannot discriminate glioblastoma from solitary metastases, CNS-lymphoma, or other tumor types, new methods such as perfusion MRI may play an increasingly important role. The results of the studies available in the literature, all with relatively limited patient numbers, indicate that DSC-MRI perfusion has proven to be a very useful diagnostic tool in the pretherapeutic workup of gliomas (▶ Fig. 3.4), CNS lymphomas, and solitary metastases, as well as in the differentiation of these neoplastic lesions from infections and tumorlike manifestations of demyelinating disease.[15,17,18,19] Quite a large number of studies on brain tumor differentiation have found that PWI has superior diagnostic performance in predicting glioma grade (▶ Fig. 3.4), providing follow-up information (▶ Fig. 3.5), and differentiating gliomas from other primary or secondary tumor entities when compared with spectroscopic imaging and dynamic contrast-enhanced (DCE) PWI.[19]

Because of a significantly higher tumor perfusion in glioblastomas compared with CNS lymphomas, a threshold value of

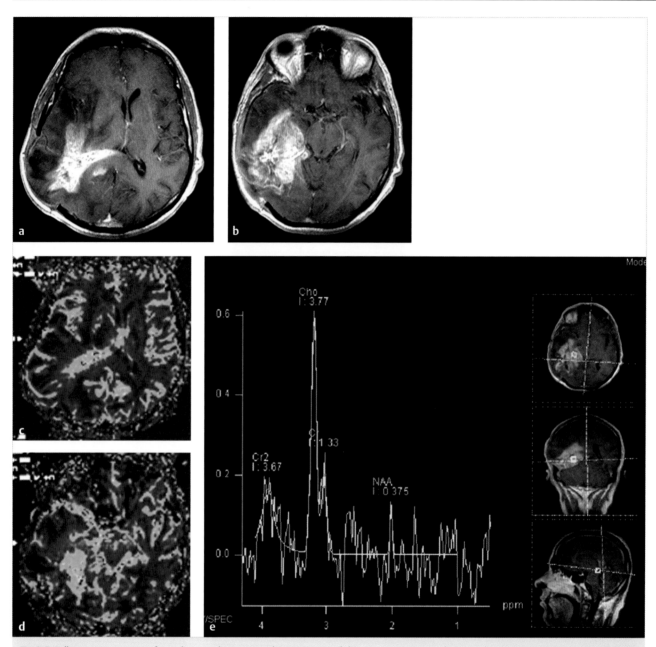

Fig. 3.5 Follow-up assessment of a malignant glioma using dynamic susceptibility contrast (DSC) perfusion and magnetic resonance spectroscopy (MRS). Postcontrast T1-weighted images (**a,b**) show prominently enhancing areas at the right hemisphere. DSC perfusion-weighted imaging (PWI) relative cerebral blood volume (rCBV) images from the corresponding slice levels (**c,d**) demonstrate both high and low perfusion areas in the contrast-enhancing lesion. High perfusion areas represent the recurrent tumor, whereas contrast-enhancing low perfusion areas represent the therapy-related changes. MRS from the high-perfusion voxels reveals a prominent increase in choline (Cho) and a prominent decrease in N-acetylaspartate (NAA) levels compatible with tumor recurrence (**e**).

about 1.4 for relative cerebral blood volume (rCBV) provided sensitivity, specificity, positive predictive value (PPV), and negative predictive values (NPVs) of 100, 50, 90, and 100% according to several publications.[15,18] Using ASL, the relative cerebral blood flow (rCBF) of lymphomas proved to be significantly lower than for high-grade gliomas (▶ Fig. 3.6).

Although conventional MRI characteristics of solitary metastases and primary high-grade gliomas may sometimes be similar, MRI perfusion and MRS enable distinction between the two.[19,20] Although both intratumoral metabolite ratios, rCBV or rCBF values did not allow for discrimination between the two

entities, analyzing the peritumoral T2-weighted hyperintense region enables discrimination between high-grade gliomas and metastases, given that CBV was significantly higher in peritumoral nonenhancing T2-weighted hyperintense regions of glioblastomas compared with metastases. Thus elevated perfusion in the peritumoral region of the lesion represents with high-specificity glioma in differentiation of gliomas from metastasis or grade one when differentiating World Health Organization (WHO) grade III meningioma. Hence PWI allows us to readily appreciate tumor extension past obvious gross anatomical boundaries on conventional MRI.

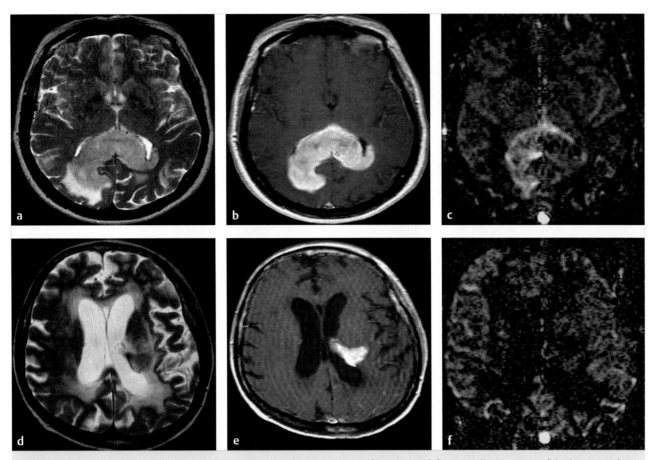

Fig. 3.6 Magnetic resonance imaging studies of a patient with glioblastoma (**a–c**) and lymphoma (**d–f**). T2-weighted images (**a,d**) both present a large tumor area with edema and infiltrative nature. Both tumors present with a marked homogeneous tumor enhancement (**b,e**). In the arterial spin labeling (ASL) perfusion both tumors are significantly different, with the glioblastoma presenting a high perfusion (**c**) and a low/normal enhancement on the lymphoma (**f**).

Correct grading of gliomas has a significant clinical impact because adjuvant therapy postsurgery is usually administered to high-grade but not to low-grade gliomas. Histopathology as the gold standard based on biopsy samples is limited due to the inherent sampling error in these heterogeneous tumors. Several studies reported that high-grade gliomas had higher relative regional CBV[17] and CBF than low-grade gliomas, and glioblastomas have the highest tumor perfusion among all other glioma grades. However, there is a significant overlap of tumor perfusion between high- and low-grade gliomas, which may be explained by the inherent glioma heterogeneity and the sampling error of biopsy samples. This overlap leads to a low specificity, especially when differentiating grade III from grade II gliomas on the WHO scale. Thus PWI has limited utility for an individual patient in making a specific diagnosis, but it may be of great clinical value for biopsy guidance because of the potential glioma heterogeneity with high-grade components that might be interspersed among low-grade components. Although PWI has a better diagnostic performance than conventional MRI techniques in distinguishing different tumor entities, PWI cannot eliminate the need for a biopsy and histological confirmation because modern treatment regimens also consider genetic mutations of tumor cells.

PWI has a tremendous impact on treatment monitoring of low-grade gliomas, besides the advantages in biopsy planning

(▶ Fig. 3.5). Because of the intact BBB, valid quantification of perfusion is possible in these entities. In case of a disrupted BBB, leakage of contrast agents from tumor vessels may cause an underestimation of tumor CBV.[20] In low-grade gliomas, determination of relative regional CBV measurements can be used to predict clinical response. In a recent study, low-grade gliomas that had progressed more rapidly (mean time to progression of 245 days) had significantly higher CBV than those with stable tumor volumes at follow-up (mean time to progression of 4,620 days). The authors proposed a threshold value of relative regional CBV (> 1.75) to indicate a propensity for malignant transformation.[21] The reason for this finding is presumably—as in biopsy planning—that PWI depicts focal anaplastic areas in low-grade gliomas that have not yet led to a disruption of the BBB and therefore to a contrast enhancement on conventional MRI. The same applies for low-grade gliomas after radiotherapy. PWI also detects a subset of patients with higher tumor CBV and shorter progression-free survival.[22] Thus PWI enables a better prediction of prognosis after radiotherapy than conventional MRI. But also, after antiangiogenic chemotherapy of gliomas, PWI has shown its potential to better predict treatment outcome than tumor volume determined on conventional MRI.[23] For other intra-axial lesions, such as brain metastases,[24,25] PWI has also shown its potential to better predict treatment outcome than tumor volume. In this context, a

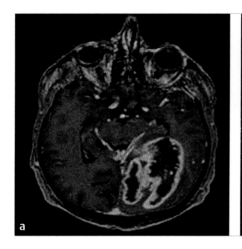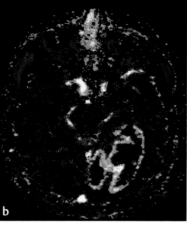

Fig. 3.7 Dynamic contrast-enhanced magnetic resonance imaging (DCE-MRI) perfusion study in a patient with malignant glioma. T1 contrast-enhanced MRI (**a**) presents a central necrotic tumor with a homogeneous rim enhancement in the occipital and parietal lobe. The pharmaco-kinetic map of DCE-MRI (**b**) presents the tumor as more heterogeneous, with areas of higher and lower proliferation and vascularity.

reduction of CBV was highly predictive of treatment response, whereas an increase in CBV was a hint for nonresponse. In extra-axial lesions, such as meningiomas, DCE-MRI might be a good alternative to DSC-MRI for treatment monitoring because the technique is not as susceptible as DSC-MRI to susceptibility artifacts arising from bone and air.

In summary, PWI delivers higher predicting values than conventional MRI by providing maps of the regional variations in cerebral microvasculature of normal and diseased brains. PWI can easily be incorporated as part of the routine clinical evaluation of intracranial mass lesions due to the relatively short imaging and data processing times and the use of a standard dose of contrast agent. Thus PWI together with conventional MRI should be regarded as the test of choice to diagnose and monitor brain tumors before, during, and after therapy. In some cases it might be beneficial to combine different perfusion MRI techniques—mainly DCE-MRI with DSC-MRI perfusion—to obtain a comprehensive picture of the pathology.

3.4 Dynamic Contrast-Enhanced Magnetic Resonance Imaging

DCE-MRI is the second most commonly used method for assessing perfusion by the acquisition of serial images before, during, and after the administration of extracellular low-molecular weighted MRI contrast media. The resulting signal intensity measurements of the tumor reflect a composite of tumor perfusion, vessel permeability, and the extravascular/extracellular space.[26,27]

The method has been investigated for a range of clinical oncological questions, including the detection and characterization of brain tumors, the exact staging and assessment of treatment response,[28,30] and the follow-up, especially after modern antiangiogenic therapy. The DCE-MRI measures permeability and its aberrations, whereas microvascular density (MVD) measures only the histopathologically partial picture of the tissue microvasculature. Furthermore, MVD is a heterogeneous property of tumors and is limited by histopathological sampling and represents generally hot spot values. In the diagnostic workup of tumors, the microvascularity has been found to correlate with prognostic factors such as tumor grade, MVD, and vascular endothelial growth factor (VEGF) expression, and with recurrence and survival outcomes.[31]

In addition, changes of DCE-MRI in follow-up studies during therapeutic intervention have been shown to correlate with outcome,[32] suggesting a role for DCE-MRI as a predictive marker.

In contrast to conventional (static postcontrast T1-weighted) enhanced MRI, which simply presents a snapshot of enhancement at one time point, DCE-MRI permits a fuller depiction of the wash-in and wash-out contrast kinetics within tumors, and this provides insight into the nature of the bulk tissue properties on its microvascular level.

With the strong demand in drug development (especially with the introduction of antiangiogenic trials) to identify a biomarker that can assess tumor microvascular properties noninvasively in animal as well as in human studies, this technique seems to be most appealing as a possible imaging biomarker.

This information can be used for improved biopsy and treatment planning (▶ Fig. 3.7). The gained information can also be used for monitoring therapeutic interventions (e.g., chemo- or radiotherapy). This is supported by the fact that the dynamic information reflects the angiogenic profile and heterogeneity of a tumor (▶ Fig. 3.8).

Shiroishi et al described that prior and during radiotherapy DCE-MRI is helpful to characterize lesion changes prior to structural changes and predict therapeutic response.[32]

Furthermore DCE-MRI in combination with DSC-MRI is helpful to assess functional tumor response, which is in concordance with WHO glioma grading, and it is also helpful to differentiate gliomas from other brain tumors.[34]

Based on the knowledge that vascular permeability and the presence of VEGF/vascular permeability factor (VEGF/VPF) are important mediators of brain tumor growth in addition to angiogenesis, combining the different perfusion and permeability measures with MRI can provide a minimally invasive measure of these pathophysiologically important parameters and be correlated with such important markers as VEGF. Because DSC-MRI T2*-weighted PWI technique is easier to acquire and to post-process, most clinicians and investigators currentlyl prefer to use this technique for brain tumor perfusion MRI.

The method also proved to be of value in the assessment of meningiomas as the most common nonglial primary tumor and the most common intracranial extra-anaplastic astrocytomaxial neoplasm. Almost all meningiomas are characterized with a rapid and intense contrast enhancement after the application of contrast media.[35] However, the intensity of enhancement

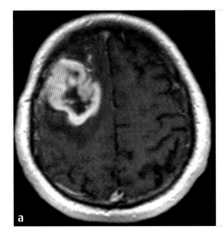
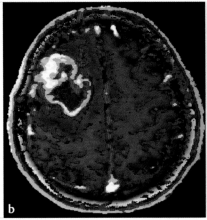

Fig. 3.8 Dynamic contrast-enhanced magnetic resonance imaging (DCE-MRI) perfusion study in a patient with malignant glioma. T1 contrast-enhanced MRI (**a**) presents a central necrotic tumor with a homogeneous rim enhancement in the right frontal lobe. In a targeted biopsy study, tissue was sampled from different areas of the tumor based on the pharmacokinetic maps (**b**). Histology shows a higher vascular density in the anterior parts, associated with a higher expression of angiogenic factors such as vascular endothelial growth factor and hepatocyte growth factor (HGF).

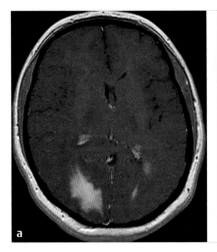
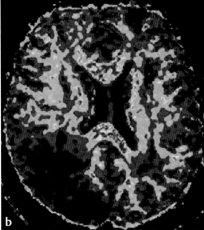

Fig. 3.9 Diffusion-weighted imaging (DWI) in a patient with malignant glioma. Inhomogeneous enhancing tumor in the right occipito-parietal region (**a**) is represented with low signal on the apparent diffusion coefficient (ADC) map from DWI (**b**). The low ADC correlates with a high cellular density.

does not differentiate typical from atypical tumors. Yang et al[34] reported that the exchange rate parameter from DCE studies allowed them to distinguish atypical from typical meningiomas, independent of the contrast behavior. Other assessed parameters have not been able to show a statistically significant difference. Though meningiomas are usually slow-growing lesions, their response to radiotherapy is often difficult to assess, and DCE-MRI techniques showed promising results during radiotherapy. Changes of tumor volume are easily measured after therapy and demonstrate possible changes but do not provide information about the tumor microcirculation. This additional information could be assessed and evaluated by pharmacokinetic analysis on the basis of DCE-MRI technique.

3.5 Diffusion- and Diffusion Tensor–Weighted MRI

Diffusion-weighted imaging (DWI) is used routinely in the assessment of cerebral infarction and infectious diseases. Both DWI and diffusion tensor-imaging (DTI) play an important role in the diagnostic workup and monitoring of patients with cerebral tumors.[36] The signal intensity of gliomas varies from hyper- over iso- to hypointense. The diffusion signal mainly depends on the cellularity of the lesion, with some influence from the amount of necrosis, water content, and hemorrhage.

The "normal" glioma appears hyperintense in DWI with a reduced apparent diffusion coefficient (ADC) (▶ Fig. 3.9). ADC values cannot be used in individual cases to differentiate glioma types reliably.[37,38,39] However, in the study by Kono et al,[36] the combination of routine image interpretation and ADC values had the highest predictive value. Gauvain et al[39] found a clear distinction between the low-grade gliomas and the embryonal tumors but were unable to differentiate between glioma and peritumoral edema based on ADC measurements. In patients with metastases the signal intensity of the nonnecrotic components was highly variably on DWI.[41] The necrotic components of metastases show a marked signal suppression on DWI and increased ADC values, which may be related to increased free water. Increased signal intensity on DWI and a low ADC value are unusual but possible in lesions with hemorrhage.[41]

In other cerebral tumors the signal intensities on DWI were also found to be highly variable and did not allow a differentiation in respect to malignancy. Some studies, however, report on a more intense signal in atypical or malignant meningiomas compared with the typical tumors.[42]

Lymphomas have a typical hyperintense signal on DWI.[43] However, due to the high variability in other tumor entities, a differential diagnosis of lymphoma from metastases or glial tumors is not possible.

A clear role, however, exists for DWI in the assessment of epidermoid tumors. Because these tumors are difficult to

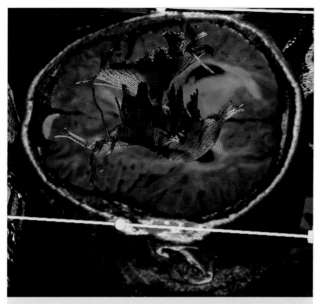

Fig. 3.10 Tractography derived from diffusion tensor imaging (DTI). Corticospinal tracts (CSTs) on both sides are shown and placed on three-dimensional anatomical imaging data. The tumor in one hemisphere displaces the ipsilateral CST bundles anteriorly. There is no destruction of the CST fibers.

exquisite details on tissue microstructure. The most advanced application is certainly that of fiber tracking in the brain (▶ Fig. 3.10), which, in combination with other functional MRI techniques, might open a window on the important issue of connectivity. DTI has also been used to demonstrate subtle abnormalities in a variety of diseases (including stroke, multiple sclerosis, dyslexia, and schizophrenia) and is currently being included in many routine clinical protocols.

DTI has recently proved to be a valuable diagnostic tool in the assessment of intracranial neoplasm.[45,46] In a recent study by Lu et al,[44] peritumoral diffusion tensor metrics could not be used to distinguish intra-axial from extra-axial lesions or to determine the grade of gliomas preoperatively. However, peritumoral DTI values were reported to be helpful in distinguishing solitary intra-axial metastatic lesions from gliomas. In addition, the method enables one to distinguish presumed tumor-infiltrated edema from vasogenic edema composed purely of extracellular water. These capabilities of diffusion tensor MRI are helpful in current diagnostic scenarios and conceivably will be useful for broader applications in the future.

Stieltjes et al[45] used a model based on probabilistic voxel classification for a user-independent analysis of DTI-derived parameters. The proposed quantification method proved to be highly reproducible in both healthy controls and patients. Fiber integrity in the corpus callosum was measured using this quantification method, and the profiles of fractional anisotropy provided additional information of the possible extent of infiltration of primary brain tumors when compared with conventional imaging (▶ Fig. 3.11). This yielded additional information on the nature of ambiguous contralateral lesions in patients with primary brain tumors. The results show that DTI-derived parameters can be determined reproducibly and may have a strong impact on evaluation of contralateral extent of primary brain tumors. A recent study also proved that the method enables investigators to predict the patterns of glioma recurrence.[47]

accurately detect and delineate based on conventional imaging techniques, they present with a very bright signal on DWI and are easily differentiated from other lesions, especially from arachnoid cysts.[44] The differential diagnosis of epidermoid and arachnoid cyst is straightforward on DWI. The epidermoid cyst is bright, whereas the arachnoid cyst is dark.

Because diffusion is truly a three-dimensional process, molecular mobility in tissues may be anisotropic, as in brain white matter. With DTI, diffusion anisotropy effects can be fully extracted, characterized, and exploited, providing even more

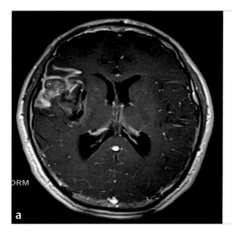
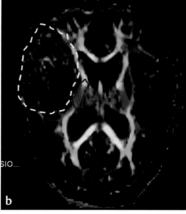

Fig. 3.11 Tractography for surgical planning. Axial contrast-enhanced T1-weighted image shows a heterogeneously enhancing tumor (bordered with the white line in **b**) on the right frontal lobe, which looks very close to the posterior limb of the internal capsule (**a**). Axial color-coded fractional anisotropy (FA) map image derived from the diffusion tensor imaging (DTI) data shows that the CST passing though the posterior limb of the internal capsule is intact (bordered with the red line) (**b**), but very close to the tumor, which is important for surgical strategy.

References

[1] Alger JR, Frank JA, Bizzi A et al. Metabolism of human gliomas: assessment with H-1 MR spectroscopy and F-18 fluorodeoxyglucose PET. Radiology 1990; 177: 633–641

[2] Negendank WG, Sauter R, Brown TR et al. Proton magnetic resonance spectroscopy in patients with glial tumors: a multicenter study. J Neurosurg 1996; 84: 449–458

[3] Meyerand ME, Pipas JM, Mamourian A, Tosteson TD, Dunn JF. Classification of biopsy-confirmed brain tumors using single-voxel MR spectroscopy. AJNR Am J Neuroradiol 1999; 20: 117–123

[4] Dowling C, Bollen AW, Noworolski SM et al. Preoperative proton MR spectroscopic imaging of brain tumors: correlation with histopathologic analysis of resection specimens. AJNR Am J Neuroradiol 2001; 22: 604–612

[5] Demaerel P, Johannik K, Van Hecke P et al. Localized 1 H NMR spectroscopy in fifty cases of newly diagnosed intracranial tumors. J Comput Assist Tomogr 1991; 15: 67–76

[6] Vuori K, Kankaanranta L, Häkkinen AM et al. Low-grade gliomas and focal cortical developmental malformations: differentiation with proton MR spectroscopy. Radiology 2004; 230: 703–708

[7] Wilson M, Cummins CL, Macpherson L et al. Magnetic resonance spectroscopy metabolite profiles predict survival in paediatric brain tumours. Eur J Cancer 2013; 49: 457–464

[8] Norfray JF, Darling C, Byrd S et al. Short TE proton MRS and neurofibromatosis type 1 intracranial lesions. J Comput Assist Tomogr 1999; 23: 994–1003

[9] Law M. MR spectroscopy of brain tumors. Top Magn Reson Imaging 2004; 15: 291–313

[10] Delorme S, Weber MA. Applications of MRS in the evaluation of focal malignant brain lesions. Cancer Imaging 2006; 6: 95–99

[11] Galanaud D, Nicoli F, Chinot O et al. Noninvasive diagnostic assessment of brain tumors using combined in vivo MR imaging and spectroscopy. Magn Reson Med 2006; 55: 1236–1245

[12] Majós C, Julià-Sapé M, Alonso J et al. Brain tumor classification by proton MR spectroscopy: comparison of diagnostic accuracy at short and long TE. AJNR Am J Neuroradiol 2004; 25: 1696–1704

[13] Provenzale JM, Mukundan S, Barboriak DP. Diffusion-weighted and perfusion MR imaging for brain tumor characterization and assessment of treatment response. Radiology 2006; 239: 632–649

[14] Cha S, Knopp EA, Johnson G, Wetzel SG, Litt AW, Zagzag D. Intracranial mass lesions: dynamic contrast-enhanced susceptibility-weighted echo-planar perfusion MR imaging. Radiology 2002; 223: 11–29

[15] Essig M, Nguyen TB, Shiroishi MS et al. Perfusion MRI: the five most frequently asked clinical questions. AJR Am J Roentgenol 2013; 201: W495–510

[16] Barbier EL, Lamalle L, Décorps M. Methodology of brain perfusion imaging. J Magn Reson Imaging 2001; 13: 496–520

[17] Law M, Yang S, Wang H et al. Glioma grading: sensitivity, specificity, and predictive values of perfusion MR imaging and proton MR spectroscopic imaging compared with conventional MR imaging. AJNR Am J Neuroradiol 2003; 24: 1989–1998

[18] Weber MA, Zoubaa S, Schlieter M et al. Diagnostic performance of spectroscopic and perfusion MRI for distinction of brain tumors. Neurology 2006; 66: 1899–1906

[19] Uematsu H, Maeda M. Double-echo perfusion-weighted MR imaging: basic concepts and application in brain tumors for the assessment of tumor blood volume and vascular permeability. Eur Radiol 2006; 16: 180–186

[20] Law M, Oh S, Babb JS et al. Low-grade gliomas: dynamic susceptibility-weighted contrast-enhanced perfusion MR imaging—prediction of patient clinical response. Radiology 2006; 238: 658–667

[21] Fuss M, Wenz F, Essig M et al. Tumor angiogenesis of low-grade astrocytomas measured by dynamic susceptibility contrast-enhanced MRI (DSC-MRI) is predictive of local tumor control after radiation therapy. Int J Radiat Oncol Biol Phys 2001; 51: 478–482

[22] Thompson EM, Guillaume DJ, Dósa E et al. Dual contrast perfusion MRI in a single imaging session for assessment of pediatric brain tumors. J Neurooncol 2012; 109: 105–114

[23] Essig M, Waschkies M, Wenz F, Debus J, Hentrich HR, Knopp MV. Assessment of brain metastases with dynamic susceptibility-weighted contrast-enhanced MR imaging: initial results. Radiology 2003; 228: 193–199

[24] Weber MA, Thilmann C, Lichy MP et al. Assessment of irradiated brain metastases by means of arterial spin-labeling and dynamic susceptibility-weighted contrast-enhanced perfusion MRI: initial results. Invest Radiol 2004; 39: 277–287

[25] Brix G, Semmler W, Port R, Schad LR, Layer G, Lorenz WJ. Pharmacokinetic parameters in CNS Gd-DTPA enhanced MR imaging. J Comput Assist Tomogr 1991; 15: 621–628

[26] Tofts PS, Kermode AG. Measurement of the blood-brain barrier permeability and leakage space using dynamic MR imaging. 1. Fundamental concepts. Magn Reson Med 1991; 17: 357–367

[27] Padhani AR, Husband JE. Dynamic contrast-enhanced MRI studies in oncology with an emphasis on quantification, validation and human studies. Clin Radiol 2001; 56: 607–620

[28] Awasthi R, Rathore RK, Soni P et al. Discriminant analysis to classify glioma grading using dynamic contrast-enhanced MRI and immunohistochemical markers. Neuroradiology 2012; 54: 205–213

[29] Weber MA, Henze M, Tüttenberg J et al. Biopsy targeting gliomas: do functional imaging techniques identify similar target areas? Invest Radiol 2010; 45: 755–768

[30] de Lussanet QG, Langereis S, Beets-Tan RG et al. Dynamic contrast-enhanced MR imaging kinetic parameters and molecular weight of dendritic contrast agents in tumor angiogenesis in mice. Radiology 2005; 235: 65–72

[31] Giesel FL, Bischoff H, von Tengg-Kobligk H et al. Dynamic contrast-enhanced MRI of malignant pleural mesothelioma: a feasibility study of noninvasive assessment, therapeutic follow-up, and possible predictor of improved outcome. Chest 2006; 129: 1570–1576

[32] Shiroishi MS, Booker MT, Agarwal M et al. Posttreatment evaluation of central nervous system gliomas. Magn Reson Imaging Clin N Am 2013; 21: 241–268

[33] Lacerda S, Law M. Magnetic resonance perfusion and permeability imaging in brain tumors. Neuroimaging Clin N Am 2009; 19: 527–557

[34] Yang S, Law M, Zagzag D et al. Dynamic contrast-enhanced perfusion MR imaging measurements of endothelial permeability: differentiation between atypical and typical meningiomas. AJNR Am J Neuroradiol 2003; 24: 1554–1559

[35] Stadnik TW, Demaerel P, Luypaert RR et al. Imaging tutorial: differential diagnosis of bright lesions on diffusion-weighted MR images. Radiographics 2003; 23: e7

[36] Kono K, Inoue Y, Nakayama K et al. The role of diffusion-weighted imaging in patients with brain tumors. AJNR Am J Neuroradiol 2001; 22: 1081–1088

[37] Stadnik TW, Chaskis C, Michotte A et al. Diffusion-weighted MR imaging of intracerebral masses: comparison with conventional MR imaging and histologic findings. AJNR Am J Neuroradiol 2001; 22: 969–976

[38] Sugahara T, Korogi Y, Kochi M et al. Usefulness of diffusion-weighted MRI with echo-planar technique in the evaluation of cellularity in gliomas. J Magn Reson Imaging 1999; 9: 53–60

[39] Gauvain KM, McKinstry RC, Mukherjee P et al. Evaluating pediatric brain tumor cellularity with diffusion-tensor imaging. AJR Am J Roentgenol 2001; 177: 449–454

[40] Krabbe K, Gideon P, Wagn P, Hansen U, Thomsen C, Madsen F. MR diffusion imaging of human intracranial tumours. Neuroradiology 1997; 39: 483–489

[41] Hartmann M, Jansen O, Heiland S, Sommer C, Münkel K, Sartor K. Restricted diffusion within ring enhancement is not pathognomonic for brain abscess. AJNR Am J Neuroradiol 2001; 22: 1738–1742

[42] Johnson BA, Fram EK, Johnson PC, Jacobowitz R. The variable MR appearance of primary lymphoma of the central nervous system: comparison with histopathologic features. AJNR Am J Neuroradiol 1997; 18: 563–572

[43] Chen S, Ikawa F, Kurisu K, Arita K, Takaba J, Kanou Y. Quantitative MR evaluation of intracranial epidermoid tumors by fast fluid-attenuated inversion recovery imaging and echo-planar diffusion-weighted imaging. AJNR Am J Neuroradiol 2001; 22: 1089–1096

[44] Lu S, Ahn D, Johnson G, Law M, Zagzag D, Grossman RI. Diffusion-tensor MR imaging of intracranial neoplasia and associated peritumoral edema: introduction of the tumor infiltration index. Radiology 2004; 232: 221–228

[45] Stieltjes B, Schlüter M, Didinger B et al. Diffusion tensor imaging in primary brain tumors: reproducible quantitative analysis of corpus callosum infiltration and contralateral involvement using a probabilistic mixture model. Neuroimage 2006; 31: 531–542

[46] Price SJ, Jena R, Burnet NG, Carpenter TA, Pickard JD, Gillard JH. Predicting patterns of glioma recurrence using diffusion tensor imaging. Eur Radiol 2007; 17: 1675–1684

[47] Fink JR, Carr RB, Matsusue E et al. Comparison of 3 Tesla proton MR spectroscopy, MR perfusion and MR diffusion for distinguishing glioma recurrence from posttreatment effects. J Magn Reson Imaging 2012; 35: 56–63

4 Perfusion Imaging: Dynamic Susceptibility Contrast Magnetic Resonance Perfusion

Marco Essig, Josep Puig, and Cem Calli

4.1 Introduction

Magnetic resonance imaging (MRI) is the imaging method of choice in the management of patients with cerebral tumors. In the diagnostic workup, including detection and differential diagnosis of central nervous system (CNS) tumors, MRI is essential because of its outstanding anatomical detail and tissue contrast. Characterization of a tumor's malignant potential, however, can be more difficult using conventional techniques only, particularly because characteristics related to tumor vascularity as well as the integrity of the blood–brain barrier (BBB) of neoplastic tissue that are assessable by conventional imaging are only moderately specific indicators of tumor malignancy or malignant potential. Other characteristics can only be assessed using modern functional or physiological imaging techniques. The degree of angiogenesis, for example, has been linked to tumor grade in human gliomas, with high-grade lesions to show increased angiogenic markers and neovasculature.

This information can also be used for an improved treatment decision and planning, especially in respect to modulated treatment regimens.

After therapy, functional imaging techniques can be used for monitoring and to differentiate treatment-related from tumor-related changes; the later present with neoangiogenesis, whereas treatment-related effects present with a leakage of the BBB but no neovasculature.

Of the available functional imaging techniques described in the previous chapters, perfusion MRI is best suited to assess specific pathophysiological parameters related to the angiogenic characteristics in tumors.[1,2]

In general, perfusion can be assessed with three different MRI techniques, namely dynamic susceptibility contrast (DSC), dynamic contrast-enhanced (DCE), and arterial spin labeling (ASL) magnetic resonance perfusion (MRP).

4.1.1 DSC-MRP

DSC-MRP is based on a dynamic acquisition in which the first pass of a bolus of gadolinium-based contrast agent through the area of interest is monitored by a series of heavily T2- or T2*-weighted MRI scans.

The signal aberration from the exogenous tracer leads to a temporal significant signal loss. Using the principles first described by Rempp et al in 1994[3] the signal information can be converted into a contrast medium–concentration time curve on a pixel by pixel basis.

Based on the indicator dilution theory, parametric maps of cerebral blood volume (CBV) and flow (CBF) can be derived from this concentration information. Regional CBF and CBV values can be obtained by region-of-interest analysis or using other postprocessing methods.[4]

4.1.2 DCE-MRP

DCE-MRP or pharmacokinetic MRI is based on the acquisition of series of T1-weighted images before, during, and after administration of gadolinium-based contrast agents. Two- or three-dimensional (2D or 3D) gradient echo imaging is usually performed. The resulting signal intensity–time curve reflects a composite of tissue perfusion, vessel permeability, and the extravascular–extracellular space.[5,6]

The method allows for a time-resolved analysis of the contrast enhancement, which gives insight into the integrity of the BBB on its microvascular level. Using pharmacokinetic modeling, clinically most often based on a two-compartment model (plasma space and extravascular–extracellular space), several characteristics can be derived: the transfer constant (K^{trans}), the fractional volume of the extravascular–extracellular space (v_e), the rate constant (k_{ev}, where $k_{ev} = K^{trans}/v_e$), and the fractional volume of the plasma space (V_p).[7,8]

4.1.3 ASL-MRP

ASL is a perfusion method that, rather than using an exogenous tracer, uses magnetically labeled blood as an endogenous tracer. Multiple ASL variants have been described.

The best tissue contrast can be reached with a specific subtype, the continuous ASL that uses a prolonged radiofrequency pulse, which continuously labels arterial blood water below the area of interest until a steady state of tissue magnetization has been reached.[9]

Pulsed ASL is technically less demanding.[10,11] A short radiofrequency pulse is used to label a thick slab of arterial blood at a single point in time, and imaging is performed following an inflow delay into the tissue of interest. Both ASL methods only allow to extract values of CBF instead of the in tumors most often used CBV.

This chapter focuses on the use of DSC-MRP in the clinical management of patients with brain tumors.

4.1.4 DSC-MRP Protocol Recommendations

There are no specific hardware requirements to acquire imaging data that can be used for a DSC-MRP analysis.

The field strength does not substantially influence the perfusion imaging quality. However, the scanner needs to be capable of echoplanar imaging. The susceptibility effect of the contrast media is field strength dependent, which might require a higher contrast media dose when using field strength below 1.5 T.

Bolus injection of the gadolinium-based contrast agent should commence after about a 20 s delay (range, 5–30 s) from the start of the dynamic susceptibility contrast MRP sequence. A minimum of 4 mL/s (range, 3–5 mL/s) bolus injection rate of gadolinium-based contrast agent was previously recommended to allow for a robust and compact bolus arrival in the cerebral tissue.[12] This should be followed by a 25 mL (minimum 10 mL, maximum 30 mL) saline flush at the same rate to push the bolus toward the heart. A contrast media dose of 0.1 mmol/kg has been described as sufficient with modern MRI contrast media.[2] Higher doses are recommended only if older MRI technology is used. In cases where the perfusion study is combined with other contrast-enhanced techniques such as contrast-enhanced magnetic resonance angiography or DCE-MRP, the overall contrast media dose can exceed the single dose.

As newer publications proposed,[1,2] for a combined DSC and DCE perfusion protocol, which can be achieved in a single MRI protocol, it is recommended to start with the DSC, followed by the DCE sequence. The first injection serves two functions, first as a preload of gadolinium-based contrast agent to help compensate for leakage correction for DSC imaging, and, secondly, to provide dynamic data for calculation of permeability metrics. Because there is an approximate 5 to 8 min interval recommended between the two injections, an intervening sequence, such as diffusion-weighted imaging or fluid-attenuated inversion recovery (FLAIR) acquisition, can be performed between the two. If combined DCE- and DSC-MRP is being performed, one should split the contrast amount into two equivalent injections followed by a minimum 10 mL saline flush for each.

4.1.5 Postprocessing of Perfusion MRI Studies

There are many different methods for analyzing perfusion data; unfortunately, there is no standardization of postprocessing.[7,13,15] However, some general recommendations can be made. The method chosen depends on whether the focus is on a routine clinical question versus one posed in the setting of clinical research, where more semiquantitative or even quantitative approaches are needed. For routine clinical practice, simple visual inspection of the parametric color maps can be sufficient to detect areas of normal versus abnormal regions. Although this type of analysis does not provide quantitative assessment of perfusion metrics, it can be very useful in the clinical setting.[16]

If semiquantitative data are desired, most often user-defined regions of interest (ROIs) can be placed in the tissue of interest as well as in the contralateral normal-appearing region, either normal-appearing white matter (NAWM) or gray matter depending on the location of the lesion.[17]

Although placement of multiple ROIs is the most common method of analysis, this method still carries with it an unavoidable component of subjectivity; thus alternative methods such as histogram analysis have been examined that appear to provide meaningful perfusion metrics.[18,19] Histograms have the ability to demonstrate the heterogeneity of the ROI; however, there is loss of spatial specificity.[20] Parametric response mapping (PRM) is another advanced method of analysis in which parametric maps are coregistered over serial exams

and compared on a voxel-wise comparison before and after treatment.[21,22]

Calculation of a summary statistic such as relative CBV (rCBV) normalized to an internal control such as NAWM does not require the determination of the arterial input function (AIF) and simplifies postprocessing. According to work by Wetzel and Weber and their colleagues, the placement of a minimum of four small ROIs in the areas thought to contain the highest rCBV values based on color maps and recording the maximal rCBV (rCBV$_{max}$) demonstrated the highest intra- and interobserver reproducibility.[23,24] Visual inspection of the signal intensity–time curves resulting from ROI placement can be examined for qualitative interpretation as well. Increased area under the curve can be consistent with tumor, whereas decreased area can be consistent with radiation necrosis or non-neoplasm. Deconvolution of the concentration of tissue tracer by the AIF is required for absolute quantification of DSC-MRI-derived CBF and CBV. This, however, is technically challenging and is the focus of intense research.[25,26,27]

4.2 Added Value of Perfusion in Brain Tumor Imaging Protocols

In recent years considerable clinical experience has been gained with perfusion MRI of tumors. Perfusion MRI can play an important role at the major clinical decision points: detection, differential diagnosis, intervention, and posttreatment monitoring.

This is based on the fact that rCBV values correlate with conventional angiographic evaluation of tumor vascular density as well as with histological measures of tumor neovascularity and grading.[17,24,28,29]

DSC-MRI-derived metrics other than rCBV have been proposed in brain tumor assessment. Percentage of signal intensity recovery is a less complex alternative measure of microvascular permeability that can be derived from the DSC-MRI signal intensity–time curve.[30,31] Peak height is another alternative metric that can be derived from the DSC-MRI signal intensity–time curve that has been highly correlated with rCBV.[32]

4.3 DSC Perfusion MRI for Differential Diagnostics and Diagnostic Workup of Patients with Brain Tumors

4.3.1 Glioma Grading

Besides the differential diagnosis between malignant and non-malignant brain lesions (► Fig. 4.1), multiple studies show that there is a strong correlation between glioma grade and CBV from DSC-MRI (► Fig. 4.2 and ► Fig. 4.3).[18,24,28] DCE perfusion MRI markers also appear to be correlated with glioma grade; however, the correlation with rCBV and grade appears stronger.[33] Values and thresholds vary in the literature, likely

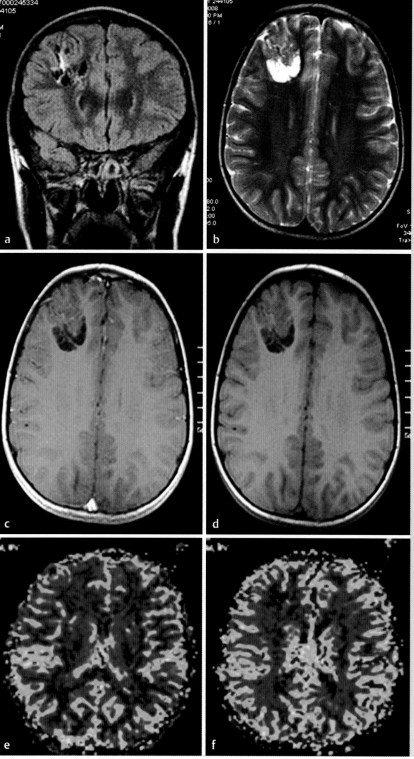

Fig. 4.1 Dynamic susceptibility contrast magnetic resonance perfusion (DSC-MRP) for differential diagnosis. Coronal fluid-attenuated inversion recovery (FLAIR) (**a**) and axial T2-weighted (**b**) sequences show a right frontal mass with cystic components. On T1-weighted image (**c**) the mass depicts heterogeneous low signals and does not enhance after intravenous gadolinium injection (**d**). On DSC perfusion cerebral blood volume maps (**e,f**) the lesion has either iso- or hypoperfusion compared with the contralateral normal-appearing white matter. Surgery revealed a focal cortical dysplasia.

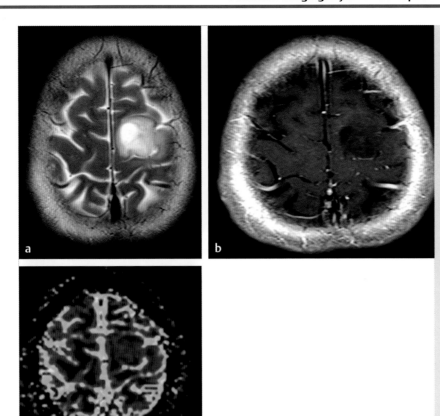

Fig. 4.2 Dynamic susceptibility contrast magnetic resonance perfusion (DSC-MRP) in low-grade astrocytoma. Patient with a left frontoparietal mass lesion suspicious for an astrocytoma. Homogeneous signal changes on T2 (**a**) and T1 (**b**) with no signs of pathological enhancement or hypervascularity. DSC-MRP (**c**) shows no elevated blood volume compared with the contralateral side or in relation to the normal-appearing gray and white matter. Histology confirmed a fibrillary astrocytoma World Health Organization grade II.

stemming from differences in image acquisition, postprocessing, and interpretation.

Bisdas et al showed that $rCBV_{max} > 4.2$ was predictive of recurrence and $rCBV_{max} \leq 3.8$ was predictive of 1 year survival in astrocytomas, excluding those with oligodendroglial components.[34] Theses values are higher than those previously reported by Lev et al (1.5) and Law et al (1.75), which could be due to differences in imaging technique, differences in tumor types, and methodology.[33,35] Law et al demonstrated that an rCBV threshold of 1.75 could predict median time to progression independent of histopathological findings.[36] rCBV has also been shown to increase up to 12 months prior to contrast enhancement being noted on conventional MRI in low-grade gliomas undergoing malignant transformation.[37]

4.3.2 Differential Diagnosis: Primary Glioma versus Solitary Metastatic Brain Tumor

The conventional imaging appearances of a primary glioma and solitary brain metastatic tumor can appear quite similar, and it can be difficult to differentiate between them. Examination of the rCBV in the peritumoral region surrounding a mass may improve differentiation between these lesions. The rCBV surrounding high-grade gliomas appears to be higher compared to a solitary metastatic tumor (▶ Fig. 4.4 and ▶ Fig. 4.5).[17,38] On the other hand, the peritumoral region of a high-grade glioma is composed of both vasogenic edema and infiltrative tumor,

which can extend far beyond the T2 hyperintense margins of the peritumoral region.[39,40]

Other perfusion techniques such as ASL have also demonstrated that CBF was significantly elevated in the peritumoral region of glioblastomas compared with metastases.[24]

4.3.3 Primary Glioma versus Lymphoma

Primary cerebral lymphoma can appear similar to a high-grade glioma or other high-grade tumors on conventional contrast-enhanced MRI (▶ Fig. 4.6).[17] Because of a lack of the striking angiogenesis usually seen in high-grade glioma, lymphomas demonstrate lower rCBV than high-grade glioma.[41,42]

4.3.4 Meningiomas, Tumefactive Demyelinating Lesions, and Infection

Although, in general, meningiomas are benign, they can have much higher rCBVs than intra-axial tumors. This is likely due to their marked vascularity and complete absence of a BBB in these tumors, which can produce erroneously high or low rCBV values.[17]

Tumefactive demyelinating lesions (TDLs) can be difficult to differentiate from an intra-axial tumor on conventional imaging. TDLs possess lower rCBV than high-grade tumors because they lack significant angiogenesis (▶ Fig. 4.7).[17] Studies that have examined the use of rCBV to differentiate pyogenic abscesses from cystic tumors have shown that rCBV is lower in

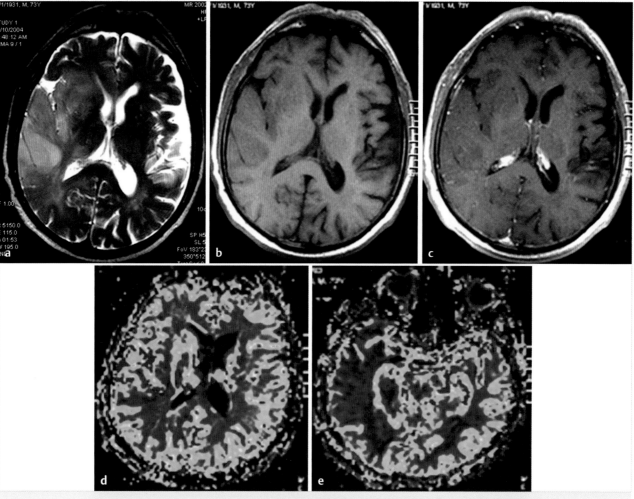

Fig. 4.3 Role of dynamic susceptibility contrast magnetic resonance perfusion (DSC-MRP) in nonenhancing high-grade astrocytoma. On axial T2-weighted image (**a**) there is a hyperintense infiltrating lesion on the right hemisphere. The lesion is mildly hypointense on T1-weighted image (**b**) and does not show enhancement (**c**). Although the conventional magnetic resonance imaging findings are suggestive of a low-grade infiltrating glioma, the DSC perfusion cerebral blood volume map (**d**) depicts highly perfused areas in that region (represented by green and red colors) indicative of a high-grade glioma. The inferior part shows low perfusion (**e**) indicated by a blue color, which is a very good example of the heterogeneous structure of gliomas (they may contain both high- and low-grade cells in a single tumor). Surgery revealed a grade III astrocytoma.

the rim-enhancing portion of abscesses compared to cystic tumors.[43,44]

4.4 DSC Perfusion MRI for Treatment Planning

Besides their use in treatment decision, functional imaging techniques such as DSC-MRP can also be used in the treatment planning process. They can be used either to guide selection of the sites for biopsy or for neuronavigation or radiation treatment planning.

4.4.1 Biopsy Guidance

The biopsy of brain tumors is guided with either contrast-enhanced computed tomography (CT) or contrast-enhanced MRI.[45] Sampling error is a major pitfall with this method because the most malignant portion of the tumor may not

necessarily enhance. It has been estimated that 38% of anaplastic astrocytomas do not significantly enhance, and up to 25% of brain tumors are likely undergraded as a result.[46] In some institutions, rCBV maps can be used to better select the highest-grade regions for biopsy targets of both enhancing and nonenhancing tumors.[17,47]

4.5 DSC-MRI for Treatment Monitoring

4.5.1 Differentiation of Recurrent Tumor and Delayed Treatment-Related Changes

Distinguishing between recurrent tumor and radiation necrosis is critical because of their vastly different management strategies. Patients with recurrent tumor may undergo further surgery and chemo-/radiation therapy, whereas those with

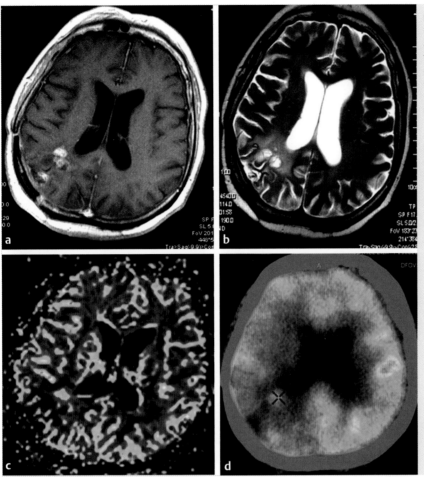

Fig. 4.4 Dynamic susceptibility contrast magnetic resonance perfusion (DSC-MRP) in anaplastic astrocytoma. A 60-year-old patient with histologically confirmed anaplastic astrocytoma. The tumor presented with two strong enhancing nodules on the contrast-enhanced T1 sequences (**a**) that are surrounded by an inhomogeneous delineated area of T2 hyperintensity (**b**). The DSC-MRP (**c**) shows only the anterior of the two nodules with a high relative cerebral blood volume, which correlates with a high activity uptake on the positron-emission tomography images. This area has a higher metabolism and represents the more aggressive part of the tumor. This information is used to improve targeting of the biopsy or can be integrated into the intensity modulation for radiotherapy.

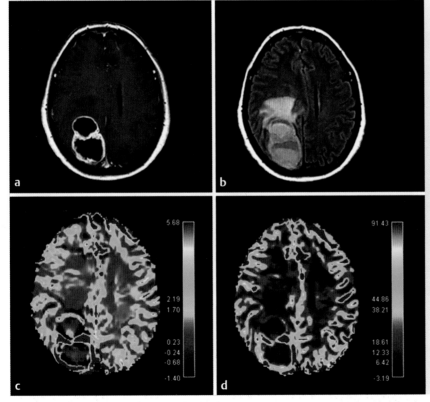

Fig. 4.5 Dynamic susceptibility contrast magnetic resonance perfusion (DSC-MRP) in a patient with cerebral metastasis. A 67-year-old woman presented with left hemiparesis. (**a**) Axial postgadolinium T1-weighted image shows irregular ringlike enhancement of the tumor, located in the right parietal lobe. (**b**) On fluid-attenuated inversion recovery image the cavitary necrosis shows high signal intensity, and the solid component of the tumor appears heterogeneous. Note also the high signal peritumoral edema. Perfusion color maps demonstrate increased relative cerebral blood volume (**c**) and relative cerebral blood flow (**d**) at the margin of the tumor. Biopsy proved lung metastasis.

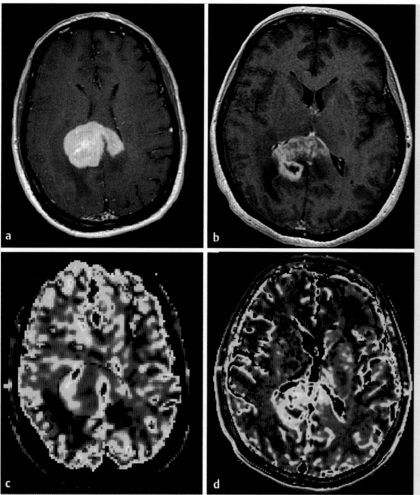

Fig. 4.6 Dynamic susceptibility contrast magnetic resonance perfusion (DSC-MRP) to differentiate cerebral lymphoma from high-grade glioma. Two patients with strong enhancing intra-axial tumors are presented (**a,b**). Lesion A presents with a more homogeneous enhancement and a low relative cerebral blood volume (rCBV) of 1.3 on DSC-MRP (**c**). Lesion B presents with a more rim-shaped enhancement but a high rCBV of 3.9 (**d**). The combination of strong enhancement representing a high permeability but low rCBV is typical for primary central nervous system lymphomas. The combination of strong enhancement and high rCBV is a typical finding in anaplastic or malignant glioma.

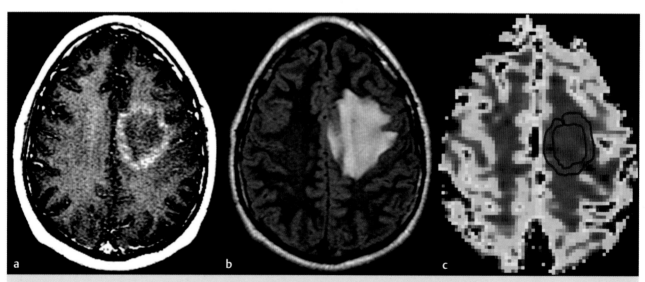

Fig. 4.7 Dynamic susceptibility contrast magnetic resonance perfusion (DSC-MRP) to differentiate tumefactive demyelination. A 45-year-old patient with a ring-enhancing (**a**) lesion associated with mass effect and surrounding edema (**b**). Even though the intensity of the enhancement is low, it is impossible to differentiate between high-grade glioma, metastasis, or nontumor lesion based on the anatomical imaging. DSC-MRP (**c**) shows a low perfusion of the tumor in total; the average CBV value in the outlined region of interest was 1.1. Histology confirmed a tumefactive demyelinating lesion.

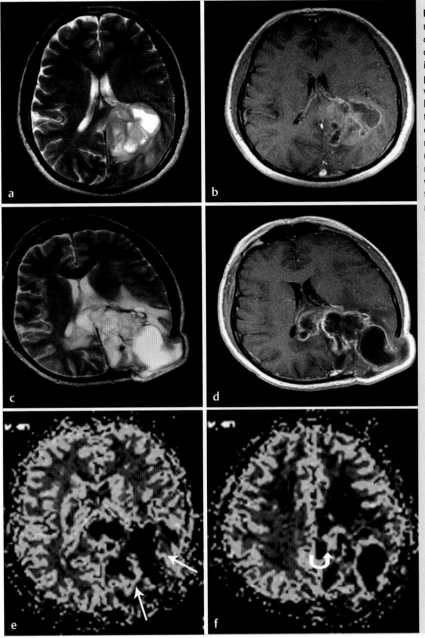

Fig. 4.8 Dynamic susceptibility contrast magnetic resonance perfusion (DSC-MRP) for differentiation of tumor recurrence. A 49-year-old man with grade IV astrocytoma–glioblastoma in left parieto-occipital region (**a,b**). Six months postresection and combined radiochemotherapy with temozolomide, a cystic tumorlike mass lesion presents within the original tumor bed and toward the resection cavity (**c,d**). Although most of the enhancement in the original tumor bed is not associated with a high perfusion on DSC-MRP (**e,f**) (arrows), some areas present with high relative cerebral blood volume (curved arrows), which could be confirmed by positron-emission tomography and later histology as tumor recurrence.

delayed radiation necrosis may be managed conservatively with steroids. On conventional contrast-enhanced MRI treatment-related changes cannot be reliably distinguished from recurrent tumor because both can appear as a contrast-enhancing mass with surrounding edema.[48] rCBV appears to be elevated in patients with recurrent tumor compared to patients with treatment-related changes such as radiation necrosis, likely reflective of the increased vascular proliferation and leaky capillaries of recurrent tumor, whereas treatment-related changes such as radionecrosis are composed of extensive fibrinoid necrosis, vascular dilation, and endothelial injury (▶ Fig. 4.8 and ▶ Fig. 4.9).[30,32,49,50] Barajas et al recently reported increased rCBV as well as lower relative PSR in recurrent glioblastoma compared with treatment changes.[30]

4.5.2 Posttherapeutic Evaluation of Glioblastoma

Changes in the two-dimensional area of contrast enhancement known as the Macdonald criteria or lately the Response Assessment in Neuro-Oncology (RANO) criteria are the most commonly used methods to evaluate therapeutic response of high-grade gliomas.[51] However, reliance on contrast enhancement is problematic because it is a nonspecific finding that reflects breakdown of the BBB, which may also occur following treatment-related BBB damage. Contrast-enhancing lesions following therapy may be due to tumor, but also to other processes, such as radiation necrosis, postsurgical changes, postictal changes, and changes in steroid dosage.[48,52,53] In the

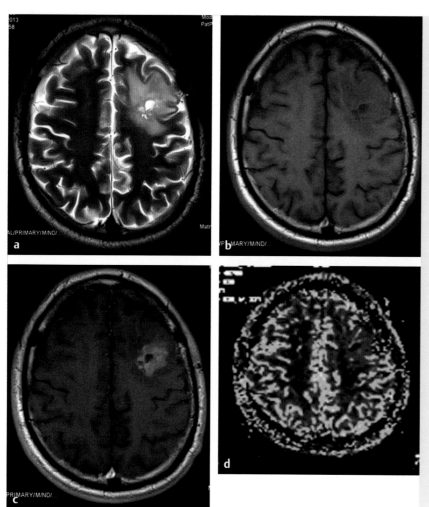

Fig. 4.9 A patient with glioblastoma multiforme who received radiotherapy. One year follow-up magnetic resonance imaging. Axial T2-weighted image (**a**) shows a hyperintense lesion at the left frontal lobe. There is contrast enhancement after intravenous gadolinium injection (**b,c**), suggesting a recurrent tumor. However, the dynamic susceptibility cerebral blood volume map (**d**) depicts hypoperfusion at the contrast-enhancing areas consistent with radiation necrosis.

glioblastoma literature, both pseudoprogression and pseudoresponse are two major concerns that have gained attention. In pseudoprogression (▶ Fig. 4.10), a transient increase in contrast enhancement is noted in the first 3 to 6 months after completion of radiation therapy as part of the standard regimen of chemoradiation with temozolomide.[54,55] The use of conventional contrast-enhanced MRI is not adequate to distinguish between pseudoprogression and true early progression, and no other imaging technique has been validated to differentiate between the two entities. Recent data appear to show that rCBV is significantly elevated in true tumor progression compared with pseudoprogression (▶ Fig. 4.10).[56,57]

Reliance on conventional contrast-enhanced MRI can also be problematic with the use of antiangiogenic agents such as bevacizumab in recurrent glioblastoma patients. These agents produce high response rates and 6 month progression-free survival; however, they appear to have modest effects on overall survival.[58]

The term *pseudoresponse* refers to the rapid decrease in contrast enhancement without significant tumor reduction following treatment with antiangiogenic agents.[59] This phenomenon has been attributed to a decrease in vascular permeability due to "normalization" of the BBB induced by these agents.[60] In addition, this vascular normalization has been shown to be reversible in patients who required a "drug holiday."[58] First results using perfusion MRI techniques proposed a "vascular normalization index" composed of changes in K^{trans}, rCBV, and circulating collagen IV that appeared to be correlated with progression-free and overall survival as early as 1 day after treatment with some of those agents.[61]

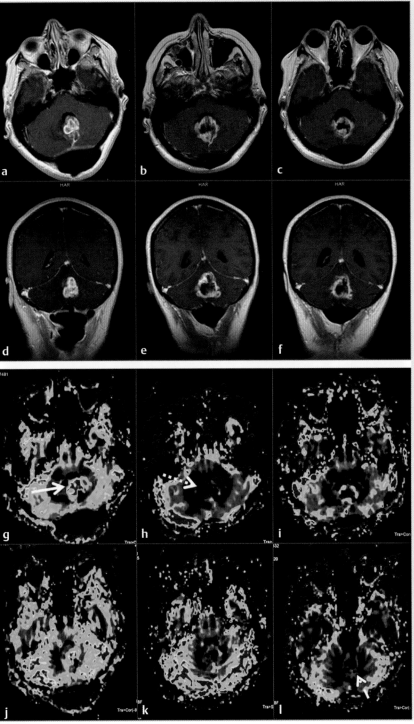

Fig. 4.10 Dynamic susceptibility contrast magnetic resonance perfusion (DSC-MRP) for identification of pseudoprogression after radiochemotherapy. After combined radiochemotherapy with temozolomide, the initial tumor in the posterior fossa (grade IV astrocytoma) (**a,b**) presented with a substantial size increase (**c,d**). These findings remained stable on the 3-month follow-up scan (**e,f**) confirming pseudoprogression on the initial follow-up. Using perfusion imaging, the initially well perfused tumor (**g,h**, arrow) showed, despite the volume increase, a significant reduction of perfusion (**i,j**, dotted arrow), confirming the treatment response already at that time point. On the 3-month follow-up, the tumor remained stable from the enhancement patterns and size (**e,f**). The perfusion pattern remains also stable with low perfusion values (**k,l**, arrowhead).

4.6 Conclusions

Many studies have documented the ability of DSC-MRP to differentiate tumor from nontumor changes, to predict tumor grade and prognosis, or to distinguish tumor recurrence from treatment-related changes.

However, at the same time, despite its existence for more than 20 years, perfusion MRI has not yet fully reached the routine clinical environment and in many institutions remains essentially a research tool and not the standard of care for the evaluation of brain tumor patients. There are several potential reasons for this. First, no specific reimbursement for perfusion MRI exists. Second, there is no specific gadolinium-based contrast agent approved for brain perfusion MRI. There is a lack of standardization for the acquisition and the postprocessing of perfusion data, and, perhaps most importantly, there is a paucity of high-quality data to demonstrate an actual clinical impact in the care of neuro-oncology patients.

Recently, a single-center prospective study of glioma patients was reported to address this issue.[62] In this study, 59 consecutive patients with gliomas were evaluated by three neuroradiologists in consensus, first using conventional MRI sequences, and afterward with incorporation of qualitative analysis of perfusion imaging (which included both DSC as well as ASL perfusion MRI techniques). These imaging data were evaluated in conjunction with clinical data and were assessed in a multidisciplinary fashion with a clinical neuro-oncology team. Hypothetical treatment plans were created for each patient prospectively, first using conventional MRI and then using conventional MRI combined with perfusion MRI. Overall, it was concluded that the addition of perfusion imaging appeared to have a significant effect on neuroradiologists' and clinicians' confidence in tumor status as well as the course of clinical management. This study concept leads the way, and larger, preferably multicenter, confirmatory studies are needed.

References

[1] Essig M, Anzalone N, Combs SE et al. MR imaging of neoplastic central nervous system lesions: review and recommendations for current practice. AJNR Am J Neuroradiol 2012; 33: 803–817

[2] Essig M, Shiroishi MS, Nguyen TB et al. Perfusion MRI: the five most frequently asked technical questions. AJR Am J Roentgenol 2013; 200: 24–34

[3] Rempp KA, Brix G, Wenz F, Becker CR, Gückel F, Lorenz WJ. Quantification of regional cerebral blood flow and volume with dynamic susceptibility contrast-enhanced MR imaging. Radiology 1994; 193: 637–641

[4] Lacerda S, Law M. Magnetic resonance perfusion and permeability imaging in brain tumors. Neuroimaging Clin N Am 2009; 19: 527–557

[5] Brix G, Semmler W, Port R, Schad LR, Layer G, Lorenz WJ. Pharmacokinetic parameters in CNS Gd-DTPA enhanced MR imaging. J Comput Assist Tomogr 1991; 15: 621–628

[6] Tofts PS, Kermode AG. Measurement of the blood-brain barrier permeability and leakage space using dynamic MR imaging. 1. Fundamental concepts. Magn Reson Med 1991; 17: 357–367

[7] Paldino MJ, Barboriak DP. Fundamentals of quantitative dynamic contrast-enhanced MR imaging. Magn Reson Imaging Clin N Am 2009; 17: 277–289

[8] Tofts PS, Brix G, Buckley DL et al. Estimating kinetic parameters from dynamic contrast-enhanced T(1)-weighted MRI of a diffusable tracer: standardized quantities and symbols. J Magn Reson Imaging 1999; 10: 223–232

[9] Petersen ET, Zimine I, Ho YC, Golay X. Non-invasive measurement of perfusion: a critical review of arterial spin labelling techniques. Br J Radiol 2006; 79: 688–701

[10] Golay X, Hendrikse J, Lim TC. Perfusion imaging using arterial spin labeling. Top Magn Reson Imaging 2004; 15: 10–27

[11] Wang J, Alsop DC, Li L et al. Comparison of quantitative perfusion imaging using arterial spin labeling at 1.5 and 4.0 tesla. Magn Reson Med 2002; 48: 242–254

[12] Essig M, Nguyen TB, Shiroishi MS et al. Perfusion MRI: the five most frequently asked clinical questions. AJR Am J Roentgenol 2013; 201: W495–510

[13] Thompson G, Mills SJ, Stivaros SM, Jackson A. Imaging of brain tumors: perfusion/permeability. Neuroimaging Clin N Am 2010; 20: 337–353

[14] Shiroishi MS, Habibi M, Rajderkar D et al. Perfusion and permeability MR imaging of gliomas. Technol Cancer Res Treat 2011; 10: 59–71

[15] Quarles CC. Dynamic susceptibility MRI: data acquisition and analysis. In: Yankeelov TE, Pickens D, Price RR, eds. Quantatative MRI in Cancer. Boca Raton, FL: CRC Press; 2012

[16] Wintermark M, Sesay M, Barbier E et al. Comparative overview of brain perfusion imaging techniques. Stroke 2005; 36: e83–e99

[17] Cha S, Knopp EA, Johnson G, Wetzel SG, Litt AW, Zagzag D. Intracranial mass lesions: dynamic contrast-enhanced susceptibility-weighted echo-planar perfusion MR imaging. Radiology 2002; 223: 11–29

[18] Law M, Young R, Babb J, Pollack E, Johnson G. Histogram analysis versus region of interest analysis of dynamic susceptibility contrast perfusion MR imaging data in the grading of cerebral gliomas. AJNR Am J Neuroradiol 2007; 28: 761–766

[19] Emblem KE, Scheie D, Due-Tonnessen P et al. Histogram analysis of MR imaging-derived cerebral blood volume maps: combined glioma grading and identification of low-grade oligodendroglial subtypes. AJNR Am J Neuroradiol 2008; 29: 1664–1670

[20] Arlinghous L, Yankeelov TE. Diffusion-weighted MRI. In: Yankeelov TE, ed. Quantitative MRI in Cancer. London, England: Taylor & Francis; 2011

[21] Galbán CJ, Chenevert TL, Meyer CR et al. The parametric response map is an imaging biomarker for early cancer treatment outcome. Nat Med 2009; 15: 572–576

[22] Moffat BA, Chenevert TL, Lawrence TS et al. Functional diffusion map: a non-invasive MRI biomarker for early stratification of clinical brain tumor response. Proc Natl Acad Sci U S A 2005; 102: 5524–5529

[23] Wetzel SG, Cha S, Johnson G et al. Relative cerebral blood volume measurements in intracranial mass lesions: interobserver and intraobserver reproducibility study. Radiology 2002; 224: 797–803

[24] Weber MA, Zoubaa S, Schlieter M et al. Diagnostic performance of spectroscopic and perfusion MRI for distinction of brain tumors. Neurology 2006; 66: 1899–1906

[25] Bleeker EJ, van Buchem MA, van Osch MJ. Optimal location for arterial input function measurements near the middle cerebral artery in first-pass perfusion MRI. J Cereb Blood Flow Metab 2009; 29: 840–852

[26] Calamante F, Mørup M, Hansen LK. Defining a local arterial input function for perfusion MRI using independent component analysis. Magn Reson Med 2004; 52: 789–797

[27] Østergaard L. Principles of cerebral perfusion imaging by bolus tracking. J Magn Reson Imaging 2005; 22: 710–717

[28] Aronen HJ, Gazit IE, Louis DN et al. Cerebral blood volume maps of gliomas: comparison with tumor grade and histologic findings. Radiology 1994; 191: 41–51

[29] Sugahara T, Korogi Y, Kochi M, Ushio Y, Takahashi M. Perfusion-sensitive MR imaging of gliomas: comparison between gradient-echo and spin-echo echo-planar imaging techniques. AJNR Am J Neuroradiol 2001; 22: 1306–1315

[30] Barajas RF, Jr, Chang JS, Segal MR et al. Differentiation of recurrent glioblastoma multiforme from radiation necrosis after external beam radiation therapy with dynamic susceptibility-weighted contrast-enhanced perfusion MR imaging. Radiology 2009; 253: 486–496

[31] Cha S. Perfusion MR imaging of brain tumors. Top Magn Reson Imaging 2004; 15: 279–289

[32] Barajas RF, Chang JS, Sneed PK, Segal MR, McDermott MW, Cha S. Distinguishing recurrent intra-axial metastatic tumor from radiation necrosis following gamma knife radiosurgery using dynamic susceptibility-weighted contrast-enhanced perfusion MR imaging. AJNR Am J Neuroradiol 2009; 30: 367–372

[33] Law M, Yang S, Babb JS et al. Comparison of cerebral blood volume and vascular permeability from dynamic susceptibility contrast-enhanced perfusion MR imaging with glioma grade. AJNR Am J Neuroradiol 2004; 25: 746–755

[34] Bisdas S, Kirkpatrick M, Giglio P, Welsh C, Spampinato MV, Rumboldt Z. Cerebral blood volume measurements by perfusion-weighted MR imaging in gliomas: ready for prime time in predicting short-term outcome and recurrent disease? AJNR Am J Neuroradiol 2009; 30: 681–688

[35] Lev MH, Ozsunar Y, Henson JW et al. Glial tumor grading and outcome prediction using dynamic spin-echo MR susceptibility mapping compared with

conventional contrast-enhanced MR: confounding effect of elevated rCBV of oligodendrogliomas [corrected]. AJNR Am J Neuroradiol 2004; 25: 214–221

[36] Law M, Young RJ, Babb JS et al. Gliomas: predicting time to progression or survival with cerebral blood volume measurements at dynamic susceptibility-weighted contrast-enhanced perfusion MR imaging. Radiology 2008; 247: 490–498

[37] Danchaivijitr N, Waldman AD, Tozer DJ et al. Low-grade gliomas: do changes in rCBV measurements at longitudinal perfusion-weighted MR imaging predict malignant transformation? Radiology 2008; 247: 170–178

[38] Law M, Oh S, Babb JS et al. Low-grade gliomas: dynamic susceptibility-weighted contrast-enhanced perfusion MR imaging—prediction of patient clinical response. Radiology 2006; 238: 658–667

[39] Strugar J, Rothbart D, Harrington W, Criscuolo GR. Vascular permeability factor in brain metastases: correlation with vasogenic brain edema and tumor angiogenesis. J Neurosurg 1994; 81: 560–566

[40] Strugar JG, Criscuolo GR, Rothbart D, Harrington WN. Vascular endothelial growth/permeability factor expression in human glioma specimens: correlation with vasogenic brain edema and tumor-associated cysts. J Neurosurg 1995; 83: 682–689

[41] Calli C, Kitis O, Yunten N, Yurtseven T, Islekel S, Akalin T. Perfusion and diffusion MR imaging in enhancing malignant cerebral tumors. Eur J Radiol 2006; 58: 394–403

[42] Sugahara T, Korogi Y, Shigematsu Y et al. Perfusion-sensitive MRI of cerebral lymphomas: a preliminary report. J Comput Assist Tomogr 1999; 23: 232–237

[43] Erdogan C, Hakyemez B, Yildirim N, Parlak M. Brain abscess and cystic brain tumor: discrimination with dynamic susceptibility contrast perfusion-weighted MRI. J Comput Assist Tomogr 2005; 29: 663–667

[44] Chan JH, Tsui EY, Chau LF et al. Discrimination of an infected brain tumor from a cerebral abscess by combined MR perfusion and diffusion imaging. Comput Med Imaging Graph 2002; 26: 19–23

[45] Kelly PJ, Daumas-Duport C, Kispert DB, Kall BA, Scheithauer BW, Illig JJ. Imaging-based stereotaxic serial biopsies in untreated intracranial glial neoplasms. J Neurosurg 1987; 66: 865–874

[46] Lev MH, Rosen BR. Clinical applications of intracranial perfusion MR imaging. Neuroimaging Clin N Am 1999; 9: 309–331

[47] Essig M, Anzalone N, Combs SE , et al. MR Imaging of Neoplastic Central Nervous System Lesions: Review and Recommendations for Current Practice. AJNR Am J Neuroradiol 2012; 33: 803–817

[48] Kumar AJ, Leeds NE, Fuller GN et al. Malignant gliomas: MR imaging spectrum of radiation therapy- and chemotherapy-induced necrosis of the brain after treatment. Radiology 2000; 217: 377–384

[49] Hu LS, Baxter LC, Smith KA et al. Relative cerebral blood volume values to differentiate high-grade glioma recurrence from posttreatment radiation effect:

direct correlation between image-guided tissue histopathology and localized dynamic susceptibility-weighted contrast-enhanced perfusion MR imaging measurements. AJNR Am J Neuroradiol 2009; 30: 552–558

[50] Oh BC, Pagnini PG, Wang MY et al. Stereotactic radiosurgery: adjacent tissue injury and response after high-dose single fraction radiation: Part I—Histology, imaging, and molecular events. Neurosurgery 2007; 60: 31–44, discussion 44–45

[51] Macdonald DR, Cascino TL, Schold SC, Jr, Cairncross JG. Response criteria for phase II studies of supratentorial malignant glioma. J Clin Oncol 1990; 8: 1277–1280

[52] Clarke JL, Chang S. Pseudoprogression and pseudoresponse: challenges in brain tumor imaging. Curr Neurol Neurosci Rep 2009; 9: 241–246

[53] Finn MA, Blumenthal DT, Salzman KL, Jensen RL. Transient postictal MRI changes in patients with brain tumors may mimic disease progression. Surg Neurol 2007; 67: 246–250, discussion 250

[54] Brandsma D, Stalpers L, Taal W, Sminia P, van den Bent MJ. Clinical features, mechanisms, and management of pseudoprogression in malignant gliomas. Lancet Oncol 2008; 9: 453–461

[55] Brandes AA, Franceschi E, Tosoni A et al. MGMT promoter methylation status can predict the incidence and outcome of pseudoprogression after concomitant radiochemotherapy in newly diagnosed glioblastoma patients. J Clin Oncol 2008; 26: 2192–2197

[56] Kong DS, Kim ST, Kim EH et al. Diagnostic dilemma of pseudoprogression in the treatment of newly diagnosed glioblastomas: the role of assessing relative cerebral blood flow volume and oxygen-6-methylguanine-DNA methyltransferase promoter methylation status. AJNR Am J Neuroradiol 2011; 32: 382–387

[57] Mangla R, Singh G, Ziegelitz D et al. Changes in relative cerebral blood volume 1 month after radiation-temozolomide therapy can help predict overall survival in patients with glioblastoma. Radiology 2010; 256: 575–584

[58] Batchelor TT, Sorensen AG, di Tomaso E et al. AZD2171, a pan-VEGF receptor tyrosine kinase inhibitor, normalizes tumor vasculature and alleviates edema in glioblastoma patients. Cancer Cell 2007; 11: 83–95

[59] Brandsma D, van den Bent MJ. Pseudoprogression and pseudoresponse in the treatment of gliomas. Curr Opin Neurol 2009; 22: 633–638

[60] Gerstner ER, Sorensen AG. Diffusion and diffusion tensor imaging in brain cancer. Semin Radiat Oncol 2011; 21: 141–146

[61] Sorensen AG, Batchelor TT, Zhang WT et al. A "vascular normalization index" as potential mechanistic biomarker to predict survival after a single dose of cediranib in recurrent glioblastoma patients. Cancer Res 2009; 69: 5296–5300

[62] Geer CP, Simonds J, Anvery A et al. Does MR perfusion imaging impact management decisions for patients with brain tumors? A prospective study. AJNR Am J Neuroradiol 2012; 33: 556–562

5 Perfusion Imaging: Dynamic Contrast-Enhanced T1-Weighted MRI (DCE-MRI) Perfusion

David Fussell and Robert J. Young

5.1 Introduction

Magnetic resonance perfusion imaging aims to derive hemodynamic information from magnetic resonance imaging (MRI) scans. Perfusion techniques include dynamic susceptibility-weighted contrast (DSC), arterial spin labeled (ASL), and dynamic contrast-enhanced T1-weighted perfusion MRI (DCE-MRI), the subject of this chapter. Because it does not require infusion of intravenous contrast material, ASL perfusion MRI can be performed entirely noninvasively and can be repeated at short intervals, without waiting for the subject to clear administered gadolinium. DSC-MRI begins with infusion of a rapidly administered bolus of contrast, after which repeated T2*-weighted acquisitions are made of the tissue of interest. DSC perfusion (Chapter 4) and ASL perfusion (Chapter 6) are discussed further in this volume.

DCE-MRI perfusion uses multiple T1-weighted images obtained at short intervals before and after intravenous administration of a bolus of gadolinium-diethylenetriamine pentaacetate (DTPA) contrast material to estimate, among other parameters, cerebral plasma volume and K^{trans}, a calculated coefficient meant to reflect capillary leakiness. Repeated short-time-to-echo (TE) magnetic resonance (MR) images are obtained through the region of interest. Then, using MR signal intensity as a measure of intravoxel gadolinium concentration, data are fitted to one of the many available models of tracer kinetics to estimate metrics such as plasma volume and K^{trans}.

Tissue hemodynamics are deranged in a wide variety of pathological states,[1] including primary and secondary neoplasm; inflammatory conditions such as multiple sclerosis; infection; and epilepsy. Perfusion imaging facilitates the diagnosis of these entities. For example, a common clinical problem is to distinguish a tumefactive demyelinating lesion from a brain tumor. Perfusion imaging consistently yields tumor plasma volume measurements in tumors higher than those found in tumefactive demyelinating lesions.[2] When the etiology of a primary brain tumor is uncertain, perfusion measurements are useful to predict the histological grade of a tumor, with higher-grade gliomas showing greater perfusion and capillary permeability.[3] On this basis, some investigators have used MR perfusion to direct brain biopsy to the most aggressive component of the brain glioma. As new treatments for brain tumors have been developed, perfusion imaging has proved instrumental in separating complications along the radiation injury spectrum from progression of disease.[4] Similarly, DCE-MRI perfusion has shown promise in assessing response to novel antiangiogenic therapies and as a tool in tailoring the chemotherapy regimen to the individual patient.

5.2 DCE-MRI Technique

5.2.1 General Principles

The goal of DCE perfusion imaging is to characterize the microvascular environment in the tissue of interest. Many different parameters can be assessed (► Fig. 5.1, ► Table 5.1).[5] Estimation of these parameters relies on accurate determination of the concentration of intravenous contrast (referred to as tracer in bolus tracking paradigms) at multiple time points as it moves through the voxel of interest. The link between the MR signal intensity of a voxel and the actual concentration of tracer within that voxel is more complex for DCE-MRI than for DSC-MRI, which assumes a linear relationship between tracer concentration and signal intensity.[6] In the case of DCE-MRI, while the relationship of relaxivity (1/T1) with gadolinium concentration is linear, the relationship between observed signal intensity and relaxivity depends on precontrast tissue relaxivity, flip angle, repetition time (TR), and proton density.[7] The dependence on precontrast relaxivity necessitates that imaging begin before the injection of intravenous contrast material to establish baseline T1 values.

Table 5.1 Common dynamic contrast-enhanced magnetic resonance imaging parameters

Parameter	Definition	Units
Perfusion curve	Dynamic dose response perfusion curve of signal intensity over time	–
AUC	Area under the perfusion curve	–
K_{ep}	K21, the volume transfer constant of contrast from the EES to the blood plasma	min^{-1}
K^{trans}	K12, the volume transfer constant of contrast from the blood plasma to the EES	min^{-1}
PE	Peak enhancement	–
TTP	Time to peak enhancement	s
V_e	Volume of EES	–
VP	Blood plasma volume per unit volume of tissue	mL/100 g or %
Wash-in	Initial upslope of perfusion curve	–
Wash-out	Downslope of perfusion curve	–

Abbreviation: EES, extravascular extracellular space.

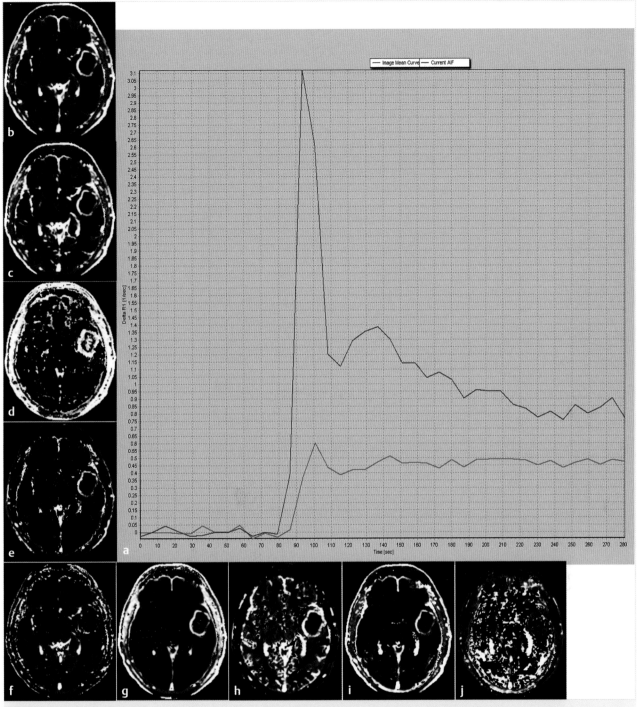

Fig. 5.1 Dynamic contrast-enhanced magnetic resonance imaging (DCE-MRI) perfusion maps. (**a**) Dynamic dose–response curve, (**b**) area under the curve (AUC), (**c**) peak enhancement, (**d**) time to peak (TTP), (**e**) wash-in, (**f**) wash-out, (**g**) V_e, (**h**) VP, (**i**) K^{trans}, and (**j**) K_{ep}. Terms are defined in ▶ Table 5.1.

5.2.2 Theory and Pharmacokinetic Models

Various hemodynamic data can be extracted from a series of contrast concentrations that change over time. The simplest and most straightforward approach is to make observations directly about the contrast versus time curve, without fitting data to any kind of model.[8] So-called non-model-based measurements include time to peak enhancement (TTP), peak enhancement or maximum signal intensity, wash-in rate, and wash-out rate.[9] Another approach is to obtain the integrated area under the signal intensity curve (IAUC or AUC). The signal intensity curve is integrated from the arrival of contrast material to a predetermined end point in time, such as 60 seconds after contrast arrival.[10] Although non-model-based measurements have been used with some success to differentiate gliomas of different histological grades[11] and to differentiate treatment-induced necrosis from tumor progression,[12] they represent descriptive indices that lack definite physical meaning. For example, which model parameter is the closest correlate of the IAUC measurement depends on primary hemodynamic variables, such as blood flow.[13] Thus the most accurate understanding of the IAUC is that it represents simply the quantity of contrast material delivered to and retained by the tissue of interest over the measured time interval.[14]

In contrast, model-based parameters result from fitting of the observed changes in tracer concentration to a mathematical model of the local tissue microenvironment. Most commonly, a simplified two-compartment model is employed.[15] Tracer flows in from a large artery and passes over time into the capillary system. From there, if there is disruption of the blood–brain barrier, it can move across the endothelium and into the surrounding tissue. The two compartments are the blood plasma space or intravascular plasma space (IVPS), which represents the fraction of whole blood within which tracer is distributed (the plasma), and the extravascular extracellular space (EES), which represents the fraction of tissue to which the tracer has access. Because gadolinium-based compounds are not thought to cross the cell membrane, the intracellular compartment is not considered in the model. With the two-compartment model in mind, tissue concentration of tracer depends on flow from the IVPS into the EES as well as flow from the EES back to the IVPS, each of which depends on the concentration gradient between the two spaces. This yields the following differential equation:

$$\frac{dC_t}{dt} = K^{trans} * C_p - K_{ep} * C_t$$

where C_p represents the plasma concentration of tracer (IVPS) and C_t represents the tracer concentration in tissue. V_e is the tracer concentration in tissue used to estimate the fractional volume of the EES. K^{trans} and K_{ep} (= K^{trans}/V_e) are the transfer constants. A solution to the differential equation is given by the extended Tofts and Kermode model, which includes a term for estimating the contribution of capillary plasma tracer.[16]

$$C_t(t) = v_p C_p(t) + K^{trans} \int_0^t C_p(\tau) \exp\left(\frac{-K^{trans}}{v_e}(t-\tau)\right) d\tau$$

Estimation of model-based parameters amounts to finding parameters V_p, K^{trans}, and V_e such that the difference between calculated and observed measurements of C_t is minimized. Bagher-Ebadian et al[17] also advocate performing a voxel-by-voxel model selection based on the single capillary model or its nested reduced models for estimation of K^{trans}.

Because model-based parameters rely on precise determination of tissue tracer concentration C_t, an allowance for the inflow of tracer at each time point must be made. This quantity is known as the arterial input function (AIF) and may be measured directly from a large artery at the base of the brain, such as the internal carotid or middle cerebral artery. This is ideal for model fitting because per-patient measurement accounts for patient-specific factors, such as cardiac output, that affect contrast delivery to tissue. However, measurement of arterial signal intensity is fraught with difficulties, including imaging artifacts related to saturation effects and arterial orientation within the slice. A very high temporal resolution is required for accurate sampling, on the order of one image per second.[10] An alternative is to use a standardized AIF, though this may be a poor representation of individual arterial blood flow and can generate large errors in tracer concentration measurement.[18]

5.2.3 DCE-MRI Limitations

Primary limitations common to all advanced MRI techniques, including DCE-MRI, involve the lack of standardization for image acquisition, postprocessing, analysis, and interpretation. Differences in the conversion of MRI signal to contrast concentration, temporal resolution, and estimations of contrast exchange between the intravascular space and the EES potentially affect both the accuracy and the precision of the perfusion results.[19] Lack of whole brain coverage is another issue in patients with large or multifocal tumors. In addition to the many choices available for model and non-model-based data analysis, the relative novelty of DCE-MRI also presents a lack of consensus of the optimal imaging metrics to be measured in tumors. Notwithstanding these potential technical limitations, and the imperfect comparisons and generalization of results among different institutions, we have been using DCE-MRI to measure VP and K^{trans} in our tumor patients to take advantage of the purported benefits in measuring perfusion and leakiness with promising early results.

5.3 Clinical Applications

Conventional MRI is the most useful radiographic modality in the localization and differential diagnosis of space-occupying cerebral lesions. Unfortunately, lesions of very different primary etiologies can overlap considerably in MRI appearance. Neoplastic, infectious, and demyelinating lesions, to name just a few, may all manifest as nondescript ring-enhancing masses. Determination of the perfusion characteristics of a lesion can aid in separating these entities; in general, brain tumors show marked central hyperperfusion, and other lesions, such as abscesses, do not.[20]

To date, most studies evaluating the utility of perfusion MRI in the characterization of brain lesions have employed DSC perfusion techniques. As described in depth in a separate chapter of this book, DSC perfusion relies on gadolinium contrast-induced decrease in signal intensity on T2*-weighted images to estimate perfusion parameters such as blood flow, blood volume, and mean transit time. Such studies have highlighted the usefulness of perfusion-weighted imaging in distinguishing abscess from infected neoplasm or cystic tumor and in characterizing demyelinating lesions and normal-appearing white matter in patients with multiple sclerosis.[21,22,23] A few studies of DCE-MRI have investigated perfusion and capillary leakiness in infectious and demyelinating diseases. DCE-MRI has proved most useful, however, in the diagnosis and grading of primary neoplasms of the brain, and as a problem-solving tool in cases of suspected treatment-related change or radiation injury.

5.3.1 DCE-MRI Perfusion in Glioma Diagnosis and Characterization

DCE-MRI has found its broadest application in the diagnosis and characterization of neoplasms of the central nervous system, primarily gliomas. Malignant gliomas account for approximately 70% of the 22,500 new cases of primary brain tumor diagnosed in the United States each year, of which approximately 14,000 are glioblastoma.[24] The World Health Organization (WHO) classification divides gliomas into four grades, with grades III and IV considered malignant. Pathologically, higher grades of tumor are characterized by increased cellularity, more numerous atypical nuclei, and greater mitotic activity. Clinically, gliomas of higher grade carry a worse prognosis: WHO grade II astrocytoma confers a 6- to 8-year median survival, whereas WHO grade IV tumors are usually fatal within about a year.[25] At present, although conventional MRI can suggest the tumor grade, only biopsy, which is extremely invasive in the brain, provides a definitive diagnosis. For the purposes of patient counseling and for the selection of appropriate therapy, a noninvasive means to assess tumor grade and aggressiveness is highly desirable.

The link between glioma grade and density of tumoral vessels is well established,[26,27] with more advanced tumors having greater vascularity. Oxygen and other vital nutrients are only able to diffuse over a relatively short distance in tissue (1–2 mm). For a tumor to grow larger than a few millimeters in size, it must induce the creation of new vessels to supply it in a process referred to as neovascularization or neoangiogenesis.[28] This complex cascade is stimulated by hypoxia and mediated by a host of vascular growth factors and other molecules.[29] Of these, vascular endothelial growth factor (VEGF) has emerged as the most important for angiogenesis in gliomas.[30] VEGF has been shown to stimulate capillary growth from host vessels,[31] increase microvascular permeability,[32] and cause vasodilatation in normal host vessels.[33] Expression of the *VEGF* gene correlates directly with tumor grade.[34] As will be discussed in a subsequent section, VEGF and other vascular growth factors have become primary targets for novel antiangiogenic chemotherapies.

In contrast to the new vessels produced by nonpathological angiogenesis, for example, as a step in normal development or in wound healing, tumor vessels are heterogeneous, fragile, and

arranged in a chaotic pattern.[35] In the brain, this means that the blood–brain barrier, which relies on tight junctions between endothelial cells, is not maintained. Absence of the normal blood–brain barrier is expected to lead to increased K^{trans} at DCE-MRI. Similarly, the greater vascular density of gliomas is expected to manifest as increased plasma volume. A primary goal of DCE-MRI is to complement conventional MRI by quantifying microcapillary perfusion and leakiness.

Hyperperfusion has been shown to correlate with increased tumor grade and more aggressive tumor biology. To date, most investigators have employed T2*-weighted dynamic susceptibility contrast (DSC) perfusion techniques, with cerebral blood volume (CBV) or relative CBV (rCBV) usually the best predictor for glioma grade.[36,37,38,39,40] DSC perfusion-derived rCBV and K^{trans} have performed well as the best set of independent measures to predict glioma grade.[39] Computed tomographic (CT) perfusion-derived metrics have also been correlated with WHO grade and microvascular density.[41,42,43,44,45] Early DCE-MRI literature has described similar success in predicting glioma grade. Nguyen et al[46] examined DCE-MRI in 46 patients with newly diagnosed gliomas using a phase-derived vascular input function and bookend T1 measurements before and after contrast injection. They found that the median plasma volume increased from grade II (0.64 mL/100 g, $n = 9$) to grade III (0.98 mL/100 g, $n = 9$) to grade IV (2.16 mL/100 g, $n = 28$), with significant differences between grades III and IV ($p = 0.015$) but not between grades II and III ($p = 0.15$). Median K^{trans} values also increased from grade II (0.0041 min^{-1}) to grade III (0.031 min^{-1}) to grade IV (0.088 min^{-1}), with significant differences between grades III and IV ($p = 0.04$) but not grades II and III ($p = 0.05$). In our experience, DCE-MRI–derived plasma volume (analogous to CBV) and K^{trans} also show good correlations, with both metrics increasing with increasing glioma grade (▶ Fig. 5.2).

Several other studies have investigated the relationship between glioma grade and capillary leakiness determined by DCE-MRI. Early studies[3,47,48] provided conflicting results, possibly because of the large number of different models used to derive perfusion parameters. A 2005 study by Pantakar et al,[49] using three-dimensional (3D) T1-weighted spoiled gradient recalled (SPGR) images and a first-pass method of analysis described by Li et al,[50] studied K^{trans} and CBV in 39 patients with WHO grade II through IV gliomas. They found a significant correlation between K^{trans} and CBV ($r = 0.688$) and significant differences between tumor grades for both K^{trans} and CBV. Pairwise comparisons between grades revealed significant differences in CBV and K^{trans} in all cases except the grade III versus IV comparison. Ultimately, the model was able to classify tumor grade with an overall accuracy of 74.4% and to distinguish between low-grade (WHO grade II) and high-grade (WHO III and IV) gliomas with sensitivity and specificity both greater than 90%. The authors suggested that their model was less successful at separating grade III from grade IV gliomas because many patients with grade IV gliomas had already been treated with steroids at the time of imaging, a therapy that is known to decrease capillary leakiness.

A more recent study of DCE-MRI in gliomas by Zhang et al[51] used the extended two-compartment Tofts model to analyze five perfusion parameters in 28 patients with histopathologically

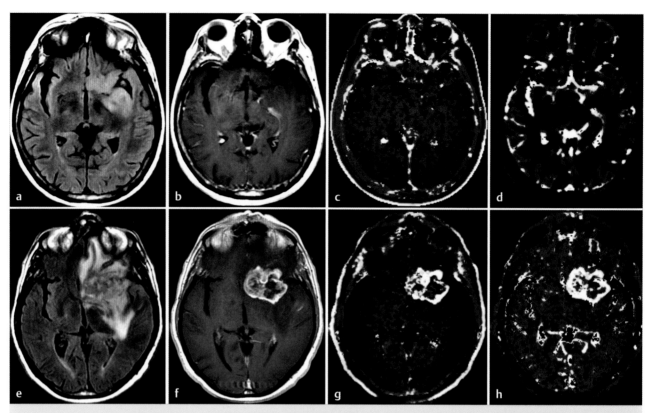

Fig. 5.2 Low-grade glioma (LGG) and high-grade glioma (HGG). (**a**) Axial fluid-attenuated inversion recovery (FLAIR) image and (**b**) contrast T1-weighted image shows an expansile FLAIR hyperintense nonenhancing tumor in the left insula, basal ganglia, and frontal lobe base. (**c**) K^{trans} and (**d**) plasma volume maps show no increase in permeability or perfusion in this diffusely infiltrating World Health Organization (WHO) grade II low-grade astrocytoma. Corresponding images (**e–h**) in another patient demonstrate a heterogeneously enhancing cystic/necrotic tumor with marked increases in permeability and perfusion and was proven to be an unmethylated, isocitrate dehydrogenase-1 (IDH-1) negative glioblastoma at histology.

graded gliomas. K^{trans} and V_e (fractional volume of the EES) showed significant differences among tumor grades. As in the Pantakar study, K^{trans} was a significant independent discriminator of grade II from grade III and grade IV tumors but not of grade III from grade IV lesions. K^{trans} distinguished low- from high-grade gliomas with sensitivity of 0.92 and specificity of 0.85. The superiority of K^{trans} compared with CBV for separating tumor grades has been reported elsewhere as well.[52]

If DCE-MRI is useful in distinguishing different grades of tumor, it should also be useful for identifying regions of higher grade within an individual lesion. Because histological grade reflects the most anaplastic portion of the tumor, and gliomas are notoriously heterogeneous, biopsy should ideally be directed at the most advanced portion of the neoplasm. Conventional MRI has been used to guide biopsy but in many cases does not provide adequate lesion characterization, especially in cases of nonenhancing tumor.[53,54,55] A recent study by Weber et al[56] applied DCE-MRI, DSC-MRI, and ASL perfusion imaging as well as fludeoxyglucose positron-emission tomography (FDG PET) and MR spectroscopy to 61 patients with gliomas that were subsequently either resected or biopsied. K_{ep} (= K^{trans}/V_e, the rate constant for diffusion of contrast from the EES to the blood plasma) was estimated with the Tofts two-compartment pharmacokinetic model. The amplitude of the enhancement curve was also measured. The authors found a significant correlation of both K^{trans} and enhancement amplitude with tumor grade. With regard to selection of the most advanced portion of tumors for biopsy, the authors found good agreement between the different advanced MR techniques in identifying the tumor areas most biologically active and thus most appropriate as biopsy targets.

5.3.2 DCE-MRI Perfusion in Monitoring Response to Therapy

Initial therapy for malignant glioma depends on grade. Standard therapy for a patient with a new diagnosis of glioblastoma (WHO grade IV) consists of surgical resection, radiotherapy, and adjuvant chemotherapy with temozolomide.[57] Anaplastic astrocytoma, anaplastic oligodendroglioma, and anaplastic mixed glioma or oligoastrocytoma (WHO grade III) may undergo surgical resection, radiotherapy with or without concomitant chemotherapy, or chemotherapy alone. Recurrent tumors may require reoperation and/or one or more antiangiogenic or experimental agents.[58,59,60,61] Now that multiple chemotherapeutic agents are available for treatment, accurate assessment of response to therapy is critical because a patient who fails to respond to one agent may be switched to an alternative therapy.[62]

Diagnosis of recurrence has traditionally relied on an increase in size of the enhancing portion of a mass lesion and/or the presence of new contrast-enhancing mass lesions.[63] Imaging criteria for response have recently been updated, however, to reflect a number of new challenges brought about by novel therapies.[64,65] Chief among these is the difficulty of accurately diagnosing tumor progression (and therefore treatment failure) when increasing or new enhancement may represent recurrent tumor, radiation injury, or both. Distinguishing the two entities may have profound effects on treatment decisions and on outcome characterization, for example, in clinical trials that use progression-free survival as a primary end point.

Radiation injury suggests a complication of treatment (i.e., radiation necrosis) or effective treatment (i.e., pseudoprogression). Radiation injury in the brain has classically been divided, according to the time after therapy at which it occurs, into three categories: acute reaction, early-delayed reaction, and late-delayed reaction.[66] Among many other factors, total dose and schedule of administration (fractionation) are important determinants of radiation injury. Acute reactions occur during radiation therapy. Early-delayed reaction occurs a few weeks to 3 months after completion of radiotherapy, is thought to represent demyelination following injury to oligodendrocytes, and is usually transient in nature.[67] Late-delayed radiation necrosis, on the other hand, typically develops 6 months to 3 years or longer after cessation of radiation therapy and is often irreversible.[68]

A fourth entity termed pseudoprogression consists of radiographic worsening in the early-delayed radiation injury time window that spontaneously stabilizes or resolves and is often asymptomatic.[69,70] The term is usually reserved for recently treated high-grade gliomas. Pseudoprogression is potentiated by temozolomide therapy, occurring in up to 30% of such patients,[71,72,73,74] but has been described in conjunction with other chemotherapy agents as well. The imaging changes are thought to represent desirable chemoradiation-related tumor necrosis; there is evidence that pseudoprogression is a good prognostic sign.[75,76,77] The benefits presented by pseudoprogression are probably related to its increased incidence in patients with methylated O(6)-methylguanine-DNA methyltransferase (MGMT) promoter status gliomas.[77]

5.3.3 DCE-MRI Perfusion in Tumor Progression

Modern response criteria used in most clinical trials do not include any advanced imaging metrics to determine progression.[64,65,78,79] Instead, progression is often defined as $\geq 25\%$ increase in diameter of the contrast-enhancing portion of a mass lesion or any new enhancing mass lesion, and may incorporate information about increasing nonenhancing disease, increasing steroid requirements, or clinical worsening. Although still considered "investigational," tools such as DCE-MRI, T2*-DSC perfusion, spectroscopy, diffusion, and PET/CT are commonly used in clinical practice to guide treatment decisions. Among the potential limitations of these techniques is the lack of consensus on the optimal imaging acquisition parameters, postprocessing analysis methods, and perfusion metrics. Tumor progression usually involves neovascularity, with the new, immature, leaky tumor blood vessels measurable by DCE-MRI. Among the numerous metrics available (► Fig. 5.1), our institution analyzes just two maps for clinical

use: K^{trans} and plasma volume. The volume transfer coefficient K^{trans} is a measure of contrast passage from the plasma to the EES, and as such is affected by both blood flow and permeability–surface area product. Plasma volume is a measure of blood volume or perfusion. K^{trans} and plasma volume are considered independent markers and typically both are elevated in tumor progression, unless directly modulated by antiangiogenic therapy (► Fig. 5.3). Of these two metrics, K^{trans} may also be elevated in radiation injury due to disruption of the blood–brain barrier, so we consider elevated plasma volume the most reliable single metric. As we and others gain experience, it is likely that our understanding and use of DCE-MRI metrics will continue to evolve.

5.3.4 DCE-MRI Perfusion in Radiation Injury

Pseudoprogression may be indistinguishable from true disease progression at conventional MRI because both manifest with increased masslike enhancement.[69] As already discussed, differentiation of the two entities is critical for informed decision making because they represent opposite responses to therapy. Indeed, pseudoprogression is likely to occur at the time when clinicians would be most inclined to change a regimen that had proved ineffective.[4] The role of DSC perfusion in identifying pseudoprogression has been fairly well established, with progressive tumor demonstrating relatively higher CBV.[4,80,81,82] The utility of T1-weighted DCE-MRI studies has not been as well studied. A recent report[83] applied DCE-MRI to seven pediatric patients with a variety of brain tumors and identified pseudoprogression in four. Calculated CBV and K^{trans} values were variable in this small sample and heterogeneous within individual tumors, though patients with medulloblastoma did demonstrate increased CBV.

Some recent papers have applied DCE-MRI to the identification of treatment-induced necrosis, an umbrella term that includes pseudoprogression as well as late-delayed radiation necrosis. Larsen et al[84] investigated DCE-MRI in 19 glioma patients, of whom 18 had WHO grade III or IV tumors treated with maximal resection, radiation, and temozolomide. Patients with new enhancing lesions identified during the follow-up period that could not be diagnosed confidently as either tumor progression or radiation necrosis were referred for DCE-MRI and FDG PET brain scans. CBV, CBF, and K^{trans} were all lower in the nonprogressive lesions, and the authors concluded that an absolute volume threshold of 2.0 mL/100 g brain parenchyma could be used to identify true progressive disease. DCE-MRI performed as well or better than FDG PET.

Narang et al[12] performed a similar long-term follow-up study of 29 glioma patients with new enhancing lesions following maximal therapy (25/29 treated with resection and chemoradiation). Using either histological confirmation or clinical/radiographic follow-up, 9 were ultimately found to have treatment-related necrosis and 20 to have recurrent tumor. A non-model-based analysis was used to extract DCE-MRI parameters, including area under the enhancement curve (IAUC), maximal slope of the enhancement curve in the initial vascular phase (MSIVP), and slope of the enhancement curve in the delayed equilibrium phase (SDEP). All calculated perfusion parameters were significantly different in patients with treatment-induced

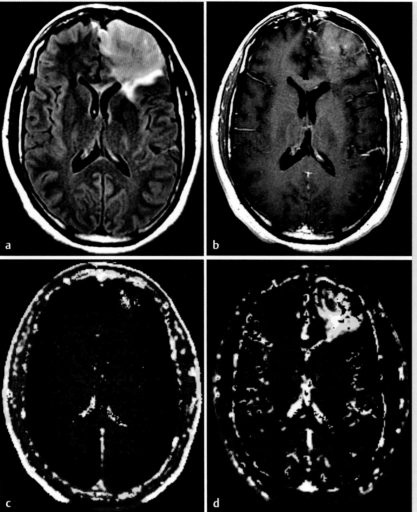

Fig. 5.3 Tumor progression. Anaplastic oligodendroglioma with 1p19q co-deletions, 1 month after completion of 12 months of adjuvant temozolomide. (**a**) Fluid-attenuated inversion recovery (FLAIR) image reveals an expansile heterogeneously hypointense to isointense tumor in the left frontal lobe with mild, more hyperintense peritumoral abnormality. (**b**) Contrast T1-weighted image shows mild heterogeneous enhancement. (**c**) K^{trans} map demonstrates only mild increase in permeability, whereas (**d**) plasma volume (VP) map shows marked disproportionate increase in perfusion of the entire lesion. Repeat resection showed recurrent anaplastic oligodendroglioma with more than 5 mitoses per 10 high-power fields.

necrosis versus recurrent tumor, showing increased perfusion in the recurrent tumor group. The authors reported 85% sensitivity and 100% specificity using SDEP and a 90% sensitivity/ 100% specificity using MSIVP to distinguish treatment-induced necrosis from recurrent tumor.

At our institution, we routinely perform DCE-MRI before surgery, at each follow-up for high-grade gliomas, and as a problem-solving tool in suspected radiation injury. Analysis is conducted using a two-compartment model with reconstruction of a dynamic dose–response curve measured on a voxel-by-voxel basis. Deconvolution of the dynamic tissue response curves is performed using an AIF based on the work of Murase et al,[85] and estimation of the contrast concentration is performed from observed dynamic changes in MRI signal intensity. We qualitatively interpret the K^{trans} and plasma volume maps for clinical cases. K^{trans} is often greater in recurrent tumor than in radiation injury, although it may be increased in both entities. The plasma volume is usually increased in recurrent tumor and normal or decreased in radiation injury. Several characteristic patterns have been observed in DCE-MRI perfusion maps of radiation injury, which most commonly manifests as decreased plasma volume with variable K^{trans} or as slightly increased plasma volume with disproportionately marked increase in K^{trans}. These patterns have been observed in cases of both early pseudoprogression and more delayed radiation necrosis (▶ Fig. 5.4, ▶ Fig. 5.5, and ▶ Fig. 5.6). A prospective clinical trial comparing DCE-MRI and 18F-fludeoxyglucose PET/CT in the diagnosis of radiation injury is ongoing at our institution.

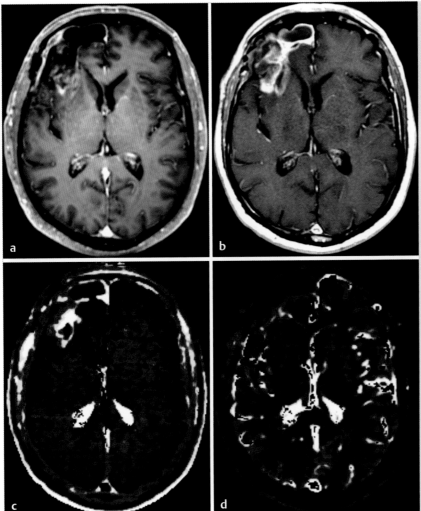

Fig. 5.4 Pseudoprogression. Axial contrast T1-weighted imaging immediately (**a**) and 4 months after (**b**) completion of combination radiation therapy and temozolomide for glioblastoma shows a new, ill-defined heterogeneously enhancing mass lesion in the frontal lobe, insula, subinsula, and basal ganglia. (**c**) K^{trans} map reveals moderately increased permeability, whereas (**d**) plasma volume shows no increased perfusion. Persistent growth over the next 3 months led to re-resection, which demonstrated extensive necrotizing treatment effects with no tumor.

5.3.5 DCE-MRI Perfusion in Patients Treated with Novel Therapeutic Agents

A number of new drugs have recently been developed to target the neoangiogenesis cascade in malignant glioma. The two most common treatments are the anti-VEGF agents bevacizumab (Avastin, Genentech, South San Francisco, CA), a monoclonal antibody, and cediranib (AZD2171), a VEGF inhibitor. Bevacizumab recently achieved accelerated Food and Drug Administration (FDA) approval for treatment of recurrent glioblastoma.[86] These agents have been shown to decrease tumor enhancement at conventional MRI as little as 24 hours after initiation of therapy.[87,88] The clinical significance of decreased volume and intensity of enhancement remains uncertain, however, because the overall survival benefit in patients treated with bevacizumab has been fairly modest despite improved progression-free survival.[89] In some patients, despite the decreased enhancement, there is continued growth of the infiltrative, nonenhancing portion of the tumor,[90] which often demonstrates restricted diffusion and intermediate T2 hyperintensity.[91,92] This appearance, which represents a new challenge

for imaging, has been termed a pseudoresponse because the older Macdonald criteria relying simply on changes in size of the enhancing component would often classify these cases as a partial or complete response. The newer Response Assessment in Neuro-Oncology (RANO) criteria[64,65] include increased fluid-attenuated inversion recovery (FLAIR) hyperintense nonenhancing disease as a criterion for progression, although the increase is described only as "significant," without any percentage increase, unlike the older enhancement-based criteria.

Investigators are just beginning to apply perfusion imaging in cases of pseudoresponse. Early studies of DSC perfusion suggest that lower CBV correlates with longer progression-free survival in patients treated with cediranib.[93,94] Rapid decreases in perfusion and permeability metrics may occur as soon as 24 hours after initiation of antiangiogenic therapy, although the DCE-MRI changes in pseudoresponse have not been well characterized in the literature. At our institution, where bevacizumab patients are routinely followed with DCE-MRI, we have observed that K^{trans} and plasma volume are usually both decreased or only slightly increased in patients with pseudoresponse. If increased, they are usually still less than before

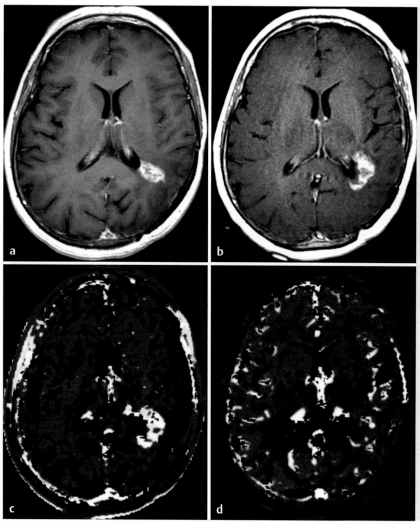

Fig. 5.5 Radiation necrosis in metastatic lung cancer. Axial contrast T1-weighted imaging before (**a**) and 6 months after (**b**) hypofractionated radiation therapy (2,500 cGy in five fractions) to recurrent tumor in the left parietal lobe shows an increasing, ill-defined, heterogeneously enhancing mass lesion. (**c**) K^{trans} map demonstrated moderately increased permeability, whereas (**d**) plasma volume (VP) reveals mostly low perfusion aside from a few small foci of slightly increased perfusion. Resection showed necrosis, fibrosis, and old hemorrhage without tumor.

beginning antiangiogenic therapy (▶ Fig. 5.7 and ▶ Fig. 5.8). Imaging of pseudoresponse is likely to develop as an active area of research as additional new antiangiogenic agents are developed and brought to market.

5.3.6 DCE-MRI Perfusion in Nonglial Neoplasms

Of the nonglial brain neoplasms, meningioma is perhaps the best studied with regard to perfusion imaging. Several early papers included perfusion findings in meningiomas primarily as part of the validation process for different perfusion techniques.[95] Because extra-axial tumors lack a blood–brain barrier at all stages of growth, they demonstrate expected high blood volume and capillary leakiness. Zhu et al[96] used a Tofts model to study five meningiomas, five vestibular schwannomas, and five gliomas, noting generally higher K^{trans} and CBV in the extra-axial tumors. Perfusion parameters alone, however, were unable to distinguish types of tumor.

Lüdemann et al[97] reported DCE-MRI results in 41 gliomas, 6 meningiomas, and 8 metastases using a novel, three-compartment model. In this model, the EES was split into two subcompartments based on different plasma space exchange constants. The "fast" compartment was thought to represent early extravasation into viable tissue, whereas the "slow" compartment was thought to represent leakage into necrotic areas, which typically occurred over a longer time. Measures of blood volume were obtained in addition to separate measures of permeability and fractional volume for each compartment. Significant differences were found in blood volume between all three groups, with meningiomas having the highest and gliomas the lowest CBV. Slow permeability was nearly the same for all tumors, a result thought to reflect the fact that all of the tumors studied were known to have large necrotic components. Fast permeability, on the other hand, was significantly greater in meningiomas (▶ Fig. 5.9).

5.3.7 DCE-MRI Perfusion in Non-neoplastic Lesions

Conventional MRI is the radiographic test of choice for diagnosis and characterization of the demyelinating plaques of multiple sclerosis (MS). The initial diagnosis of MS is in most cases

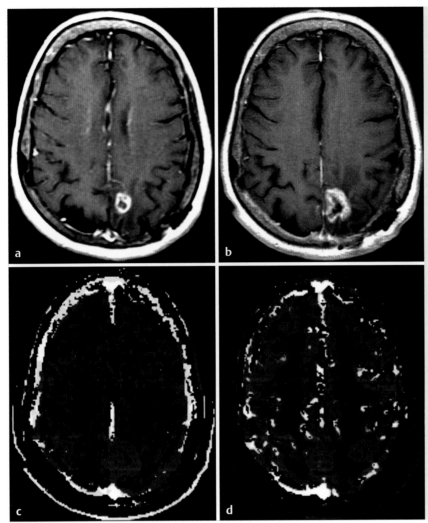

Fig. 5.6 Radiation necrosis in metastatic breast cancer. Axial contrast T1-weighted imaging before (**a**) and 4 years after (**b**) partial brain radiation (3,500 cGy in 14 fractions) to the surgical cavity show increasing heterogeneously enhancing mass lesion in the left parietal lobe. (**c**) K^{trans} map demonstrates mild increase in permeability of the enhancing periphery, whereas (**d**) plasma volume (VP) map reveals no increase in perfusion. Repeat resection showed only necrosis and reactive brain tissue without tumor. Note subtle enhancement in the contralateral paramedian parietal lobe in (**b**) is an additional clue to indicate radiation necrosis.

straightforward using conventional MRI, with individual lesions having a characteristic and often asymmetric distribution. However, the relationship between the severity of the imaging appearance and of clinical manifestations is complex.[98] Traditionally, enhancement is used as a measure of lesion activity because it indicates breakdown of the blood–brain barrier.[99] A recent study by Ingrisch et al[100] identified early changes in perfusion in demyelinating plaques, which are known to precede breakdown of the blood–brain barrier and thus contrast enhancement at conventional MRI. The study used parallel imaging to obtain 3D, T1-weighted images at high temporal resolution of the whole brain, which is desirable in patients with MS because demyelinating plaques occur both supra- and infratentorially. Permeability, blood flow, and blood volume were calculated using a two-compartment model in 19 patients. Significantly higher CBF, CBV, and permeability were observed in contrast-enhancing lesions relative to normal-appearing white matter. Significantly increased CBV was observed in nonenhancing lesions as well.

DCE-MRI has also been used to evaluate cerebral infections (▶ Fig. 5.10). In a study of 5 tuberculomas and 10 gliomas, Singh et al[101] found a trend toward increased K^{trans} in tuberculomas compared to gliomas, and toward increased CBV in

tuberculoma intermediate between low-grade and high-grade gliomas. Haris et al[102] used DCE-MRI and found a strong correlation ($r = 0.918$) between K^{trans} and the percentage of individual high-powered fields over which matrix metalloproteinase 9 (MMP-9) was expressed in brain tuberculomas. A weak correlation ($r = 0.232$) was found between K^{trans} and VEGF expression. These results suggest that, in tuberculoma, MMP-9 plays a greater role in blood–brain barrier disruption than does VEGF. A second study[103] applied DCE-MRI to 26 patients with infection, 52 with high-grade glioma, and 25 with low-grade glioma and correlated the findings with VEGF expression and microvascular density (MVD) noted in pathological slides. The authors found that CBV, CBF, and K^{trans} showed significant differences across the three patient groups, again with infectious lesions demonstrating perfusion intermediate between low- and high-grade gliomas. MVD and expression of VEGF were also significantly different and ranked the entities in the same order. CBV measurements in all patients showed a statistically significant correlation with MVD.

The same group used perfusion imaging to monitor response to therapy in patients with brain tuberculoma,[104] demonstrating a significant decrease in CBV, CBF, and K^{trans} over time in patients with clinical and radiological response to therapy. In

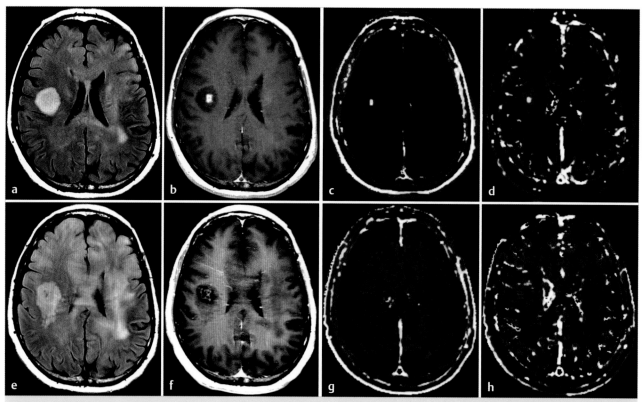

Fig. 5.7 Pseudoresponse. Glioblastoma in left frontal lobe (not shown) with methylated O(6)-methylguanine-DNA methyltransferase (MGMT) promoter status, receiving adjuvant temozolomide 13 months after completion of concurrent radiation therapy. (**a**) Axial fluid-attenuated inversion recovery (FLAIR) shows a new expansile hyperintense mass lesion in the right corona radiata, and (**b**) contrast T1-weighted imaging shows new central enhancement, with (**c**) K^{trans} and (**d**) plasma volume showing increased permeability and perfusion, respectively. Patient began antiangiogenic therapy with bevacizumab (a vascular endothelial growth factor antibody) and RO4929097 (a gamma-secretase inhibitor important for Notch activation). Two months later, corresponding images (**e–h**) demonstrate decreased, albeit more irregular and diffuse, enhancing lesion in the right corona radiata (**f**) with smaller increases in K^{trans} (**g**) and plasma volume (**h**). Despite the apparent improvement in enhancement, however, the nonenhancing changes in bilateral hemispheres and corpus callosum (**e**) continue to increase, consistent with antiangiogenic therapy–mediated pseudoresponse. The patient had worsening leg weakness, dysarthria, and dysphagia, and succumbed to his disease 3 months later.

patients whose lesions ultimately required surgical excision, K^{trans} increased significantly over time. A similar study of DCE-MRI findings in patients with neurocysticercosis[105] also found a strong correlation between K^{trans} and MMP-9 expression ($r = 0.71$). K_{ep} was significantly different in the colloidal, granular-nodular, and calcified stages of cysticercosis. These findings highlight the role of DCE-MRI in the characterization and monitoring of intracranial infectious lesions.

5.4 Conclusions

Perfusion MRI provides noninvasive characterization of the microvascular environment in a tissue of interest. DCE-MRI in particular offers quantification of capillary leakiness and plasma volume at high spatial resolution. These measures complement conventional MRI in the differential diagnosis and characterization of newly discovered brain lesions and in the monitoring of these lesions during treatment. As new chemotherapies are incorporated into standard treatment regimens for central nervous system malignancy, perfusion and other advanced imaging techniques have growing roles for characterizing the individual response to therapy and guiding the course of treatment. Improvements in the standardization of acquisition techniques, analysis algorithms, and interpretation experience are expected to further improve the importance of DCE-MRI perfusion as an essential research and clinical tool in the years ahead.

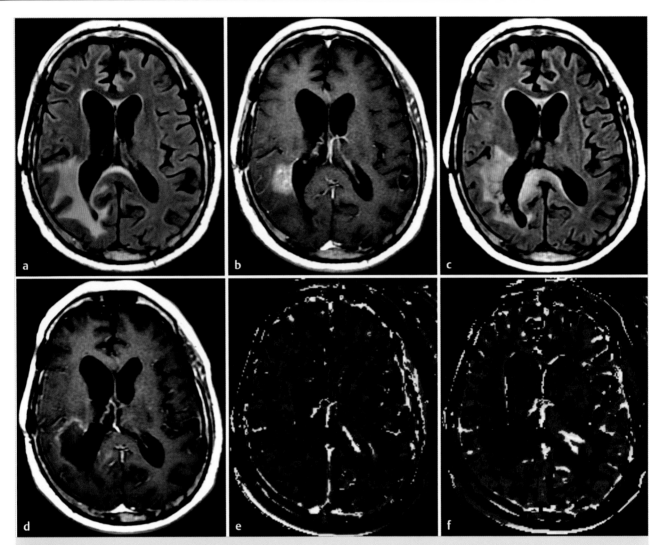

Fig. 5.8 Pseudoresponse. (**a**) Axial fluid-attenuated inversion recovery (FLAIR) image reveals moderate hyperintense changes, and (**b**) contrast T1-weighted imaging (T1WI) shows a recurrent ill-defined enhancing glioblastoma with subependymal spread. Six months after beginning bevacizumab, (**c**) FLAIR image reveals increased expansile hyperintense changes in the splenium of the corpus callosum, and (**d**) contrast T1WI demonstrates a thin enhancing periphery around the increased, mostly nonenhancing tumor. (**e**) K^{trans} and (**f**) plasma volume (VP) maps show no increase in permeability or perfusion.

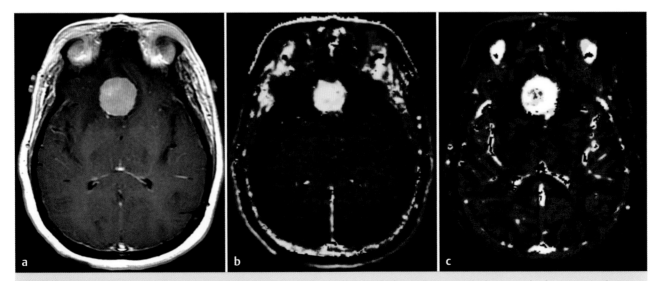

Fig. 5.9 Planum sphenoidale meningioma. (**a**) Axial contrast T1-weighted imaging reveals a well-circumscribed extra-axial enhancing mass lesion projecting superiorly from the planum sphenoidale into the base of the frontal lobes. (**b**) K^{trans} and (**c**) plasma volume maps show markedly increased permeability and perfusion typical for these tumors that lie outside the blood–brain barrier.

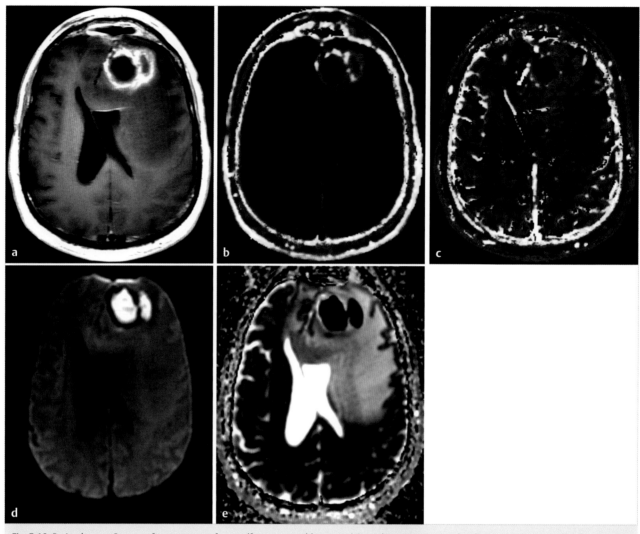

Fig. 5.10 Brain abscess, 3 years after treatment for an olfactory neuroblastoma. (**a**) Axial contrast T1-weighted imaging shows an ill-defined peripherally enhancing mass in the left frontal lobe with a small lateral daughter lesion and extensive surrounding edema. (**b**) K^{trans} map reveals heterogeneous increase in permeability of the enhancing periphery, whereas (**c**) plasma volume map shows no increase in perfusion. (**d**) Diffusion-weighted imaging and (**e**) apparent diffusion coefficient map confirm central diffusion restriction in this abscess. Pathology showed pus with necrotic and inflammatory debris.

References

[1] Lacerda S, Shiroishi MS, Law M. Clinical applications of dynamic contrast-enhanced (DCE) permeability imaging. In: Faro SH, Mohamed FB, Law M, Ulmer JT, eds. Functional Neuroradiology: Principles and Clinical Applications. New York, NY: Springer; 2011:117–137

[2] Al-Okaili RN, Krejza J, Woo JH et al. Intraaxial brain masses: MR imaging-based diagnostic strategy—initial experience. Radiology 2007; 243: 539–550

[3] Roberts HC, Roberts TPL, Brasch RC, Dillon WP. Quantitative measurement of microvascular permeability in human brain tumors achieved using dynamic contrast-enhanced MR imaging: correlation with histologic grade. AJNR Am J Neuroradiol 2000; 21: 891–899

[4] Young RJ, Gupta A, Shah AD et al. MRI perfusion in determining pseudoprogression in patients with glioblastoma. Clin Imaging 2013; 37: 41–49

[5] Tofts PS, Brix G, Buckley DL et al. Estimating kinetic parameters from dynamic contrast-enhanced T(1)-weighted MRI of a diffusable tracer: standardized quantities and symbols. J Magn Reson Imaging 1999; 10: 223–232

[6] Jackson A, O'Connor JP, Parker GJ, Jayson GC. Imaging tumor vascular heterogeneity and angiogenesis using dynamic contrast-enhanced magnetic resonance imaging. Clin Cancer Res 2007; 13: 3449–3459

[7] Evelhoch JL. Key factors in the acquisition of contrast kinetic data for oncology. J Magn Reson Imaging 1999; 10: 254–259

[8] Cheng HL. Improved correlation to quantitative DCE-MRI pharmacokinetic parameters using a modified initial area under the uptake curve (mIAUC) approach. J Magn Reson Imaging 2009; 30: 864–872

[9] Mazzetti S, Gliozzi AS, Bracco C, Russo F, Regge D, Stasi M. Comparison between PUN and Tofts models in the quantification of dynamic contrast-enhanced MR imaging. Phys Med Biol 2012; 57: 8443–8453

[10] Cheng HL. Investigation and optimization of parameter accuracy in dynamic contrast-enhanced MRI. J Magn Reson Imaging 2008; 28: 736–743

[11] Mills SJ, Soh C, O'Connor JP et al. Enhancing fraction in glioma and its relationship to the tumoral vascular microenvironment: A dynamic contrast-enhanced MR imaging study. AJNR Am J Neuroradiol 2010; 31: 726–731

[12] Narang J, Jain R, Arbab AS et al. Differentiating treatment-induced necrosis from recurrent/progressive brain tumor using nonmodel-based semiquantitative indices derived from dynamic contrast-enhanced T1-weighted MR perfusion. Neuro-oncol 2011; 13: 1037–1046

[13] Walker-Samuel S, Leach MO, Collins DJ. Evaluation of response to treatment using DCE-MRI: the relationship between initial area under the gadolinium curve (IAUGC) and quantitative pharmacokinetic analysis. Phys Med Biol 2006; 51: 3593–3602

[14] O'Connor JP, Jackson A, Parker GJ, Jayson GC. DCE-MRI biomarkers in the clinical evaluation of antiangiogenic and vascular disrupting agents. Br J Cancer 2007; 96: 189–195

[15] Koh TS, Bisdas S, Koh DM, Thng CH. Fundamentals of tracer kinetics for dynamic contrast-enhanced MRI. J Magn Reson Imaging 2011; 34: 1262–1276

[16] Tofts PS. Modeling tracer kinetics in dynamic Gd-DTPA MR imaging. J Magn Reson Imaging 1997; 7: 91–101

[17] Bagher-Ebadian H, Jain R, Nejad-Davarani SP et al. Model selection for DCE-T1 studies in glioblastoma. Magn Reson Med 2012; 68: 241–251

[18] Parker G, Tanner S, Leach M. Pitfalls in the measurement of tissue permeability over short time-scales using multi-compartment models with a low temporal resolution blood input function. Presented at: 4th Meeting of the International Society for Magnetic Resonance in Medicine; New York, New York, April 27-May 3, 1996

[19] Zhang Y, Wang J, Wang X, Zhang J, Fang J, Jiang X. Feasibility study of exploring a T$_1$-weighted dynamic contrast-enhanced MR approach for brain perfusion imaging. J Magn Reson Imaging 2012; 35: 1322–1331

[20] Wolf RL. Clinical Applications of MR Perfusion Imaging. In: Faro SH, Mohamed FB, Law M, Ulmer JT, eds. Functional Neuroradiology: Principles and Clinical Applications. New York, NY: Springer; 2011:71–105

[21] Chan JH, Tsui EY, Chau LF et al. Discrimination of an infected brain tumor from a cerebral abscess by combined MR perfusion and diffusion imaging. Comput Med Imaging Graph 2002; 26: 19–23

[22] Erdogan C, Hakyemez B, Yildirim N, Parlak M. Brain abscess and cystic brain tumor: discrimination with dynamic susceptibility contrast perfusion-weighted MRI. J Comput Assist Tomogr 2005; 29: 663–667

[23] Ge Y, Law M, Johnson G et al. Dynamic susceptibility contrast perfusion MR imaging of multiple sclerosis lesions: characterizing hemodynamic impairment and inflammatory activity. AJNR Am J Neuroradiol 2005; 26: 1539–1547

[24] Wen PY, Kesari S. Malignant gliomas in adults. N Engl J Med 2008; 359: 492–507

[25] Krex D, Klink B, Hartmann C et al. German Glioma Network. Long-term survival with glioblastoma multiforme. Brain 2007; 130: 2596–2606

[26] Brem S, Cotran R, Folkman J. Tumor angiogenesis: a quantitative method for histologic grading. J Natl Cancer Inst 1972; 48: 347–356

[27] Cheng SY, Huang HJ, Nagane M et al. Suppression of glioblastoma angigenicity and tumorigenicity by inhibition of endogenous expression of vascular endothelial growth factor. Proc Natl Acad Sci U S A 1996; 93: 8502–8507

[28] Russell D, Rubinstein L. Tumors of central neuroepithelial origin. In: Russell D, Rubinstein L, eds. Pathology of Tumours of the Central Nervous System. Baltimore, MD: Williams & Wilkins; 1989:53–350

[29] Li WW. Tumor angiogenesis: molecular pathology, therapeutic targeting, and imaging. Acad Radiol 2000; 7: 800–811

[30] Kargiotis O, Rao JS, Kyritsis AP. Mechanisms of angiogenesis in gliomas. J Neurooncol 2006; 78: 281–293

[31] Dvorak HF, Nagy JA, Feng D, Brown LF, Dvorak AM. Vascular permeability factor/vascular endothelial growth factor and the significance of microvascular hyperpermeability in angiogenesis. Curr Top Microbiol Immunol 1999; 237: 97–132

[32] Senger DR, Van de Water L, Brown LF et al. Vascular permeability factor (VPF, VEGF) in tumor biology. Cancer Metastasis Rev 1993; 12: 303–324

[33] Wei W, Chen ZW, Yang Q et al. Vasorelaxation induced by vascular endothelial growth factor in the human internal mammary artery and radial artery. Vascul Pharmacol 2007; 46: 253–259

[34] Erdamar S, Bagci P, Oz B, Dirican A. Correlation of endothelial nitric oxide synthase and vascular endothelial growth factor expression with malignancy in patients with astrocytic tumors. J BUON 2006; 11: 213–216

[35] Padhani AR, Husband JE. Dynamic contrast-enhanced MRI studies in oncology with an emphasis on quantification, validation and human studies. Clin Radiol 2001; 56: 607–620

[36] Shin JH, Lee HK, Kwun BD et al. Using relative cerebral blood flow and volume to evaluate the histopathologic grade of cerebral gliomas: preliminary results. AJR Am J Roentgenol 2002; 179: 783–789

[37] Sugahara T, Korogi Y, Kochi M et al. Correlation of MR imaging-determined cerebral blood volume maps with histologic and angiographic determination of vascularity of gliomas. AJR Am J Roentgenol 1998; 171: 1479–1486

[38] Wong ET, Jackson EF, Hess KR et al. Correlation between dynamic MRI and outcome in patients with malignant gliomas. Neurology 1998; 50: 777–781

[39] Law M, Young R, Babb J et al. Comparing perfusion metrics obtained from a single compartment versus pharmacokinetic modeling methods using dynamic susceptibility contrast-enhanced perfusion MR imaging with glioma grade. AJNR Am J Neuroradiol 2006; 27: 1975–1982

[40] Young R, Babb J, Law M, Pollack E, Johnson G. Comparison of region-of-interest analysis with three different histogram analysis methods in the determination of perfusion metrics in patients with brain gliomas. J Magn Reson Imaging 2007; 26: 1053–1063

[41] Jain R, Gutierrez J, Narang J et al. In vivo correlation of tumor blood volume and permeability with histologic and molecular angiogenic markers in gliomas. AJNR Am J Neuroradiol 2011; 32: 388–394

[42] Jain R, Narang J, Gutierrez J et al. Correlation of immunohistologic and perfusion vascular parameters with MR contrast enhancement using image-guided biopsy specimens in gliomas. Acad Radiol 2011; 18: 955–962

[43] Jain R. Perfusion CT imaging of brain tumors: an overview. AJNR Am J Neuroradiol 2011; 32: 1570–1577

[44] Narang J, Jain R, Scarpace L et al. Tumor vascular leakiness and blood volume estimates in oligodendrogliomas using perfusion CT: an analysis of perfusion parameters helping further characterize genetic subtypes as well as differentiate from astroglial tumors. J Neurooncol 2011; 102: 287–293

[45] Ellika SK, Jain R, Patel SC et al. Role of perfusion CT in glioma grading and comparison with conventional MR imaging features. AJNR Am J Neuroradiol 2007; 28: 1981–1987

[46] Nguyen TB, Cron GO, Mercier JF et al. Diagnostic accuracy of dynamic contrast-enhanced MR imaging using a phase-derived vascular input function in the preoperative grading of gliomas. AJNR Am J Neuroradiol 2012; 33: 1539–1545

[47] Lüdemann L, Grieger W, Wurm R, Budzisch M, Hamm B, Zimmer C. Comparison of dynamic contrast-enhanced MRI with WHO tumor grading for gliomas. Eur Radiol 2001; 11: 1231–1241

[48] Lüdemann L, Hamm B, Zimmer C. Pharmacokinetic analysis of glioma compartments with dynamic Gd-DTPA-enhanced magnetic resonance imaging. Magn Reson Imaging 2000; 18: 1201–1214

[49] Patankar TF, Haroon HA, Mills SJ et al. Is volume transfer coefficient (K(trans)) related to histologic grade in human gliomas? AJNR Am J Neuroradiol 2005; 26: 2455–2465

[50] Li KL, Zhu XP, Waterton J, Jackson A. Improved 3D quantitative mapping of blood volume and endothelial permeability in brain tumors. J Magn Reson Imaging 2000; 12: 347–357

[51] Zhang N, Zhang L, Qiu B, Meng L, Wang X, Hou BL. Correlation of volume transfer coefficient Ktrans with histopathologic grades of gliomas. J Magn Reson Imaging 2012; 36: 355–363

[52] Cha S, Yang L, Johnson G et al. Comparison of microvascular permeability measurements, K(trans), determined with conventional steady-state T1-weighted and first-pass T2*-weighted MR imaging methods in gliomas and meningiomas. AJNR Am J Neuroradiol 2006; 27: 409–417

[53] Henson JW, Gaviani P, Gonzalez RG. MRI in treatment of adult gliomas. Lancet Oncol 2005; 6: 167–175

[54] Jacobs AH, Kracht LW, Gossmann A et al. Imaging in neurooncology. NeuroRx 2005; 2: 333–347

[55] Weber MA, Giesel FL, Stieltjes B. MRI for identification of progression in brain tumors: from morphology to function. Expert Rev Neurother 2008; 8: 1507–1525

[56] Weber MA, Henze M, Tüttenberg J et al. Biopsy targeting gliomas: do functional imaging techniques identify similar target areas? Invest Radiol 2010; 45: 755–768

[57] Stupp R, Mason WP, van den Bent MJ et al. European Organisation for Research and Treatment of Cancer Brain Tumor and Radiotherapy Groups, National Cancer Institute of Canada Clinical Trials Group. Radiotherapy plus concomitant and adjuvant temozolomide for glioblastoma. N Engl J Med 2005; 352: 987–996

[58] Chi AS, Wen PY. Inhibiting kinases in malignant gliomas. Expert Opin Ther Targets 2007; 11: 473–496

[59] Furnari FB, Fenton T, Bachoo RM et al. Malignant astrocytic glioma: genetics, biology, and paths to treatment. Genes Dev 2007; 21: 2683–2710

[60] Sathornsumetee S, Reardon DA, Desjardins A, Quinn JA, Vredenburgh JJ, Rich JN. Molecularly targeted therapy for malignant glioma. Cancer 2007; 110: 13–24

[61] Sathornsumetee S, Rich JN, Reardon DA. Diagnosis and treatment of high-grade astrocytoma. Neurol Clin 2007; 25: 1111–1139, x

[62] Lamborn KR, Yung WK, Chang SM et al. North American Brain Tumor Consortium. Progression-free survival: an important end point in evaluating therapy for recurrent high-grade gliomas. Neuro-oncol 2008; 10: 162–170

[63] Macdonald DR, Cascino TL, Schold SC, Jr, Cairncross JG. Response criteria for phase II studies of supratentorial malignant glioma. J Clin Oncol 1990; 8: 1277–1280

[64] Wen PY, Macdonald DR, Reardon DA et al. Updated response assessment criteria for high-grade gliomas: response assessment in neuro-oncology working group. J Clin Oncol 2010; 28: 1963–1972

[65] Gállego Pérez-Larraya J, Lahutte M, Petrirena G et al. Response assessment in recurrent glioblastoma treated with irinotecan-bevacizumab: comparative analysis of the Macdonald, RECIST, RANO, and RECIST+F criteria. Neuro-oncol 2012; 14: 667–673

[66] Leibel S, Sheline G. Tolerance of the brain and spinal cord to conventional irradiation. In: Gutin P, Sheline G, eds. Radiation injury to the nervous system. New York, NY: Raven; 1991:239–256

[67] Hoffman WF, Levin VA, Wilson CB. Evaluation of malignant glioma patients during the postirradiation period. J Neurosurg 1979; 50: 624–628

[68] Martins AN, Johnston JS, Henry JM, Stoffel TJ, Di Chiro G. Delayed radiation necrosis of the brain. J Neurosurg 1977; 47: 336–345

[69] de Wit MC, de Bruin HG, Eijkenboom W, Sillevis Smitt PA, van den Bent MJ. Immediate post-radiotherapy changes in malignant glioma can mimic tumor progression. Neurology 2004; 63: 535–537

[70] Brandsma D, Stalpers L, Taal W, Sminia P, van den Bent MJ. Clinical features, mechanisms, and management of pseudoprogression in malignant gliomas. Lancet Oncol 2008; 9: 453–461

[71] Brandes AA, Franceschi E, Tosoni A et al. MGMT promoter methylation status can predict the incidence and outcome of pseudoprogression after concomitant radiochemotherapy in newly diagnosed glioblastoma patients. J Clin Oncol 2008; 26: 2192–2197

[72] Chamberlain MC, Glantz MJ, Chalmers L, Van Horn A, Sloan AE. Early necrosis following concurrent Temodar and radiotherapy in patients with glioblastoma. J Neurooncol 2007; 82: 81–83

[73] Taal W, Brandsma D, de Bruin HG et al. Incidence of early pseudo-progression in a cohort of malignant glioma patients treated with chemoirradiation with temozolomide. Cancer 2008; 113: 405–410

[74] Young RJ, Gupta A, Shah AD et al. Potential utility of conventional MRI signs in diagnosing pseudoprogression in glioblastoma. Neurology 2011; 76: 1918–1924

[75] Eoli M, Menghi F, Bruzzone MG et al. Methylation of O6-methylguanine DNA methyltransferase and loss of heterozygosity on 19q and/or 17p are overlapping features of secondary glioblastomas with prolonged survival. Clin Cancer Res 2007; 13: 2606–2613

[76] Chaskis C, Neyns B, Michotte A, De Ridder M, Everaert H. Pseudoprogression after radiotherapy with concurrent temozolomide for high-grade glioma: clinical observations and working recommendations. Surg Neurol 2009; 72: 423–428

[77] Brandes AA, Franceschi E, Tosoni A et al. MGMT promoter methylation status can predict the incidence and outcome of pseudoprogression after concomitant radiochemotherapy in newly diagnosed glioblastoma patients. J Clin Oncol 2008; 26: 2192–2197

[78] Reardon DA, Galanis E, DeGroot JF et al. Clinical trial end points for high-grade glioma: the evolving landscape. Neuro-oncol 2011; 13: 353–361

[79] Henson JW, Ulmer S, Harris GJ. Brain tumor imaging in clinical trials. AJNR Am J Neuroradiol 2008; 29: 419–424

[80] Hygino da Cruz LC, Jr, Rodriguez I, Domingues RC, Gasparetto EL, Sorensen AG. Pseudoprogression and pseudoresponse: imaging challenges in the assessment of posttreatment glioma. AJNR Am J Neuroradiol 2011; 32: 1978–1985

[81] Mangla R, Singh G, Ziegelitz D et al. Changes in relative cerebral blood volume 1 month after radiation-temozolomide therapy can help predict overall survival in patients with glioblastoma. Radiology 2010; 256: 575–584

[82] Tsien C, Galbán CJ, Chenevert TL et al. Parametric response map as an imaging biomarker to distinguish progression from pseudoprogression in high-grade glioma. J Clin Oncol 2010; 28: 2293–2299

[83] Thompson EM, Guillaume DJ, Dósa E et al. Dual contrast perfusion MRI in a single imaging session for assessment of pediatric brain tumors. J Neurooncol 2012; 109: 105–114

[84] Larsen VA, Simonsen HJ, Law I, Larsson HB, Hansen AE. Evaluation of dynamic contrast-enhanced T1-weighted perfusion MRI in the differentiation of tumor recurrence from radiation necrosis. Neuroradiology 201 3; 55: 361–369

[85] Murase K. Efficient method for calculating kinetic parameters using T1-weighted dynamic contrast-enhanced magnetic resonance imaging. Magn Reson Med 2004; 51: 858–862

[86] Cohen MH, Shen YL, Keegan P, Pazdur R. FDA drug approval summary: bevacizumab (Avastin) as treatment of recurrent glioblastoma multiforme. Oncologist 2009; 14: 1131–1138

[87] Kreisl TN, Kim L, Moore K et al. Phase II trial of single-agent bevacizumab followed by bevacizumab plus irinotecan at tumor progression in recurrent glioblastoma. J Clin Oncol 2009; 27: 740–745

[88] Schiff D, Purow B. Bevacizumab in combination with irinotecan for patients with recurrent glioblastoma multiforme. Nat Clin Pract Oncol 2008; 5: 186–187

[89] Brandsma D, van den Bent MJ. Pseudoprogression and pseudoresponse in the treatment of gliomas. Curr Opin Neurol 2009; 22: 633–638

[90] Norden AD, Young GS, Setayesh K et al. Bevacizumab for recurrent malignant gliomas: efficacy, toxicity, and patterns of recurrence. Neurology 2008; 70: 779–787

[91] Pope WB, Kim HJ, Huo J et al. Recurrent glioblastoma multiforme: ADC histogram analysis predicts response to bevacizumab treatment. Radiology 2009; 252: 182–189

[92] Gerstner ER, Chen PJ, Wen PY, Jain RK, Batchelor TT, Sorensen G. Infiltrative patterns of glioblastoma spread detected via diffusion MRI after treatment with cediranib. Neuro-oncol 2010; 12: 466–472

[93] Sorensen AG, Batchelor TT, Zhang WT et al. A "vascular normalization index" as potential mechanistic biomarker to predict survival after a single dose of cediranib in recurrent glioblastoma patients. Cancer Res 2009; 69: 5296–5300

[94] Emblem KE, Bjornerud A, Mouridsen K et al. T(1)- and T(2)(*)-dominant extravasation correction in DSC-MRI: part II-predicting patient outcome after a single dose of cediranib in recurrent glioblastoma patients. J Cereb Blood Flow Metab 2011; 31: 2054–2064

[95] Hawighorst H, Engenhart R, Knopp MV et al. Intracranial meningeomas: time- and dose-dependent effects of irradiation on tumor microcirculation monitored by dynamic MR imaging. Magn Reson Imaging 1997; 15: 423–432

[96] Zhu XP, Li KL, Kamaly-Asl ID et al. Quantification of endothelial permeability, leakage space, and blood volume in brain tumors using combined T1 and T2* contrast-enhanced dynamic MR imaging. J Magn Reson Imaging 2000; 11: 575–585

[97] Lüdemann L, Grieger W, Wurm R, Wust P, Zimmer C. Quantitative measurement of leakage volume and permeability in gliomas, meningiomas and brain metastases with dynamic contrast-enhanced MRI. Magn Reson Imaging 2005; 23: 833–841

[98] Rocca MA, Messina R, Filippi M. Multiple sclerosis imaging: recent advances. J Neurol 201 3; 260: 929–935

[99] Neema M, Stankiewicz J, Arora A, Guss ZD, Bakshi R. MRI in multiple sclerosis: what's inside the toolbox? Neurotherapeutics 2007; 4: 602–617

[100] Ingrisch M, Sourbron S, Morhard D et al. Quantification of perfusion and permeability in multiple sclerosis: dynamic contrast-enhanced MRI in 3D at 3 T. Invest Radiol 2012; 47: 252–258

[101] Singh A, Haris M, Rathore D et al. Quantification of physiological and hemodynamic indices using T(1) dynamic contrast-enhanced MRI in intracranial mass lesions. J Magn Reson Imaging 2007; 26: 871–880

[102] Haris M, Husain N, Singh A et al. Dynamic contrast-enhanced (DCE) derived transfer coefficient (ktrans) is a surrogate marker of matrix metalloproteinase 9 (MMP-9) expression in brain tuberculomas. J Magn Reson Imaging 2008; 28: 588–597

[103] Haris M, Gupta RK, Singh A et al. Differentiation of infective from neoplastic brain lesions by dynamic contrast-enhanced MRI. Neuroradiology 2008; 50: 531–540

[104] Haris M, Gupta RK, Husain M et al. Assessment of therapeutic response in brain tuberculomas using serial dynamic contrast-enhanced MRI. Clin Radiol 2008; 63: 562–574

[105] Gupta RK, Awasthi R, Garg RK et al. T1-weighted dynamic contrast-enhanced MR evaluation of different stages of neurocysticercosis and its relationship with serum MMP-9 expression. AJNR Am J Neuroradiol 2013; 34: 997–1003

6 Perfusion Imaging: Arterial Spin Labeling

S. Ali Nabavizadeh, Suyash Mohan, and Jeffrey M. Pollock

6.1 Introduction

Over the last 20 years, magnetic resonance (MR) perfusion imaging techniques have been used for evaluation of tumor vasculature in various settings such as tumor grading, biopsy guidance, recurrence versus radiation necrosis, response assessment, and prognostication. Perfusion MR techniques can be divided into two general categories: those that employ exogenous tracer (gadolinium-based contrast agents) and those that use endogenous tracers, such as arterial spin labeling (ASL). Contrast-based methods can be further divided into T1-weighted steady-state dynamic contrast-enhanced magnetic resonance imaging (DCE-MRI) and T2*-weighted dynamic susceptibility weighted contrast-enhanced MRI (DSC-MRI). Of these methods, DSC-MRI has been of more widespread use in the clinical setting, and many investigators have compared this method with ASL in various aspects of brain tumor imaging.

ASL perfusion has become more widespread in recent years secondary to emergence of higher magnetic field MR scanners, refinement and development of improved and more robust pulse sequences, and the clinical release of the ASL pulse sequences by most major MRI vendors. This chapter discusses ASL perfusion MRI for evaluation of various aspects of brain tumors.

6.2 General Principles of ASL Imaging

In order to measure the blood flow delivered to the brain tissue, water molecules in the inflowing arterial blood are labeled by inverting the magnetization outside the imaging plane. After a postlabeling delay (PLD), during which time there is T1 decay of the label, labeled blood water reaches the target tissue by crossing the blood–brain barrier, and an image is acquired, which is called the label image. A control image is then acquired without labeling of arterial blood. The subtraction of label and control image will be proportional to amount of cerebral blood flow.[1]

There are three major classes of ASL based on different tagging techniques as described in the following section. Detailed discussion about methodology and advantages/disadvantages is beyond the scope of this chapter, and interested readers are referred to excellent reviews on this subject.[2,3]

6.2.1 Pulsed Arterial Spin Labeling

In pulsed ASL (PASL), short (5–20 ms) inversion pulses are applied[4] in a thick slab located next to the slice of interest. There are different types of PASL based on the location of the tagging plane and the magnetic state of labeled spins for the control and labeled images. In echoplanar imaging and signal targeting with alternating radiofrequency (EPISTAR) the magnetization is inverted in a thick slab proximal to the imaging slab, whereas for the control image, inversion pulse is applied

in a symmetrical slab distal to the imaging slice.[5] Proximal inversion with a control for off-resonance effects (PICORE) is a derivative of EPISTAR, which uses the same label, but, to compensate for magnetization effect without inverting the magnetization, an off-resonance inversion pulse is applied in the control image at the same frequency offset relative to the imaging slice as the label.[6] Another PASL method, which is called flow-sensitive alternating inversion recovery (FAIR), consists of imaging with two sets of inversion recovery pulses, one being slice selective and another non–slice selective.[7] Several refinements have also been made to optimize PASL sequence. Inversion efficiency has been improved by adiabatic hyperbolic secant (AHS) radiofrequency (RF) pulses, which are insensitive to B1 field inhomogeneity.[5,8] Labeling plane slice profile was also achieved with frequency offset correction inversion AHS RF pulses.[9] Other methods known as quantitative imaging of perfusion using a single subtraction (QUIPSS), QUIPSS II, and Q2TIPS (QUIPSS II with thin-slice inversion time [TI1] periodic saturation) apply a saturation between the labeling pulse and image acquisition[10] to sharply define the distal edge of the tagging plane and prevent systematic bias resulting from spatially varying delay in the transit of blood from the tagging region to the imaging slice. Overall, the advantage of PASL is high labeling efficiency and lower RF power deposition, but it has lower perfusion sensitivity. Recently Petersen et al developed a new version of the PASL sequence, named quantitative signal targeting by alternating radiofrequency (STAR) labeling of arterial regions (QUASAR).[11] They acquired images at different inversion times after labeling, to determine whole signal difference curve over time. Voxel-by-voxel arterial input functions were then estimated by subtracting two perfusion-weighted images acquired with and without crusher gradients, respectively, leading to calculation of a parameter named arterial blood volume (aBV) based on a velocity exceeding a predefined threshold.

6.2.2 Continuous Arterial Spin Labeling

In continuous ASL (CASL), long and continuous RF pulses (1–2 s) are applied to continuously label the blood, below the imaging plane, usually at the base of the brain, to induce a flow-driven adiabatic inversion in a narrow plane of spins.[12] Continuous inversion led to higher perfusion sensitivity in CASL compared with PASL; however, it also partially excited the imaging plane through the magnetization transfer (MT) effect, which must be compensated for to avoid overestimation of perfusion.[12] In addition, long labeling pulses and techniques that are used to compensate the magnetization transfer (MT) effect deposit high levels of RF energies to the patient, which may exceed the specific absorption rate (SAR), limiting the use of CASL, especially in high-field MR. The MT effect can be avoided by the use of two RF coils, but this technique also requires special hardware that is not commonly available on commercial scanners.

6.2.3 Pseudocontinuous Arterial Spin Labeling

In pseudocontinuous ASL (PCASL) a train of discrete RF pulses are applied in conjunction with a synchronous gradient field to mimic a flow-driven adiabatic inversion seen in CASL.[13] This technique creates a better balance between the labeling efficiency and the perfusion signal to noise ratio, in addition to reducing MT effects and RF power deposition compared with CASL methods. In addition, a standard body coil can be used for transmission in PCASL, which eliminates the need for a dedicated transmit coil. The disadvantage of PCASL is that it may be susceptible to B0 inhomogeneity and eddy currents, depending on implementation.[14] Of the three leading ASL techniques, PCASL will likely emerge as the most robust clinically available pulse sequence.

6.2.4 Strategies to Improve Arterial Spin Labeling

Magnetic Field

Due to the intrinsic low signal-to-noise ratio (SNR) of ASL techniques, using a high magnetic field strength can improve the SNR.[15,16] In addition, lengthening of T1 is another factor that allows more spins to reach and accumulate in the image slab. Previous studies have shown doubling of signal performing CASL/PASL at 3 and 4 T, compared to 1.5 T.[15,16]

Phased Array Receiver Coils and Parallel Imaging

Another approach to increase SNR is to use a phased array of receiver coils. Use of these coils is associated with inhomogeneity of received signal; however, calibration steps involved in perfusion quantification leave the final cerebral blood flow (CBF) maps unaffected,[17] and SNR will be increased not only in the regions close to the coil but in the entire image. Another advantage of phase array coils is the potential for using parallel imaging, which can also be helpful by shortening the imaging time and reducing image distortion from susceptibility artifacts.[17]

Crusher Gradients

Crusher gradients are an option with most clinical releases, but they have a significant influence on the appearance of pathology with ASL. Crusher gradients are applied prior to image acquisition to null the signal from intravascular moving spins. If these spins are not eliminated, quantification of CBF derived from ASL will be artificially high in slow-flow states where the ASL signal is predominantly intravascular. Ye et al[18] proposed the use of bipolar crusher gradients to eliminate the signal from large arteries by dephasing the moving spins. These crusher gradients have more significant implications with stroke or slow-flow imaging; however, when quantification of CBF in tumors is considered, a consistent technique should be employed to decrease variability when tracking blood flow in tumors over time, especially in regard to tumor response.

Readout Strategies

A two-dimensional (2D) echoplanar imaging (EPI) readout is commonly used in ASL imaging due to high SNR and rapid acquisition time; however, EPI suffers from susceptibility artifact with the potential for signal loss and image distortion, especially when the lesion is near the skull base, orbit, or sinuses, or in the presence of blood products. Three-dimensional (3D) techniques with spin-echo (GRASE) or rapid acquisition with relaxation enhancement (RARE)-based readout strategies for ASL can be of particular benefit to improve the image quality for several reasons. They improve SNR secondary to slab excitation and a prolonged image acquisition window and are also associated with less image distortion and susceptibility artifact. Furthermore, 3D imaging is associated with more effective background suppression,[19] which can significantly increase the measured signal.[20] 3D techniques such as GRACE or RARE-based readout strategies are also less affected by susceptibility artifacts.[21,22,23]

Absolute versus Relative Cerebral Blood Flow

The absolute CBF value could be theoretically determined by using ASL[24,25]; however, there are several factors that can potentially affect quantitative CBF measurement. These include dependence on transit time of the labeled blood, the local relaxation times of tissue and blood, and the assumption of a constant T1 relaxation time of arterial blood regardless of variable factors, such as vessel size or level of oxygenation.[26] In addition there are large interindividual differences in perfusion[27] that can affect estimation of CBF. The accuracy of absolute perfusion measurement by using Q2TIPS has not been fully established, especially in pathological conditions[28,29]; therefore most of the authors used relative perfusion index rather than the absolute blood flow value. In most of the studies, the average signal intensity of gray matter was used as a reference for relative perfusion instead of white matter. This is mainly because the arterial transit time of white matter is much longer than that of gray matter, resulting in a substantial underestimation of the blood flow in white matter.[30,31]

Comparison of ASL to Contrast-Based MR Perfusion Methods

Numerous studies demonstrated positive correlation of relative cerebral blood volume (rCBV) measured by DSC-MRI with histological measurements of tumor neovascularization.[32,33,34] Compared to MR perfusion methods based on contrast injection (DSC and DCE), ASL is capable of measuring absolute CBF values. Other advantages of ASL include noninvasiveness, repeatability, utility in patients with renal failure who are at risk of related nephrogenic systemic fibrosis, and utility in young children in whom the rapid bolus injection of contrast materials into the vein may be problematic. Despite these advantages, ASL suffers from lower SNR and requires multiple signal acquisitions, which increase the imaging time.

Numerous studies have compared ASL and DSC perfusion in various aspects of brain tumor imaging. Weber et al evaluated normal brain tissue in 62 patients with brain metastases who were treated with stereotactic radiosurgery using PASL and

DSC perfusion and demonstrated good correlation between perfusion values, which remained unchanged after stereotactic radiosurgery.[35] A study by Lehmann et al[36] that evaluated 27 patients included 9 gliomas, 10 metastases, and 8 meningiomas. They used PASL and DSC T2* perfusion sequence and found a significant correlation between rCBF calculated from the two perfusion sequences. Warmuth et al showed a high correlation for rCBF measurements on ASL and DSC perfusion maps using 1.5 T using single TI PASL.[26] Lüdemann et al[37] used different perfusion techniques (DCE-MRI/DSC-MRI, PASL, and $H_2^{15}O$ positron-emission tomography) in 12 patients with brain tumors, and demonstrated a linear relationship between all five imaging modalities regarding the perfusion signal of normal brain tissue and tumor; however, the perfusion ratios between tumor and brain differed significantly with the method applied. This suggested that relative tumor perfusion values determined with different techniques cannot be directly compared.[37] Hirai et al compared ASL MRI using QUASAR and DSC-MRI on 3 T scanners [38] in 24 patients with histologically proved glioma. They demonstrated good to excellent intermodality agreement for maximum rCBF between ASL and DSC.

Very few studies have been performed to compare ASL with DCE-MRI. Roy et al evaluated 64 patients with glioma using 3D-PCASL and DCE-MRI and demonstrated a weak correlation in rCBF values between the two methods. They also did not find a significant difference in absolute or relative CBF values between high- and low-grade gliomas using ASL, whereas DCE indices were significantly higher in high-grade gliomas.[39]

Van Westen et al[40] used the QUASAR method at 3 T to measure aBV in 11 brain tumors (grade III gliomas, glioblastomas, and meningiomas), and compared measurement of aBV from arterial spin labeling with CBV from DSC-MRI. They demonstrated a positive correlation between ASL-based aBV tumor-to-gray matter(GM) ratios and DSC-MRI-based CBV tumor-to-GM ratios.

Diagnostic Impact

A few studies have evaluated the diagnostic impact of adding ASL imaging in patients with brain tumors. Geer et al[41] evaluated 59 patients with glial tumors and demonstrated that the addition of perfusion to the standard imaging protocol was associated with a change in management plan in 8.5% of patients and an increase in the treatment team's confidence in their management plan in 57.6% of patients. Kim et al in a prospective study evaluated the added value of pulsed ASL and apparent diffusion coefficients in the grading of gliomas. In this study, two observers made the correct diagnosis in 23 of 33 (70%) lesions in the first review and in 29 of 33 (88%) of lesions in the second review.[42]

Quantitative vs. Qualitative Techniques of ASL Image Interpretation in Brain Tumors

Although quantitative analysis of ASL imaging is more valuable and gives investigators the potential to compare perfusion values between patients and during the course of the disease, quantitative analysis is more practical in the research setting with a limited number of patients. On the other hand qualitative methods are very fast and more applicable in routine clinical practice. In a prospective study, Järnum et al used PCASL and DSC perfusion to evaluate 28 patients with contrast-enhancing brain tumors at 3 T with whole-brain coverage.[43] They used a qualitative scoring system to evaluate signal enhancement and susceptibility artifact in the tumor. They also performed a quantitative analysis with normalized tumor blood flow (TBF) values. Results of this study showed no difference in total visual score for signal enhancement between PCASL and DSC relative to CBF, and a good correlation between normalized CBF between both perfusion methods. Not surprisingly, ASL had a lower susceptibility-artifact score than DSC-MRI. Studies using ASL imaging in distinguishing predominantly recurrent high-grade glioma from radiation necrosis also demonstrated that both qualitative (based on visual inspection) and quantitative techniques were effective in differentiation of radiation necrosis from tumor recurrence.[44] Kim and Kim also did not find a significant difference between the quantitative and qualitative ASL parameters in glioma grading.[42]

6.3 ASL Clinical Diagnostic Applications

6.3.1 Extra-axial Tumors

One advantage of ASL over contrast-enhanced methods is reliability on a theoretically freely diffusible tracer, which makes it less sensitive to abnormal blood–brain barrier (BBB) permeability.[45] This can be particularly helpful in the setting of extra-axial lesions. Due to lack of BBB permeability in extra-axial masses, gadolinium can potentially cause T1 shortening and mask the T2* effect with resultant underestimation of rCBV. Despite less susceptibility to abnormal permeability compared to DSC, however, ASL quantification methods are also based on an intact BBB,[46] and a leaky BBB may also potentially affect ASL, causing overestimation of CBF. In order to evaluate this, Wolf et al[47] used a simulation two-compartment single-pass approximation (SPA) model accounting for T1/T2 effects, blood volume, and permeability suggested by St Lawrence and Wang,[48] to simulate the change in CASL signal at 3 T and demonstrated that an increase in permeability reduces the CASL signal by 2%, even if permeability is tripled. In another study, Parkes and Tofts showed that there should be a 100% change in permeability per capillary volume to achieve a 5% change in ASL signal.[49] Another relevant feature of extra-axial brain tumors is their potential to have dual arterial supply from external and internal carotid arteries. Sasao et al demonstrated that ASL can provide important information about the vascular supply of meningiomas by selective labeling of the external carotid artery.[50] In addition to PASL, based on magnetic resonance angiography (MRA) anatomy analysis, the external carotid artery was selectively labeled followed by a regional perfusion imaging (RPI) sequence in eight patients with meningiomas. In this study, a meningioma that was mainly supplied by the internal carotid and ophthalmic arteries showed entirely different perfusion maps on PASL and RPI images. Results of this study suggested that selective labeling of the external carotid artery can accurately predict the vascular supply in extra-axial brain tumors.

One of the advantages of contrast-based MR perfusion methods is the ability to measure permeability either with DCE

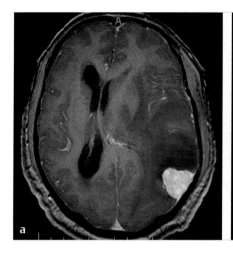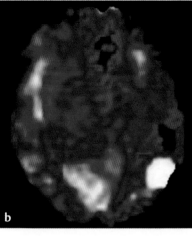

Fig. 6.1 Meningioma. (**a**) Axial postcontrast T1 image shows avid homogeneous enhancement of a left parietal extra-axial mass with surrounding vasogenic edema. (**b**) Quantitative pulsed arterial spin labeling image shows dramatic hyperperfusion of the known meningioma and hypoperfusion in the edematous brain tissue.

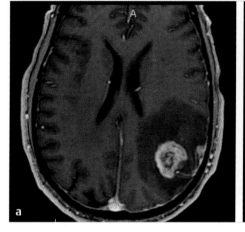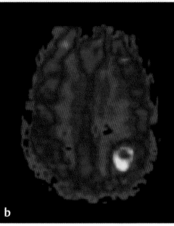

Fig. 6.2 Glioblastoma multiforme. (**a**) Axial postcontrast T1 image shows a peripherally enhancing left parietal mass. (**b**) Pulsed arterial spin labeling shows significant hyperperfusion in the periphery of the mass with relative central hypoperfusion. The mass was a grade IV glioblastoma multiforme at pathology.

T1-based methods[51] or first pass T2-DSC acquisition[52] in addition to perfusion. Because increased permeability can occur in tumoral vessels even before neovascularization,[53] it may provide important information in primary diagnosis[51] as well as following treatment efficiency with antiangiogenic drugs.[54] Measurement of permeability with ASL was not possible until recently when Wang et al combined CASL with a twice-refocused spin-echo diffusion sequence[55] and separated the signal contributions from capillaries and brain tissue. This ASL-based permeability has the potential to estimate water permeability of brain tumors.

6.3.2 Meningioma and Schwannoma

Kimura et al[56] used CASL and DSC perfusion for characterization of meningioma by MR perfusion imaging with histopathological correlation. They demonstrated a significant correlation between CASL-% signal intensity change and microvessel area determined by immunostaining specimens with anti-CD31. They also demonstrated a significant correlation between CASL-rCBF and T2DSC-rCBF. Noguchi et al[57] used PASL to evaluate 35 patients with brain tumors including gliomas, meningiomas, schwannomas, diffuse large B-cell lymphoma, hemangioblastomas, and metastatic brain tumor, and demonstrated that signal intensity was significantly higher in hemangioblastomas compared to meningiomas and schwannomas.

They did not find a significant difference between signal intensity of meningioma and schwannomas. Anecdotally, meningiomas are one of the most homogeneously hyperperfused tumors encountered in clinical practice (▶ Fig. 6.1).

6.3.3 Intra-Axial Tumors

Gliomas

Neovascularization is one of the hallmarks of malignancy along with mitosis, pleomorphism, and necrosis.[58] A direct correlation between glioma grade and angiogenesis has been well established.[59,60] DSC perfusion has been proved to increase the sensitivity in determining glioma grade, compared with conventional MRI.[61] In addition, DSC perfusion has been shown to be a better predictor of tumor progression and patient outcome compared with initial histopathological interpretation.[62] ASL was first used in 1996 to evaluate perfusion in a heterogeneous group of brain tumors, and demonstrated elevated perfusion in high-grade astrocytomas with marked regional heterogeneity compared with low perfusion in low-grade astrocytomas and lymphomas.[63] More recently Wolf et al using CASL at 3 T demonstrated that maximum CBF normalized to the global mean CBF in the brain provided the best distinction between high- and low-grade gliomas (▶ Fig. 6.2).[47] They also showed that low-grade gliomas with oligodendroglial components

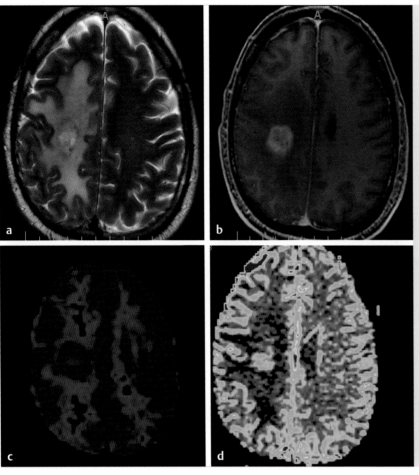

Fig. 6.3 Anaplastic oligodendroglioma. (**a**) Axial T2 shows a right posterior frontal T2 hyperintense mass with surrounding vasogenic edema. (**b**) Axial postcontrast T1 shows some peripheral enhancement of the mass. (**c**) Axial pulsed arterial spin labeling (PASL) shows mild hyperperfusion of the mass with a background of surrounding hypoperfusion in the region of vasogenic edema. The mass is much less hyperperfused than the glioblastoma multiforme in (**d**). Cerebral blood volume from a dynamic susceptibility weighted contrast-enhanced perfusion analysis shows increased cerebral blood volume in the enhancing component of the mass similar in appearance to the PASL image (**d**).

demonstrated high CBF. This confounding effect of oligodendrogliomas in glioma grading has also been encountered in DSC perfusion imaging.[64] As a solution Chawla et al showed that ASL-guided voxelwise analysis of proton MR spectroscopy of regions of high blood flow may be helpful in distinguishing low-grade from high-grade oligodendrogliomas (▶ Fig. 6.3).[65]

Different thresholds have been proposed for glioma grading. Weber et al,[29] using a relative CBF of 1.4 for discrimination of glioblastomas from grade III gliomas, showed sensitivity was 97%, specificity was 50%, positive predictive value (PPV) was 84%, and negative predictive value (NPV) was 86%. In the same study, using an rCBF value of 1.6 for discrimination of glioblastomas from grade II gliomas, sensitivity was 94%, specificity was 78%, PPV was 94%, and NPV was 78%. In Warmuth et al's study, the mean rCBF values in high- and low-grade gliomas were 1.54 and 0.64, respectively.[26]

Typically, based on T1 decay of blood, ASL measurements are acquired at an inversion time, which is approximately 1,200 ms at 1.5 T and 1,600 ms at 3 T.[66,67] In a study of healthy volunteers MacIntosh et al[68] showed that the mean arterial transit time is approximately 641 to 935 ms, depending on the brain region. Furtner et al used PASL at eight different inversion times from 370 ms to 2,114 ms in order to find the largest difference in normalized intratumoral signal intensity between high-grade and low-grade astrocytomas, and demonstrated that inversion time of 370 ms best differentiated high-grade and low-grade astrocytomas. They suggested that, at this short inversion time, the

labeled spins are located primarily within the vessel and mainly reflect the labeled intra-arterial blood bolus, and they called it normalized vascular intratumoral signal intensity (nVITS).[69]

Hemangioblastoma and Subependymal Giant Cell Astrocytoma

Yamashita evaluated 19 patients with posterior fossa tumors including 5 hemangioblastomas and 14 metastatic tumors (lung cancer, breast cancer, renal cell carcinoma [RCC], gastric cancer, and metastases of unknown origin) with PASL, and demonstrated that both absolute and relative CBF values were significantly higher in hemangioblastomas compared with metastatic brain tumors, although a metastasis from RCC showed very high CBF.[70] Anecdotal reports of subependymal giant cell astrocytoma (SGCA) also revealed significant elevation of CBF compared to mean gray matter.[71]

Metastatic Tumors

There are very few studies dedicated to evaluating the ASL characteristics of metastatic brain lesions; however, metastatic brain tumors were frequently included in the heterogeneous population of brain tumors in ASL studies. In a study of posterior fossa tumors, hemangioblastomas showed significantly higher CBF values compared to metastasis, with the exception of a metastatic RCC, which showed very high CBF.[70] Another

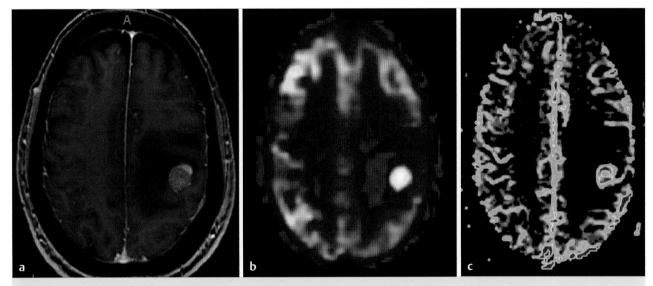

Fig. 6.4 Metastatic breast carcinoma. (**a**) A relatively solid left posterior frontal mass shows homogeneous discrete enhancement with local mass effect and vasogenic edema on the postcontrast T1 image. (**b**) Pulsed arterial spin labeling (PASL) shows homogeneous hyperperfusion on the cerebral blood flow map. (**c**) Cerebral blood volume (CBV) map derived from a dynamic susceptibility weighted contrast-enhanced (DSC) perfusion study shows that the periphery of the mass has higher CBV than the core. This physiology is less well seen on the PASL image in this case. The margins of the mass on both PASL and DSC perfusion are very sharply demarcated.

study of 25 brain metastases from various primaries, including lung, stomach, melanoma, RCC, breast, testis, and colon, demonstrated a wide range of rCBF ranging from 0.28 in a patient with metastatic breast cancer to 5.92 in metastatic RCC.[28]

6.3.4 Differentiation of High-Grade Glioma from Metastasis

Based on the well-known concept that gliomas are infiltrating the surrounding brain compared to metastasis, ASL perfusion has been used to evaluate the T2 hyperintensity surrounding the enhancing intra-axial lesions to differentiate high-grade glioma and metastasis. Using a threshold value of 0.5 for CBF, Weber et al[29] were able to differentiate high-grade glioma from metastasis with sensitivity of 100% and 71%.

In clinical practice the solid components of the metastatic lesion will tend to show hyperperfusion, whereas the cystic or necrotic components will show hypoperfusion. Similarly to the margin of a metastatic lesion, the hyperperfusion will appear more discrete as compared with an infiltrative primary glioma (▶ Fig. 6.4).

6.3.5 Lymphoma

Yamashita et al evaluated 19 patients with PCNSL and 37 with glioblastoma multiforme (GBM) using ASL, diffusion-weighted imaging (DWI), and ^{18}F-fluorodeoxyglucose positron-emission tomography (FDG-PET). They demonstrated that absolute and relative CBF were significantly higher in GBMs compared to PCNSLs.[72] In this study ASL perfusion imaging was as efficient as DWI and FDG-PET to differentiate PCNSLs from GBMs,[72] which is consistent with CBV results from DSC perfusion studies.[73] Using PASL perfusion, Weber et al[29] showed that glioblastomas show significantly higher TBF compared with central nervous system (CNS) lymphomas, and a threshold value of 1.2

for CBF provided sensitivity of 97% and specificity of 80% (▶ Fig. 6.5). Another diagnostic dilemma in the immuno-compromised patient is differentiating primary CNS lymphoma from toxoplasmosis. Small studies using DSC and PASL have shown that CNS lymphoma is hyperperfused, whereas toxoplasmosis is hypoperfused.[3,74]

6.4 ASL Clinical Therapeutic Applications

6.4.1 Guiding Biopsy

Due to the heterogeneous nature of brain tumors, numerous advanced imaging techniques have been used to increase the diagnostic yield by targeting the most pathological region of the tumor. The key advantage of perfusion methods is to show tumoral hyperperfusion in the areas that do not enhance on conventional postcontrast T1 imaging. This phenomenon can be very important in nonenhancing high-grade gliomas and also in gliomatosis cerebri (▶ Fig. 6.6)[66] because it can show areas of higher histological grade, which can be crucial in biopsy planning. Failure to recognize these foci may result in undergrading of a high-grade tumor, which can result in incorrect treatment and poor patient outcome. Several studies have shown that ASL is able to show heterogeneity in blood flow distribution of a tumor.[26,27,28,29]

Weber et al[75] evaluated 61 patients with suspected glioma who had either gross total resection or stereotactic biopsy with ^{18}F-fluorothymidine-PET, and FDG-PET, and proton spectroscopic imaging (1H-MRSI [magnetic proton spectroscopic imaging], point-resolved spectroscopy), ASL perfusion MRI, DCE-MRI, and DSC perfusion MRI and demonstrated that there was good correlation between ASL CBF and CBF/CBV derived from DSC in vascular areas of tumor (▶ Fig. 6.7).

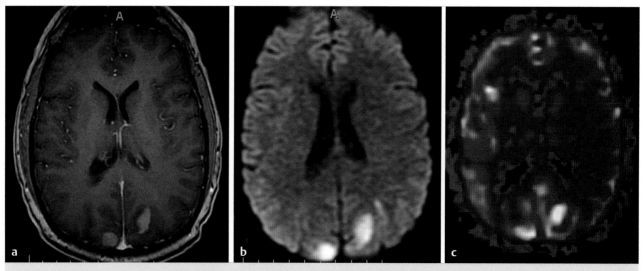

Fig. 6.5 Lymphoma. (**a**) Bilateral homogeneously enhancing masses are seen in the medial parietal lobes. (**b**) The masses have diffuse diffusion restriction. (**c**) Mild hyperperfusion is seen on pulsed arterial spin labeling corresponding to the masses.

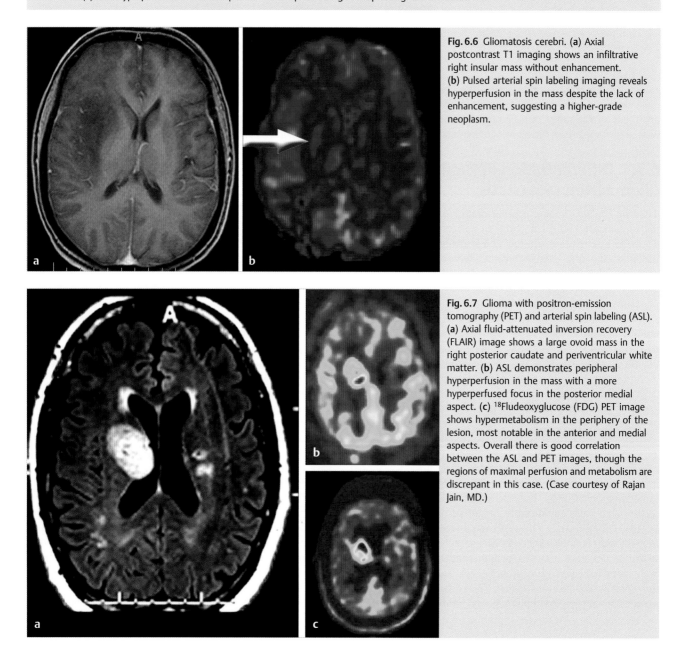

Fig. 6.6 Gliomatosis cerebri. (**a**) Axial postcontrast T1 imaging shows an infiltrative right insular mass without enhancement. (**b**) Pulsed arterial spin labeling imaging reveals hyperperfusion in the mass despite the lack of enhancement, suggesting a higher-grade neoplasm.

Fig. 6.7 Glioma with positron-emission tomography (PET) and arterial spin labeling (ASL). (**a**) Axial fluid-attenuated inversion recovery (FLAIR) image shows a large ovoid mass in the right posterior caudate and periventricular white matter. (**b**) ASL demonstrates peripheral hyperperfusion in the mass with a more hyperperfused focus in the posterior medial aspect. (**c**) ^{18}Fludeoxyglucose (FDG) PET image shows hypermetabolism in the periphery of the lesion, most notable in the anterior and medial aspects. Overall there is good correlation between the ASL and PET images, though the regions of maximal perfusion and metabolism are discrepant in this case. (Case courtesy of Rajan Jain, MD.)

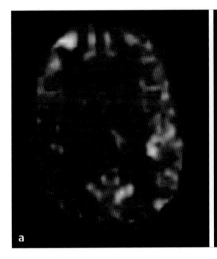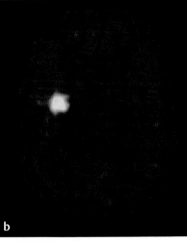

Fig. 6.8 Glioblastoma recurrence. (**a**) Axial pulsed arterial spin labeling (PASL) imaging after a right frontal glioblastoma multiforme (GBM) resection shows no hyperperfusion 8 weeks postsurgery. (**b**) Axial PASL imaging at 18 weeks postsurgery reveals significant new hyperperfusion corresponding to disease recurrence confirmed on subsequent biopsy.

6.4.2 ASL Perfusion in Monitoring Response to Therapy

Yamamoto et al evaluated six consecutive patients with PCASL before and after treatment with extra-axial brain tumors that were treated only with radiotherapy (RT). They demonstrated a strong correlation between the tumor volume ratio (defined as percentage change in volume before and after RT) and the maximum TBF (mTBF) before and after RT; however, no significant correlation was identified between changes in enhancement and volume ratio or between changes in enhancement and mTBF ratio.[23] According to this study, pretreatment TBF can be an important index that may determine the choice of RT by predicting the potential response. Weber et al evaluated 25 patients with a total of 28 brain metastases, using DSC-MRI and ASL perfusion, prior to radiosurgery and at 6 weeks, 12 weeks, and 24 weeks after stereotactic radiosurgery. This study suggested that both ASL and DSC-MRI techniques are able to predict the treatment outcome by showing a decrease in rCBF at the 6 week follow-up in all metastases for ASL and in 13 of 16 metastases for DSC-MRI.[28]

Sedlacik evaluated 35 patients with newly diagnosed diffuse infiltrative pontine glioma (DIPG) who were treated with RT and vandetanib, a vascular endothelial growth factor receptor 2 inhibitor, with both PASL and DSC perfusion, and demonstrated that increased tumor perfusion and decreased tumor volume during combined therapy were associated with longer progression-free survival.[76] In this study, CBF and CBV linearly increased during RT followed by a gradual linear decrease.

Outside the brain, ASL has also been successfully used as a surrogate parameter for early assessment of response to novel antiangiogenic therapy in patients with multiple myeloma[77] and has been shown to provide clinically relevant information in renal cell cancer's response to antiangiogenic therapy.[78]

6.4.3 ASL Perfusion in Tumor Progression/Pseudoprogression

Currently chemoradiotherapy with temozolomide is considered the standard of care for patients with GBM.[79,80] A recently described phenomenon is the progressive enhancement of a new lesion immediately after the end of treatment, which later involutes or stabilizes without further treatment. This phenomenon is known as pseudoprogression, and it occurs in up to 20% of patients.[80] Pseudoprogression is likely secondary to extensive necrosis of tumor cells, which elicits secondary reactions, such as edema and abnormal vascular permeability, and presents as new or increased contrast enhancement, which can be interpreted as disease progression based on conventional MR criteria for worsening disease.[81]

Using ASL and DSC perfusion, Choi et al evaluated 62 patients with newly diagnosed GBM who developed contrast-enhancing lesions following surgical resection and concurrent chemoradiotherapy to distinguish early tumor progression (▶ Fig. 6.8) from pseudoprogression.[82] In this study, there was no significant difference between diagnostic accuracy of ASL and DSC perfusion in isolation; however, addition of ASL to DSC produced more accurate results than DSC perfusion MRI alone. The authors used a semiquantitative grading system based on tumor perfusion signal intensity relative to equal signal intensity to white matter (grade I), gray matter (grade II), and blood vessels (grade III), and pseudoprogression was observed in 15 (53.6%) patients with ASL grade I, 13 (46.4%) with grade II, and 0 (0%) with grade III lesions.

6.4.4 ASL Perfusion in Radiation Injury

Differentiation of recurrent tumor from treatment-induced radiation necrosis has important implications for a patient. Both of these entities enhance with conventional imaging; however, unlike recurrent brain tumors, radiation necrosis is associated with extensive vascular injury without significant neovascularity. Several studies demonstrated the efficacy of DSC[83,84] and DCE[85] perfusion MRI to differentiate tumor progression from radiation necrosis.[83,84] Ozsunar et al evaluated 30 patients with grade II to IV gliomas with new enhancing nodules or masses who were previously treated with surgery and proton-beam therapy to differentiate tumor recurrence versus radiation necrosis using ASL, DSC perfusion, and PET examinations. They showed using a normalized cutoff ratio of 1.3, ASL has the highest sensitivity (94%) compared to PET and DSC imaging.[44]

Effect of RT on normal brain tissue perfusion has also been evaluated. Yamamoto et al demonstrated that CBF in normal

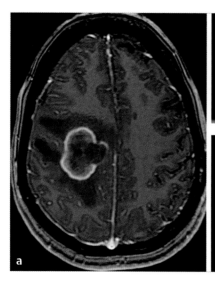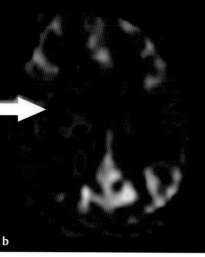

Fig. 6.9 Tumefactive multiple sclerosis (MS). **(a)** Axial postcontrast T1 image of a large right frontal tumefactive demyelinating lesion with surrounding edema. The lesion demonstrates a classic incomplete ring and enhancement like a propagating wave. **(b)** Axial pulsed arterial spin labeling perfusion imaging shows minimal hyperperfusion in the ring of the lesion relative to the adjacent white matter (arrow). (Case courtesy of Justin Simonds, MD.)

brain tissue was relatively constant before and after RT.[23] Weber et al also showed that rCBF values in normal brain tissue affected by radiation doses less than 0.5 Gy remained unchanged after therapy.[28] These studies are important because they show that normal brain tissue can be reliably used as a reference standard for normalized CBF measurements before and after treatment.

6.4.5 ASL in Tumor Mimics

There are many pathologies, such as tumefactive demyelination, subacute infarction, and infectious pathologies, that can mimic brain tumors. The BBB can be disrupted in these pathologies, leading to enhancement on conventional imaging; however, unlike brain tumors, they are not as hypervascular as neoplasms on perfusion imaging (▸ Fig. 6.9). Many studies have shown that DSC is helpful to differentiate tumors from tumor mimics[86]; however, dedicated ASL studies are still in progress.

6.4.6 Pediatric Brain Tumors

ASL has distinct advantages for use in children: no need for contrast, high SNR, labeling efficiency, and the potential for CBF quantification. Also, ASL can be repeated in cases of failed sedation or patient motion, a frequent problem in children with brain tumors. In a study of pediatric brain tumors, Yeom et al[22] showed that the maximal relative TBF of high-grade tumors (grades III and IV) was significantly higher than that of low-grade tumors (grades I and II). In addition, among posterior fossa tumors, relative TBF was significantly higher for medulloblastoma compared with pilocytic astrocytoma.[22]

6.4.7 ASL and Vascular Density

Noguchi et al compared ASL signal intensity with histopathological vascular density and demonstrated a positive correlation in 35 patients with brain tumors, including six gliomas, meningiomas, schwannomas, lymphoma, hemangioblastomas, and metastatic brain tumors. They also showed ASL signal intensity to be significantly higher in hemangioblastomas compared to gliomas, meningiomas, and schwannomas.[57] In this study, CBF

was significantly increased for high-grade compared with low-grade tumors. Kimura et al[56] also reported a significant correlation in meningiomas between the relative mean TBF and the microvessel area; however, Weber et al[29] failed to show a significant correlation between the cell proliferation index and the microvessel area, although their study was limited by a high rate of stereotactic biopsy in their series (23/79 patients) with the potential for sampling error.

Sakai et al investigated the relationship between the normalized blood flow of nonfunctioning pituitary macroadenomas, measured by ASL and the microvessel attenuation which was determined as the total microvessel wall area divided by the entire tissue area on CD-31-stained specimens. They demonstrated a significant correlation between normalized TBF values and relative microvessel attenuation; howevers, the degree of enhancement was not correlated with relative microvessel attenuation.[87] Preoperative knowledge of degree of vascularity of pituitary macroadenomas can be important for surgeons to avoid vascular complications of transsphenoidal surgery.[88]

6.4.8 Vessel Reactivity

ASL has been used to measure autoregulation of cerebral perfusion in various disease states, including anoxic injury,[89] migraine,[90] and hypercapnia,[91] as well as physiological states such as hyperoxia.[92] Pollock et al evaluated 45 patients with altered mental status, metastasis, or suspected stroke and demonstrated a significant positive linear relationship between global gray matter cerebral perfusion and the partial pressure of carbon dioxide determined by arterial blood gas.[91]

The concept of vessel reactivity can potentially be used in brain tumors. The cerebrovascular reserve (CVR), which is a measure of the degree of cerebral perfusion increase in response to a cerebral vasodilator, may be different between high- and low-grade tumors due to various factors such as dissimilar metabolic demand and degree of differentiation of vessel neovascularity. Lee et al used acetazolamide, a carbonic anhydrase inhibitor that is a known cerebral vasodilator, to evaluate CBF changes in four patients with nonenhancing brain tumors using a PCASL sequence.[93] In this study, one patient with grade II oligodendroglioma demonstrated a modest increase of CBF after acetazolamide administration; however, the remaining three patients with grade III astrocytomas demonstrated no significant difference in CBF. This study suggested that low-grade gliomas may have a higher cerebrovascular reactivity compared with high-grade gliomas.

6.5 Conclusions and Future Direction

The absence of radiation, the lack of an exogenous contrast agent, as well as indefinite repeatability and reproducible quantification, make ASL an optimum technique for brain tumor imaging. As 3 T MRI scanners are increasingly available at many neuroimaging centers, high-field ASL is expected to become a standard clinically available pulse sequence. In addition, recent developments and further standardization in ASL sequences and postprocessing will likely result in widespread use of this technique in various aspects of brain tumor imaging, which can potentially improve our knowledge of brain tumor pathology, physiology, and treatment effects, which will ultimately improve patient outcomes.

6.5.1 Acknowledgments

JMP: I owe much of my knowledge and understanding of ASL to my prior research team collaborators from Wake Forest University. Without their mentorship, friendship, and guidance over the years, this chapter and much of my career would not have been possible. Thank you for all your contributions: Joe Maldjian, MD; Robert Kraft, PhD; Huan Tan, PhD; Jonathan Burdette, MD; Andrew Deibler, MD; Christopher Whitlow, MD; Blake McGehee, MD; Tom West, MD; and Justin Simonds, MD.

SAN, SM: The authors would also like to acknowledge the seminal work of John A. Detre, MD, University of Pennsylvania, and David C. Alsop, PhD, Harvard Medical School, in the development of ASL technique, and the efforts of Ron Wolf, MD, PhD, University of Pennsylvania, and JJ Wang, PhD, UCLA, in further refinements of ASL and implementation in the clinical arena.

References

[1] Alsop DC. Perfusion MR imaging. In: Atlas SW, ed. Magnetic Resonance Imaging of the Brain and Spine. Philadelphia, PA: Lippincott Williams and Wilkins; 2002:215–238

[2] Deibler AR, Pollock JM, Kraft RA, Tan H, Burdette JH, Maldjian JA. Arterial spin-labeling in routine clinical practice, part 1: technique and artifacts. AJNR Am J Neuroradiol 2008; 29: 1228–1234

[3] Pollock JM, Tan H, Kraft RA, Whitlow CT, Burdette JH, Maldjian JA. Arterial spin-labeled MR perfusion imaging: clinical applications. Magn Reson Imaging Clin N Am 2009; 17: 315–338

[4] Liu TT, Brown GG. Measurement of cerebral perfusion with arterial spin labeling: Part 1. Methods. J Int Neuropsychol Soc 2007; 13: 517–525

[5] Edelman RR, Siewert B, Darby DG et al. Qualitative mapping of cerebral blood flow and functional localization with echo-planar MR imaging and signal targeting with alternating radio frequency. Radiology 1994; 192: 513–520

[6] Wong EC, Buxton RB, Frank LR. Implementation of quantitative perfusion imaging techniques for functional brain mapping using pulsed arterial spin labeling. NMR Biomed 1997; 10: 237–249

[7] Kim SG. Quantification of relative cerebral blood flow change by flow-sensitive alternating inversion recovery (FAIR) technique: application to functional mapping. Magn Reson Med 1995; 34: 293–301

[8] Kim SG, Tsekos NV. Perfusion imaging by a flow-sensitive alternating inversion recovery (FAIR) technique: application to functional brain imaging. Magn Reson Med 1997; 37: 425–435

[9] Yongbi MN, Yang Y, Frank JA, Duyn JH. Multislice perfusion imaging in human brain using the C-FOCI inversion pulse: comparison with hyperbolic secant. Magn Reson Med 1999; 42: 1098–1105

[10] Wong EC, Buxton RB, Frank LR. Quantitative imaging of perfusion using a single subtraction (QUIPSS and QUIPSS II). Magn Reson Med 1998; 39: 702–708

[11] Petersen ET, Lim T, Golay X. Model-free arterial spin labeling quantification approach for perfusion MRI. Magn Reson Med 2006; 55: 219–232

[12] Alsop DC, Detre JA. Multisection cerebral blood flow MR imaging with continuous arterial spin labeling. Radiology 1998; 208: 410–416

[13] Garcia DM, Bazelaire CD, Alsop D. Pseudo-continuous Flow Driven Adiabatic Inversion for Arterial Spin Labeling. ISMRM. May 2005. Miami Beach, Florida, USA

[14] Wu WC, Fernández-Seara M, Detre JA, Wehrli FW, Wang J. A theoretical and experimental investigation of the tagging efficiency of pseudocontinuous arterial spin labeling. Magn Reson Med 2007; 58: 1020–1027

[15] Wang J, Alsop DC, Li L et al. Comparison of quantitative perfusion imaging using arterial spin labeling at 1.5 and 4.0 tesla. Magn Reson Med 2002; 48: 242–254

[16] Yongbi MN, Fera F, Yang Y, Frank JA, Duyn JH. Pulsed arterial spin labeling: comparison of multisection baseline and functional MR imaging perfusion signal at 1.5 and 3.0 T: initial results in six subjects. Radiology 2002; 222: 569–575

[17] Wang Z, Wang J, Connick TJ, Wetmore GS, Detre JA. Continuous ASL (CASL) perfusion MRI with an array coil and parallel imaging at 3 T. Magn Reson Med 2005; 54: 732–737

[18] Ye FQ, Mattay VS, Jezzard P, Frank JA, Weinberger DR, McLaughlin AC. Correction for vascular artifacts in cerebral blood flow values measured by using arterial spin tagging techniques. Magn Reson Med 1997; 37: 226–235

[19] Ye FQ, Frank JA, Weinberger DR, McLaughlin AC. Noise reduction in 3D perfusion imaging by attenuating the static signal in arterial spin tagging (ASSIST). Magn Reson Med 2000; 44: 92–100

[20] Fernández-Seara MA, Wang J, Wang Z et al. Imaging mesial temporal lobe activation during scene encoding: comparison of fMRI using BOLD and arterial spin labeling. Hum Brain Mapp 2007; 28: 1391–1400

[21] Fernández-Seara MA, Wang Z, Wang J et al. Continuous arterial spin labeling perfusion measurements using single shot 3D GRASE at 3 T. Magn Reson Med 2005; 54: 1241–1247

[22] Yeom KW, Mitchell LA, Lober RM et al. Arterial spin-labeled perfusion of pediatric brain tumors. AJNR Am J Neuroradiol 201 4; 35: 395–401

[23] Yamamoto T, Kinoshita K, Kosaka N et al. Monitoring of extra-axial brain tumor response to radiotherapy using pseudo-continuous arterial spin labeling images: preliminary results. Magn Reson Imaging 2013; 31: 1271–1277

[24] Luh WM, Wong EC, Bandettini PA, Hyde JS. QUIPSS II with thin-slice TI1 periodic saturation: a method for improving accuracy of quantitative perfusion imaging using pulsed arterial spin labeling. Magn Reson Med 1999; 41: 1246–1254

[25] Noguchi T, Yoshiura T, Hiwatashi A et al. Quantitative perfusion imaging with pulsed arterial spin labeling: a phantom study. Magn Reson Med Sci 2007; 6: 91–97

[26] Warmuth C, Gunther M, Zimmer C. Quantification of blood flow in brain tumors: comparison of arterial spin labeling and dynamic susceptibility-weighted contrast-enhanced MR imaging. Radiology 2003; 228: 523–532

[27] Parkes LM, Rashid W, Chard DT, Tofts PS. Normal cerebral perfusion measurements using arterial spin labeling: reproducibility, stability, and age and gender effects. Magn Reson Med 2004; 51: 736–743

[28] Weber MA, Thilmann C, Lichy MP et al. Assessment of irradiated brain metastases by means of arterial spin-labeling and dynamic susceptibility-weighted contrast-enhanced perfusion MRI: initial results. Invest Radiol 2004; 39: 277–287

[29] Weber MA, Zoubaa S, Schlieter M et al. Diagnostic performance of spectroscopic and perfusion MRI for distinction of brain tumors. Neurology 2006; 66: 1899–1906

[30] Donahue MJ, Lu H, Jones CK, Pekar JJ, van Zijl PC. An account of the discrepancy between MRI and PET cerebral blood flow measures. A high-field MRI investigation. NMR Biomed 2006; 19: 1043–1054

[31] Ye FQ, Berman KF, Ellmore T et al. H(2)(15)O PET validation of steady-state arterial spin tagging cerebral blood flow measurements in humans. Magn Reson Med 2000; 44: 450–456

[32] Aronen HJ, Gazit IE, Louis DN et al. Cerebral blood volume maps of gliomas: comparison with tumor grade and histologic findings. Radiology 1994; 191: 41–51

[33] Knopp EA, Cha S, Johnson G et al. Glial neoplasms: dynamic contrast-enhanced T2*-weighted MR imaging. Radiology 1999; 211: 791–798

[34] Sugahara T, Korogi Y, Kochi M et al. Correlation of MR imaging-determined cerebral blood volume maps with histologic and angiographic determination of vascularity of gliomas. AJR Am J Roentgenol 1998; 171: 1479–1486

[35] Weber MA, Günther M, Lichy MP et al. Comparison of arterial spin-labeling techniques and dynamic susceptibility-weighted contrast-enhanced MRI in perfusion imaging of normal brain tissue. Invest Radiol 2003; 38: 712–718

[36] Lehmann P, Monet P, de Marco G et al. A comparative study of perfusion measurement in brain tumours at 3 Tesla MR: Arterial spin labeling versus dynamic susceptibility contrast-enhanced MRI. Eur Neurol 2010; 64: 21–26

[37] Lüdemann L, Warmuth C, Plotkin M et al. Brain tumor perfusion: comparison of dynamic contrast enhanced magnetic resonance imaging using T1, T2, and T2* contrast, pulsed arterial spin labeling, and H2(15)O positron emission tomography. Eur J Radiol 2009; 70: 465–474

[38] Hirai T, Kitajima M, Nakamura H et al. Quantitative blood flow measurements in gliomas using arterial spin-labeling at 3T: intermodality agreement and inter- and intraobserver reproducibility study. AJNR Am J Neuroradiol 2011; 32: 2073–2079

[39] Roy B, Awasthi R, Bindal A et al. Comparative evaluation of 3-dimensional pseudocontinuous arterial spin labeling with dynamic contrast-enhanced perfusion magnetic resonance imaging in grading of human glioma. J Comput Assist Tomogr 2013; 37: 321–326

[40] van Westen D, Petersen ET, Wirestam R et al. Correlation between arterial blood volume obtained by arterial spin labelling and cerebral blood volume in intracranial tumours. MAGMA 2011; 24: 211–223

[41] Geer CP, Simonds J, Anvery A et al. Does MR perfusion imaging impact management decisions for patients with brain tumors? A prospective study. AJNR Am J Neuroradiol 2012; 33: 556–562

[42] Kim HS, Kim SY. A prospective study on the added value of pulsed arterial spin-labeling and apparent diffusion coefficients in the grading of gliomas. AJNR Am J Neuroradiol 2007; 28: 1693–1699

[43] Järnum H, Steffensen EG, Knutsson L et al. Perfusion MRI of brain tumours: a comparative study of pseudo-continuous arterial spin labelling and dynamic susceptibility contrast imaging. Neuroradiology 2010; 52: 307–317

[44] Ozsunar Y, Mullins ME, Kwong K et al. Glioma recurrence versus radiation necrosis? A pilot comparison of arterial spin-labeled, dynamic susceptibility contrast enhanced MRI, and FDG-PET imaging. Acad Radiol 2010; 17: 282–290

[45] St Lawrence KS, Frank JA, McLaughlin AC. Effect of restricted water exchange on cerebral blood flow values calculated with arterial spin tagging: a theoretical investigation. Magn Reson Med 2000; 44: 440–449

[46] Tanaka Y, Nagaoka T, Nair G, Ohno K, Duong TQ. Arterial spin labeling and dynamic susceptibility contrast CBF MRI in postischemic hyperperfusion, hypercapnia, and after mannitol injection. J Cereb Blood Flow Metab 2011; 31: 1403–1411

[47] Wolf RL, Wang J, Wang S et al. Grading of CNS neoplasms using continuous arterial spin labeled perfusion MR imaging at 3 Tesla. J Magn Reson Imaging 2005; 22: 475–482

[48] St Lawrence KS, Wang J. Effects of the apparent transverse relaxation time on cerebral blood flow measurements obtained by arterial spin labeling. Magn Reson Med 2005; 53: 425–433

[49] Parkes LM, Tofts PS. Improved accuracy of human cerebral blood perfusion measurements using arterial spin labeling: accounting for capillary water permeability. Magn Reson Med 2002; 48: 27–41

[50] Sasao A, Hirai T, Nishimura S et al. Assessment of vascular supply of hypervascular extra-axial brain tumors with 3 T MR regional perfusion imaging. AJNR Am J Neuroradiol 2010; 31: 554–558

[51] Roberts HC, Roberts TP, Bollen AW, Ley S, Brasch RC, Dillon WP. Correlation of microvascular permeability derived from dynamic contrast-enhanced MR imaging with histologic grade and tumor labeling index: a study in human brain tumors. Acad Radiol 2001; 8: 384–391

[52] Boxerman JL, Schmainda KM, Weisskoff RM. Relative cerebral blood volume maps corrected for contrast agent extravasation significantly correlate with glioma tumor grade, whereas uncorrected maps do not. AJNR Am J Neuroradiol 2006; 27: 859–867

[53] Cha S, Johnson G, Wadghiri YZ et al. Dynamic, contrast-enhanced perfusion MRI in mouse gliomas: correlation with histopathology. Magn Reson Med 2003; 49: 848–855

[54] Batchelor TT, Sorensen AG, di Tomaso E et al. AZD2171, a pan-VEGF receptor tyrosine kinase inhibitor, normalizes tumor vasculature and alleviates edema in glioblastoma patients. Cancer Cell 2007; 11: 83–95

[55] Wang J, Fernández-Seara MA, Wang S, St Lawrence KS. When perfusion meets diffusion: in vivo measurement of water permeability in human brain. J Cereb Blood Flow Metab 2007; 27: 839–849

[56] Kimura H, Takeuchi H, Koshimoto Y et al. Perfusion imaging of meningioma by using continuous arterial spin-labeling: comparison with dynamic susceptibility-weighted contrast-enhanced MR images and histopathologic features. AJNR Am J Neuroradiol 2006; 27: 85–93

[57] Noguchi T, Yoshiura T, Hiwatashi A et al. Perfusion imaging of brain tumors using arterial spin-labeling: correlation with histopathologic vascular density. AJNR Am J Neuroradiol 2008; 29: 688–693

[58] Louis DN, Ohgaki H, Wiestler OD et al. The 2007 WHO classification of tumours of the central nervous system. Acta Neuropathol 2007; 114: 97–109

[59] Leon SP, Folkerth RD, Black PM. Microvessel density is a prognostic indicator for patients with astroglial brain tumors. Cancer 1996; 77: 362–372

[60] Folkerth RD. Descriptive analysis and quantification of angiogenesis in human brain tumors. J Neurooncol 2000; 50: 165–172

[61] Law M, Yang S, Wang H et al. Glioma grading: sensitivity, specificity, and predictive values of perfusion MR imaging and proton MR spectroscopic imaging compared with conventional MR imaging. AJNR Am J Neuroradiol 2003; 24: 1989–1998

[62] Law M, Oh S, Babb JS et al. Low-grade gliomas: dynamic susceptibility-weighted contrast-enhanced perfusion MR imaging—prediction of patient clinical response. Radiology 2006; 238: 658–667

[63] Gaa J, Warach S, Wen P, Thangaraj V, Wielopolski P, Edelman RR. Noninvasive perfusion imaging of human brain tumors with EPISTAR. Eur Radiol 1996; 6: 518–522

[64] Lev MH, Ozsunar Y, Henson JW et al. Glial tumor grading and outcome prediction using dynamic spin-echo MR susceptibility mapping compared with conventional contrast-enhanced MR: confounding effect of elevated rCBV of oligodendrogliomas [corrected]. AJNR Am J Neuroradiol 2004; 25: 214–221

[65] Chawla S, Wang S, Wolf RL et al. Arterial spin-labeling and MR spectroscopy in the differentiation of gliomas. AJNR Am J Neuroradiol 2007; 28: 1683–1689

[66] Deibler AR, Pollock JM, Kraft RA, Tan H, Burdette JH, Maldjian JA. Arterial spin-labeling in routine clinical practice, part 3: hyperperfusion patterns. AJNR Am J Neuroradiol 2008; 29: 1428–1435

[67] Lu H, Clingman C, Golay X, van Zijl PC. Determining the longitudinal relaxation time (T1) of blood at 3.0 Tesla. Magn Reson Med 2004; 52: 679–682

[68] MacIntosh BJ, Filippini N, Chappell MA, Woolrich MW, Mackay CE, Jezzard P. Assessment of arterial arrival times derived from multiple inversion time pulsed arterial spin labeling MRI. Magn Reson Med 2010; 63: 641–647

[69] Furtner J, Schöpf V, Schewzow K et al. Arterial Spin-Labeling Assessment of Normalized Vascular Intratumoral Signal Intensity as a Predictor of Histologic Grade of Astrocytic Neoplasms. AJNR Am J Neuroradiol 201 4; 35: 482–489

[70] Yamashita K, Yoshiura T, Hiwatashi A et al. Arterial spin labeling of hemangioblastoma: differentiation from metastatic brain tumors based on quantitative blood flow measurement. Neuroradiology 2012; 54: 809–813

[71] Pollock JM, Whitlow CT, Tan H, Kraft RA, Burdette JH, Maldjian JA. Pulsed arterial spin-labeled MR imaging evaluation of tuberous sclerosis. AJNR Am J Neuroradiol 2009; 30: 815–820

[72] Yamashita K, Yoshiura T, Hiwatashi A et al. Differentiating primary CNS lymphoma from glioblastoma multiforme: assessment using arterial spin labeling, diffusion-weighted imaging, and ^{18}F-fluorodeoxyglucose positron emission tomography. Neuroradiology 2013; 55: 135–143

[73] Hartmann M, Heiland S, Harting I et al. Distinguishing of primary cerebral lymphoma from high-grade glioma with perfusion-weighted magnetic resonance imaging. Neurosci Lett 2003; 338: 119–122

[74] Ernst TM, Chang L, Witt MD et al. Cerebral toxoplasmosis and lymphoma in AIDS: perfusion MR imaging experience in 13 patients. Radiology 1998; 208: 663–669

[75] Weber MA, Henze M, Tüttenberg J et al. Biopsy targeting gliomas: do functional imaging techniques identify similar target areas? Invest Radiol 2010; 45: 755–768

[76] Sedlacik J, Winchell A, Kocak M, Loeffler RB, Broniscer A, Hillenbrand CM. MR imaging assessment of tumor perfusion and 3D segmented volume at baseline, during treatment, and at tumor progression in children with newly diagnosed diffuse intrinsic pontine glioma. AJNR Am J Neuroradiol 2013; 34: 1450–1455

[77] Fenchel M, Konaktchieva M, Weisel K et al. Early response assessment in patients with multiple myeloma during anti-angiogenic therapy using arterial spin labelling: first clinical results. Eur Radiol 2010; 20: 2899–2906

[78] Schor-Bardach R, Alsop DC, Pedrosa I et al. Does arterial spin-labeling MR imaging-measured tumor perfusion correlate with renal cell cancer response to antiangiogenic therapy in a mouse model? Radiology 2009; 251: 731–742

[79] Brandsma D, Stalpers L, Taal W, Sminia P, van den Bent MJ. Clinical features, mechanisms, and management of pseudoprogression in malignant gliomas. Lancet Oncol 2008; 9: 453–461

[80] Taal W, Brandsma D, de Bruin HG et al. Incidence of early pseudo-progression in a cohort of malignant glioma patients treated with chemoirradiation with temozolomide. Cancer 2008; 113: 405–410

[81] Wen PY, Macdonald DR, Reardon DA et al. Updated response assessment criteria for high-grade gliomas: response assessment in neuro-oncology working group. J Clin Oncol 2010; 28: 1963–1972

[82] Choi YJ, Kim HS, Jahng GH, Kim SJ, Suh DC. Pseudoprogression in patients with glioblastoma: added value of arterial spin labeling to dynamic susceptibility contrast perfusion MR imaging. Acta Radiol 2013; 54: 448–454

[83] Barajas RF, Jr, Chang JS, Segal MR et al. Differentiation of recurrent glioblastoma multiforme from radiation necrosis after external beam radiation therapy with dynamic susceptibility-weighted contrast-enhanced perfusion MR imaging. Radiology 2009; 253: 486–496

[84] Kim HS, Kim JH, Kim SH, Cho KG, Kim SY. Posttreatment high-grade glioma: usefulness of peak height position with semiquantitative MR perfusion histogram analysis in an entire contrast-enhanced lesion for predicting volume fraction of recurrence. Radiology 2010; 256: 906–915

[85] Paldino MJ, Barboriak DP. Fundamentals of quantitative dynamic contrast-enhanced MR imaging. Magn Reson Imaging Clin N Am 2009; 17: 277–289

[86] Cha S, Knopp EA, Johnson G, Wetzel SG, Litt AW, Zagzag D. Intracranial mass lesions: dynamic contrast-enhanced susceptibility-weighted echo-planar perfusion MR imaging. Radiology 2002; 223: 11–29

[87] Sakai N, Koizumi S, Yamashita S et al. Arterial spin-labeled perfusion imaging reflects vascular density in nonfunctioning pituitary macroadenomas. AJNR Am J Neuroradiol 2013; 34: 2139–2143

[88] Berker M, Aghayev K, Saatci I, Palaoğlu S, Onerci M. Overview of vascular complications of pituitary surgery with special emphasis on unexpected abnormality. Pituitary 2010; 13: 160–167

[89] Pollock JM, Whitlow CT, Deibler AR et al. Anoxic injury-associated cerebral hyperperfusion identified with arterial spin-labeled MR imaging. AJNR Am J Neuroradiol 2008; 29: 1302–1307

[90] Pollock JM, Deibler AR, Burdette JH et al. Migraine associated cerebral hyperperfusion with arterial spin-labeled MR imaging. AJNR Am J Neuroradiol 2008; 29: 1494–1497

[91] Pollock JM, Deibler AR, Whitlow CT et al. Hypercapnia-induced cerebral hyperperfusion: an underrecognized clinical entity. AJNR Am J Neuroradiol 2009; 30: 378–385

[92] Zaharchuk G, Martin AJ, Dillon WP. Noninvasive imaging of quantitative cerebral blood flow changes during 100% oxygen inhalation using arterial spin-labeling MR imaging. AJNR Am J Neuroradiol 2008; 29: 663–667

[93] Lee J, Wang S, Mohan S, Melhem ER. Differentiating Grade II from Grade III Nonenhancing Astrocytomas and Oligodendrogliomas Using Arterial Spin Labeling Perfusion MR: Comparison of Cerebrovascular Reactivity to Acetazolamide - Initial Experience. ASNR. 2013. San Diego, CA, USA. eP-26

7 Perfusion Imaging: Perfusion CT

Brent Griffith and Rajan Jain

7.1 Introduction

Perfusion computed tomography (PCT) is a well established modality for acute stroke assessment[1,2] and has been used sporadically for assessing postsubarachnoid hemorrhage vasospasm,[3] as well as for the evaluation of cerebrovascular reserve in patients with major vessel steno-occlusive disease.[4] Traditionally, perfusion imaging of brain tumors has been performed with magnetic resonance imaging (MRI) with the goal of estimating tumor vascular parameters.[5,6,7] However, given its ease of availability, faster scan times, and low cost when compared with magnetic resonance (MR) perfusion, PCT also may be well suited for brain tumor evaluation[8,9]—potentially offering a robust tool for the quantitative estimation of tumor vascular parameters and opening the door for their potential use as imaging biomarkers.

In recent years, PCT has been used for glioma grading,[6,7] for differentiating recurrent or progressive tumor from treatment-induced effects (e.g., radiation necrosis),[10] as well as in differentiating nonneoplastic tumefactive lesions from neoplasms.[11] One of the advantages of PCT is the linear relationship between tissue attenuation and concentration of contrast agent, in contradistinction to MR perfusion techniques. This, in turn, leads to a less biased estimation of tumor vascular parameters when compared with MR perfusion techniques. However, one of PCT's biggest limitations, apart from radiation exposure concerns, is the need to obtain an entirely separate PCT examination, rather than simply obtaining additional MR perfusion sequences at the time of the routine contrast-enhanced MRI, which is the standard of care for the imaging evaluation of brain tumor patients. Yet, despite these limitations, PCT has potential as a very useful tool for brain tumor assessment, especially in those patients unable to undergo MRI due to a variety of contraindications.

7.2 Perfusion CT Tracer Kinetics and Vascular Parameters

Dynamic contrast-enhanced imaging attempts to observe the distribution of contrast agent within tissues over time. To be successful, the correct mathematical tracer kinetic model to the dynamic data set must be implemented in order to obtain an accurate estimate of contrast agent distribution between the intravascular and extravascular compartments. Each kinetic model makes a number of assumptions and, as such, may have limitations in particular experimental situations and also be dependent on tissue physiology.

A fundamental difference between the various kinetic models stems from the assumption of *homogeneous* (well-mixed) or *distributed* compartments. A *homogeneous* compartment assumes instantaneous mixing of tracer within the compartment such that tracer concentration is uniform throughout, whereas a *distributed* compartment attempts to account for spatial differences in tracer concentration within the compartment. The generalized kinetic and conventional compartmental[12,13] models assume

homogeneous compartments, whereas the adiabatic tissue homogeneity[14,15,16,17] and distributed parameter[18,19] models assume a distributed vascular compartment.[19] The applicability of a particular model depends on the underlying tissue physiology (i.e., tracer transit, distribution, and exchange rates), as well as the imaging protocol and noise condition of the dynamic contrast-enhanced imaging data set.

Due to the complex tissue characteristics of brain tumors, and also the fact that temporal resolution of image sampling is on the order of 1 second when using multislice fast CT scanners, compartment models are best suited for assessing dynamic data when evaluating brain tumors with PCT. The two-compartment model, based on the adiabatic approximation of the John and Wilson model,[15] has been used in the past at our institution with good success.[8,9,10,11,20,21,22] These compartment models can simultaneously measure four independent vascular parameters: two rate parameters (blood flow and permeability surface area-product [PS]) and two volume parameters (blood volume and volume of extravascular extracellular space [v_e]). Mean transit time (MTT) can be derived based on the central volume principle; blood volume = blood flow × MTT.[23]

Permeability is related to the diffusion coefficient of contrast agent in the assumed water-filled pores of the capillary endothelium. The diffusion flux of contrast agent across the capillary endothelium is dependent on both the diffusion coefficient and the total surface area of the pores. PS characterizes the diffusion of some of the contrast agent from the blood vessels into the interstitial space due to deficient or leaky blood–brain barrier (BBB) and is used as a means of quantifying the "leakiness" of the regional vasculature. PS is computed from the impulse residue function (IRF). Contrast agent diffusion appears in the IRF as a residual enhancement that occurs after the initial impulse response and that decreases exponentially with time. The IRF is used to estimate the first-pass fraction of contrast agent that remains in the tissue, the extraction fraction (E).[15] The extraction fraction is related to the rate at which contrast leaks out of the vasculature *via* the following relationship:

$$E = 1 - e^{-\frac{PS}{F}}$$

where PS is the permeability surface-area product and F is flow. The PS product has the same dimensions as flow (mL/100 g/min), and thus the ratio

$$\frac{PS}{F}$$

is dimensionless. In physiological terms, PS is the rate at which contrast agent flows into the extravascular tissues; it is related to another commonly stated parameter of vascular leakage, the forward transfer constant (K^{trans}) by the following: $K^{trans} = E \times F$, where K^{trans} is the forward transfer constant with, again, the same dimensions as flow (units commonly employed min^{-1}). It is easily demonstrated that, if

$$\frac{PS}{F}$$

$\ll 1$ (or $F \gg PS$) then $K^{trans} \approx PS$. In normal cerebral vasculature, PS is negligible for all contrast agents presently in clinical use.

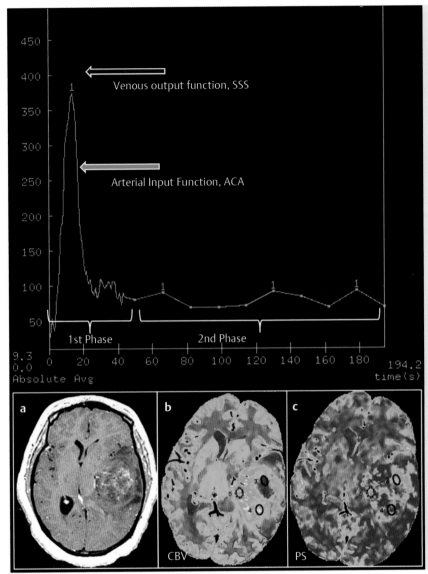

Fig. 7.1 Perfusion computed tomography (PCT) time concentration curve showing arterial input function (AIF) selected from anterior cerebral artery and venous output function selected from superior sagittal sinus in a patient with grade III glioma. PCT done with a two-phase study: First vascular phase followed by delayed or parenchyma back flux phase. (**a**) Postcontrast T1-weighted magnetic resonance imaging axial image showing heterogeneous enhancement within a large left temporal lobe tumor. Corresponding PCT (**b**) cerebral blood volume and (**c**) permeability surface area-product (PS) parametric maps.

7.3 Perfusion CT Protocol

Perfusion studies can be performed using multidetector row CT (MDCT) scanners. Currently available 16-slice CT scanners can cover 2 cm of the brain, which is increased to 4 cm using a 64-slice CT scanner. Prior to obtaining the perfusion scan, a low radiation dose noncontrast CT head study is usually performed to localize the tumor region. For the perfusion scan, 50 mL of nonionic contrast is injected at a rate of 4 to 5 mL/s through an intravenous (IV) line using an automatic power injector. The brain tumor PCT protocol at our institution includes two phases: (1) First pass or vascular phase—cine (continuous) scan initiated 5 seconds into the injection with the following technique: 80 kVp, 100 to 120 mA, 1 second per rotation for a duration of 50 seconds, matrix size 512 × 512, and 24 cm field of view; and (2) delayed or parenchyma back flux phase—following the initial 50-second vascular phase, eight additional axial images are acquired, one image every 15 seconds for an additional 2 minutes, giving a total acquisition time of 170 seconds to assess for

delayed permeability.[9] With the use of the 16-slice CT scanner, four 5-mm thick axial slices are acquired for a total coverage of 2 cm, whereas with the 64-slice CT scanner, eight 5-mm thick axial slices are acquired, resulting in a total coverage area of 4 cm. Perfusion maps of vascular parameters can then be obtained using many of the commercially available software packages. Our institution uses an Advantage Windows workstation and CT perfusion software (General Electric Medical Systems, Milwaukee, WI), which uses a two-compartment model based on the adiabatic approximation of the John and Wilson model[15] to generate cerebral blood volume (CBV), cerebral blood flow (CBF), MTT, and PS parametric maps. The superior sagittal sinus is generally used as the venous output function, and the artery with the greatest peak and slope on time-attenuation curves is used as the arterial input function (AIF) (▶ Fig. 7.1). In selecting the AIF, a region of interest (ROI) is drawn within the confines of a large vessel, and the automatic function of the software selects the pixels with the greatest peak and slope on the time-attenuation curve for analysis.

7.4 Perfusion CT: Technical Considerations

Permeability estimates can be affected by a number of factors that must be taken into consideration when performing PCT. One such technical factor—which affects permeability estimates regardless of the perfusion imaging technique—is the *scanning* or *acquisition time.* Although no definite consensus exists regarding optimal acquisition time, it is understood that delayed permeability caused by slow leakage of contrast from leaky blood vessels may be inaccurately measured with the first pass of the contrast agent using a 45 or 60 s scanning time[24,25,26] and can be accurately measured only with longer acquisition times. Our institution uses an extended acquisition time of 170 s for brain tumor patients (▶ Fig. 7.1), and a recent publication supports this use of longer scanning times as a means of reducing random errors.[27] A second factor that can influence permeability estimates relates to the nature of the tumors themselves, particularly high-grade gliomas, which can have extremely variable and heterogeneous blood flow due to the complex tumor vasculature.[28,29,30] Other factors also influencing permeability include blood vessel luminal surface area, as well as interstitial, hydrostatic, and osmotic pressure gradients across the endothelium. For example, slow blood flow or low osmotic gradients, which can occur in high-grade tumors with a lot of vasogenic edema, as well as in the central parts of large tumors, can lead to a larger component of delayed permeability, requiring longer acquisition times.

Selection of an accurate AIF is also an important aspect of the postprocessing of dynamic data sets. Although AIF selection is relatively easier with PCT, yet to be discussed here, it still requires particular attention as absolute values of vascular parameters may be affected by the choice of AIF. Although there is literature in acute stroke patients in which laterality of AIF did not affect the measurements,[31,32] as with acquisition time, there is no consensus in brain tumor patients. It should be noted though that this pitfall is less severe with deconvolution-based software programs using a delay insensitive technique than with those using a standard deconvolution method.[32]

7.5 Comparison with MR Perfusion Techniques for Brain Tumor Assessment

7.5.1 Limitations of PCT

MRI-based perfusion techniques have been at the forefront of brain tumor assessment due to the role of contrast-enhanced MRI as the standard of care in evaluation of brain tumor patients. Therefore, obtaining an additional perfusion sequence, whether using dynamic contrast-enhanced T1-weighted imaging (DCE-T1 MRI) or dynamic susceptibility contrast-enhanced T2- or T2*-weighted imaging (DSC), with bolus injection of contrast agent is relatively easy. On the contrary, PCT requires a *separate and additional examination* with an *additional iodinated contrast agent* injection. Hence, using PCT as a routine diagnostic tool or as a routine follow-up tool in patients treated

with various combinations of therapy is impractical. However, PCT may still be useful if MRI is contraindicated, whether due to MRI compatibility issues, patient choice, or the limitations of MR perfusion techniques described later in the chapter.

Another major concern with PCT, as compared to MR perfusion techniques, is *radiation exposure.* However, low radiation dose protocols, which can be obtained using 100 to 120 mA (as presently done at our center) as compared to 200 mA, have reduced the mean effective dose of PCT to 3 to 4 mSv, offering nearly a 50 to 60% reduction in radiation dose (our unpublished data) without affecting the image quality of perfusion parametric maps. In addition, some of the advanced image reconstruction techniques, such as adaptive statistical iterative reconstruction, can further reduce image noise and improve low contrast detection and image quality with up to 32 to 65% CT dose index reductions.[30] Wider availability and implementation of these new techniques could further reduce the radiation dose for PCT studies, making them more attractive for routine use.

An additional relative limitation of PCT in the past was *limited coverage* of the brain, particularly with the use of 16-slice CT scanners, which covered only 2 cm. However, the use of 64-slice CT scanners, which can cover up to 4 cm of brain, allows for coverage of most of the tumors in our clinical experience. In addition, brain coverage has been increased to include the whole brain with the use of 128-, 256-, or 320-slice CT scanners.

7.5.2 Advantages of PCT

Despite the aforementioned limitations, PCT has certain advantages over MR perfusion techniques. Two of the most important advantages, the *linear relationship between tissue attenuation and concentration of contrast agent* and the ease of obtaining a robust *AIF,* both have led to less biased estimation of tumor vascular parameters compared to MR perfusion techniques. Regarding the relationship between tissue attenuation and concentration, contrast agent bolus-based MR perfusion techniques have a nonlinear relationship of the signal intensity with the contrast agent concentration whether using DCE-T1 MRI or DSC imaging, which are the two most commonly employed techniques. In the latter case, when the contrast agent remains intravascular, the method is widely accepted as a relative estimate of CBF and CBV, although there is a possibility of artifacts due to difficulties in assessing the shape and timing of the arterial input function.[28] In the event that substantial leakage of a contrast agent from intra- to extravascular space takes place, which is a common occurrence in brain tumors (especially high-grade tumors), a strong and competing T1 contrast effect is often noticed in the areas of pathology because of the short (~ 1 s) repetition times needed to estimate CBF. As a first-order tactic to minimize the competing T1 contrast, preloading with contrast agent has been proposed with some success.[29] However, this approach does not allow an estimate of K[trans]. An alternative has also been proposed,[33] which aimed to decrease the T1 effect by using a slower repetition time, lengthening the acquisition time of the experiment, and undermining the estimation of CBF, thus yielding estimates of only CBV and K[trans]. A further refinement, allowing the estimate of blood volume and

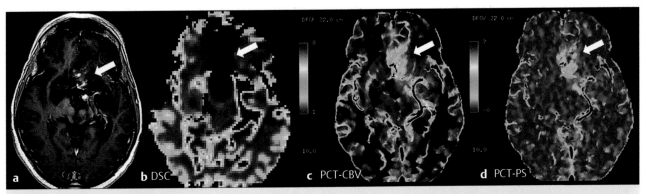

Fig. 7.2 (a) Postcontrast T1-weighted axial magnetic resonance imaging (MRI) and (b) dynamic susceptibility contrast-enhanced (DSC)-MRI cerebral blood volume (CBV) map in patient with a grade III glioma (arrow) close to the skull base showing obscuration of the medial portion of the tumor on DSC-MRI maps due to susceptibility artifacts as a result of close approximation to the skull base. (c) Perfusion computed tomography (PCT) CBV and (d) permeability surface area-product (PS) parametric maps showing a more detailed evaluation of the tumor with increased CBV and PS in the obscured part of the tumor.

producing an index of transfer constant, has been suggested,[29] and a dual-echo gradient echo sequence[25] also shows potential for an index of blood volume and transfer constant. Despite the partial success of these rapid imaging studies, in contrast to PCT, there does not appear to be an MRI technique that will *reliably quantify CBF, CBV, and K^{trans} in one single experiment*.

Selection of an appropriate *AIF* is also difficult with MR-based techniques due to susceptibility and flow artifacts, whereas it is very robust with PCT. With the advent of faster helical CT scanners, *temporal sampling* of image acquisition could be on the order of 1 s or less (which may not be possible even with the latest MR scanners), and could be an important consideration for both pharmacokinetic modeling (distributed compartment models), as well as for obtaining a robust AIF.

Another disadvantage of MR perfusion, particularly with DSC MR perfusion, is the presence of *susceptibility artifacts* related to hemorrhage and various mineral depositions, which can be a major issue in brain tumor patients following surgery and chemoradiation therapy combination regimens. Brain tumors along the skull base also could be difficult to assess with DSC imaging due to susceptibility artifacts (▸ Fig. 7.2), though susceptibility is not an issue with DCE-T1 MRI. On the other hand, PCT could be very useful in these scenarios. DCE-T1 MRI also has its own drawbacks, such as those associated with the need to calculate baseline T1 values as well as magnetic field inhomogeneity issues, making it much more technically challenging than PCT.

7.6 Tumor Vascular Parameters: Relevance to Angiogenesis

As already discussed, various tumor vascular parameters, which can be measured using perfusion techniques, have a specific physiological basis and have been correlated with tumor grade, aggressiveness, and prognosis.[5,7,9,34] Of the available parameters, tumor blood volume and leakiness (permeability), which have been shown to be associated with tumor angiogenesis and can be measured with PCT in one single experiment, are two of the most important and commonly used parameters. Tumor blood volume and permeability have also been shown to

correlate with genes regulating angiogenesis[35] and hence support a molecular basis for these two imaging parameters, which has importance in attempting to establish these parameters as imaging biomarkers.

7.6.1 Tumor Blood Volume

Regional tumor blood volume (CBV) measurements reflect an assessment of tumor vasculature and perfusion and have been correlated with glioma grading as well as prognosis. Measurement of tumor blood volume is a good surrogate marker for microvascular density (MVD), a measure of angiogenesis and an important prognostic indicator[24,36,37] in many human cancers. The association between MVD and tumor aggressiveness can be explained by the following: (1) solid tumors are composed of two interdependent components, which include the malignant cells and the stroma that they induce, and MVD could be a measure of the success that a tumor has in forming this stromal component; (2) endothelial cells in this stromal component stimulate the growth of tumor cells, thus the more intratumoral vessels there are, the more endothelial cells present and therefore the more paracrine growth stimulation; and, finally, (3) intratumoral MVD is a direct measure of the vascular window through which tumor cells pass to spread to distant sites.[37] Tumoral MVD, however, does not distinguish neoangiogenic vessels from native ones, and hence, probably does not identify active sites of angiogenesis. Jain et al, using image-guided biopsy specimens and correlation of PCT parameters with immune-histological markers, demonstrated correlation between CBV and MVD (▸ Fig. 7.3), but not microvascular cellular proliferation (MVCP), which is a histological surrogate marker of angiogenesis.[20] However, these limitations do not diminish the clinical value of this measure. Cha et al[38] showed a strong correlation of CBV measurements in mouse gliomas with MVD and suggested that rCBV may be elevated due to increase in vessel size or total number of vessels or both. Aronen et al[39] also showed a strong correlation of CBV and tumor energy metabolism with MVD using MR perfusion and[40] F-fluorodeoxyglucose positron-emission tomography (FDG-PET) imaging, respectively.

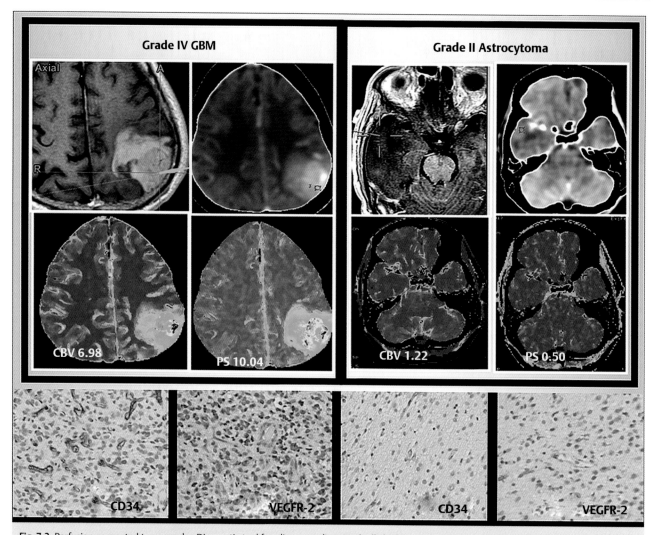

Fig. 7.3 Perfusion computed tomography. Diagnostic tool for glioma grading. Markedly higher cerebral blood volume (CBV) and permeability surface area-product (PS) in a grade IV glioblastoma multiforme (GBM) as compared to a low-grade astrocytoma (grade II). Bottom row: cluster of differentiation 34 (CD34) and vascular endothelial growth factor receptor 2 (VEGFR-2) staining from image-guided biopsy specimens from both tumors showing much higher microvascular density (MVD) as well as VEGFR-2 immunoreactivity in GBM specimen as compared to low-grade glioma.

7.6.2 Tumor Vascular Leakiness

It is a fact that tumor blood vessels have defective and leaky endothelium. Tumor growth leads to hypoxia and increased expression of vascular endothelial growth factor (VEGF), which is both a potent proangiogenic factor and a potent permeability factor.[41,42] VEGF leads to the development of neoangiogenic vessels that are immature, tortuous,[43] and have increased leakiness to macromolecules due to large endothelial cell gaps, incomplete basement membrane, and absence of smooth muscles. Jain et al[20] have shown that tumor vascular leakiness permeability surface area-product (PS) shows correlation with MVCP and also shows a trend with vascular endothelial growth factor receptor-2 (VEGFR-2) expression, suggesting that tumor leakiness could be a better measure of active sites of angiogenesis than CBV and MVD. Thus in vivo measurement of tumor vessel permeability is important for various reasons: (1) it can be used for tumor grading because increased permeability is associated with immature blood vessels, which is seen with

angiogenesis; (2) it can be used to study the response of tumors to various therapies, especially antiangiogenic therapy[40,44]; (3) understanding the concept of leakiness can help in understanding the mechanism of entry of therapeutic agents into the central nervous system; and (4) it assists in the development of methods to selectively alter the BBB to enhance drug delivery.[45]

7.6.3 Correlation between Tumor Blood Volume and Tumor Leakiness

The concept of angiogenesis in tumor growth picked up in the early 1960s and has continued to expand over the last 5 decades, spearheaded by researchers such as Judah Folkman.[46,47] It has been convincingly shown that growth of new capillary blood vessels, or angiogenesis, is required for growth of solid tumors and metastasis. Tumor growth starts as an avascular mass, especially in well-vascularized tissues like brain and lung. Tumor cells can then grow along existing vessels without

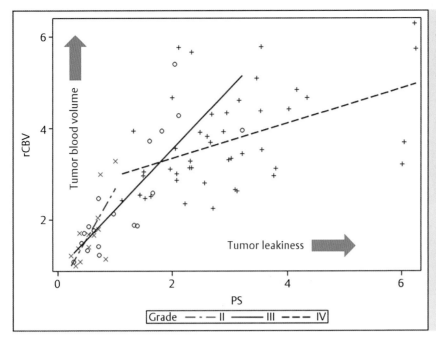

Fig. 7.4 Correlation between cerebral blood volume (CBV) and permeability surface area-product (PS). Scatter plot showing a much higher relative CBV:PS ratio (rCBV:PS) in grade II gliomas compared to grade IV gliomas.

invoking an angiogenic response, a process that has been defined as vessel co-option. Initial co-opted vessels undergo dramatic regression as a host defense mechanism with tumor cell death in the center of the tumor. However, remaining tumor cells are rescued by robust angiogenesis at the periphery of the tumor. Angiogenesis has also been proposed to be required by in situ tumors to convert from those having low metastatic activity, or quiescent phenotype, to those having an aggressive or invasive phenotype.[48,49] This conversion and acquisition of angiogenic properties has also been referred to as angiogenic switch. This whole process of recruiting native vessels (co-option) to formation of neovessels (intussusceptive and sprouting angiogenesis) is essential for tumor growth and can in fact occur as gliomas transform from lower to higher grades. Jain et al[50] have shown that CBV and PS values increase with increasing glioma grade, although their relationship changes as the tumor grade increases (▶ Fig. 7.4). Grade II gliomas show a much larger increase of CBV compared to PS (correlating with the vessel co-option stage of tumor vascularization), and grade IV gliomas show a much larger increase of PS compared to CBV (correlating with the intussusceptive and sprouting angiogenesis stage). This implies that the tumor vasculature undergoes angiogenic switch from lower- to higher-grade gliomas, which can be appreciated noninvasively using these vascular parameters. This can provide imaging insight into tumor angiogenesis and angiogenic switch.

7.7 Perfusion CT: Clinical Utility

7.7.1 Diagnostic Tool and Glioma Grading

Most of the literature regarding the utility of perfusion imaging for glioma grading is based on various MR perfusion techniques. Previous studies using MR perfusion have described various relative CBV (rCBV) threshold values for glioma grading. Lev et al[51] described a threshold of 1.5 in discriminating between patients with low- and high-grade gliomas with a sensitivity and specificity of 100% and 69%, respectively. Law et al[52] showed a sensitivity and specificity of 95% and 57.5%, respectively, by using a threshold value of 1.75 for rCBV. Recently, PCT has also been used for glioma grading based on perfusion parameters.[8,9,53] Ding et al[53] demonstrated that PCT can provide useful information about glioma grading, and low-grade gliomas showed low rCBV and relative permeability surfacea area-product (rPS) compared to high-grade gliomas. Ellika et al[8] were able to differentiate low- and high-grade gliomas with a high sensitivity (85.7%) and specificity (100%) using PCT and a normalized CBV (nCBV) threshold of 1.92. This relationship between CBV and histological grade is intuitive because pathology studies show higher MVD in higher-grade tumors (▶ Fig. 7.3). Jain et al,[9] in addition to differentiating low- and high-grade gliomas, were also able to differentiate high-grade tumors into grade III and grade IV, particularly enhancing grade III from grade IV, based on the differences in PS using PCT. This is in keeping with the current World Health Organization (WHO) guidelines of including MVCP as a diagnostic criterion of grade IV, but not for grade III astrocytic tumors, suggesting that PS measurements could show better correlation with MVCP[20] and hence could be an imaging surrogate marker of more immature and leaky blood vessels. Increased angiogenesis in grade IV tumors is characterized not only by an increased number of vessels as compared to grade III astrocytic tumors, but also by association with disproportionate lengthening, increased pliability, endothelial cell proliferation, and irregular shape, which can explain the difference in perfusion parameters for grade IV as compared to grade III tumors. Nonenhancing grade III tumors have also been shown to have lower mean PS, CBV, and CBF as compared to the enhancing grade III group.[9] This difference is probably due to higher tumor vascular density and more leaky vessels seen in enhancing tumors as compared

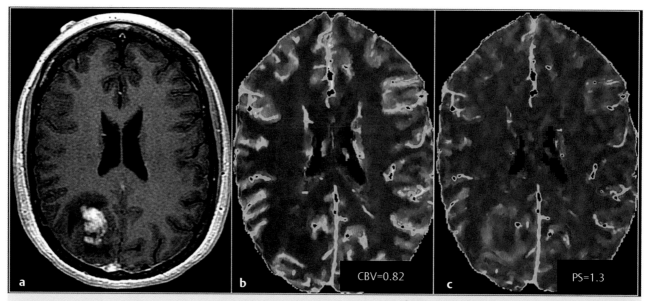

Fig. 7.5 Perfusion computed tomography (PCT). Diagnostic tool. (**a**) Postcontrast T1-weighted axial magnetic resonance imaging (MRI) in a 45-year-old woman presenting with a single solid enhancing lesion in the right parietal lobe demonstrating a tumefactive demyelinating lesion (TDL) mimicking a high-grade glioma. PCT parametric maps showed (**b**) low cerebral blood volume (CBV) and (**c**) low permeability surface area-product (PS) suggesting a nonneoplastic lesion and histology revealed a TDL.

to the nonenhancing group. This could have prognostic implications because grade III tumors with higher PS and CBV may be more aggressive with higher recurrence rates and shorter patient survival as compared to grade III tumors with lower perfusion parameters.[54] In a more recent study, Xyda et al[55] used whole brain perfusion CT and showed that K[trans] demonstrated the highest sensitivity, specificity, and positive predictive value, for both the comparisons between high-grade versus low-grade gliomas and low-grade versus primary cerebral lymphomas.

7.7.2 Diagnostic Tool and Differentiating Neoplasms from Nonneoplastic Lesion/Mimics

Tumefactive demyelinating lesions (TDLs) are usually solitary lesions that can mimic intracranial neoplasms on initial presentation due to their atypical morphological MRI features. The situation can be confounded by the fact that TDLs occasionally simulate neoplasms on histopathological examination,[56,57] although this has been attributed mostly to limited tissue samples, such as those obtained from stereotactic brain biopsy. For example, biopsy of the gliotic margin at the edge of a glioma may be pathologically misinterpreted, and biopsy of the center of a TDL lesion may lead to the erroneous diagnosis of an infarct or necrotic neoplasm.[57] Furthermore, the numerous macrophages and reactive astrocytes usually present in TDL biopsies may appear atypical and mimic a hypercellular lesion consistent with glioma, particularly on intraoperative smear preparations. One of the important biological differences between TDL and high-grade intracranial tumors is the presence of neoangiogenesis and vascular endothelial proliferation in the latter, whereas TDLs are characterized by intrinsically normal or inflamed vessels without evidence of neovascularity.[56,58,59] As

expected, given these histological differences, TDLs show lower PS and CBV (▶ Fig. 7.5) as compared to high-grade gliomas, and perfusion CT can be used to differentiate the two entities.[11] Similarly, various vasculitides and angiopathies, and even uncommonly abscesses can present as solitary or multiple masslike lesions mimicking neoplasm on morphological imaging. PCT can be used to exclude neoplasm by demonstrating low blood volume in these nonneoplastic lesions.

7.7.3 Prognostic Tool

Tumor blood volume measured alone has been used in the past as a prognostic marker.[5,51,60,63] Aronen et al[61] showed that glial tumors with rCBV > 1.5 were more likely to develop into high-grade gliomas. In a study by Law et al,[62] low-grade gliomas with rCBV < 1.75 had a much longer median time to progression compared to those with rCBV > 1.75. In another study involving both low- and high-grade gliomas, Law et al[5] showed that gliomas with rCBV > 1.75 had more rapid time to progression than those with low rCBV independent of pathological findings; however, these authors did not perform a similar analysis for their high-grade glioma group separating grade III and grade IV gliomas. Bisdas et al[63] also showed rCBV being predictive for recurrence and 1-year survival and it may be more accurate than histopathological grading in astrocytomas, but only after tumors with oligodendroglial components are excluded.[63] Hirai et al[64] is the only study about the prognostic value of rCBV in high-grade gliomas, showing that high-grade gliomas with higher rCBV (> 2.3) had significantly lower 2-year overall survival (OS) compared to those with lower rCBV. Only a few studies have explored the use of tumor leakiness estimates as a prognostic factor,[60,65,66] and only one study measured both CBV and K[trans] in a single experiment.[60] However, Mills et al found that patients with higher K[trans] showed better survival,[60] contrary to the other published literature and the results from a

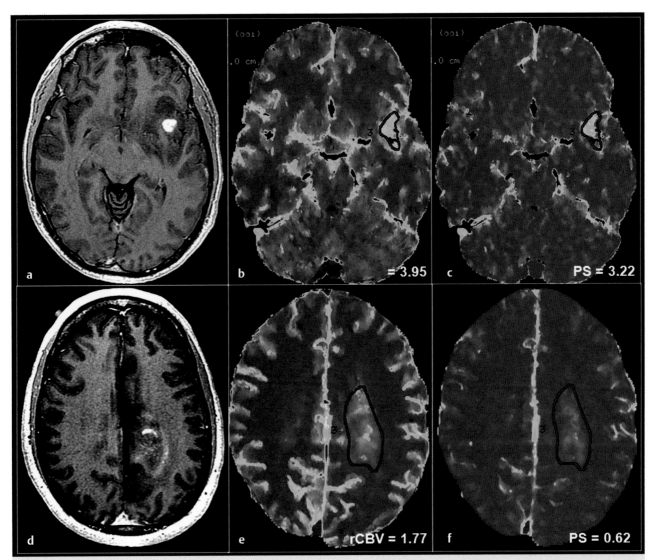

Fig. 7.6 Perfusion computed tomography (PCT). Prognostic tool. Grade III glioma: (**a**) postcontrast T1-weighted axial magnetic resonance imaging (MRI), (**b**) relative cerebral blood volume (rCBV), and (**c**) permeability surface area-product (PS) map in a patient with a heterogeneously enhancing solid mass showing higher rCBV (3.95) and higher PS (3.22 mL/100 g/min). (**d**) Postcontrast T1-weighted axial MRI, (**e**) rCBV, and (**f**) PS maps in another patient showing a similar heterogeneously enhancing solid mass with lower rCBV (1.77) and PS (0.62 mL/100 g/min). The patient in the top row (higher rCBV and higher PS) had a worse overall survival (519 days) as compared to the patient in the bottom row (alive at 1,015 days). (Used with permission from Jain R, Narang J, Griffith B, et al. Prognostic vascular imaging biomarkers in high-grade gliomas: tumor permeability as an adjunct to blood volume estimates. Acad Radiol 2013;20(4):483.)

recent study by Jain et al.[54] Cao et al demonstrated that both tumor vascular leakage volume and vascular leakiness were copredictors of time to progression in high-grade gliomas, along with the surgical status[65] even though they did not adjust their analyses for WHO grade (grade III and grade IV) of the tumors. Dhermain et al recently demonstrated that low-grade gliomas with microvascular leakage and contrast enhancement show worse progression-free survival (PFS) as compared to those without,[66] but did not quantify the leakage. In a more recent study, Jain et al[54] evaluated tumor leakiness (PS) in addition to tumor rCBV using PCT. This study demonstrated that high-grade gliomas with high PCT parameters (rCBV, PS, and rCBV + PS) have poor overall survival compared to those with low PCT parameters (▶ Fig. 7.6 and ▶ Fig. 7.7). rCBV and rCBV + PS estimates also predicted survival irrespective of the

histological grade in these patients, suggesting that in vivo assessment of vascular parameters could potentially be more accurate than histological grading in predicting survival.[54]

7.7.4 Follow-up Tool in Differentiating Recurrent Tumor from Treatment-Induced Necrosis

Recent advances in brain tumor treatment have led to aggressive management strategies with combinations of surgery, chemotherapy, and radiation therapy based on the location and histological type of the tumor. In particular, various forms of radiation therapy, including stereotactic radiosurgery, high-dose external beam radiation, and brachytherapy, have become

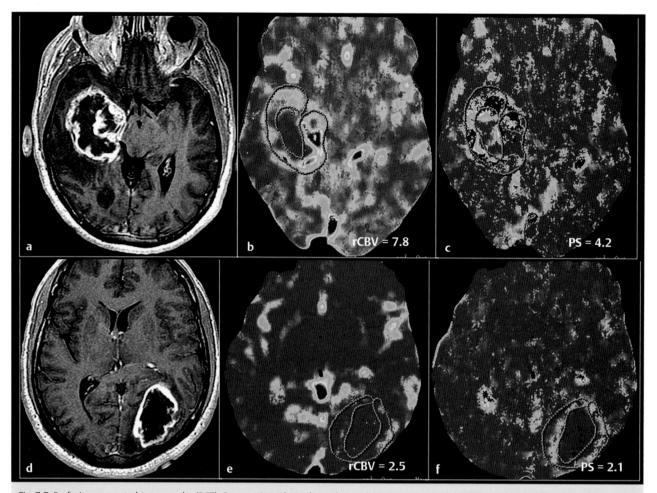

Fig. 7.7 Perfusion computed tomography (PCT). Prognostic tool. Grade IV glioma: (**a**) postcontrast T1-weighted axial magnetic resonance imaging (MRI), (**b**) relative cerebral blood volume (rCBV), and (**c**) permeability surface area-product (PS) map in a patient with an enhancing necrotic mass showing higher rCBV (7.8) and higher PS (4.2 mL/100 g/min) who had worse overall survival (OS) (268 days) as compared to another patient with a (**d**) similar necrotic mass with (**e**) relatively lower rCBV (2.5) and (**f**) lower PS (2.1 mL/100 g/min) with a better OS (1,185 days). (Used with permission from Jain R, Narang J, Griffith B, et al. Prognostic vascular imaging biomarkers in high-grade gliomas: tumor permeability as an adjunct to blood volume estimates. Acad Radiol 2013;20(4):484.)

important therapeutic adjuncts. Patient survival and quality of life are correlated with response to therapy, tumor recurrence, and adverse effects of therapy such as radiation necrosis. As a result, the imaging differentiation of recurrent tumor from treatment effects, such as radiation necrosis, is an important clinical imperative given the vastly different clinical management of these entities.

Unfortunately, the problem of differentiating tumor recurrence from treatment effect is further confounded by the frequent mixture of tumor cells with necrosis. Conventional MRI features and MR spectroscopic imaging have been used to differentiate radiation necrosis from recurrent tumors with mixed success.[67,68] Various forms of metabolic imaging techniques have also been used in the past with limited results. FDG-PET,[69] which is based on tumor glucose metabolism, has shown variable sensitivity and specificity in differentiating recurrent tumors from radiation necrosis and also has limited spatial resolution. Posttreatment recurrent enhancing lesions have also been evaluated with MR perfusion imaging, showing increased CBV in recurrent tumors as compared to nonneoplastic

lesions.[10,70] Jain et al[10] used perfusion CT to successfully differentiate the two entities with recurrent tumors showing higher CBV and CBF, and lower MTT as compared to radiation necrosis. PCT could have a slight edge because most of these patients, after having undergone multiple various combination therapies, have some components of hemorrhage and mineralization, which could produce susceptibility artifacts complicating the perfusion analysis by MR, especially when using dynamic susceptibility weighted imaging.[10]

Previous authors have successfully used relative percentage signal intensity recovery (rPSR) or signal enhancement–time curves as an indirect measure of vascular leakiness using MR perfusion techniques; however, absolute quantitative estimates of permeability have not yet been used for this very important clinical scenario. Kamiryo et al[71] have also demonstrated that BBB architecture of capillaries within previously irradiated brain tissue remains intact despite a decrease in the mean capillary density, as well as increased capillary diameter. Barajas et al[72] showed lower relative PSR in recurrent GBM as compared to radiation necrosis using DSC MR perfusion

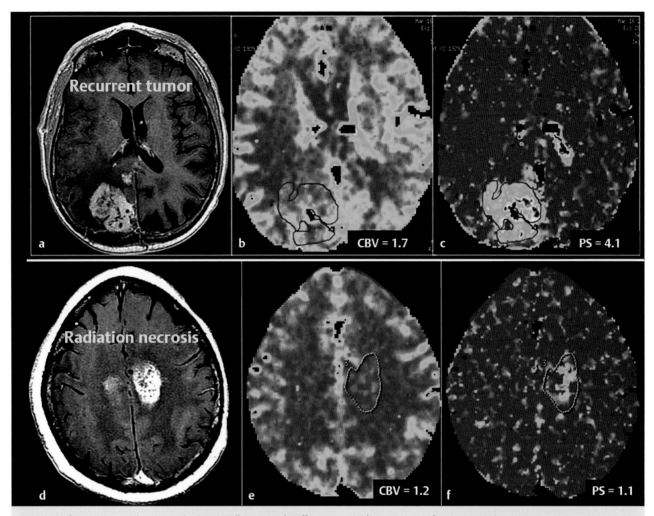

Fig. 7.8 Perfusion computed tomography (PCT). Follow-up tool. Differentiating radiation necrosis from recurrent/progressive tumor. Similar-appearing recurrent enhancing lesions in two different patients previously treated with surgery, chemotherapy, and radiation treatment. Top row shows (**a**), recurrent tumor (**b**) higher cerebral blood volume (CBV) and (**c**) permeability surface area-product (PS) compared to bottom row showing (**d**) radiation necrosis and (**e**) much lower CBV and (**f**) PS. (Used with permission from Jain R, Narang J, Schultz L, et al. Permeability estimates in histopathology-proved treatment-induced necrosis using perfusion CT: can these add to other perfusion parameters in differentiating from recurrent/progressive tumors? AJNR Am J Neuroradiol 2011;32(4):661.)

imaging, suggesting a disrupted BBB that was more permeable to macromolecular contrast agents; however, their measurements were not a direct estimate of lesion leakiness. They also noted a large degree of overlap between the two groups, making rPSR a less robust predictor of recurrent tumor. The same group[73] recently demonstrated significantly lower percentage signal intensity recovery in radiation necrosis as compared to recurrent metastatic intra-axial tumors; however, they also noted a major limitation of susceptibility artifacts resulting in image degradation making DSC measurements difficult to obtain. Quantitative estimates of PS obtained using PCT are not affected by susceptibility artifacts and can help differentiate radiation necrosis from recurrent tumors. Radiation necrosis shows lower PS in addition to lower CBV as compared to recurrent tumors (▶ Fig. 7.8), probably due to the fact that recurrent tumors have much higher expression of VEGF leading to much leakier blood vessels as compared to radiation necrosis.[21]

7.8 Conclusions

Despite the limited role PCT currently plays in the evaluation and management of brain tumors, it does have a number of particular advantages over MR perfusion, including a linear relationship of tissue attenuation with contrast agent concentration, faster temporal resolution, and the availability of a robust arterial input function. These factors, although not the only advantages of PCT, help reduce the biases involved with in vivo estimation of vascular parameters, which is especially important for assessment of complex tumor vasculature and regional heterogeneity, a common feature of many brain tumors. In addition, the ability to estimate both tumor blood volume and leakiness in a single experiment could be particularly advantageous because it not only betters our understanding of tumor angiogenesis, it also provides useful diagnostic and prognostic information, paving the way for further integration of these vascular parameters into clinical practice as potential imaging biomarkers.

References

[1] Hoeffner EG, Case I, Jain R et al. Cerebral perfusion CT: technique and clinical applications. Radiology 2004; 231: 632–644

[2] Wintermark M, Flanders AE, Velthuis B et al. Perfusion-CT assessment of infarct core and penumbra: receiver operating characteristic curve analysis in 130 patients suspected of acute hemispheric stroke. Stroke 2006; 37: 979–985

[3] Wintermark M, Ko NU, Smith WS, Liu S, Higashida RT, Dillon WP. Vasospasm after subarachnoid hemorrhage: utility of perfusion CT and CT angiography on diagnosis and management. AJNR Am J Neuroradiol 2006; 27: 26–34

[4] Rim NJ, Kim HS, Shin YS, Kim SY. Which CT perfusion parameter best reflects cerebrovascular reserve?: correlation of acetazolamide-challenged CT perfusion with single-photon emission CT in Moyamoya patients. AJNR Am J Neuroradiol 2008; 29: 1658–1663

[5] Law M, Young RJ, Babb JS et al. Gliomas: predicting time to progression or survival with cerebral blood volume measurements at dynamic susceptibility-weighted contrast-enhanced perfusion MR imaging. Radiology 2008; 247: 490–498

[6] Roberts HC, Roberts TP, Brasch RC, Dillon WP. Quantitative measurement of microvascular permeability in human brain tumors achieved using dynamic contrast-enhanced MR imaging: correlation with histologic grade. AJNR Am J Neuroradiol 2000; 21: 891–899

[7] Law M, Yang S, Babb JS et al. Comparison of cerebral blood volume and vascular permeability from dynamic susceptibility contrast-enhanced perfusion MR imaging with glioma grade. AJNR Am J Neuroradiol 2004; 25: 746–755

[8] Ellika SK, Jain R, Patel SC et al. Role of perfusion CT in glioma grading and comparison with conventional MR imaging features. AJNR Am J Neuroradiol 2007; 28: 1981–1987

[9] Jain R, Ellika SK, Scarpace L et al. Quantitative estimation of permeability surface-area product in astroglial brain tumors using perfusion CT and correlation with histopathologic grade. AJNR Am J Neuroradiol 2008; 29: 694–700

[10] Jain R, Scarpace L, Ellika S et al. First-pass perfusion computed tomography: initial experience in differentiating recurrent brain tumors from radiation effects and radiation necrosis. Neurosurgery 2007; 61: 778–786, discussion 786–787

[11] Jain R, Ellika S, Lehman NL et al. Can permeability measurements add to blood volume measurements in differentiating tumefactive demyelinating lesions from high grade gliomas using perfusion CT? J Neurooncol 2010; 97: 383–388

[12] Brix G, Bahner ML, Hoffmann U, Horvath A, Schreiber W. Regional blood flow, capillary permeability, and compartmental volumes: measurement with dynamic CT—initial experience. Radiology 1999; 210: 269–276

[13] Hayton P, Brady M, Tarassenko L, Moore N. Analysis of dynamic MR breast images using a model of contrast enhancement. Med Image Anal 1997; 1: 207–224

[14] Johnson JA, Wilson TA. A model for capillary exchange. Am J Physiol 1966; 210: 1299–1303

[15] St Lawrence KS, Lee TY. An adiabatic approximation to the tissue homogeneity model for water exchange in the brain: I. Theoretical derivation. J Cereb Blood Flow Metab 1998; 18: 1365–1377

[16] St Lawrence KS, Lee TY. An adiabatic approximation to the tissue homogeneity model for water exchange in the brain: II. Experimental validation. J Cereb Blood Flow Metab 1998; 18: 1378–1385

[17] Lee TY, Purdie TG, Stewart E. CT imaging of angiogenesis. Q J Nucl Med 2003; 47: 171–187

[18] Larson KB, Markham J, Raichle ME. Tracer-kinetic models for measuring cerebral blood flow using externally detected radiotracers. J Cereb Blood Flow Metab 1987; 7: 443–463

[19] Koh TS, Bisdas S, Koh DM, Thng CH. Fundamentals of tracer kinetics for dynamic contrast-enhanced MRI. J Magn Reson Imaging 2011; 34: 1262–1276

[20] Jain R, Gutierrez J, Narang J et al. In vivo correlation of tumor blood volume and permeability with histologic and molecular angiogenic markers in gliomas. AJNR Am J Neuroradiol 2011; 32: 388–394

[21] Jain R, Narang J, Schultz L et al. Permeability estimates in histopathology-proved treatment-induced necrosis using perfusion CT: can these add to other perfusion parameters in differentiating from recurrent/progressive tumors? AJNR Am J Neuroradiol 2011; 32: 658–663

[22] Jain R. Perfusion CT imaging of brain tumors: an overview. AJNR Am J Neuroradiol 2011; 32: 1570–1577

[23] TY L. Functional CT: physiological models. Trends Biotechnol 2002; 20: S3–S10

[24] Leon SP, Folkerth RD, Black PM. Microvessel density is a prognostic indicator for patients with astroglial brain tumors. Cancer 1996; 77: 362–372

[25] Uematsu H, Maeda M. Double-echo perfusion-weighted MR imaging: basic concepts and application in brain tumors for the assessment of tumor blood volume and vascular permeability. Eur Radiol 2006; 16: 180–186

[26] Miles KA. Perfusion CT for the assessment of tumour vascularity: which protocol? Br J Radiol 2003; 76: S36–S42

[27] Yeung TP, Yartsev S, Bauman G, He W, Fainardi E, Lee TY. The effect of scan duration on the measurement of perfusion parameters in CT perfusion studies of brain tumors. Acad Radiol 2013; 20: 59–65

[28] Conturo TE, Akbudak E, Kotys MS et al. Arterial input functions for dynamic susceptibility contrast MRI: requirements and signal options. J Magn Reson Imaging 2005; 22: 697–703

[29] Boxerman JL, Schmainda KM, Weisskoff RM. Relative cerebral blood volume maps corrected for contrast agent extravasation significantly correlate with glioma tumor grade, whereas uncorrected maps do not. AJNR Am J Neuroradiol 2006; 27: 859–867

[30] Hara AK, Paden RG, Silva AC, Kujak JL, Lawder HJ, Pavlicek W. Iterative reconstruction technique for reducing body radiation dose at CT: feasibility study. AJR Am J Roentgenol 2009; 193: 764–771

[31] Bisdas S, Konstantinou GN, Gurung J et al. Effect of the arterial input function on the measured perfusion values and infarct volumetric in acute cerebral ischemia evaluated by perfusion computed tomography. Invest Radiol 2007; 42: 147–156

[32] Ferreira RM, Lev MH, Goldmakher GV et al. Arterial input function placement for accurate CT perfusion map construction in acute stroke. AJR Am J Roentgenol 2010; 194: 1330–1336

[33] Johnson G, Wetzel SG, Cha S, Babb J, Tofts PS. Measuring blood volume and vascular transfer constant from dynamic, T(2)*-weighted contrast-enhanced MRI. Magn Reson Med 2004; 51: 961–968

[34] Law M, Oh S, Johnson G et al. Perfusion magnetic resonance imaging predicts patient outcome as an adjunct to histopathology: a second reference standard in the surgical and nonsurgical treatment of low-grade gliomas. Neurosurgery 2006; 58: 1099–1107, discussion 1099–1107

[35] Jain R, Poisson L, Narang J et al. Correlation of perfusion parameters with genes related to angiogenesis regulation in glioblastoma: a feasibility study. AJNR Am J Neuroradiol 2012; 33: 1343–1348

[36] Li VW, Folkerth RD, Watanabe H et al. Microvessel count and cerebrospinal fluid basic fibroblast growth factor in children with brain tumours. Lancet 1994; 344: 82–86

[37] Weidner N. Intratumor microvessel density as a prognostic factor in cancer. Am J Pathol 1995; 147: 9–19

[38] Cha S, Johnson G, Wadghiri YZ et al. Dynamic, contrast-enhanced perfusion MRI in mouse gliomas: correlation with histopathology. Magn Reson Med 2003; 49: 848–855

[39] Aronen HJ, Pardo FS, Kennedy DN et al. High microvascular blood volume is associated with high glucose uptake and tumor angiogenesis in human gliomas. Clin Cancer Res 2000; 6: 2189–2200

[40] Raatschen HJ, Simon GH, Fu Y et al. Vascular permeability during antiangiogenesis treatment: MR imaging assay results as biomarker for subsequent tumor growth in rats. Radiology 2008; 247: 391–399

[41] Plate KH, Breier G, Weich HA, Risau W. Vascular endothelial growth factor is a potential tumour angiogenesis factor in human gliomas in vivo. Nature 1992; 359: 845–848

[42] Shweiki D, Itin A, Soffer D, Keshet E. Vascular endothelial growth factor induced by hypoxia may mediate hypoxia-initiated angiogenesis. Nature 1992; 359: 843–845

[43] Jain RK, Munn LL, Fukumura D. Dissecting tumour pathophysiology using intravital microscopy. Nat Rev Cancer 2002; 2: 266–276

[44] Bhujwalla ZM, Artemov D, Natarajan K, Solaiyappan M, Kollars P, Kristjansen PE. Reduction of vascular and permeable regions in solid tumors detected by macromolecular contrast magnetic resonance imaging after treatment with antiangiogenic agent TNP-470. Clin Cancer Res 2003; 9: 355–362

[45] Provenzale JM, Mukundan S, Dewhirst M. The role of blood-brain barrier permeability in brain tumor imaging and therapeutics. AJR Am J Roentgenol 2005; 185: 763–767

[46] Folkman J, Cole P, Zimmerman S. Tumor behavior in isolated perfused organs: in vitro growth and metastases of biopsy material in rabbit thyroid and canine intestinal segment. Ann Surg 1966; 164: 491–502

[47] Folkman J. Tumor angiogenesis: therapeutic implications. N Engl J Med 1971; 285: 1182–1186

[48] Folkman J. The role of angiogenesis in tumor growth. Semin Cancer Biol 1992; 3: 65–71

[49] Folkman J. Role of angiogenesis in tumor growth and metastasis. Semin Oncol 2002; 29 Suppl 16: 15–18

[50] Jain R, Griffith B, Khalil K, Scarpace L, Mikkelsen T, Schultz L. Glioma angiogenesis and angiogenic switch: through the eyes of perfusion imaging. Presented at: 7th Annual Meeting of American Society of Functional Neuroradiology; Charleston, SC; March 12, 2013

[51] Lev MH, Ozsunar Y, Henson JW et al. Glial tumor grading and outcome prediction using dynamic spin-echo MR susceptibility mapping compared with conventional contrast-enhanced MR: confounding effect of elevated rCBV of oligodendrogliomas [corrected]. AJNR Am J Neuroradiol 2004; 25: 214–221

[52] Law M, Yang S, Wang H et al. Glioma grading: sensitivity, specificity, and predictive values of perfusion MR imaging and proton MR spectroscopic imaging compared with conventional MR imaging. AJNR Am J Neuroradiol 2003; 24: 1989–1998

[53] Ding B, Ling HW, Chen KM, Jiang H, Zhu YB. Comparison of cerebral blood volume and permeability in preoperative grading of intracranial glioma using CT perfusion imaging. Neuroradiology 2006; 48: 773–781

[54] Jain R, Narang J, Griffith B et al. Prognostic vascular imaging biomarkers in high-grade gliomas: tumor permeability as an adjunct to blood volume estimates. Acad Radiol 2013; 20: 478–485

[55] Xyda A, Haberland U, Klotz E et al. Diagnostic performance of whole brain volume perfusion CT in intra-axial brain tumors: preoperative classification accuracy and histopathologic correlation. Eur J Radiol 2012; 81: 4105–4111

[56] Sugita Y, Terasaki M, Shigemori M, Sakata K, Morimatsu M. Acute focal demyelinating disease simulating brain tumors: histopathologic guidelines for an accurate diagnosis. Neuropathology 2001; 21: 25–31

[57] Annesley-Williams D, Farrell MA, Staunton H, Brett FM. Acute demyelination, neuropathological diagnosis, and clinical evolution. J Neuropathol Exp Neurol 2000; 59: 477–489

[58] Zagzag D, Miller DC, Kleinman GM, Abati A, Donnenfeld H, Budzilovich GN. Demyelinating disease versus tumor in surgical neuropathology. Clues to a correct pathological diagnosis. Am J Surg Pathol 1993; 17: 537–545

[59] Prineas JW, MacDonald WI. Demyelinating diseases. In: Graham DI, Lantos PL, eds. Greenfield's Neuropathology. 6th ed. London, UK: Oxford University Press; 1997:814–846

[60] Mills SJ, Patankar TA, Haroon HA, Balériaux D, Swindell R, Jackson A. Do cerebral blood volume and contrast transfer coefficient predict prognosis in human glioma? AJNR Am J Neuroradiol 2006; 27: 853–858

[61] Aronen HJ, Gazit IE, Louis DN et al. Cerebral blood volume maps of gliomas: comparison with tumor grade and histologic findings. Radiology 1994; 191: 41–51

[62] Law M, Oh S, Babb JS et al. Low-grade gliomas: dynamic susceptibility-weighted contrast-enhanced perfusion MR imaging—prediction of patient clinical response. Radiology 2006; 238: 658–667

[63] Bisdas S, Kirkpatrick M, Giglio P, Welsh C, Spampinato MV, Rumboldt Z. Cerebral blood volume measurements by perfusion-weighted MR imaging in gliomas: ready for prime time in predicting short-term outcome and recurrent disease? AJNR Am J Neuroradiol 2009; 30: 681–688

[64] Hirai T, Murakami R, Nakamura H et al. Prognostic value of perfusion MR imaging of high-grade astrocytomas: long-term follow-up study. AJNR Am J Neuroradiol 2008; 29: 1505–1510

[65] Cao Y, Nagesh V, Hamstra D et al. The extent and severity of vascular leakage as evidence of tumor aggressiveness in high-grade gliomas. Cancer Res 2006; 66: 8912–8917

[66] Dhermain F, Saliou G, Parker F et al. Microvascular leakage and contrast enhancement as prognostic factors for recurrence in unfavorable low-grade gliomas. J Neurooncol 2010; 97: 81–88

[67] Kumar AJ, Leeds NE, Fuller GN et al. Malignant gliomas: MR imaging spectrum of radiation therapy- and chemotherapy-induced necrosis of the brain after treatment. Radiology 2000; 217: 377–384

[68] Chernov M, Hayashi M, Izawa M et al. Differentiation of the radiation-induced necrosis and tumor recurrence after gamma knife radiosurgery for brain metastases: importance of multi-voxel proton MRS. Minim Invasive Neurosurg 2005; 48: 228–234

[69] Langleben DD, Segall GM. PET in differentiation of recurrent brain tumor from radiation injury. J Nucl Med 2000; 41: 1861–1867

[70] Covarrubias DJ, Rosen BR, Lev MH. Dynamic magnetic resonance perfusion imaging of brain tumors. Oncologist 2004; 9: 528–537

[71] Kamiryo T, Lopes MB, Kassell NF, Steiner L, Lee KS. Radiosurgery-induced microvascular alterations precede necrosis of the brain neuropil. Neurosurgery 2001; 49: 409–414, discussion 414–415

[72] Barajas RF, Jr, Chang JS, Segal MR et al. Differentiation of recurrent glioblastoma multiforme from radiation necrosis after external beam radiation therapy with dynamic susceptibility-weighted contrast-enhanced perfusion MR imaging. Radiology 2009; 253: 486–496

[73] Barajas RF, Chang JS, Sneed PK, Segal MR, McDermott MW, Cha S. Distinguishing recurrent intra-axial metastatic tumor from radiation necrosis following gamma knife radiosurgery using dynamic susceptibility-weighted contrast-enhanced perfusion MR imaging. AJNR Am J Neuroradiol 2009; 30: 367–372

8 Diffusion-Weighted Imaging for Gliomas

Benjamin M. Ellingson, Bryan Yoo, and Whitney B. Pope

8.1 Introduction

Diffusion-weighted magnetic resonance imaging (DWI or DW-MRI) is a magnetic resonance imaging (MRI) technique that is sensitive to the Brownian, random motion of water molecules. More specifically, DWI measures the attenuation of the magnetic resonance (MR) signal due to incoherent motion from unbound water molecules. DWI was first used as a method to analyze diffusion-induced signal attenuation in chemical samples using nuclear magnetic resonance (NMR) spectroscopy[1,2] and later to analyze restricted diffusion and flow in MRI experiments.[3] Since the early 1990s, DWI has shown to be a valuable microstructural, molecular imaging tool in many aspects of neuroscience and cancer. For example, DWI has shown exquisite sensitivity to detect acute stroke,[4,5,6] has shown value as a biomarker for the assessment of early cancer treatment response,[7,8] and has even been used to identify patient subtypes that will eventually benefit from specific therapies before treatment.[9,10,11] To aid in understanding how DWI reflects specific biological changes in the microenvironment, basic principles of diffusion physics and the DWI experiment must first be described.

8.2 Diffusion Physics

8.2.1 General

Net Brownian movement of water molecules (e.g., spins, protons, or, more correctly, "water protons") can be characterized by a diffusion coefficient, D, a variable relating the concentration gradient to the rate of transfer of water molecules through a unit of area.[12] In the brain, no appreciable water concentration gradients exist (i.e., no net flux of water); however, the concentration gradients of water in the DWI experiment can be thought of in terms of the concentration of "tagged" water molecules, similar to diffusion tracer experiments where dye is used to quantify random motion of substances. For non-restricted diffusion, the mean displacement of a water molecule in a single dimension during time t follows Einstein's equation.[12,13]

$$(r - r_0) = \sqrt{6Dt} \qquad (8.1)$$

resulting in a Gaussian probability of displacement for a given water molecule:

$$P(r_0 | r, t) = \frac{1}{\sqrt{(4\pi Dt)}} e^{-\frac{(r-r_0)}{4Dt}} \qquad (8.2)$$

where r_0 is the initial position of a specific water molecule, r is the current position, D is the diffusion coefficient, and t is time. The Gaussian probability distribution of water molecule displacement forms the basis of conventional DWI quantification.

8.2.2 Diffusion Nuclear Magnetic Resonance

The time-evolving magnetization density including non-restricted self-diffusion of a single NMR species was first described by Torrey in 1956.[14] The solution is conveniently expressed in the following form:

$$\overline{M}(t) = \underbrace{\overline{M}(0)}_{\substack{\text{Initial} \\ \text{Magnetization}}} \cdot \underbrace{1 - e^{-\frac{t}{T_1}}}_{\substack{\text{Spin–Lattice} \\ \text{Relaxation}}} \cdot \underbrace{e^{-\frac{t}{T_2}}}_{\substack{\text{Spin–Spin} \\ \text{Relaxation}}} \cdot \underbrace{e^{-b \cdot D}}_{\substack{\text{Diffusion} \\ \text{Weighting}}} \qquad (8.3)$$

where the b-value represents the "level of diffusion weighting," or attenuation, of the MR signal for a given set of DWI experimental parameters (▶ Fig. 8.1). From Equation 8.3, we see that attenuation of the MR signal from nonrestricted diffusion of a single NMR species having a specific T_1 and T_2 characteristic follows a monoexponential decay that is dependent on the experimental parameters (b-value) and diffusion coefficient, D.

8.2.3 Biexponential Diffusion MR Signal Attenuation

For two NMR species with similar T1 and T2 characteristics and differing diffusion coefficients (e.g., intra- and extracellular free water), MR signal attenuation is slightly more complicated. If the diffusion time, τ, the time between "tagging" and "untagging" water molecules in the DWI experiment, is slow such that there is perfect mixing between the compartments, then the MR signal attenuation is monoexponential, with a single apparent diffusion coefficient (ADC) (▶ Fig. 8.2):

$$\frac{S(b)}{S_0} = e^{-b(f_{in}D_{in} + f_{ex}D_{ex})} \qquad (8.4)$$

and

$$ADC = f_{in}D_{in} + f_{ex}D_{ex} \qquad (8.5)$$

Here, $S(b)$ represents the MR signal intensity as a function of b-value for a given echo time and repetition time, S_0 is the MR signal intensity without diffusion weighting (i.e., $b = 0 \, \text{s/mm}^2$), f_{in} is the intracellular volume fraction, f_{ex} is the extracellular volume fraction, D_{in} is the intracellular volume fraction, and D_{ex} is the extracellular water fraction. For short diffusion times where minimal mixing between compartments occurs, MR attenuation is *biexponential* (▶ Fig. 8.2b):

$$\frac{S(b)}{S_0} = f_{in}e^{-bD_{in}} + f_{ex}e^{-bD_{ex}} \qquad (8.6)$$

In the human brain, $f_{in} \approx 0.8$, $f_{ex} \approx 0.2$, and $D_{in} < D_{ex}$ due to higher protein concentration and viscosity within the cytosol. For

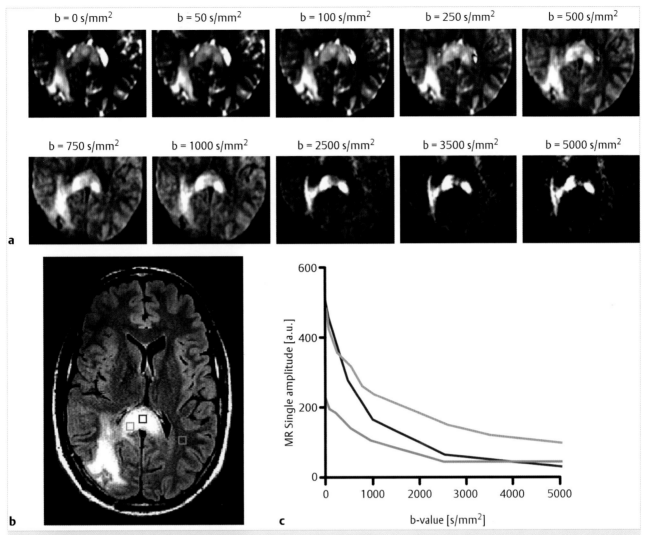

Fig. 8.1 Diffusion-weighted images (DWIs) of a glioblastoma with various levels of diffusion weighting (b-values). **(a)** DWIs with b-values ranging from 0 to 5,000 s/mm². **(b)** Regions of interest for normal-appearing contralateral white matter (green), highly dense tumor (blue), and infiltrating, less dense tumor (red). **(c)** Magnetic resonance signal intensity versus b-value for the three regions of interest. DWIs were collected with each time (TE) = 105 ms, repetition time (TR) = 13.5 s, 128 × 128 matrix size, Generalized Autocalibrating Partially Parallel Acquisition (GRAPPA) = 2, slice thickness = 3 mm (no skip), and 6/8 partial Fourier encoding.

intermediate mixing times and compartment permeability, the solution becomes increasingly complex as described by Kärger et al.[15] As such, investigators have chosen to fit "apparent" biexponential parameters to experimental data:

$$\frac{S(b)}{S_0} = f \cdot e^{-bD_{fast}} + (1-f) \cdot e^{-bD_{slow}} \qquad (8.7)$$

where f is the volume fraction of the "fast" diffusion component, D_{fast} is the larger of the two diffusion coefficients typically dominating signal attenuation at low b-values, and D_{slow} is the lower of the two diffusion coefficients typically used to explain the residual signal intensity at high b-values. The biological basis and interpretation of biexponential diffusion, however, is still a topic of controversy.[16,17]

8.2.4 Stretched-Exponential Diffusion Imaging

These early DWI experiments in the brain resulted in new exploration of diffusion models to explain nonmonoexponential diffusion behavior. In malignant brain tumors the microenvironment is highly heterogeneous, containing a variety of cell sizes and cell shapes, having highly complex and tortuous extracellular space, and containing a wide range of water concentrations from vasogenic edema and necrosis. This can result in complex patterns of signal attenuation, such that a simple mono- or biexponential model may not be as valuable. To explain this complexity, Bennett et al[18,19] demonstrated the utility of a continuously distributed, or "stretched," exponential diffusion model (also known as the Kohlrausch-Williams-Watts

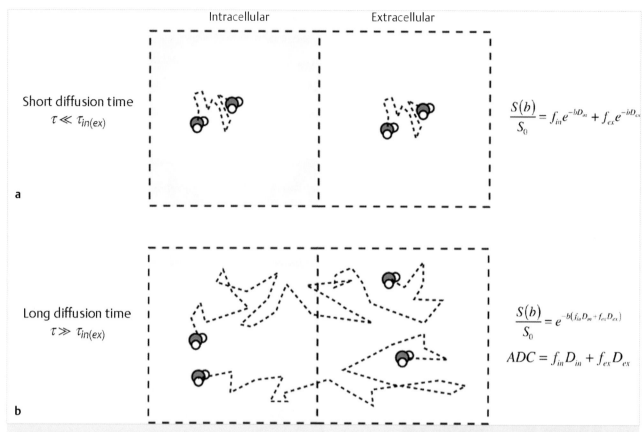

Fig. 8.2 (a) Mono- and (b) biexponential magnetic resonance signal attenuation from two water species compartment as measured with short or long diffusion times, respectively.

[KWW] function, ▶ Fig. 8.3) to explain nonmonoexponential diffusion in the human brain and brain tumors. This model is described as follows:

$$\frac{S(b)}{S_0} = e^{-(b \cdot DDC)^{\alpha}}$$ (8.8)

Here, DDC is a distributed diffusion coefficient, and α is a heterogeneity index that ranges from 0 (highly heterogeneous) to 1 (low heterogeneity, i.e., monoexponential decay). Investigations by Kwee et al[20] further suggested the heterogeneity index may be sensitive to early microscopic tumor invasion, although histological validation has not yet been performed.

8.2.5 Diffusion Kurtosis Imaging (Isotropic)

Similar to the stretched-exponential model, Jensen et al[21] described a "diffusion kurtosis model," in which the first two terms of a Taylor series expansion of the logarithm of the signal with respect to b is performed, resulting in the following description of diffusion-induced MR signal attenuation:

$$\frac{S(b)}{S_0} = e^{-b \cdot D + \frac{K \cdot b^2 \cdot D^2}{6}}$$ (8.9)

where D is the kurtosis-corrected estimate of the diffusion coefficient and K is the "kurtosis excess," or "peakedness of the

diffusion distribution." A recent study by Van Cauter et al[22] has suggested increasing diffusion kurtosis with increasing malignancy in gliomas. Additionally, a statistical model for diffusion-attenuated MR signal was proposed by Yablonskiy et al,[23] in which the total MR signal is described in terms of a probability distribution of ADC values arising from multiple water species. The model is described by the following:

$$\frac{S(b)}{S_0} = e^{-b \cdot D + \frac{\sigma^2 \cdot b^2}{2}}$$ (8.10)

where σ is the width of the ADC distribution estimate and has been shown to be on the order of 36% of ADC magnitude.

8.2.6 Quantitative Q-Space Imaging

Although probing the subvoxel environment using multiple b-value DWI can elicit important information about the complex tumor microstructure, many of these models assume water undergoes free, nonrestricted movement within the tissue environment. Using a technique in many ways analogous to X-ray crystallography, q-space imaging (QSI) or diffusion spectral imaging (DSI) is a molecular imaging technique that uses the properties of restricted diffusion to quantify a water displacement profile. Simply stated, water molecules will diffuse a mean distance for a given diffusion time and diffusion coefficient according to Einstein's equation. If this distance is longer than the boundaries of a compartment restricting

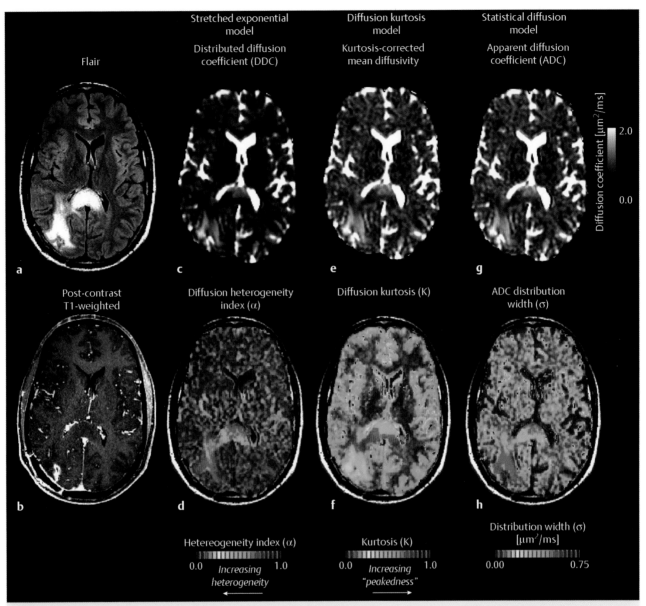

Fig. 8.3 Various diffusion models applied to multiple b-value diffusion-weighted imaging (DWI) data in a patient with glioblastoma. (a) Fluid-attenuated inversion recovery (FLAIR) and (b) postcontrast T1-weighted images showing tumor crossing the corpus callosum. (c) Distributed diffusion coefficient (DDC) and (d) diffusion heterogeneity index (α) maps showing restricted diffusion and increasing diffusion heterogeneity, respectively, within the regions of suspected infiltrating tumor. (e) Kurtosis-corrected mean diffusivity and (f) diffusion kurtosis (K) showing restricted diffusion and increased kurtosis or "peakedness," respectively, within regions of suspected tumor. (g) Apparent diffusion coefficient (ADC) and (h) ADC distribution width (σ) showing restricted diffusion and decreased width within the lesion. Model fits were created using the Analysis of Functional NeuroImages (AFNI) 3dNLfim nonlinear regression tool applied to motion and eddy current corrected DWI data with $b = 0$, 50, 100, 250, 500, 750, 1,000, 2,500, 3,500, and 5,000 s/mm², echo time (TE) = 105 ms, repetition time (TR) = 13.5 s, 128 × 128 matrix size, Generalize Autocalibrating Partially Parallel Acquisition (GRAPPA) = 2, slice thickness = 3 mm (no skip), and 6/8 partial Fourier encoding.

diffusion of the water molecule, these molecules will reflect off the boundaries and result in an increase in MR signal amplitude as water molecules approach their original position (▶ Fig. 8.4). If the MR signal amplitude is recorded for increasingly longer diffusion times, harmonics appear in intervals related to the mean compartment size. Taking the Fourier transform of the resulting q-space spectrum results in a water displacement probability density function for each image voxel, typically on the order of micrometers. ▶ Fig. 8.5 illustrates this phenomenon.

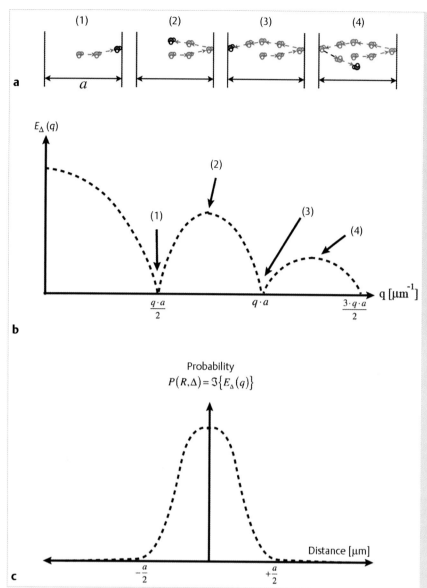

Fig. 8.4 Physical principles of q-space imaging. (a) As water molecules diffuse across a compartment, (1) the magnetic resonance (MR) signal continues to attenuate until the boundary is reached at a/2. At longer diffusion times, (2) water molecules reflect off the boundaries of the compartment and approach their original position, resulting in an increase in signal intensity. Water molecules will then continue to reflect off other boundaries (3–4). (b) This results in harmonics in the MR signal with respect to q. (c) Performing the Fourier transform of the resulting signal attenuation with respect to q results in a water displacement probability density function for a given voxel.

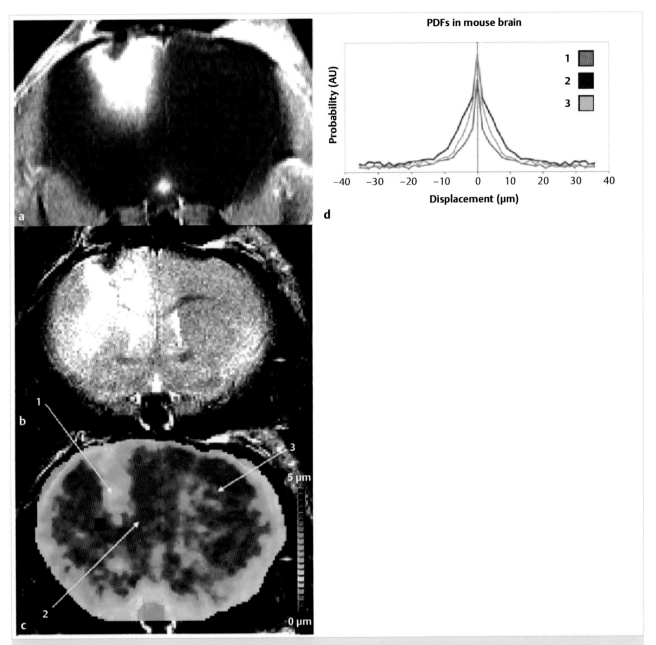

Fig. 8.5 (**a**) T1-weighted contrast-enhancing and (**b**) T2-weighted image of a GL261 glioblastoma tumor in a mouse at 7 T. (**c**) Full-width, half-maximum (FMHM) maps generated from the q-space spectrum. (**d**) Water displacement probability density functions (PDFs) for three regions of interest. Green, areas of injected tumor; red, fluidlike edematous tissue surrounding the tumor; blue, normal-appearing contralateral brain. Note that the compartment size is smaller in tumor regions compared with edematous tissue and contralateral brain tissue. Q-space data were acquired in a single-slice one-directional q-space spectrum with 49 q-values ranging from 0 to 674.3 mm⁻¹, corresponding to a maximum b-value of 34,560 s/mm², a resolution of 1.48 µm, and a maximum displacement of 35.6 µm.

8.3 Clinical Diffusion-Weighted Imaging Methodology

8.3.1 Diffusion Measurement with NMR

At the most fundamental level, diffusion weighting of MR images requires phase labeling of water molecules at an initial time point using magnetic field gradients, followed by phase refocusing after a certain diffusion time later using the same gradients. The simplest method of employing diffusion sensitivity is through the use of bipolar diffusion sensitizing gradients applied to a gradient-recalled echo (GRE) experiment. A monopolar continuous gradient can be applied to a spin-echo (SE) experiment, resulting in the same expression for b-value. In 1965, Stejskal and Tanner introduced the pulsed gradient spin-echo (PGSE) diffusion encoding scheme,[1,2] which is still one of the most popular sequences used in clinical DWI. The PGSE experiment differed from previous techniques in that a *diffusion mixing time*, Δ, was introduced into the experiment. More exotic diffusion encoding schemes have also been developed for use in clinical DWI. For example, Reese et al[24] recently developed the twice-refocused spin-echo method for diffusion preparation, which reduces eddy-current-related artifacts by introducing additional refocusing pulse and reversed polarity gradients. This sequence is now widely available on clinical scanners, but it has the disadvantage of relatively long echo times compared to other PGSE sequences. Another example of a rather common, more advanced diffusion encoding scheme is a stimulated echo acquisition mode (STEAM) PGSE, which is useful for reducing the long echo time requirements for long diffusion mixing times (Δ). In the STEAM-PGSE encoding scheme, transverse magnetization from the initial excitation pulse is tipped 90 degrees into the longitudinal orientation, where the magnetization vector decays according to the T1 relaxation instead of the shorter T2. At some later time, τ, the magnetization is tipped back into the transverse plane, the spins are refocused using the diffusion sensitizing gradients, then the spin-echo is acquired. Yet another example of an exotic diffusion encoding scheme that is clinically useful is the oscillating-gradient spin-echo (OGSE) sequence, which can be used to probe very small diffusion times while maintaining relatively large b-values.

8.3.2 Acquisition Techniques

Traditional PGSE diffusion MRI requires a single diffusion preparation per line of k-space. Although this is the simplest method of performing diffusion MRI and the method that results in the highest overall signal-to-noise ratio, it is not clinically feasible due to long acquisition times and high sensitivity to bulk motion between acquisitions. Scan time for traditional PGSE DWI can be approximated by the following:

$$t_{acq} = (\#b - values) \times (NEX) \times (\#PE) \times (TR) \times (\#Slices) \quad (8.11)$$

where #b-*values* is the total number of b-values acquired for the experiment (e.g., $b = 0$ and 1,000 s/mm^2), NEX is the number of excitations (averages), #PE is the number of phase encode lines per image slice (e.g., 64 or 128), *TR* is the repetition time, and #*Slices* are the total number of slices acquired. A single PGSE diffusion experiment for 10 slices, 2 b-values, a single average, 128 phase-encoding lines, and a TR of 4 seconds requires more than 2.8 hours (and this is measuring diffusion in only a single direction!). Thus fast acquisition strategies are crucial for overcoming challenges associated with these long scan times and making DWI clinically feasible.

Single-shot diffusion-weighted spin-echo echoplanar imaging (SS-DW-EPI) is now the most common, easy to use method for acquiring DWI data. EPI has the fastest acquisition time, allowing sampling of all of k-space in a single diffusion preparation. EPI works by using activating a rapidly switching gradient in the frequency-encoding while using another gradient to "blip" a small pulse in the phase-encoding direction. Each rapidly switching gradient in the frequency-encode direction allows for acquisition of k-space from right to left or left to right, depending on the polarity, while the blipped phase-encoding gradient moves k-space trajectory sequentially from one line to the next. Because all of k-space is acquired in a single excitation, the time for SS-DW-EPI can be approximated by the following:

$$t_{acq} = (\#b - values) \times (NEX) \times (TR) \quad (8.12)$$

Note that the number of slices is limited by the chosen TR, where longer TR values allow for more k-space coverage and thereby more slices. Note that DWI acquisition for a single PGSE diffusion experiment for 10 slices, 2 b-values, a single average, 128 phase-encoding lines, and a TR of 4 seconds is only 8 seconds, compared with 2.8 hours without EPI! (Note that this is only for a single direction.) Despite SS-DW-EPI being the fastest and most common sequence for clinical DWI, comparatively it has relatively low image quality and high sensitivity to image artifacts, including susceptibility-related geometric distortions and chemical shift artifacts.

Segmented or multishot EPI acquisition is a compromise between the high signal-to-noise traditional PGSE acquisition and the fast SS-DW-EPI. Multishot EPI allows for acquisition of k-space by dividing it into a specific number of segments.[25] Thus multishot EPI allows for a shorter echo train and effective echo time compared to SS-DW-EPI, resulting in reduction of geometric distortions and higher physical resolutions (▶ Fig. 8.6). The acquisition time, however, increases proportional to the number of segments when directly compared to SS-DW-EPI acquisition. Multishot EPI, however, is highly sensitive to phase errors between shots resulting from motion,[26] which results in image ghosting and other artifacts. Correction of these phase errors is typically performed through the use of navigator echoes that measure the phase errors and retrospectively correct them prior to reconstruction.[27,28]

Diffusion-weighted turbo spin-echo (TSE) and fast spin-echo (FSE) are acquisition with rapid acquisition with relaxation enhancement (RARE) sequences involving refocusing radiofrequency (RF) excitation pulses between each line or multiple lines of k-space acquisition. RF refocusing results in formation of spin-echoes, which, when used to fill k-space, decreases the observed relaxation time (T2* decay effects), echo train length, and geometric distortions while increasing signal-to-noise in resulting DWIs. RARE sequences are commonly employed in hybrid with EPI, where multiple lines of k-space are sampled between each RF refocusing pulse. In this way, RARE sequences can be very fast while reducing effective echo train length and

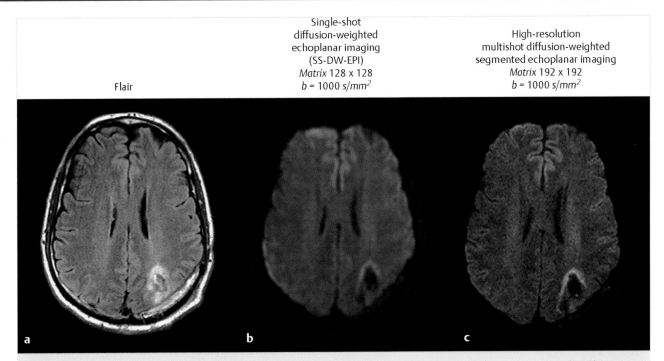

| Flair | Single-shot diffusion-weighted echoplanar imaging (SS-DW-EPI) Matrix 128 x 128 $b = 1000 \, s/mm^2$ | High-resolution multishot diffusion-weighted segmented echoplanar imaging Matrix 192 x 192 $b = 1000 \, s/mm^2$ |

Fig. 8.6 Comparison of echoplanar acquisition techniques in a patient with glioblastoma. **(a)** Fluid-attenuated inversion recovery (FLAIR) image showing a left parietal lesion. **(b)** Standard single-shot diffusion-weighted echoplanar image showing restricted diffusion along the resection cavity. **(c)** High-resolution, multishot (nine excitations) diffusion-weighted segmented echoplanar image.

reducing chemical shift artifacts. Unfortunately, RARE sequences also increase the specific absorption rate (SAR) and tissue heating compared with other sequences from administration of additional RF energy.

Radial or spiral acquisition techniques can be advantageous when patient head motion is problematic. Unlike Cartesian sampling of k-space, radial acquisition techniques traverse through the center of k-space at least once in each excitation (similar to the orientation of spokes on a bicycle), while spiral acquisition techniques consist of a curved k-space trajectory typically moving from the center to the periphery of k-space (or less commonly the periphery to the center of k-space). This results in a high sampling density in center k-space regions compared to the periphery. Since the center of k-space is highly sampled, radial acquisition techniques are less prone to issues related to data acquisition and corruption, have relatively high signal-to-noise, and can be easily compensated for patient motion through phase-error correction. Unfortunately, azimuthal regions of k-space are highly undersampled; therefore, radial or spiral acquisition techniques can result in unique "aura"-like artifacts.[29] Radial EPI techniques, including periodically rotated overlapping parallel lines with enhanced reconstruction (PROPELLER) and BLADE sequences, involve acquisition of multiple lines of central k-space using echoplanar encoding techniques separated by periodic rotations of k-space trajectories[30,31] and are also commonly implemented clinical DWI techniques.

8.4 Postprocessing Techniques

There are numerous postprocessing techniques that can be used to improve accuracy of diffusion measurements and expand the biological insight of diffusion MR images in brain tumors. Some techniques are basic and easy to implement, whereas others require a more advanced knowledge of computer programming and MR physics.

8.4.1 Eddy Current Correction

Dielectric properties of biological tissues combined with the large, rapidly changing magnetic field gradients can result in eddy currents that form residual magnetic fields during the acquisition portion of the DWI experiment. EPI readout during the time-varying eddy current–induced magnetic fields results in geometric distortions depending on the direction of the diffusion-encoding gradients. Eddy current distortions can be corrected post hoc[32] either by B_0-field correction[33]; by dual echo blip-reversed EPI correction,[34] where an EPI image is collected without diffusion weighting then another EPI images is collected with the same acquisition parameters but with the frequency directions swapped; or by affine-based registration of diffusion-weighted images to a non-diffusion-weighted image (e.g., $b = 0 \, s/mm^2$ images).[35] Software for B_0 and eddy current correction is currently not implemented on most MR system consoles, but it is available from offline from various research laboratories (e.g., methods from Chen et al[33] can be found at: http://www.nitrc.org/projects/dtic/). A comprehensive review article is available from Andersson et al,[36] which outlines practical implementation of eddy current correction using B_0 field and gradient characteristic information. Additionally, software code for affine-based registration is available from the FMRIB Software Library (FSL's *eddy_correct* script; http://fsl.fmrib.ox.ac.uk/fsl/).

8.4.2 Diffusion Parameter Estimation

Estimation of quantitative diffusion parameters from diffusion-weighted images can be performed in a number of ways. For isotropic diffusion measurements, the DWI experiment is repeated in three orthogonal directions with diffusion sensitizing gradients applied in the *x*, *y*, and *z* directions. For single, monoexponential ADC estimation from two DWIs with different b-values, ADC is directly calculated:

$$\text{ADC} = -\frac{1}{(b_2 - b_1)} \ln \frac{(S_{b_2})}{(S_{b_1})} \qquad (8.13)$$

where b_2 is the larger b-value (e.g., $b = 1{,}000\,\text{s/mm}^2$), b_1 is the smaller b-value (e.g., $b = 0\,\text{s/mm}^2$), S_{b1} is the MR signal intensity in an image voxel with b-value = b_1, S_{b2} is the MR signal intensity in an image voxel with b-value = b_2, and *ln* denotes the natural logarithm. When more than one b-value is collected, linear regression can be used to fit Equation 8.13 across multiple b-values. Alternatively, nonlinear least squares regression can be used to fit the model:

$$S(b) = A \cdot e^{-b \cdot \text{ADC}} \qquad (8.14)$$

where *S(b)* is the MR signal intensity for a particular b-value, and *A* is a free parameter corresponding to the estimated signal intensity for $b = 0\,\text{s/mm}^2$. Estimation of parameters from sophisticated diffusion models, including biexponential, kurtosis, and stretched-exponential diffusion imaging models, can be performed using a similar nonlinear regression approach. Nonlinear regression optimizers are available through a variety of freely available software packages, including the Analysis of Functional NeuroImages from the National Institutes of Health (AFNI 3dNLfim; http://afni.nimh.nih.gov/afni/) and MATLAB (matrix laboratory) toolboxes (MathWorks, Inc., Natick, MA).

8.4.3 ADC Histogram Analyses

Tissue microstructure within brain tumors is very spatially heterogeneous. Therefore, techniques aimed at quantifying global tumor characteristics and heterogeneity provide rich information regarding tumor composition. ADC histogram analysis, broadly speaking, involves extraction of diffusion measurements from well-defined regions of interest (ROIs) obtained from structural MRI datasets (typically contrast-enhancing or T2 hyperintense regions), then parameterization of these ADC characteristics within the ROIs. Mean, median, minimum, standard deviation, and skewness can all be considered various parameters extracted from ADC histogram analysis. Mean and standard deviation of ADC characteristics within an ROI are considered parameters relating to a single-compartment Gaussian model. More sophisticated models of multiple tissue compartments, such as the two-compartment Gaussian mixed model, are defined as follows:

$$p(\text{ADC}) = f \cdot N(\mu_{\text{ADC}_L}, \sigma_{\text{ADC}_L}) + (1 - f) \cdot N(\mu_{\text{ADC}_H}, \sigma_{\text{ADC}_H}) \qquad (8.15)$$

where *p(ADC)* is the probability of a voxel having a particular ADC value within the ROI, *f* is the fraction of all voxels in the lower of the two Gaussian distributions, *N(μ,σ)* represents a normal (Gaussian) distribution with mean μ and standard deviation σ, and ADC_L represents the lower and ADC_H represents the larger of the two Gaussian distributions.

8.4.4 Functional Diffusion Mapping

Functional diffusion mapping (fDM) is a voxel-wise subtraction technique that quantifies regional changes in ADC after treatment or during clinical follow-up.[37,38,39,40,41,42,43,44,45,46] More specifically, fDMs involve image registration of ADC maps from subsequent days to a single, baseline (e.g., pretreatment) ADC map. Voxels are then characterized according to the degree of change in ADC between the two scan dates based on empirical or a priori data. The typical threshold for a change in ADC using traditional fDM analysis is $0.4\,\mu\text{m}^2/\text{ms}$, measured as the 95% confidence interval for a 50% mixture of normal-appearing white and gray matter in 69 brain tumor patients with follow-up times ranging from 1 week to 5 years.[45] Voxels with decreasing ADC are typically thought to reflect regions where tumor cells are becoming more concentrated, either by proliferation or by reduction in vasogenic edema, whereas voxels with increasing ADC are thought to reflect regions with decreasing cell density, either from tumor destruction, necrosis, or edema.

Traditional (Linear) fDM Analysis. Linear fDM analysis first involves conversion of diffusion MR data into ADC maps for each respective day. Next, a 12-degree-of-freedom affine-based registration algorithm is used to align ADC maps from subsequent days to baseline time points. This is performed either by alignment of high-resolution anatomical scans then subsequent application of the resulting transformation matrix to ADC maps, or, alternatively, by direct registration of ADC maps at the different time points. This process can be performed using a variety of freely available software packages, including FSL's FLIRT command. Next, voxel-wise subtraction of follow-up ADC values from baseline ADC values is performed. Voxels are then labeled "blue" if they have decreased in ADC beyond $0.4\,\mu\text{m}^2/\text{ms}$, "red" if they have increased in ADC beyond $0.4\,\mu\text{m}^2/\text{ms}$, and "green" if they have not changed beyond these thresholds. The volume of tissue with increasing (red), decreasing (blue), or changing (red or blue), or the volume fraction of tumor exhibiting these changes, is then quantified in either the contrast-enhancing or the T2 hyperintense ROIs.

Nonlinear fDM Analysis. Tumor growth and response to therapy can dramatically alter the morphology of the brain; thus traditional fDM analysis may be inaccurate or difficult to interpret due to image registration errors from resulting tissue displacement. To overcome this potential issue, nonlinear registration of either anatomical images or ADC maps directly has been investigated.[43] The concept is to use an additional elastic (nonlinear) registration step after linear registration in order to better align ADC map information prior to voxel-wise classification.

Probabilistic fDM Analysis. A new technique for quantifying the uncertainty of fDM classification with respect to linear alignment of ADC maps has been described.[42] This technique involves the standard linear registration steps, with the addition of purposeful, repeated, finite perturbation of the alignment between ADC maps in translation, rotation, and/or skew. After each perturbation, fDM classification is performed according to the standard empirical thresholds ($0.4\,\mu\text{m}^2/\text{ms}$), then this process is repeated hundreds to thousands of times. The frequency in which a given voxel is classified as increasing or decreasing, or the probability of a voxel being classified as increasing or decreasing over all perturbations, is retained and used for subsequent analysis. The total probability of ADC increasing or decreasing beyond a specific threshold, over a specific ROI, is used to evaluate tumor response.

8.4.5 Cell Invasion, Motility, and Proliferation Level Estimate Maps

The observations that ADC estimates correlate with tumor cell density and changes in ADC reflect physiological changes in cell density (as measured using fDMs) has led to the formation of a comprehensive spatiotemporal model for estimation of tumor growth and invasion parameters. Specifically, this technique, termed cell invasion, motility, and proliferation level estimates (CIMPLE maps), states that the rate of change in tumor cell density within a voxel, estimated by the rate of change in ADC, is equal to the rate at which tumor cells are being generated plus the rate at which they are invading the voxel from adjacent voxels. Using ADC as a surrogate for cell density in this context, spatiotemporal changes in ADC can be modeled as follows:

$$\underbrace{\frac{d}{dt}ADC(t)}_{\substack{\text{Rate of Change} \\ \text{in Cell Density}}} = \underbrace{\rho \cdot ADC(t)}_{\text{Proliferation}} + \underbrace{\nabla \cdot (D\nabla ADC(t))}_{\text{Invasion}} \tag{8.16}$$

where ∇ is the spatial gradient operator and ∇ is the divergence operator. Using three or more ADC maps collected in the same patient, the proliferation rate estimate ρ and invasion rate estimate D at time point n can be calculated as follows:

$$\rho(n) = \frac{1}{ADC^{n-1}}\left(\frac{d}{dt}ADC^{n-1} - D\nabla^2 ADC^{n-1} - \nabla D \cdot ADC^{n-1}\right) \tag{8.17}$$

$$D(n) = \frac{\frac{d}{dt}ADC^n - \lambda \cdot \frac{d}{dt}ADC^{n-1}}{\nabla^2 ADC^n - \lambda \cdot \nabla^2 ADC^{n-1}} \tag{8.18}$$

where ∇^2 is the Laplacian, or second-order, spatial gradient, and $\lambda = ADC^n / ADC^{n-1}$.

8.5 Clinical Applications of Diffusion-Weighted Imaging

DWI in patients with glioma has been investigated as a means to add value to standard pulse sequences in determining patient prognosis and disease status. Diffusion imaging has also been employed to help distinguish glioma from other tumors and tumor mimics that can have a similar appearance on standard MRI. The goal is to improve clinical decision making, thereby improving patient outcomes. Following maximal tumor resection and concurrent chemo- and radiation therapy, a patient must be assessed for residual tumor, treatment-related injury, and treatment response and then followed for evidence of tumor recurrence or progression. The last determination

requires the ability to distinguish enhancement associated with tumor from that due to treatment effect (pseudoprogression), which remains a significant challenge in neuro-oncology. Diffusion imaging can be used to calculate the ADC, which provides information on tissue microstructure, and is thought to be mostly sensitive to the extracellular volume fraction.[47] Interpreting these data leads to improved understanding of several processes that are related to treatment effect and tumor status. For instance, vasogenic edema, as well as necrosis and disruption of cellular integrity, act to increase the extracellular water fraction and result in increased ADC. Conversely, cytotoxic edema (cell swelling) and increased tissue cell density result in decreased ADC. Extrapolating this information, it would be expected that more highly cellular tumors and regions of tumor cell proliferation would exhibit lower ADC values (unless counteracted by vasogenic edema related to opening of the blood–brain barrier). Agents that reduce vasogenic edema, such as steroids and antiangiogenic treatments, reduce ADC. Ischemia, resulting in cytotoxic edema, also diminishes ADC. Conversely, treatment effect that results in cell death, whether due to cytotoxic chemotherapy or to radiation-induced necrosis, would be expected to increase ADC. Although diffusion imaging is a promising venue to improve our assessment of tumor status, most of the subsequently discussed diffusion-based analyses remain exploratory due to lack of standardization and multicenter validation among other causes.

8.5.1 Distinguishing Glioma from Other Masses

Gliomas and other mass lesions can have a similar appearance on MRI, oftentimes resulting in a differential, rather than a specific, diagnosis. The ability to distinguish glioblastoma multiforme (GBM) from other ring-enhancing lesions (abscess, single metastasis, tumefactive multiple sclerosis) remains a common diagnostic challenge. An important advance came from studies dating back to 1996,[48] which showed that well-formed abscesses typically demonstrate "restricted diffusion" with corresponding low ADC values, whereas areas of tumor-induced necrosis, either related to GBM or to metastases, are usually increased in ADC (▶ Fig. 8.7). More recently several groups have used diffusion imaging to try to reliably differentiate GBM from metastasis. For instance, Lee et al[49] assessed minimum ADC values in tumor and peritumoral regions in 38 GBM patients compared to 35 patients with metastases. They found that the peritumoral minimum ADC (normalized against contralateral normal-appearing white matter) was significantly lower in GBM compared to metastatic disease. Using a receiver operating characteristic (ROC) curve analysis and a cutoff value of 1.3×10^{-3} mm^2/s for the minimum peritumoral ADC value, they achieved a sensitivity of 83% and specificity of 79% for distinguishing GBM from metastases in this retrospective analysis. They (and others) hypothesize that peritumoral edema is infiltrated by tumor cells in patients with GBM, but not metastases, and, because there is an inverse correlation between cell density and ADC,[45,50] it would be expected that peritumoral edema in GBM would have diminished ADC values, unlike the peritumoral edema of metastases.

In an attempt to further improve diagnostic certainty, diffusion tensor imaging (DTI) metrics have been tested for the

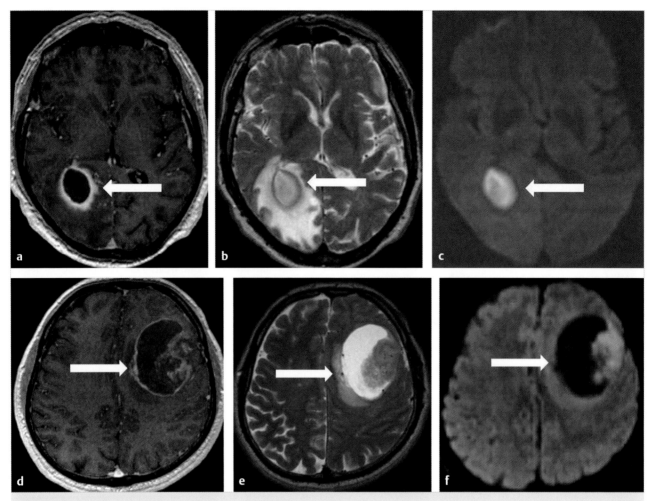

Fig. 8.7 Diffusion imaging in cerebral abscess (**a-c**) and GBM (**d-f**). Cerebral abscesses and GBM can both present as ring-enhancing lesions on post-contrast T1-weighted imaging (**a,d**) with perilesional edema best seen on T2-weighted images (**b,e**). However abscesses, as in this case, often show restricted diffusion and are very bright on DWI (**c**). In contrast, the GBM shows only mild DWI hyperintensity (**f**) in the enhancing nodule along the lateral margin of the necrotic region, but the necrotic area itself (arrows) shows no diffusion signal hyperintensity.

ability to improve upon standard diffusion imaging for the differentiation of abscess, GBM, and cystic metastases. Toh et al[51] analyzed multiple DTI metrics in 15 abscesses, 15 necrotic GBM, and 26 cystic metastases and found that, using an area under the curve (AUC) analysis, the fractional anisotropy, linear tensor, and spheric tensor outperformed ADC in discriminating these lesions from one another. In fact, fractional anisotropy (FA) was 100% accurate in differentiating abscess from GBM/cystic metastases. However, differentiating GBM from single metastases is typically the more challenging issue, because abscesses, as mentioned, can usually be identified based on diffusion restriction. Unfortunately FA does not appear to be able to accurately separate metastases from high-grade gliomas.[52] Thus further development of these and other techniques will be required before patients can be confidently diagnosed with glioma based on these imaging findings.

8.5.2 Predicting Tumor Grade and Histology

Conventional interpretation of tumor MRI has relied on contrast enhancement as a marker for malignancy, where high-grade gliomas typically demonstrate moderate to strong contrast enhancement, and low-grade gliomas have minimal or no enhancement.[53] However, a broad spectrum of tumor histological types and grades may present as nonenhancing lesions. For instance, it has been shown that nonenhancing gliomas are malignant (grade III and IV) in up to 20 to 33% of cases.[54,55] Even a small portion of glioblastomas do not enhance on presentation scans.[56] Additional imaging characteristics such as mass effect and necrosis are correlated with tumor aggressiveness.[56,57] A high-grade glioma may be mistaken for a low-grade glioma when it demonstrates minimal edema, no contrast enhancement, and no necrosis, thereby presenting a diagnostic challenge and impacting treatment decisions (▶ Fig. 8.8).

Several studies have examined whether DWI and quantification of ADC values can be used to predict tumor grade.[50,58,59,60,61,62,63,64,65] Sugahara et al[50] hypothesized that highly cellular tumors should have reduced ADC values due to decreased interstitial space, thereby limiting the free diffusion of water. They evaluated 20 patients with histologically proven gliomas and showed that tumor cellularity correlated well with minimum ADC values ($r = 0.77$). They also demonstrated the mean minimum ADC values of high-grade gliomas were significantly

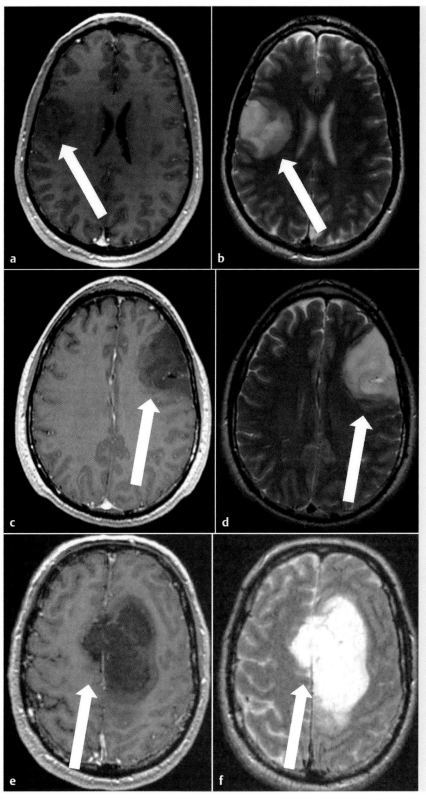

Fig. 8.8 Nonenhancing tumors (arrows) grade II, III, and IV. Postcontrast T1-weighted (**a,c,e**) and T2-weighted (**b,d,f**) images of grade II oligoastrocytoma (**a,b**), grade III oligoastrocytoma (**c,d**), and glioblastoma multiforme (**e,f**). Note the similar appearance between tumor grades with lack of contrast enhancement, and little peritumoral edema.

lower than low-grade gliomas (1.2 vs. 2.7×10^{-3} mm^2/s). This was the first demonstration of the relationship of cellularity to ADC values, and the potential to estimate tumor grade using diffusion imaging.

Later studies confirmed that ADC values were correlated with cellularity based on stereotactic image-guided biopsy specimens.[45] This was shown for gliomas grade II, III, and IV, as well as gliomatosis cerebri. An important caveat is that, although

ADC is correlated to cellularity, other tumor features also impact ADC measurements. For instance, ischemia, compression related to tumor mass effect, and edema levels, among other factors, can all affect ADC values; thus the relationship between cell density and ADC is not one to one.[66]

The population difference in ADC values between high- and low-grade gliomas has been confirmed in a number of studies.[58,59,62,63] For instance, in a larger retrospective study of 51 patients Arvinda et al[63] recorded minimum ADC tumoral values and found that 0.985×10^{-3} mm^2/s was the optimal ADC threshold to distinguish high- versus low-grade gliomas. This analysis yielded a sensitivity, specificity, positive predictive value (PPV), and negative predictive value (NPV) of 90, 87.1, 81.81, and 93.10%, respectively, representing a substantial improvement over conventional MRI. Similar results have been reported in at least one prospective analysis.[59]

The relationship between ADC values and tumor grade has also been studied, specifically in nonenhancing tumors.[62] Regions of nonenhancing grade III gliomas were found to have ADC values less than contralateral normal-appearing white matter, whereas grade I and II gliomas did not demonstrate significantly lower ADC values. Further, there was no significant difference when comparing ADC values of high- and low-grade gliomas directly.

Another area of interest is the relationship between ADC and tumor grade within a glioma subtype (i.e., tumors of astrocytic vs. oligodendrocytic lineages). As is the case for gliomas in general, ADC of grade III oligodendrogliomas is lower than that of grade II oligodendrogliomas,[65] with an optimal cutoff of 0.925×10^{-3} mm^2/s. Differences in ADC have also been evaluated by glioma subtype within the same grade (grade II)[64]: oligodendrogliomas were found to have ADC histograms shifted to the left (i.e., containing lower values) compared with astrocytomas. Using a multiple discriminant analysis based on ADC histograms, the authors were able to correctly classify 83% of subjects according to tumor subtype (oligodendroglioma, oligoastrocytoma, or astrocytoma).

One substantial limitation in the clinical applicability of these analyses is that, although population differences in ADC values by tumor grade and subtype clearly exist, there is a great deal of overlap between the patient cohorts, so that these metrics are not accurate enough for diagnosis on an individualized basis. Therefore Murakami et al[58] sought to improve differentiation of tumor grades by combining minimum ADC values with "ADC difference values" to generate a two-parameter method in the hopes of improving diagnostic accuracy. "ADC difference" is defined as the difference between the minimum and maximum region of interest (ROI) values within the solid portion of a tumor, and is thereby a reflection, to some degree, of tumor heterogeneity. The authors found that higher-grade tumors tended not only to have lower minimum ADC, as previously reported, but also had higher tumor ADC heterogeneity (increased ADC difference value). This method appeared to improve upon the use of minimum ADC alone as a way of distinguishing tumors of varying grades because it was accurate in predicting grade for 41 out of 50 tumors. Even so, some overlap between tumor groups based on these diffusion metrics remained, awaiting additional refinements of this technique.

In addition to overlapping diffusion metrics, several additional limitations must be overcome before these techniques can be used for routine patient care. Technical limitations and lack of standardization remain a challenge. For instance, there is significant variation in methods of measuring ADC values, which causes difficulties, such as the reliable establishment of thresholds for high- versus low-grade gliomas. The inclusion/exclusion of necrotic regions, areas of enhancement, and other variables affect ADC values, and even when these criteria are precisely defined, the generation of minimum ROIs has a fair degree of interobserver variability.[63] Another major issue is the method of ADC value normalization. Although this is typically performed using contralateral white matter, we, and others, have found that this can introduce additional sources of error.[63] Accurate registration of ADC maps to the anatomical images also remains a challenge because ADC images can be sensitive to distortion, resulting in significant registration errors.[42,43] The combination of diffusion imaging with adjunct physiological MR modalities such as MR spectroscopy and perfusion-weighted imaging may be helpful in improving diffusion-based biomarker performance.[59,63] Alternately, more sophisticated measures of water diffusivity such as DTI and diffusion kurtosis may overcome some limitations of conventional diffusion imaging in assessing tumor grade.[22,67,68]

8.5.3 Molecular Features of Glioma: MGMT Promoter Methylation

An important molecular feature of malignant gliomas is the methylation status of the O6-methylguanine-DNA methyltransferase (MGMT) gene promoter, which is associated with improved patient prognosis and chemotherapy (temozolomide) sensitivity.[69] However, methylation status can currently be determined only by interrogating surgical or biopsy specimens. As such, noninvasive evaluation of MGMT methylation status could be highly useful. A few studies have compared ADC values in methylated versus nonmethylated tumors. One study[70] found that methylated tumors had higher minimum ADC values (0.88 vs. 0.67×10^{-3} mm^2/s) than nonmethylated tumors. A minimum ADC value of 0.8×10^{-3} mm^2/s was proposed as the optimal cutoff to distinguish methylated versus nonmethylated tumors with a sensitivity of 94% and a specificity of 91%. Another study[71] focused on mean, instead of minimum, ADC values of GBM with similar results: methylated tumors had higher mean ADC values than nonmethylated tumors (1.3 vs. 1.1×10^{-3} mm^2/s). ADC values were correlated with progression-free survival in both studies; whether or not this is directly related to the association of ADC and MGMT promoter methylation is an interesting topic for further investigation.

8.5.4 Patient Prognosis

The relationship between tumor ADC and patient outcomes has also been an area of active investigation in recent years. For instance, Higano et al[72] compared pretreatment minimum ADC values to patient status (progressive vs. stable disease) at 2-year follow-up in a group of subjects with grade III and IV gliomas (22 GBM, 15 anaplastic astrocytoma). They found that lower ADC values were associated with a higher Ki-67 index (a proliferation marker) and with poorer outcomes. However, because GBMs have higher Ki-67 and shorter survival than anaplastic astrocytomas, the question arises as to whether these data simply reflect the association of low minimum ADC with GBM, rather than being an independent marker of prognosis. This is of concern given that within the GBM-only group there was no separation of progressors versus nonprogressors based on ADC values. Further, in another study,[73] there was no significant difference in survival of patients with GBM ($n = 21$) based on mean ADC of contrast-enhancing regions, although the analysis was performed on residual tumor following surgery, rather than on preoperative scans, as in the paper by Higano et al.[72]

To specifically address this issue of the added value of diffusion imaging in determining prognosis, a group from Kumamoto University combined analysis of ADC values with Radiation Therapy Oncology Group recursive partitioning analysis (RTOG-RPA) class (an RPA that includes clinical data such as age, extent of resection, and Karnofsky performance status). They found added value of minimum pretreatment tumor ADC in a cohort of malignant gliomas[74] and, subsequently, also in a very large ($n = 139$) group of GBM only patients.[75] In this latter study, the investigators found that, in a multivariate Cox model, low minimum ADC conferred a greater hazard ratio (HR) of dying (HR = 2.4) than either Karnofsky performance status (HR = 1.8) or tumor residual after resection (HR = 1.8). This study provides substantial evidence that ADC analyses can yield independent prognostic information that adds value to clinical data.

The imaging phenotypes of tumor features that may account for this association of outcomes with ADC are now being investigated at the molecular level. For instance, Barajas et al[76] demonstrated an inverse correlation between relative ADC and histopathological features of tumor aggressiveness (microvascular expression, hypoxia, cellular density, tumor density). It has been hypothesized that there is a link between malignant tumor phenotypes, molecular features including gene expression, and tumor physiology.[77,78,79] The latter provides an avenue for advanced MR sequences such as perfusion or diffusion imaging to provide added value in which the entire tumor is noninvasively characterized. Our recent data support this hypothesis as we have shown an association between higher ADC values and extracellular matrix gene expression including several collagen isoforms.[80] The importance of this finding is due to the relationship between collagen deposition and promotion of invasion in GBM,[81] which is a central feature of the disease and of paramount importance in its lethality. These, as well as studies linking ADC values to MGMT promoter methylation discussed earlier, are merely the first steps in characterizing the interdependent domains of imaging, molecular features, tumor biology, and clinical outcomes.

8.5.5 Predictive Biomarker of Treatment Response

In addition to development as a marker of patient prognosis (irrespective of treatment), diffusion imaging has also been investigated as a means to generate a marker of response to specific therapies, that is, as a *predictive* biomarker. In May 2009 the Food and Drug Administration (FDA) gave accelerated approval for the treatment of recurrent GBM with the antivascular endothelial growth factor (VEGF) antibody bevacizumab (Avastin, Genentech, South San Francisco, CA).[82] The response to this and other antiangiogenic therapy is highly variable; some patients do well and others show no response.[83,84]

Treatment with antiangiogenic agents can preclude a patient from being enrolled in other investigational drug studies. Therefore, it would be of potential benefit to be able to predict a patient's response to bevacizumab prior to treatment initiation. In the first paper characterizing the imaging response of malignant glioma to bevacizumab treatment, we noted that areas of highly necrotic-appearing tumor seemed to have a particularly good response to therapy.[83] We hypothesized that, because these areas of necrosis would also be expected to have high ADC values due to loss of cellular integrity, there may be a relationship between ADC and response to bevacizumab treatment. Therefore we constructed ADC histograms of enhancing tumor regions and noted that tumors with lower and narrower ADC histograms seemed to progress earlier than tumors that showed broader histograms containing higher ADC values. We analyzed this relationship in several studies, both from our own data and from data derived from multicenter trials. We found that the histograms could be well fitted with a 2-normal Gaussian distribution and that classifiers derived from the lower curve (e.g., ADC_L, corresponding to the median ADC value of the lower-curve histogram) was associated with clinical outcomes (▶ Fig. 8.9). Specifically, we found that, for bevacizumab-treated patients, low versus high ADC_L values corresponded to an HR for progression by 6 months of 4.1, and a 2.75-fold reduction in the median time to progression. For a non-bevacizumab-treated control group, there was no significant difference in the high versus low ADC_L group. Remarkably for the bevacizumab-treated group, pretreatment ADC values were more accurate at predicting progression at 6 months than were changes in enhancing tumor volume at first follow-up. Additional studies confirmed these results,[11] even when the analysis was applied to a multicenter trial with no standardization of imaging protocols.[85] It is hoped that such standardization and refinement of this ADC histogram biomarker could substantially improve its accuracy to the point where it could be reliably implemented in clinical decision making.

8.5.6 Early Assessment and Monitoring of Treatment Response

Current methods to assess tumor response are based on quantifying changes in enhancing tumor size.[86] For the Response Assessment in Neuro-Oncology (RANO) criteria,[87] the currently accepted standard, fluid-attenuated inversion recovery (FLAIR) image are also qualitatively assessed for evidence of nonenhancing tumor progression. However, it may take weeks to months before there is sufficient evidence of tumor response to therapy (either growth or regression) based on these methods, potentially delaying treatment changes.[88] Additionally, newer, antiangiogenic drugs used for salvage chemotherapy such as bevacizumab have antipermeability effects on the blood–brain barrier, decreasing the leakage of contrast agent into the interstitium and diminishing contrast enhancement.[8,9] Thus reduction in contrast enhancement may not necessarily reflect a cytotoxic or cytostatic tumor response, but rather be simply a by-product of a restored blood–brain barrier. This "pseudo-normalization" of the tumor vasculature increases the difficulty of accurately assessing tumor burden by standard imaging (▶ Fig. 8.10). Therefore two goals of neuro-oncological imaging are to (1) develop early response markers that are sensitive to

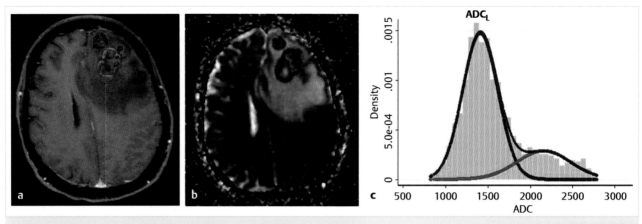

Fig. 8.9 Apparent diffusion coefficient (ADC) histogram analysis. Enhancing tumor (blue regions of interest) on postcontrast T1-weighted images (a), are segmented and mapped to the corresponding ADC image (b) for generation of an ADC histogram (c) fitted with a 2-normal distribution (red and green curves on (c)). ADC_L, corresponding to the median of the lower (red) curve is associated with better response to bevacizumab treatment if, as in this case, it is higher than 1,200 (units for (c), x-axis are $mm^2/s \times 10^{-6}$).

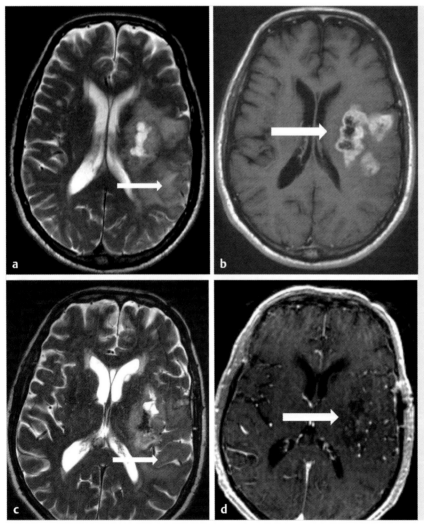

Fig. 8.10 Pseudoresponse of glioblastoma multiforme following bevacizumab therapy. T2-weighted (a,c) and postcontrast T1-weighted images of a patient with glioblastoma before (a,b) and 6 days following bevacizumab treatment (c,d). Note near complete resolution of contrast enhancement (large arrows), even though the tumor size as shown on T2-weighted image is similar before and after bevacizumab therapy. Substantial T2-hyperintense infiltrative tumor remains (small arrows).

treatment effect (or lack thereof) prior to change in tumor size and (2) develop a measure of tumor burden that is less reliant on contrast-enhancing volume. Diffusion imaging has been proposed as a method to address both these needs. For instance, initial work done in preclinical models suggesting a role for diffusion imaging as an early response marker[90,91,92,93] has been followed up with a number of human studies. In a pilot study of human patients, Mardor et al[94] evaluated diffusion MRI for detecting early tumor response to radiation therapy. They found a significant correlation between changes in diffusion parameters at 1 week postradiation therapy and later radiographic response. Although the study was limited in that most patients had metastatic brain lesions and only one had primary high-grade glioma, this was the first study to suggest the feasibility of diffusion MRI as a biomarker for early tumor response to radiation therapy.

Moffat et al[39] used a novel approach to quantify changes in ADC by developing functional diffusion maps (fDMs) that are potentially sensitive to the spatial heterogeneity of response within an individual tumor. Spatial information is preserved because these maps are based on registering follow-up to baseline ADC images to assess changes in diffusion on a voxel-by-voxel basis. In the Moffat et al[39] study, the authors used fDMs acquired 3 weeks after initiation of chemo- and/or radiotherapy to assess a heterogeneous population of malignant tumors. Voxels were color coded as red (significantly increasing ADC), blue (significantly decreasing ADC), and green (no change in ADC). ADC volumes of these regions were then correlated against subsequent tumor response (stable disease, progressive disease, and partial response), as determined by standard radiographic follow-up. fDM analysis at 3 weeks from the start of treatment was found to add value to standard imaging as a prognostic indicator of subsequent volumetric tumor response. Follow-up studies demonstrated similar results in cohorts restricted to patients with malignant glioma[37] and also showed the predictive value of fDMs in not only treatment response but also overall survival.[38] Conventional radiological response at 10 weeks had a similar prognostic value, but fDMs provided similar information 7 to 8 weeks earlier. In the largest fDM study to date, Ellingson et al[44] confirmed in 143 newly diagnosed GBM patients that the volume of tumor tissue with increasing ADC 10 weeks after initiation of radiotherapy was a significant predictor of both progression-free and overall survival, where the larger the volume the longer the survival. Additionally, this study also showed that the volume of *decreasing* ADC, thought to contain hypercellular and growing tumor, was also a significant predictor of survival. In a follow-up study with the same patients, Ellingson et al[42] implemented a "probabilistic" approach to fDM quantification and showed this technique was significantly better at predicting patient survival compared with traditional fDM techniques (▶ Fig. 8.11).

Not all studies attempting to demonstrate the utility of diffusion-based biomarkers as early response measures have been entirely successful. For instance, Khayal et al[95] assessed diffusion parameters as early response markers of progression based on disease status at 6 months in postsurgical GBM patients who received standard therapy followed by adjuvant temozolomide and an antiangiogenic agent. Midradiation therapy median normalized ADC values within the contrast-enhancing lesion were not significantly different in nonprogressors versus progressors.

Additionally both progressors and nonprogressors showed significant change in normalized ADC from pre- to postradiation therapy. Thus, for patients with this treatment protocol, changes in median ADC values may not be reflective of subsequent outcomes.

8.5.7 Diffusion Imaging following Antiangiogenic Therapy

Antiangiogenic agents such as bevacizumab, an anti-VEGF antibody, and cediranib, a VEGF receptor tyrosine kinase inhibitor, have recently been tested in clinical trials for treatment of high-grade gliomas.[85,96] These agents have been shown to produce a rapid decrease in tumor contrast enhancement with a high response rate and potential improvement in 6-month progression-free survival, but with only modest, if any, effects on overall survival. Anti-VEGF agents diminish vascular permeability resulting in a decrease in leakage of gadolinium-based contrast agents into the brain.[97] Because this regression of contrast enhancement may be due primarily to reversal of vascular hyperpermeability rather than tumor reduction (so-called pseudoresponse), the true antitumor response to this class of agent is difficult to ascertain based on contrast-enhanced images alone. Improved measures of disease burden are needed, especially methods sensitive to non- or faintly enhancing tumor following anti-VEGF therapy.

In a preclinical study,[98] correlation between changes in tumor volume and ADC were evaluated in mice with angiogenesis-dependent tumors before and after 2, 7, 14, and 21 days of treatment with the anti-angiogenic agent sunitinib maleate. The authors found a significant negative correlation between changes in ADC and tumor volume, and mice with unidirectional changes in tumor volume showed a strongly negative correlation with changes in ADC, suggesting that percent change in ADC may be a reliable and accurate biomarker for monitoring tumor response.

Diminished diffusion within areas of T2/FLAIR signal hyperintensity that lack corresponding contrast enhancement have been observed in patients with malignant glioma.[99,100,101,102] This seems to be more common in patients treated with bevacizumab or cediranib, but is also found in patients that have not received antiangiogenic therapy.[100] The majority of these lesions (85%) develop into enhancing masses at a median of 3 months later,[100] and in some cases areas of low ADC have been histopathologically shown to represent viable tumor.[101] These studies suggest that, given the link between low ADC and increased cellularity,[45,50] areas of diminished diffusion may help detect or quantify disease burden in areas lacking significant contrast enhancement.

However, there is one caveat to this approach. We and others have found that patients with malignant glioma, typically following initiation of antiangiogenic therapy, develop areas of persistent highly restricted diffusion (▶ Fig. 8.12).[103,104,105] These lesions typically evolve slowly over time but do not seem to develop into areas of active tumor growth. Further, we also found that patients with these restricted diffusion lesions had significantly greater time-to-progression, time-to-survival, and overall survival compared to matched controls. In a case where histopathology was obtained following surgical resection, there

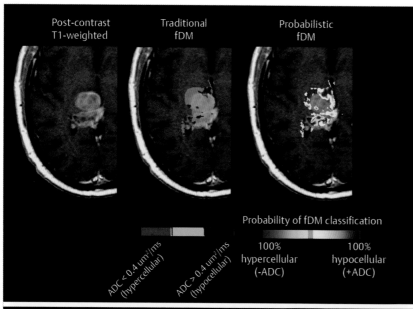

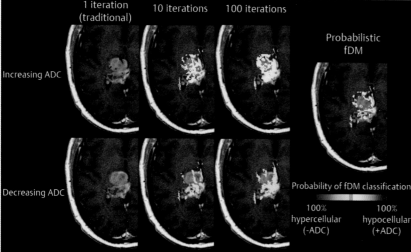

Fig. 8.11 Probabilistic functional diffusion maps. (a) Comparison between traditional and 0robabilistic functional diffusion maps (fDMs). (Left) Postcontrast T1-weighted image. (Middle) Traditional fDMs showing regions of relative increasing and decreasing apparent diffusion coefficient (ADC). (Right) Probabilistic fDMs showing likelihood of a voxel being characterized as increasing or decreasing ADC in the presence of misalignment. (b) Construction of probabilistic functional diffusion maps. (Top row) Regions of increasing ADC or (bottom row) decreasing ADC beyond the empirical threshold of $0.4\,\mu m^2/m$. (Left) Results from a single iteration, representing "traditional" fDMs where there is only linear registration/alignment between ADC maps. (Middle column) Resultant probability maps generated after application of empirical thresholds following each iteration for a total of 10 finite, random translational and rotational perturbations. (Right column) Resultant probability maps generated after application of empirical thresholds following each iteration for a total of 100 finite, random translational and rotational perturbations. (Far right) Composite probabilistic fDM after 100 iterations showing probability of both increasing (yellow/red) and decreasing (blue) ADC.

was no viable tumor, but rather only atypical gelatinous necrosis.[105] Additionally we have found a similar phenomenon in a patient with a brain metastasis treated with stereotactic radiotherapy who was placed on bevacizumab to control subsequent, histopathologically confirmed, radiation necrosis (unpublished data). Thus at least some forms of marked and persistent diffusion restriction in patients with brain tumor, particularly in the setting of bevacizumab treatment, represent quiescent or necrotic tissue, rather than actively growing tumor.

fDM analysis in glioma patients treated with antiangiogenic therapy has also been performed.[41,42,44] In patients with recurrent GBM, changes in ADC were found to be predictive of survival using fDM analysis before and after bevacizumab therapy.[41] It was suggested that the volume of tissue illustrating a subtle decrease in ADC within contrast-enhancing regions was correlated with tumor burden after therapy, but confirmation of this hypothesis will require histopathological correlation. A follow-up study[43] demonstrated the added value of fDM analysis in the context of antiangiogenic therapy by using nonlinear registration of pretreatment to posttreatment ADC maps to correct for mass effect, providing improved separation of survival curves based on fDM metrics. fDM analysis examining the changes in fDM-quantified hypercellular volume (decreasing ADC) over time tended to predict tumor recurrence several months prior to the development of new contrast enhancement. Early changes after therapy could be used to predict time to progression and overall survival.[46] CIMPLE maps, which use spatiotemporal changes in ADC to quantify tumor proliferation and invasion rates, can be used to predict survival and specify areas of future contrast enhancement (in approximately 30% of patients; ▶ Fig. 8.13).[106]

Thus several lines of evidence indicate that diffusion metrics are correlated with outcomes and may add value to enhancing tissue measurements as an indicator of tumor burden, particularly following antiangiogenic therapy. However, it is important to keep in mind the possibility that some areas of decreasing ADC may reflect atypical necrosis rather than viable tumor.

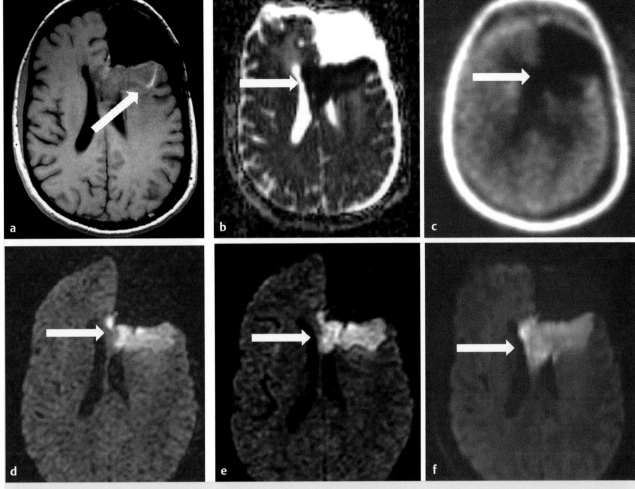

Fig. 8.12 Persistent restricted diffusion in a patient with recurrent glioblastoma multiforme (GBM). Imaging was obtained approximately 5 (**a,d**), 7 (**b,e**), and 9 (**c,f**) months after treatment with bevacizumab. Diffusion-weighted images (bottom row, arrows), show a persistent region of restricted diffusion posterior to the resection cavity and bordering the lateral ventricles. The lesion shows some spontaneous peripheral T1-weighted hyperintensity (**a**) (arrow), is low on ADC images (**b**) (arrow), and shows no uptake of tracer on ^{18}F-FDOPA (3,4-dihydroxy-6-^{18}F-fluoro-L-phenylalanine) positron-emission tomographic scans (**c**) (arrow), consistent with a lack of viable tumor.

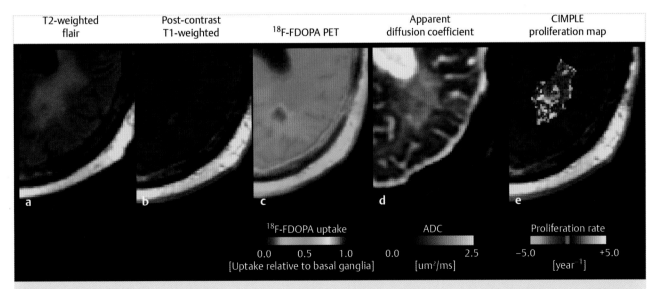

Fig. 8.13 Cell invasion, motility, and proliferation level estimate (CIMPLE) maps of tumor proliferation rate for a patient with recurrent glioblastoma. (**a**) T2-weighted fluid-attenuated inversion recovery (FLAIR) image showing hyperintensity near the posterior aspect of the left lateral ventricle. (**b**) Postcontrast T1-weighted image showing a subtle enhancing lesion. (**c**) ^{18}F-FDOPA (3,4-dihydroxy-6-^{18}F-fluoro-L-phenylalanine) positron-emission tomography (PET) illustrating elevated amino acid uptake relative to the basal ganglia, indicative of a malignant process near the areas of contrast enhancement. (**d**) Apparent diffusion coefficient (ADC) maps showing overall elevated diffusivity in the region with abnormal FLAIR hyperintensity, along with a subtle pocket of relatively low diffusivity in a region posterior to the left lateral ventricle. (**e**) CIMPLE map estimates of proliferation rate demonstrating positive proliferation (rapidly decreasing ADC) in a region near the site of contrast enhancement and 18F-FDOPA PET positivity.

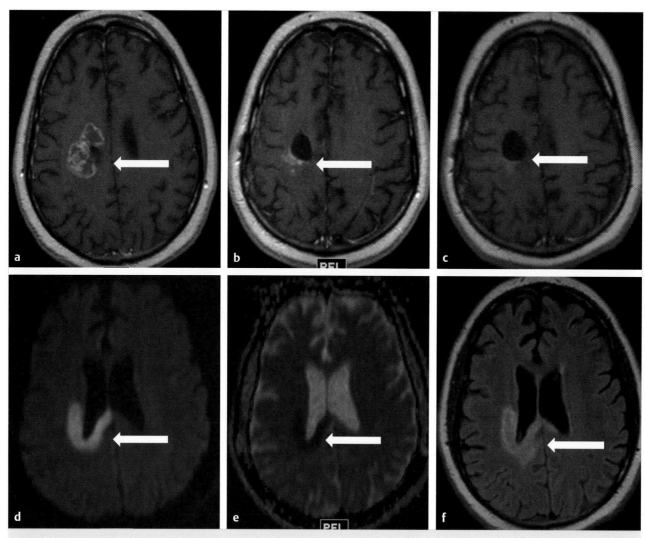

Fig. 8.14 Pseudoprogression in a patient with metastatic testicular cancer. The patient had a history of chemotherapy followed by stereotactic radiotherapy with excellent response of a right cerebral brain metastasis, but then developed new symptoms of weakness. Follow-up magnetic resonance imaging showed new enhancement. This was resected and found to be radiation necrosis. The patient's symptoms improved but then worsened again, with imaging again showing development of new enhancement (**a**) (arrow). Based on the prior resection, this was diagnosed as radiation necrosis, and the patient was started on bevacizumab, with improvement of symptoms and near resolution of contrast enhancement (**b,c**) (arrows). Approximately 1 month after the initiation of bevacizumab therapy, diffusion-weighted imaging (DWI) (**d**) and apparent diffusion coefficient (ADC) images (**e**) show a periventricular region of restricted diffusion extending along the splenium of the corpus callosum within a region of abnormal fluid-attenuated inversion recovery signal hyperintensity (**f**). This is similar to regions of atypical necrosis demonstrated in patients with recurrent glioblastoma multiforme following bevacizumab therapy.

8.5.8 Pseudoprogression

After completion of initial treatment, patients with high-grade glioma can demonstrate increased contrast enhancement, followed by subsequent improvement or stabilization without initiation of further therapies. Because this enhancement, which is thought to be a result of treatment effect, can mimic worsening tumor, the term *pseudoprogression* has been used to describe this phenomenon (▶ Fig. 8.14). Pseudoprogression most likely represents a local tissue reaction due to radiation injury, resulting in edema and abnormal vessel permeability, manifesting with increased contrast enhancement.[107] There is a link between pseudoprogression and MGMT promoter methylation status: pseudoprogression is more than twice as common

in methylated compared to unmethylated tumors.[108] Currently, the only method of differentiating pseudoprogression from true tumor progression by conventional MRI is to perform serial follow-up examinations.[109] Thus there is interest in developing imaging biomarkers for the early identification of pseudoprogression.

One of the potential causes of pseudoprogression is infarction of brain tissue due to surgical resection of adjacent tumor. Smith et al[110] evaluated the significance of periresectional diffusion abnormalities in a cohort of 44 patients and found that 64% demonstrated areas of restricted diffusion in or around the resection cavity in the postoperative period. Contrast enhancement was then observed in the region of restricted diffusion, potentially mimicking tumor residual or recurrence, but these regions ultimately demonstrated volume loss in 93% of cases as would be expected for chronic infarction. Thus diffusion imaging is an important component in the postoperative evaluation of glioma patients, and any new contrast enhancement on follow-up imaging should be evaluated in the context of the presence of restricted diffusion in the immediate postoperative period.

More commonly pseudoprogression results from radiation and chemotherapy-induced treatment effect, which can have enhancement and associated vasogenic edema similar to recurrent tumor. It is thought that this treatment-related necrosis will exhibit higher ADC values than recurrent disease because there is loss of cellular integrity in contrast to cellularity gain associated with growing tumor. Therefore, ADC, which is sensitive to cell density, could potentially help distinguish the two processes. Several studies have evaluated the potential role of diffusion imaging for this purpose. In a small retrospective study from 2004, Hein et al[111] reviewed 18 patients with areas of abnormal enhancement 1 month after completion of radiation treatment. Recurrence was determined by histological examination or by clinical course and follow-up imaging studies. The authors demonstrated that mean ADC and ADC ratios (ratio of ADC of the enhancing lesion to ADC of contralateral white matter) were significantly lower in the recurrence group (ADC mean 1.18×10^{-3} mm^2/s; ADC ratio 1.43) than the nonrecurrence group (ADC mean 1.4×10^{-3} mm^2/s; ADC ratio 1.82).

A subsequent study[112] of a larger cohort ($n = 55$) of malignant glioma patients also found that recurrent tumor has significantly lower mean ADC (taken from enhancing regions) than pseudoprogression, although, as with the previous study, there was substantial overlap between the two groups. ADC ratios generated from normalization against contralateral brain were similarly diminished in recurrence. The combination of MR spectroscopy and DWI improved the power of differentiating radiation injury from recurrent tumor compared to MR spectroscopy alone (96.4% vs. 85.5%).

Conversely, at least two papers (albeit with smaller sample sizes) did not find a significant difference in mean ADC values between recurrent tumor and pseudoprogression.[113,114] Instead, Asao et al[113] found that, for patients with radiation necrosis, enhancing lesions were heterogeneous and/or markedly hypointense on diffusion imaging, whereas in the tumor recurrence group, no marked DWI hypointensity was noted. Maximal ADC values in the recurrence group were significantly lower than in the radiation necrosis group (1.68 vs. 2.30×10^{-3} mm^2/s). Mean ADC values were not statistically different. Thus the authors suggest that heterogeneity with regions of hypointensity on DWI on visual inspection may be helpful in distinguishing between radiation necrosis and recurrent tumor, although tumor heterogeneity with regions of necrosis may be mistaken for radiation injury. Similarly Lee et al[114] reported no difference in mean ADC of recurrent tumor versus pseudoprogression, but they did find that diffusion images were increased in signal intensity in recurrent tumors compared with pseudoprogression.

A group at the University of Washington investigated the value of combining diffusion imaging with perfusion and spectroscopy to differentiate true from pseudoprogression. Matsusue et al[115] proposed a multiparametric scoring system using DWI, MR spectroscopy, and DSC acquired at 3 T to distinguish between glioma progression (grades II–IV) and pseudoprogression. In a pilot study they demonstrated that mean ADC ratios were significantly lower in tumor recurrence than pseudoprogression (1.14 vs. 1.56×10^{-3} mm^2/s), supporting the findings of Zeng et al[112] An ADC ratio threshold of 1.30 resulted in diagnostic accuracy of nearly 87% in a ROC analysis, which improved to 93% using a multiparametric scoring system based on the combination of DWI, DSC, and MR spectroscopy. The same group then extended this work to a collection of 40 patients (again gliomas grade II–IV),[116] confirming that ADC ratios were lower in recurrent tumor versus pseudoprogression. However, the authors also note that the diagnostic performance of ADC ratios was inferior to either CBV or multivoxel MR spectroscopy, similar to at least one other study that also concluded that ADC was inferior to MR spectroscopy for this task.[117]

Thus the use of diffusion imaging to distinguish true from pseudoprogression suffers from the same limitation as that for using diffusion imaging to distinguish tumor grades: although there may be population differences between groups (recurrence vs. pseudoprogression), there is a substantial overlap in values; thus the ability to diagnose an individual patient as having true versus pseudoprogression is limited. It is also likely that many areas of contrast enhancement represent a mixture of treatment-related necrosis and viable tumor, potentially explaining some of this overlap. Multimodal physiological imaging or other technical refinements are still needed to further improve diagnostic certainty.

8.6 Conclusion

In summary, diffusion imaging has the ability to provide needed insight into tumor biology. There are several stages in the treatment of glioma patients in which diffusion imaging could help aid in clinical decision making. Assuring that this promise becomes a reality requires standardization and validation of potential biomarkers against clinically meaningful end points, such as progression-free and overall survival.

References

[1] Stejskal EO, Tanner JE. Spin diffusion measurements: Spin echoes in the presence of a time-dependent field gradient. J Chem Phys 1965; 42: 288–292

[2] Stejskal EO. Use of spin echoes in a pulsed magnetic-field gradient to study anisotropic, restricted diffusion and flow. J Chem Phys 1965; 43: 3597–3603

[3] Le Bihan D, Breton E, Lallemand D, Aubin ML, Vignaud J, Laval-Jeantet M. Separation of diffusion and perfusion in intravoxel incoherent motion MR imaging. Radiology 1988; 168: 497–505

[4] Maier SE, Gudbjartsson H, Patz S et al. Line scan diffusion imaging: characterization in healthy subjects and stroke patients. AJR Am J Roentgenol 1998; 171: 85–93

[5] Warach S, Chien D, Li W, Ronthal M, Edelman RR. Fast magnetic resonance diffusion-weighted imaging of acute human stroke. Neurology 1992; 42: 1717–1723

[6] Sunshine JL, Tarr RW, Lanzieri CF, Landis DM, Selman WR, Lewin JS. Hyperacute stroke: ultrafast MR imaging to triage patients prior to therapy. Radiology 1999; 212: 325–332

[7] Chenevert TL, McKeever PE, Ross BD. Monitoring early response of experimental brain tumors to therapy using diffusion magnetic resonance imaging. Clin Cancer Res 1997; 3: 1457–1466

[8] Chenevert TL, Meyer CR, Moffat BA et al. Diffusion MRI: a new strategy for assessment of cancer therapeutic efficacy. Mol Imaging 2002; 1: 336–343

[9] Pope WB, Kim HJ, Huo J et al. Recurrent glioblastoma multiforme: ADC histogram analysis predicts response to bevacizumab treatment. Radiology 2009; 252: 182–189

[10] Pope WB, Lai A, Mehta R et al. Apparent diffusion coefficient histogram analysis stratifies progression-free survival in newly diagnosed bevacizumab-treated glioblastoma. AJNR Am J Neuroradiol 2011; 32: 882–889

[11] Pope WB, Qiao XJ, Kim HJ et al. Apparent diffusion coefficient histogram analysis stratifies progression-free and overall survival in patients with recurrent GBM treated with bevacizumab: a multi-center study. J Neurooncol 2012; 108: 491–498

[12] Crank J. The Mathematics of Diffusion. New York, NY: Oxford University Press; 1975

[13] Einstein A. Investigations on the Theory of Brownian Movement. New York, NY: Dover; 1956

[14] Torrey HC. Bloch equations with diffusion terms. Phys Rev 1956; 104: 563–565

[15] Kärger J, Pfeifer H, Heink W. Principles and application of self-diffusion measurements by nuclear magnetic resonance. Adv Magn Reson 1988; 12: 1–89

[16] Kiselev VG, Il'yasov KA. Is the "biexponential diffusion" biexponential? Magn Reson Med 2007; 57: 464–469

[17] Mulkern RV, Haker SJ, Maier SE. On high b diffusion imaging in the human brain: ruminations and experimental insights. Magn Reson Imaging 2009; 27: 1151–1162

[18] Bennett KM, Schmainda KM, Bennett RT, Rowe DB, Lu H, Hyde JS. Characterization of continuously distributed cortical water diffusion rates with a stretched-exponential model. Magn Reson Med 2003; 50: 727–734

[19] Bennett KM, Hyde JS, Rand SD et al. Intravoxel distribution of DWI decay rates reveals C6 glioma invasion in rat brain. Magn Reson Med 2004; 52: 994–1004

[20] Kwee TC, Galbán CJ, Tsien C et al. Intravoxel water diffusion heterogeneity imaging of human high-grade gliomas. NMR Biomed 2010; 23: 179–187

[21] Jensen JH, Helpern JA, Ramani A, Lu H, Kaczynski K. Diffusional kurtosis imaging: the quantification of non-gaussian water diffusion by means of magnetic resonance imaging. Magn Reson Med 2005; 53: 1432–1440

[22] Van Cauter S, Veraart J, Sijbers J et al. Gliomas: diffusion kurtosis MR imaging in grading. Radiology 2012; 263: 492–501

[23] Yablonskiy DA, Bretthorst GL, Ackerman JJ. Statistical model for diffusion attenuated MR signal. Magn Reson Med 2003; 50: 664–669

[24] Reese TG, Heid O, Weisskoff RM, Wedeen VJ. Reduction of eddy-current-induced distortion in diffusion MRI using a twice-refocused spin echo. Magn Reson Med 2003; 49: 177–182

[25] Poustchi-Amin M, Mirowitz SA, Brown JJ, McKinstry RC, Li T. Principles and applications of echo-planar imaging: a review for the general radiologist. Radiographics 2001; 21: 767–779

[26] Bammer R, Stollberger R, Augustin M et al. Diffusion-weighted imaging with navigated interleaved echo-planar imaging and a conventional gradient system. Radiology 1999; 211: 799–806

[27] de Crespigny AJ, Marks MP, Enzmann DR, Moseley ME. Navigated diffusion imaging of normal and ischemic human brain. Magn Reson Med 1995; 33: 720–728

[28] Nunes RG, Jezzard P, Behrens TE, Clare S. Self-navigated multishot echo-planar pulse sequence for high-resolution diffusion-weighted imaging. Magn Reson Med 2005; 53: 1474–1478

[29] Bernstein M, King K, Zhou X. 2004

[30] Pipe JG. Motion correction with PROPELLER MRI: application to head motion and free-breathing cardiac imaging. Magn Reson Med 1999; 42: 963–969

[31] Pipe JG, Zwart N. Turboprop: improved PROPELLER imaging. Magn Reson Med 2006; 55: 380–385

[32] Horsfield MA. Mapping eddy current induced fields for the correction of diffusion-weighted echo planar images. Magn Reson Imaging 1999; 17: 1335–1345

[33] Chen B, Guo H, Song AW. Correction for direction-dependent distortions in diffusion tensor imaging using matched magnetic field maps. Neuroimage 2006; 30: 121–129

[34] Gallichan D, Andersson JL, Jenkinson M, Robson MD, Miller KL. Reducing distortions in diffusion-weighted echo planar imaging with a dual-echo blip-reversed sequence. Magn Reson Med 2010; 64: 382–390

[35] Mohammadi S, Möller HE, Kugel H, Müller DK, Deppe M. Correcting eddy current and motion effects by affine whole-brain registrations: evaluation of three-dimensional distortion correction and comparison with slicewise correction. Magn Reson Med 2010; 64: 1047–1056

[36] Andersson JL, Skare S, Ashburner J. How to correct susceptibility distortions in spin-echo echo-planar images: application to diffusion tensor imaging. Neuroimage 2003; 20: 870–888

[37] Hamstra DA, Chenevert TL, Moffat BA et al. Evaluation of the functional diffusion map as an early biomarker of time-to-progression and overall survival in high-grade glioma. Proc Natl Acad Sci U S A 2005; 102: 16759–16764

[38] Hamstra DA, Galbán CJ, Meyer CR et al. Functional diffusion map as an early imaging biomarker for high-grade glioma: correlation with conventional radiologic response and overall survival. J Clin Oncol 2008; 26: 3387–3394

[39] Moffat BA, Chenevert TL, Lawrence TS et al. Functional diffusion map: a non-invasive MRI biomarker for early stratification of clinical brain tumor response. Proc Natl Acad Sci U S A 2005; 102: 5524–5529

[40] Moffat BA, Chenevert TL, Meyer CR et al. The functional diffusion map: an imaging biomarker for the early prediction of cancer treatment outcome. Neoplasia 2006; 8: 259–267

[41] Ellingson BM, Cloughesy TF, Lai A et al. Graded functional diffusion map-defined characteristics of apparent diffusion coefficients predict overall survival in recurrent glioblastoma treated with bevacizumab. Neuro-oncol 2011; 13: 1151–1161

[42] Ellingson BM, Cloughesy TF, Lai A, Nghiemphu PL, Liau LM, Pope WB. Quantitative probabilistic functional diffusion mapping in newly diagnosed glioblastoma treated with radiochemotherapy. Neuro-oncol 2013; 15: 382–390

[43] Ellingson BM, Cloughesy TF, Lai A, Nghiemphu PL, Pope WB. Nonlinear registration of diffusion-weighted images improves clinical sensitivity of functional diffusion maps in recurrent glioblastoma treated with bevacizumab. Magn Reson Med 2012; 67: 237–245

[44] Ellingson BM, Cloughesy TF, Zaw T et al. Functional diffusion maps (fDMs) evaluated before and after radiochemotherapy predict progression-free and overall survival in newly diagnosed glioblastoma. Neuro-oncol 2012; 14: 333–343

[45] Ellingson BM, Malkin MG, Rand SD et al. Validation of functional diffusion maps (fDMs) as a biomarker for human glioma cellularity. J Magn Reson Imaging 2010; 31: 538–548

[46] Ellingson BM, Malkin MG, Rand SD et al. Volumetric analysis of functional diffusion maps is a predictive imaging biomarker for cytotoxic and anti-angiogenic treatments in malignant gliomas. J Neurooncol 2011; 102: 95–103

[47] Latour LL, Svoboda K, Mitra PP, Sotak CH. Time-dependent diffusion of water in a biological model system. Proc Natl Acad Sci U S A 1994; 91: 1229–1233

[48] Ebisu T, Tanaka C, Umeda M et al. Discrimination of brain abscess from necrotic or cystic tumors by diffusion-weighted echo planar imaging. Magn Reson Imaging 1996; 14: 1113–1116

[49] Lee EJ, terBrugge K, Mikulis D et al. Diagnostic value of peritumoral minimum apparent diffusion coefficient for differentiation of glioblastoma multiforme from solitary metastatic lesions. AJR Am J Roentgenol 2011; 196: 71–76

[50] Sugahara T, Korogi Y, Kochi M et al. Usefulness of diffusion-weighted MRI with echo-planar technique in the evaluation of cellularity in gliomas. J Magn Reson Imaging 1999; 9: 53–60

[51] Toh CH, Wei KC, Ng SH, Wan YL, Lin CP, Castillo M. Differentiation of brain abscesses from necrotic glioblastomas and cystic metastatic brain tumors with diffusion tensor imaging. AJNR Am J Neuroradiol 2011; 32: 1646–1651

[52] Tsuchiya K, Fujikawa A, Nakajima M, Honya K. Differentiation between solitary brain metastasis and high-grade glioma by diffusion tensor imaging. Br J Radiol 2005; 78: 533–537

[53] Jenkinson MD, Du Plessis DG, Walker C, Smith TS. Advanced MRI in the management of adult gliomas. Br J Neurosurg 2007; 21: 550–561

[54] Scott JN, Brasher PM, Sevick RJ, Rewcastle NB, Forsyth PA. How often are non-enhancing supratentorial gliomas malignant? A population study. Neurology 2002; 59: 947–949

[55] Knopp EA, Cha S, Johnson G et al. Glial neoplasms: dynamic contrast-enhanced T2*-weighted MR imaging. Radiology 1999; 211: 791–798

[56] Pope WB, Sayre J, Perlina A, Villablanca JP, Mischel PS, Cloughesy TF. MR imaging correlates of survival in patients with high-grade gliomas. AJNR Am J Neuroradiol 2005; 26: 2466–2474

[57] Dean BL, Drayer BP, Bird CR et al. Gliomas: classification with MR imaging. Radiology 1990; 174: 411–415

[58] Murakami R, Hirai T, Sugahara T et al. Grading astrocytic tumors by using apparent diffusion coefficient parameters: superiority of a one- versus two-parameter pilot method. Radiology 2009; 251: 838–845

[59] Yang D, Korogi Y, Sugahara T et al. Cerebral gliomas: prospective comparison of multivoxel 2D chemical-shift imaging proton MR spectroscopy, echoplanar perfusion and diffusion-weighted MRI. Neuroradiology 2002; 44: 656–666

[60] Kono K, Inoue Y, Nakayama K et al. The role of diffusion-weighted imaging in patients with brain tumors. AJNR Am J Neuroradiol 2001; 22: 1081–1088

[61] Fan G, Zang P, Jing F, Wu Z, Guo Q. Usefulness of diffusion/perfusion-weighted MRI in rat gliomas: correlation with histopathology. Acad Radiol 2005; 12: 640–651

[62] Fan GG, Deng QL, Wu ZH, Guo QY. Usefulness of diffusion/perfusion-weighted MRI in patients with non-enhancing supratentorial brain gliomas: a valuable tool to predict tumour grading? Br J Radiol 2006; 79: 652–658

[63] Arvinda HR, Kesavadas C, Sarma PS et al. Glioma grading: sensitivity, specificity, positive and negative predictive values of diffusion and perfusion imaging. J Neurooncol 2009; 94: 87–96

[64] Tozer DJ, Jäger HR, Danchaivijitr N et al. Apparent diffusion coefficient histograms may predict low-grade glioma subtype. NMR Biomed 2007; 20: 49–57

[65] Khalid L, Carone M, Dumrongpisutikul N et al. Imaging characteristics of oligodendrogliomas that predict grade. AJNR Am J Neuroradiol 2012; 33: 852–857

[66] Rose S, Fay M, Thomas P et al. Correlation of MRI-derived apparent diffusion coefficients in newly diagnosed gliomas with [18F]-fluoro-L-dopa PET: What are we really measuring with minimum ADC? AJNR Am J Neuroradiol 201 3; 34: 758–764

[67] Jakab A, Molnár P, Emri M, Berényi E. Glioma grade assessment by using histogram analysis of diffusion tensor imaging-derived maps. Neuroradiology 2011; 53: 483–491

[68] Lee HY, Na DG, Song IC et al. Diffusion-tensor imaging for glioma grading at 3-T magnetic resonance imaging: analysis of fractional anisotropy and mean diffusivity. J Comput Assist Tomogr 2008; 32: 298–303

[69] Hegi ME, Diserens AC, Godard S et al. Clinical trial substantiates the predictive value of O-6-methylguanine-DNA methyltransferase promoter methylation in glioblastoma patients treated with temozolomide. Clin Cancer Res 2004; 10: 1871–1874

[70] Romano A, Calabria LF, Tavanti F et al. Apparent diffusion coefficient obtained by magnetic resonance imaging as a prognostic marker in glioblastomas: correlation with MGMT promoter methylation status. Eur Radiol 2013; 23: 513–520

[71] Sunwoo L, Choi SH, Park CK et al. Correlation of apparent diffusion coefficient values measured by diffusion MRI and MGMT promoter methylation semiquantitatively analyzed with MS-MLPA in patients with glioblastoma multiforme. J Magn Reson Imaging 2013; 37: 351–358

[72] Higano S, Yun X, Kumabe T et al. Malignant astrocytic tumors: clinical importance of apparent diffusion coefficient in prediction of grade and prognosis. Radiology 2006; 241: 839–846

[73] Oh J, Henry RG, Pirzkall A et al. Survival analysis in patients with glioblastoma multiforme: predictive value of choline-to-N-acetylaspartate index, apparent diffusion coefficient, and relative cerebral blood volume. J Magn Reson Imaging 2004; 19: 546–554

[74] Murakami R, Sugahara T, Nakamura H et al. Malignant supratentorial astrocytoma treated with postoperative radiation therapy: prognostic value of pretreatment quantitative diffusion-weighted MR imaging. Radiology 2007; 243: 493–499

[75] Nakamura H, Murakami R, Hirai T, Kitajima M, Yamashita Y. Can MRI-derived factors predict the survival in glioblastoma patients treated with postoperative chemoradiation therapy? Acta Radiol 201 3; 54: 214–220

[76] Barajas RF, Jr, Hodgson JG, Chang JS et al. Glioblastoma multiforme regional genetic and cellular expression patterns: influence on anatomic and physiologic MR imaging. Radiology 2010; 254: 564–576

[77] Carlson MR, Pope WB, Horvath S et al. Relationship between survival and edema in malignant gliomas: role of vascular endothelial growth factor and neuronal pentraxin 2. Clin Cancer Res 2007; 13: 2592–2598

[78] Hobbs SK, Shi G, Homer R, Harsh G, Atlas SW, Bednarski MD. Magnetic resonance image-guided proteomics of human glioblastoma multiforme. J Magn Reson Imaging 2003; 18: 530–536

[79] Van Meter T, Dumur C, Hafez N, Garrett C, Fillmore H, Broaddus WC. Microarray analysis of MRI-defined tissue samples in glioblastoma reveals differences in regional expression of therapeutic targets. Diagn Mol Pathol 2006; 15: 195–205

[80] Pope WB, Mirsadraei L, Lai A et al. Differential gene expression in glioblastoma defined by ADC histogram analysis: relationship to extracellular matrix molecules and survival. AJNR Am J Neuroradiol 2012; 33: 1059–1064

[81] Huijbers IJ, Iravani M, Popov S et al. A role for fibrillar collagen deposition and the collagen internalization receptor endo180 in glioma invasion. PLoS ONE 2010; 5: e9808

[82] Cohen MH, Shen YL, Keegan P, Pazdur R. FDA drug approval summary: bevacizumab (Avastin) as treatment of recurrent glioblastoma multiforme. Oncologist 2009; 14: 1131–1138

[83] Pope WB, Lai A, Nghiemphu P, Mischel P, Cloughesy TF. MRI in patients with high-grade gliomas treated with bevacizumab and chemotherapy. Neurology 2006; 66: 1258–1260

[84] Norden AD, Drappatz J, Wen PY. Antiangiogenic therapy in malignant gliomas. Curr Opin Oncol 2008; 20: 652–661

[85] Friedman HS, Prados MD, Wen PY et al. Bevacizumab alone and in combination with irinotecan in recurrent glioblastoma. J Clin Oncol 2009; 27: 4733–4740

[86] Macdonald DR, Cascino TL, Schold SC, Jr, Cairncross JG. Response criteria for phase II studies of supratentorial malignant glioma. J Clin Oncol 1990; 8: 1277–1280

[87] Wen PY, Macdonald DR, Reardon DA et al. Updated response assessment criteria for high-grade gliomas: response assessment in neuro-oncology working group. J Clin Oncol 2010; 28: 1963–1972

[88] Therasse P, Arbuck SG, Eisenhauer EA et al. New guidelines to evaluate the response to treatment in solid tumors. European Organization for Research and Treatment of Cancer, National Cancer Institute of the United States, National Cancer Institute of Canada. J Natl Cancer Inst 2000; 92: 205–216

[89] Gerstner ER, Duda DG, di Tomaso E, et al. VEGF inhibitors in the treatment of cerebral edema in patients with brain cancer. Nat Rev Clin Oncol 2009; 6(4): 229–236

[90] Chenevert TL, Stegman LD, Taylor JM et al. Diffusion magnetic resonance imaging: an early surrogate marker of therapeutic efficacy in brain tumors. J Natl Cancer Inst 2000; 92: 2029–2036

[91] Hamstra DA, Lee KC, Tychewicz JM et al. The use of 19F spectroscopy and diffusion-weighted MRI to evaluate differences in gene-dependent enzyme prodrug therapies. Mol Ther 2004; 10: 916–928

[92] Hall DE, Moffat BA, Stojanovska J et al. Therapeutic efficacy of DTI-015 using diffusion magnetic resonance imaging as an early surrogate marker. Clin Cancer Res 2004; 10: 7852–7859

[93] Rehemtulla A, Hall DE, Stegman LD et al. Molecular imaging of gene expression and efficacy following adenoviral-mediated brain tumor gene therapy. Mol Imaging 2002; 1: 43–55

[94] Mardor Y, Pfeffer R, Spiegelmann R et al. Early detection of response to radiation therapy in patients with brain malignancies using conventional and high b-value diffusion-weighted magnetic resonance imaging. J Clin Oncol 2003; 21: 1094–1100

[95] Khayal IS, Polley MY, Jalbert L et al. Evaluation of diffusion parameters as early biomarkers of disease progression in glioblastoma multiforme. Neuro-oncol 2010; 12: 908–916

[96] Batchelor TT, Duda DG, di Tomaso E et al. Phase II study of cediranib, an oral pan-vascular endothelial growth factor receptor tyrosine kinase inhibitor, in patients with recurrent glioblastoma. J Clin Oncol 2010; 28: 2817–2823

[97] Norden AD, Drappatz J, Wen PY. Novel anti-angiogenic therapies for malignant gliomas. Lancet Neurol 2008; 7: 1152–1160

[98] Suh JY, Cho G, Song Y et al. Is apparent diffusion coefficient reliable and accurate for monitoring effects of antiangiogenic treatment in a longitudinal study? J Magn Reson Imaging 2012; 35: 1430–1436

[99] Jain R, Scarpace LM, Ellika S et al. Imaging response criteria for recurrent gliomas treated with bevacizumab: role of diffusion weighted imaging as an imaging biomarker. J Neurooncol 2010; 96: 423–431

[100] Gupta A, Young RJ, Karimi S et al. Isolated diffusion restriction precedes the development of enhancing tumor in a subset of patients with glioblastoma. AJNR Am J Neuroradiol 2011; 32: 1301–1306

[101] Gerstner ER, Frosch MP, Batchelor TT. Diffusion magnetic resonance imaging detects pathologically confirmed, nonenhancing tumor progression in a patient with recurrent glioblastoma receiving bevacizumab. J Clin Oncol 2010; 28: e91–e93

[102] Gerstner ER, Chen PJ, Wen PY, Jain RK, Batchelor TT, Sorensen G. Infiltrative patterns of glioblastoma spread detected via diffusion MRI after treatment with cediranib. Neuro-oncol 2010; 12: 466–472

[103] Rieger J, Bähr O, Müller K, Franz K, Steinbach J, Hattingen E. Bevacizumab-induced diffusion-restricted lesions in malignant glioma patients. J Neurooncol 2010; 99: 49–56

[104] Rieger J, Bähr O, Ronellenfitsch MW, Steinbach J, Hattingen E. Bevacizumab-induced diffusion restriction in patients with glioma: tumor progression or surrogate marker of hypoxia? J Clin Oncol 2010; 28: e477–, author reply e478

[105] Mong S, Ellingson BM, Nghiemphu PL et al. Persistent diffusion-restricted lesions in bevacizumab-treated malignant gliomas are associated with improved survival compared with matched controls. AJNR Am J Neuroradiol 2012; 33: 1763–1770

[106] Ellingson BM, Cloughesy TF, Lai A, Nghiemphu PL, Pope WB. Cell invasion, motility, and proliferation level estimate (CIMPLE) maps derived from serial diffusion MR images in recurrent glioblastoma treated with bevacizumab. J Neurooncol 2011; 105: 91–101

[107] Brandsma D, Stalpers L, Taal W, Sminia P, van den Bent MJ. Clinical features, mechanisms, and management of pseudoprogression in malignant gliomas. Lancet Oncol 2008; 9: 453–461

[108] Brandes AA, Franceschi E, Tosoni A et al. MGMT promoter methylation status can predict the incidence and outcome of pseudoprogression after concomitant radiochemotherapy in newly diagnosed glioblastoma patients. J Clin Oncol 2008; 26: 2192–2197

[109] Fink J, Born D, Chamberlain MC. Pseudoprogression: relevance with respect to treatment of high-grade gliomas. Curr Treat Options Oncol 2011; 12: 240–252

[110] Smith JS, Cha S, Mayo MC et al. Serial diffusion-weighted magnetic resonance imaging in cases of glioma: distinguishing tumor recurrence from postresection injury. J Neurosurg 2005; 103: 428–438

[111] Hein PA, Eskey CJ, Dunn JF, Hug EB. Diffusion-weighted imaging in the follow-up of treated high-grade gliomas: tumor recurrence versus radiation injury. AJNR Am J Neuroradiol 2004; 25: 201–209

[112] Zeng QS, Li CF, Liu H, Zhen JH, Feng DC. Distinction between recurrent glioma and radiation injury using magnetic resonance spectroscopy in combination with diffusion-weighted imaging. Int J Radiat Oncol Biol Phys 2007; 68: 151–158

[113] Asao C, Korogi Y, Kitajima M et al. Diffusion-weighted imaging of radiation-induced brain injury for differentiation from tumor recurrence. AJNR Am J Neuroradiol 2005; 26: 1455–1460

[114] Lee WJ, Choi SH, Park CK et al. Diffusion-weighted MR imaging for the differentiation of true progression from pseudoprogression following concomitant radiotherapy with temozolomide in patients with newly diagnosed high-grade gliomas. Acad Radiol 2012; 19: 1353–1361

[115] Matsusue E, Fink JR, Rockhill JK, Ogawa T, Maravilla KR. Distinction between glioma progression and post-radiation change by combined physiologic MR imaging. Neuroradiology 2010; 52: 297–306

[116] Fink JR, Carr RB, Matsusue E et al. Comparison of 3 Tesla proton MR spectroscopy, MR perfusion and MR diffusion for distinguishing glioma recurrence from posttreatment effects. J Magn Reson Imaging 2012; 35: 56–63

[117] Rock JP, Scarpace L, Hearshen D et al. Associations among magnetic resonance spectroscopy, apparent diffusion coefficients, and image-guided histopathology with special attention to radiation necrosis. Neurosurgery 2004; 54: 1111–1117, discussion 1117–1119

9 Diffusion Tensor Imaging

Bram Stieltjes and Peter Neher

9.1 Introduction

In Chapter 8, isotropic diffusion and the related diffusion weighted-imaging (DWI) were described. This chapter introduces a special case of DWI, diffusion tensor imaging (DTI) and other diffusion magnetic resonance imaging (MRI)-derived methods that are sensitive to anisotropic diffusion. The chapter also discusses the theory of DTI and other diffusion MRI-derived methods for anisotropy modeling and their application in the human brain. Chapters 10 and 11 discuss the application of DTI in surgical planning.

The human brain forms a complex network of billions of neurons. The rapid increase in knowledge about the human brain anatomy, physiology, and pathologies was originally based primarily on invasive animal or postmortem human studies. With the development of MRI, the first tool to gain noninvasive insights into the human brain was introduced. Initially, this technique proved to be valuable for assessing the macroscopic structure of brain regions and their pathologies (e.g., by identifying volumetric abnormalities of white matter [WM] or gray matter [GM] tissue).

Nevertheless, conventional MRI does not allow inferences to be made about the microstructural organization of tissue. WM and GM are depicted as largely homogeneous regions, with no means of identifying, for example, single-fiber strands and axonal connectivity patterns, well known from invasive animal and human postmortem studies.

The development of DWI changed this dramatically. DWI is a technique that enables the noninvasive probing of molecular diffusion processes and has found a wide range of applications in material sciences and medicine. Since its introduction in 1985, DWI has developed rapidly and enables insights into the anatomical and physiological properties of human tissue on a microscopic scale that cannot be obtained with other imaging techniques. The first medical applications of DWI focused on the management of acute stroke patients by analyzing the measured diffusivity maps. Over the last 10 to 15 years technical and methodological advances in DWI—such as DTI, diffusion spectrum imaging (DSI), and high angular resolution diffusion imaging (HARDI)—shifted the focus of research toward the analysis of WM structures, its disorders, and the mapping of the human connectome using fiber tractography.

Fiber tractography on the basis of DWI enables the three-dimensional (3D) reconstruction of the major WM pathways connecting the different regions of the cortex and thus a tract-specific analysis of tissue properties reflected in the DWI signal. It proved to be of great value in the identification of specific fiber bundles in vivo, tract-specific analysis (tractometry) and diagnosis of neurodegenerative diseases and neurolog disorders, development and aging studies, as well as surgical planning.[1,2,3,4,5,6] Besides these applications for visualization, quantifying, and analyzing the WM tracts themselves, tractography is also used for automatically subdividing the cortex into areas with similar connectivity patterns. Such GM parcellations have shown to be in good agreement with histology and functional MRI (fMRI).[7]

Because fiber tractography builds on a series of other processing steps, adding multiple layers of abstract modeling, simplification, and accumulated errors to the desired information about WM fibers, it comes with a number of limitations and issues to be considered. The quality of a tractogram depends on three main factors:
1. The acquisition parameters and quality of the raw diffusion-weighted data
2. The voxel-wise mathematical modeling of diffusion of the raw data
3. The actual tractography method itself

Fiber tractography is very sensitive to image quality and acquisition parameters. Depending on the method used, a single distorted voxel can compromise the complete fiber, causing it to end prematurely or leading it astray.[8] Also, the choice of imaging parameters—such as the number of acquired diffusion directions, the strength of the applied diffusion weighting, and the voxel size—can introduce considerable changes in the final tractogram. Another limitation directly arises from the fact that many fiber tractography algorithms assume a correlation of the principal diffusion directions of water molecules, usually represented by a mathematical model, and the principal fiber direction in the corresponding image voxel.[3,9] This assumption is valid only for certain fiber configurations and can cause a considerable number of false-positive or false-negative fibers in the final tractography result. Additionally, DWI does not provide information about the position of the neuronal synapses, which is necessary for a correct determination of fiber origins and terminations, or about the distinction between afferent and efferent axonal pathways.[7] Besides relying on the accuracy and validity of the preceding processing steps, fiber tractography shows a high degree of variability across different algorithms and subjects. This is owed to the different assumptions the methods are based on as well as their sometimes complex parametrization. Many studies also observed that WM boundaries are commonly underestimated by most of the tractography methods currently available.[6,10]

Over the last couple of years a substantial effort was made to alleviate these issues on all levels, including studies for optimal acquisition sequences,[11,12,13] novel preprocessing and diffusion modeling techniques,[14,15] as well as a wide variation of fiber tractography methods,[16] ranging from local deterministic approaches through probabilistic methods to global tractography. As these novel ideas and methods were being introduced, a number of new questions became increasingly important:

Which of the methods is the best? Is there a single best method for all the tasks at hand? What does "being the best" mean in the context of tractography?

In short, how can fiber tractography be evaluated? Although these questions cannot be answered to a full extent, the current chapter aims to explain the pros and cons of different methods and describe ways and means to evaluate a complete DTI pipeline before application of the results in a patient setting (Chapters 10 and 11). This chapter discusses commonly used methods for DWI-derived signal modeling and fiber-tracking methods.

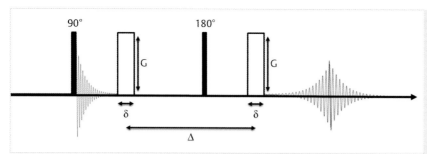

Fig. 9.1 Pulsed field gradient spin-echo sequence. After the 90-degree pulse, the first diffusion encoding gradient of amplitude G is applied. The diffusion encoding gradient pulse is applied again after the 180-degree pulse. Particles that move around during the diffusion time (Δ) will accumulate different phase shifts during each of the two diffusion gradient pulses, which leads to an incomplete rephasing of the spins and a successively weaker echo signal.

9.2 Diffusion-Weighted Imaging

In theory, every conventional MRI sequence can be sensitized for diffusion with additional strong magnetic field gradients. The basic principle of DWI is that particles moving around in a magnetic field gradient store the history of their movement as an accumulated phase gained at the different positions. Stejskal and Tanner[17] presented a DWI sequence based on a pulsed field gradient spin-echo (PFGSE). This sequence applies a strong diffusion-encoding gradient pulse of amplitude and direction G before the application of the 180-degree pulse. Particles at different positions along this direction will accumulate a different phase Φ_1 during the gradient application time δ. Here we are assuming that δ is short enough to render diffusion taking place during the application of the gradient pulse insignificant (narrow pulse approximation). After the 180-degree pulse, the diffusion encoding gradient pulse is applied a second time, resulting in a second phase shift Φ_2 (▶ Fig. 9.1).

For all stationary particles, the resulting net phase shift amounts to $\Phi_1 - \Phi_2 = \Phi_1 - \Phi_1 = 0$. The minus sign is a result of the 180 degree echo pulse. Particles that displace during the time Δ gain different phases during the first and second gradient pulse. This results in a net phase shift $\Phi_{diff} = \Phi_1 - \Phi_2 \neq 0$. Because randomly diffusing spins accumulate different phase shifts Φ_{diff} the signal measured when particles are diffusing along the direction of the gradient will be attenuated compared to a reference measurement S_0, acquired without the application of the gradient. The signal attenuation due to diffusion processes is usually expressed as follows:

$$E(q) = \frac{S(q)}{S_0} \tag{9.1}$$

with $q = \gamma G \delta$. One measurement $E(q)$ can be envisioned as one point in a three-dimensional (3D) space, further on denoted as q-space. By rewriting the net phase shift of a spin as $\Phi_{diff} = -q(x_1 - x_2)$ with the spin's start and end locations x_1 and x_2, the signal attenuation is described as follows:

$$(Eq) = \int \rho(x_1) \int P(x_1, x_2, \Delta) e^{-iq(x_2 - x_1)} dx_1 dx_2 \tag{9.2}$$

where $\rho(x_1)$ is the spin density at location x_1 and $P(x_1, x_2, \Delta)$ the diffusion propagator. In case of a Gaussian diffusion propagator, Equation 9.2 can be written as follows:

$$E(q) = e^{-q^2 \left(\Delta - \frac{\delta}{3}\right)D} = e^{-bD} \tag{9.3}$$

The factor $b = q^2\left(\Delta - \frac{\delta}{3}\right)$, first introduced by Bihan and Breton,[18] is called b-value and characterizes the strength of the diffusion

weighting. Equation 9.3 can be easily rearranged to calculate D. Because the diffusion coefficient of a fluid is constant, but the measured value varies depending on q and the tissue architecture, D is denoted as the apparent diffusion coefficient (ADC). If the shape of the diffusion propagator is not known a priori, one can either fit mathematical models that assume certain properties of the propagator to the measured data or one can directly estimate the so-called ensemble average propagator (EAP) from the q-space data. Using the net displacement variable $= x_2 - x_1$, the EAP is defined as follows:

$$-P(x, t) = \int \rho(x_1) P(x_1, x_2 + x, l) dx_1 \tag{9.4}$$

with Equation 9.4, Equation 9.2 can be simplified:

$$E(q) = \int -P(x, \Delta) e^{-iqx} dx \tag{9.5}$$

The EAP can now be obtained by inverting the Fourier transform in Equation 9.5. This technique is called q-space imaging (QSI),[19,20] or DSI.[21,22,23]

9.3 Mathematical Modeling of Anisotropic DWI Signals

The direct calculation of the EAP, as performed in QSI and DSI, requires a densely sampled q-space, which results in very long acquisition times. By fitting mathematical models to the measured data, an approximation of the EAP or a description of the underlying tissue structure can be obtained from a much more sparsely sampled q-space. A large variety of methods to reconstruct such an approximation has been introduced, and the most commonly used techniques are described in this section.

9.3.1 Diffusion Tensor Imaging

The simplest model of anisotropic diffusion is based on the so-called diffusion tensor (DT) and assumes that the EAP can be described by a, possibly anisotropic, 3D Gaussian distribution. The DT can be described by a 3×3 matrix D, containing the eigenvalues of diffusion on its diagonal. The other matrix elements describe the correlation between the diffusion along the three coordinate axes. The diffusion tensor matrix can be depicted as a 3D ellipsoid pointing in the direction of largest diffusion (▶ Fig. 9.2). Because the DT matrix is a symmetric

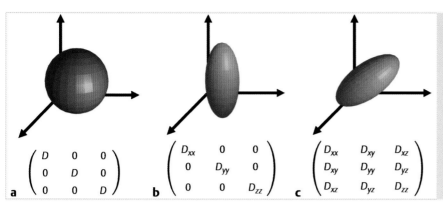

Fig. 9.2 The diffusion tensor. Diffusion tensor shapes for isotropic (**a**) and anisotropic (**b,c**) diffusion.

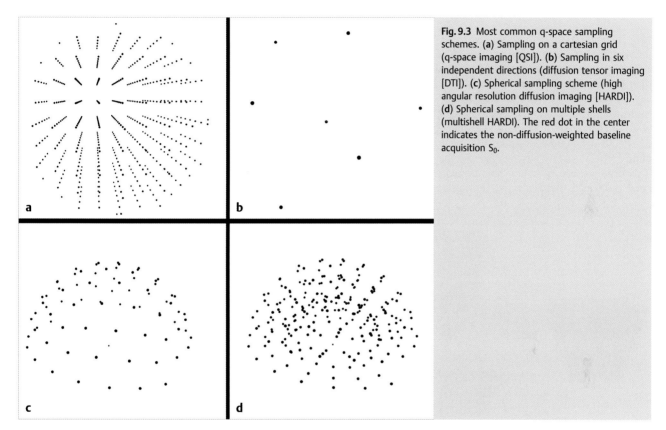

Fig. 9.3 Most common q-space sampling schemes. (**a**) Sampling on a cartesian grid (q-space imaging [QSI]). (**b**) Sampling in six independent directions (diffusion tensor imaging [DTI]). (**c**) Spherical sampling scheme (high angular resolution diffusion imaging [HARDI]). (**d**) Spherical sampling on multiple shells (multishell HARDI). The red dot in the center indicates the non-diffusion-weighted baseline acquisition S_0.

matrix, six acquisitions S(q) in different directions plus one reference acquisition S_0 without diffusion weighting are sufficient to fit a tensor to the data. To this end, Equation 9.3 can be rewritten:

$$E(q) = e^{-bq^T D q} \qquad (9.6)$$

where q = q/|q| is the normalized q-space vector, pointing in the direction of the magnetic field gradient G. Several fitting methods for the diffusion tensor have been proposed, but the most commonly used technique is a simple least squares approximation.

This imaging technique is called DTI and was first introduced by Basser et al[24] Despite its simplicity, or maybe precisely because of it, the DT is still the most commonly used model to describe the shape of the EAP, at least in clinical settings.

9.3.2 High Angular Resolution Diffusion Imaging

In many cases, the assumption of a Gaussian EAP does not hold, for example in crossing fiber configurations and for higher b-values. Thus, in such cases, the DT does not describe the diffusion process accurately in the corresponding image voxel. To resolve such complex fiber configurations, which occur in more than one third of the voxels of a typical brain image,[25] or to estimate microstructural tissue parameters, more complex modeling and thus more information is required. A commonly used approach that lies between the full q-space sampling of QSI and the six-direction acquisition scheme of DTI is the HARDI acquisition scheme. In HARDI, the sampled q-space points are distributed spherically around the q-space center, possibly over multiple shells (i.e., with multiple b-values). ▶ Fig. 9.3 illustrates the most commonly used q-space sampling schemes.

9.3.3 Multitensor Reconstruction and Multicompartment Modeling

Instead of fitting a single diffusion tensor to the acquired data, it is possible to fit a mixture of multiple tensors to account for multiple fiber populations or fiber compartments. This technique assumes that each voxel contains a distinct number of fiber clusters n, that the diffusing molecules do not exchange between these clusters, and that the diffusion tensor is an appropriate model for a directionally coherent fiber bundle. This can be written as the sum:

$$E(q) = \sum_{i=1}^{\eta} w_i e^{-bq^T D_{iq}} \tag{9.7}$$

with the compartment weights w_i. The drawback of this method is that the number of fiber clusters n needs to be known a priori. Also, nonlinear optimization is necessary to fit the parameters D_i of the model. ▶ Fig. 9.4 illustrates the method for n = 2. Several implementations of the multitensor reconstruction method have been presented, imposing different kinds of constraints to stabilize the fit, which is often difficult due to the high number of parameters required for larger values of n.[11,23,26,27]

A large variety of other multicompartment models has been developed. Besides trying to calculate the main fiber orientations in one voxel, most of these techniques try to obtain information about the volume fractions of the different cellular structures. One example of this type of signal modeling is the composite hindered and restricted model of diffusion (CHARMED) proposed by Assaf and Basser.[28] Panagiotaki et al[29] present a comprehensive taxonomy of the abundance of different compartment models currently available. These models try to explain the restricted diffusion within the axons, the hindered diffusion between the axons, and the remaining isotropically diffusing water. Other approaches try to obtain microstructural features like the axon diameter or fiber dispersion.[30,31] Nevertheless, all of these modeling techniques rely on parametric representations of the single compartments and impose a lot of assumptions and restrictions on the nature of diffusion in human tissue.

9.3.4 Spherical Deconvolution

Similar to the multitensor approach described in the previous section, this method assumes that the measured HARDI signal consists of the weighted sum of signals generated by different fiber compartments. This is equivalent to modeling the signal as a convolution of the fiber orientation distribution function (fODF), which describes the distribution of fibers within a voxel, with the signal generated by a single fiber (response function, ▶ Fig. 9.5). The method assumes that the diffusion properties of

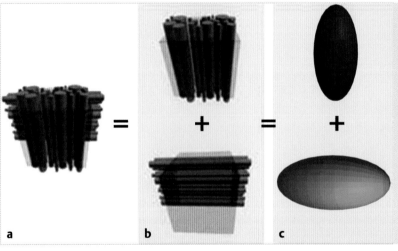

Fig. 9.4 Multitensor signal modeling. The multitensor model assumes that each voxel contains a distinct number of fiber clusters (here two), each of which can be modeled by a Gaussian distribution. The signal is modeled as the weighted sum of these distributions. (Adapted from Seunarine KK, Alexander DC. Multiple fibers: beyond the diffusion tensor. In: Johansen-Berg H, Behrens, TEJ, eds. Diffusion MRI: From Quantitative Measurement to In-Vivo Neuroanatomy. Burlington, MA: Elsevier Academic Press; 2009:55–72.)

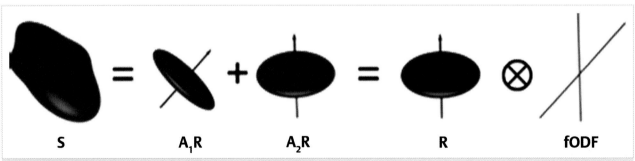

Fig. 9.5 Similar to the multitensor model, the spherical deconvolution (SD) models the signal (S) in each voxel as the weighted sum of a certain response function (R) rotated into the direction of the fiber populations with rotation matrices A_1 and A_2, which is equivalent to the convolution of R and the fiber orientation distribution function (fODF). The signal can thus be obtained by deconvolving S with R. (Adapted from Seunarine KK, Alexander DC. Multiple fibers: beyond the diffusion tensor. In: Johansen-Berg H, Behrens, TEJ, eds. Diffusion MRI: From Quantitative Measurement to In-Vivo Neuroanatomy. Burlington, MA: Elsevier Academic Press; 2009:55–72.)

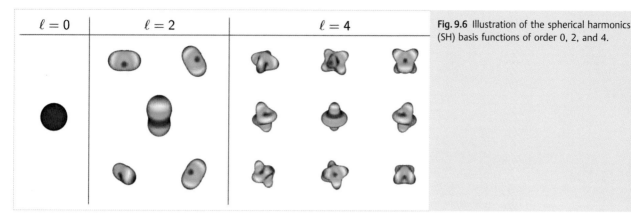

$\ell = 0$	$\ell = 2$	$\ell = 4$

Fig. 9.6 Illustration of the spherical harmonics (SH) basis functions of order 0, 2, and 4.

a single fiber are constant over the whole brain and that anisotropy differences are purely a result of partial volume effects. Furthermore, it assumes that there is no exchange of diffusing molecules between the directionally distinct fiber populations. The response function can either be modeled explicitly[9] or learned directly from the data by aligning and averaging the signal of the voxels displaying the highest anisotropy.[25] The fODF can then be obtained by deconvolving the signal with the response function. The peak size of the fODF contains the information about the volume fractions of the single-fiber populations. By using a linear basis to model the response function (e.g., the spherical harmonics [SH] basis), the deconvolution step reduces to a single matrix multiplication. Compared to the multitensor approach, one of the biggest advantages of the spherical deconvolution (SD) is that the number of fibers per voxel does not need to be known a priori.

The main drawback of this method is its dependency on the estimated deconvolution kernel and its susceptibility to noise, resulting in a large number of spurious peaks. Tournier et al[32] proposed a regularization of the SD method, which removes spurious peaks and negative lobes of the fODF while retaining a high angular resolution, called super-resolved constrained spherical deconvolution (CSD).

9.3.5 Persistent Angular Structure MRI

Jansons and Alexander[33] proposed a projection of the diffusion propagator onto a sphere, resulting in a structure similar to the fODF called persistent angular structure (PAS). The PAS is defined as the function on the sphere that, when Fourier transformed, best explains the normalized diffusion-weighted signal. The original implementation uses a maximum-entropy parametrization of the PAS that imposes very few assumptions and can therefore capture the true shape of the PAS very well. The main drawback of this method is the high computational cost of the needed nonlinear optimization and the successive long computation times of several days for a whole brain. Alternative implementations[34,35] use a linear SH basis, which speeds up the process significantly but at the same time reduces the accuracy of the PAS estimate.

9.3.6 Q-Ball Imaging

Q-ball imaging methods approximate the EAP using a diffusion orientation distribution function (dODF), which is defined as

the radial projection of the EAP onto the unit sphere. To calculate the dODF from a HARDI acquisition, a transformation defined for spherical functions, the Funk-Radon transform (FRT), is used. The FRT of a function evaluated in a direction x is calculated as the integral over the signal values $S(q)$ lying on a circle with a certain radius rq in the plane perpendicular to x. This transform is used to calculate a set of discrete dODF values:

$$dODF(x) = \int_q S(q)\delta(xq)\delta(|q| - r_q) \tag{9.8}$$

To calculate this integral, the available discrete values of $S(q)$ have to be interpolated. The original implementation, introduced by Tuch,[36] uses radial basis functions for the interpolation. Other works use an SH basis, which has the advantage that the FRT in Equation 9.8 can be calculated analytically and that the representation of the signal becomes much more compact.[37] With increasing order l of the SH basis functions, more details can be modeled at the cost of more coefficients and a successively less robust fit (▶ Fig. 9.6). A further extension of the Q-ball algorithm was presented by Aganj et al[38] The original calculation of the dODF uses a radial projection of the EAP onto the sphere, without taking the quadratic change of the volume element into account, which decreases the overall dODF sharpness and causes the need for normalization. Aganj et al[39] proposed an adaptation of the original algorithm, using the mathematically correct definition of the dODF by considering the quadratic constant solid angle factor r^2 in the radial projection of the EAP:

$$dODF(x) = \int_0^\infty -P(xr_q)r_q^2 dr_q \tag{9.9}$$

Q-ball imaging has the advantage, besides its speed and robustness, that no assumptions about the shape of the propagator are imposed. Also, extensions to integrate the information of data acquired with multiple b-values have been proposed.[39] Nevertheless, in comparison with algorithms that reconstruct the fODF, the dODF yields less sharp and accurate peaks, which is especially important for many fiber-tracking algorithms.

9.4 Fiber Tracking

Tractography algorithms try to explicitly estimate the underlying fiber pathways from the given voxel-wise information (▶ Fig. 9.7). There exists a wide variety of different tractography algorithms that can be roughly divided into the two subgroups of local and global methods. The following subsections will give

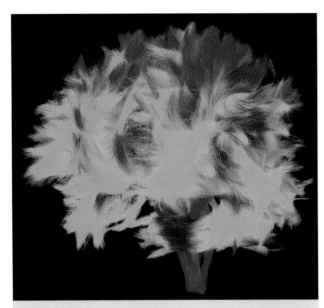

Fig. 9.7 Whole brain tractography. Fibers running left–right are colored red, anteroposterior are green, and caudocranial are blue.

a brief overview over the basic principles of some of the most common tractography methods.

9.4.1 Tracking Using Local Information

Deterministic local tracking methods try to reconstruct one fiber at a time by following the voxel-wise information about the main fiber directions and successively adding segments to the fiber (line propagation techniques).[40–45] Although most of these methods are known to be computationally performant, they often struggle with image artifacts or complex fiber configurations like crossings or kissings.[46] Probabilistic approaches take the local uncertainty of the fiber orientation into account by sampling the next propagation direction from a local probability distribution.[47–54] Such a probabilistic sampling of the fiber directions allows these methods to overcome ambiguous image regions by also including other fiber progressions besides the most likely one. Other local methods try to approach the tracing of white matter tracts as a segmentation task, for example, using hidden Markov random fields to model WM tracts as regions of coherent diffusion,[55] or using fast marching methods that model a fiber tract as a surface that is evolved depending on the local diffusivity along the surface normal.[56,57,58] Furthermore, multistage methods, in which the actual tractography is guided by connectivity information based on a previous graph search, have also been presented.[59,60] Despite these clear limitations, especially in crossing regions, line propagation techniques are still the most commonly used methods, which is owed to their relative simplicity and wide availability as well as computational performance.

9.4.2 Deterministic Streamline Tractography

One of the first deterministic streamline tractography methods —fiber assignment by continuous tracking (FACT)—was introduced by Mori et al.[44] In this line propagation technique the major DT eigenvector in the current voxel defines the direction of the next propagation step. A wide range of adaptations to the classic FACT algorithm have been presented, including different interpolation methods of the discrete tensor field (▶ Fig. 9.8) and higher-order integration methods (e.g., Euler and Runge-Kutta)[40,42] as well as extensions to multiple fiber directions per voxel, based on modeling techniques like PAS, Q-ball, and CSD.[61,62]

9.4.3 Tensorline Tractography

Image noise, partial volume effects, and complex fiber configurations influence the direction of the major DT eigenvector, which causes simple streamline techniques like FACT to accumulate an error with each propagation step of the streamline. Weinstein et al[63] and Lazar et al[64] introduced a technique called tensor deflection (TEND) that uses the entire tensor D to determine the direction v_{out} of tract propagation:

$$v_{out} = fe_1 + (1 - g)((1 - g)v_{in} + gDv_{in})(10)v_{out}$$
$$= fe_1 + (1 - f)((1 - g)v_{in} + gDv_{in}) \qquad (9.10)$$

where e_1 is the direction of the largest eigenvector, v_{in} is the direction of the last propagation step, and f and g are weighting factors between e_1, the incoming direction v_{in}, and the actual tensor deflection term Dv_{in}. D only bends the incoming vector toward the major eigenvector direction instead of simply setting $v_{out} = e_1$, which directly limits curvature, results in smoother tracts, and allows the tracking, even through anisotropic regions, where conventional tensor streamline techniques fail to follow the correct fiber trajectory (▶ Fig. 9.9). Setting f to 1 is equivalent to performing FACT tractography. Tractography methods based on TEND are referred to as tensorline tractography.

9.4.4 Tractography Using State Space Models

Another approach to overcome the limitations of simple streamline tractography is to simultaneously estimate the diffusion model parameters using state space models while propagating the streamline.[65] The method proposed by Malcolm et al[66] uses an unscented Kalman filter to nonlinearly fit a multitensor model to the data. The filter creates candidate models for the signal at the current position based on the model parameters at the last propagation step. The streamline is then propagated into the direction estimated by the candidate that is most consistent with the signal at the current position. Using causal estimation in this way yields intrinsically smooth fiber trajectories and a reduced modeling error. The drawback of this method is its high computational effort compared with other local tractography techniques.

9.4.5 Seeding and Termination

For all local tractography methods, the starting points (seed points) of the fibers need to be defined. Depending on the task, the method, and the implementation, different seeding strategies can be pursued, for example, seeding the whole brain or only a certain region of interest (ROI), placing single or multiple

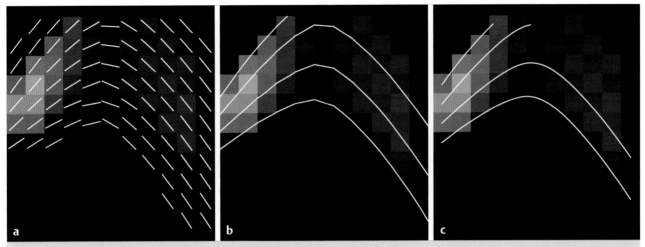

Fig. 9.8 Deterministic streamline tractography. Simple line propagation techniques based on the diffusion tensor model follow the major diffusion tensor (DT) eigenvector in the current voxel (**a**). (**b, c**) The difference between the nearest neighbor-based fiber assignment by continuous tracking (FACT) algorithm (**b**) and a line propagation technique using a linearly interpolated tensor field (**c**), which results in a much smoother tract propagation.

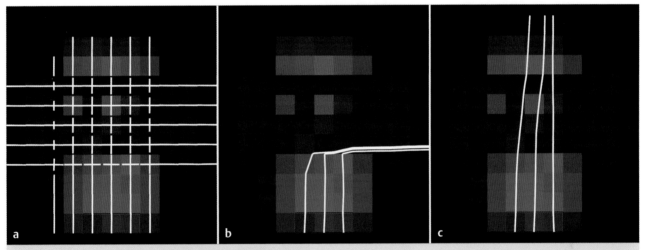

Fig. 9.9 Tensorline tractography. (**a**) The actual fiber directions in each voxel. Since the diffusion tensor cannot resolve crossing situations, the fiber assignment by continuous tracking (FACT) tractography cannot follow the fiber through the crossing but stops or goes astray (**b**). Using tensor deflection the crossing situation can be resolved successfully (**c**). The seeding area is indicated with a red frame in the lower part of the image.

seeds per voxel, and using fixed or random positions for the seeds in the image volume. Alternatively, some methods use a reverse strategy by placing seeds in the whole image volume and retaining only the fibers passing a specified ROI. Commonly used stopping criteria for the streamline propagation are thresholds on the fractional anisotropy (FA), the tract curvature and the maximum fiber length. The FA is a commonly used scalar index determining the degree of anisotropy of a tensor with values between 0 (completely isotropic) and 1 (maximally anisotropic). FA values for single fiber WM voxels are usually larger than 0.2.[67]

9.4.6 Global Tractography

Global methods try to reconstruct all fibers simultaneously, searching for a global optimum. Although computationally much more challenging, global methods promise more robust results.[68] Methods based on vector field regularization that infer information about the local fiber orientation by including information from their direct neighborhood were the first techniques working in the spirit of global tractography that did not base the fiber propagation purely on the local information gathered along its path.[69] Other methods try to reconstruct WM fibers globally by means of a random walk algorithm[70] or a voting process that assigns scores to a set of candidate trajectories provided by the Hough transform of the input image.[71] Global fiber tractography was boosted by the development of energy-based approaches and their recent computationally efficient enhancements.[72]

The basic idea of the global tractography algorithm proposed by Reisert et al[72] is to fit a model M, consisting of directed points (particles) and connections between the particles, to the image data D by minimizing two energy terms. The first energy, the so-called external energy (E_{ext}), measures the distance from an artificial signal computed from the current model configuration to the original image data (i.e., the external energy ensures that M is able to explain the signal in the best possible way). The second energy, the internal energy (E_{int}), applies certain constraints to the model itself. It is designed to enforce long and straight fibers. By minimizing E_{int} the model is shaped in a way that is consistent with structural knowledge about neuronal fibers. Each particle can connect to another particle with one of its end points. A chain of connected particles represents a fiber. The connection potential between two particles is small if the end points of two connected particles lie close together and point in the same direction. To optimize the model, the whole problem is formulated as a maximization of the posteriori probability of the model M given the image data D:

$$P(M|D) = e^{-E_{int}(M)/T - E_{ext}(M,D)/T} \qquad (9.11)$$

$P(M|D)$ is maximized via the introduction of random changes into the model M. The resulting model configuration M' is afterward accepted or rejected according to a certain ratio calculated from $P(M'|D)$ and $P(M|D)$. By successively reducing the temperature T it becomes more and more likely to converge to a steady and optimal configuration of the model.

9.5 In Vivo Evaluation of Diffusion Models in an Anisotropic Environment

In the following part, we will try to illustrate the behavior of common combinations of signal modeling and fiber tracking algorithms. To do so, the local directional fiber plausibility (LDFP) of over 13,000 tractograms was evaluated. The concept of LDFP enables the assessment of tractograms obtained from all study types including in vivo, where other automatic and quantitative evaluation concepts are usually restricted to phantom or postmortem data sets. The LDFP assesses whether a fiber configuration reconstructed by a tractography algorithm correctly represents the main underlying fiber directions. To this end, the voxel-wise directional error of a tractogram is calculated directly with respect to a reference. If no reference is available, as is the case for in vivo datasets, high-quality reference datasets that allow for a robust estimation of the local fiber architecture are employed. The reference datasets are then used to evaluate algorithms that were run only on information-reduced subsets of the reference data in order to better reflect real clinical scenarios, where the acquisition of high-quality data sets is usually unrealistic, mainly due to time constraints.

In the presented results 10 diffusion-weighted data sets included in the Q1 data release of the human connectome project (HCP) (http://humanconnectome.org) were used. All data sets were acquired on a Siemens Skyra 3T scanner (Siemens Medical Solutions USA, Inc., Malvern, PA) at Washington University in St. Louis.[73] Among other customizations, these scanners were equipped with a set of high-end gradient coils, enabling diffusion encoding gradient strengths of 100mT/m. The acquisition parameters were as follows: three b-values: 1,000, 2,000, and 3,000 s/mm², 90 gradient directions per b-value, spherically distributed over the half-shell.[74] Eighteen baseline

volumes without diffusion weighting (6 per b-value), isotropic voxel size of 1.25 mm with 111 slices covering the whole brain, TR/TE: 5,520/89.5 ms, bandwidth: 1,488 Hz/P.

All data sets were corrected for head motion, eddy currents, and susceptibility distortions and are in general of very high quality. These data sets therefore meet all preconditions to be used as a high-quality reference for evaluating the LDFP of a tractogram. The following set of tractography and local modeling methods was used to perform full-brain tractography on all 10 in vivo datasets:

Local models:
- Diffusion tensor (DT)
- Q-ball
- CSA Q-ball
- CSD

Tractography algorithm:
- Deterministic streamline
- Probabilistic streamline
- Global Gibbs tractography

The tractography was performed using all combinations of the following parameters:
- Streamline tractography:
  - Step size: 0.3, 0.6, 1, and 3 mm
  - Curvature radius: 0.3, 0.6, 1, and 3 mm
- Global Gibbs tractography:
  - Iterations: $10^6, 5 \times 10^6, 10^7, 5 \times 10^7, 10^8$
  - Curvature threshold: 45 degrees
  - Particle length: 1.25, 2.5, and 3.75 mm
  - Particle width: 0.1, 0.5, 1, 2, and 3 mm

Tractography was restricted for all data sets using a WM mask image generated by the Freesurfer recon-all command.[28]

The LDFP evaluation of each tractogram was performed in three individual ROIs inside the WM of the respective HCP dataset:
1. ROI-1 consists of all voxels inside the WM that contain crossing fibers (i.e., more than one fiber direction).
2. ROI-2 consists of all single-fiber voxels inside the WM.
3. ROI-3 consists of all WM voxels.

9.5.1 Results

Across all ROIs, the best results obtained by all algorithms in conjunction with the DT or CSD local model show the lowest variance. In crossing-fiber regions (ROI-1), all algorithms performed best using the CSD local model (► Table 9.1). In single-fiber regions (ROI-2), the smoother DT and Q-ball models performed best (► Table 9.2). If evaluated in the complete WM (ROI-3), the best probabilistic result was obtained using the DT model, the best deterministic result with the Q-ball model, and the best global result using CSD (► Table 9.3). No algorithm yielded its best result using CSA Q-ball. The deterministic method performed best in all ROIs. The tractograms yielding the lowest angular error per algorithm class in the respective ROI are depicted in ► Fig. 9.10, ► Fig. 9.11, and ► Fig. 9.12.

Since the number of single-fiber voxels exceeds the number of crossing voxels in the reference data sets by a factor of about 3, the LDFP results of ROI-3 are strongly biased toward the best

Table 9.1 Best in vivo local directional fiber plausibility (LDFP) results for all algorithms and local models obtained in region of interest-1 (ROI-1)

	Diffusion Tensor (degrees)	Q-ball (degrees)	Constant solid angle (CSA) Q-ball (degrees)	Constrained spherical deconvolution (degrees)
Deterministic Streamline	39.4	26.9	74.8	**9.2**
Global Gibbs	38.3	32.3	21.5	**11.4**
Probabilistic Streamline	39.2	41.1	36.4	**15.9**

Note: In crossing-fiber regions, all algorithms yielded the lowest angular error using constrained spherical deconvolution (CSD) as the local model (dark blue cells).

Table 9.2 Best in vivo local directional fiber plausibility (LDFP) results for all algorithms and local models obtained in region of interest-2 (ROI-2)

	Diffusion tensor (degrees)	Q-ball (degrees)	Constant solid angle (CSA) Q-ball (degrees)	Constrained spherical deconvolution (degrees)
Deterministic Streamline	6.5	**5.4**	13.5	7.8
Global Gibbs	8.4	**7.5**	7.6	8.2
Probabilistic Streamline	**6.9**	54.9	13.3	9.8

Note: In single-fiber regions all algorithms yielded their best results using smoother and more robust models such as the diffusion tensor (DT) (dark cells).

Table 9.3 Best in vivo local directional fiber plausibility (LDFP) results for all algorithms and local models obtained in region of interest-3 (ROI-3)

	Diffusion tensor (degrees)	Q-ball (degrees)	Constant solid angle (CSA) Q-ball (degrees)	Constrained spherical deconvolution (degrees)
Deterministic Streamline	11.0	**8.0**	39.1	8.5
Global Gibbs	12.7	11.2	9.9	**9.3**
Probabilistic Streamline	**11.4**	50.8	18.2	11.6

Note: Each class of algorithms yielded their lowest angular error (dark blue cells) with a different local model when evaluated in the complete white matter.

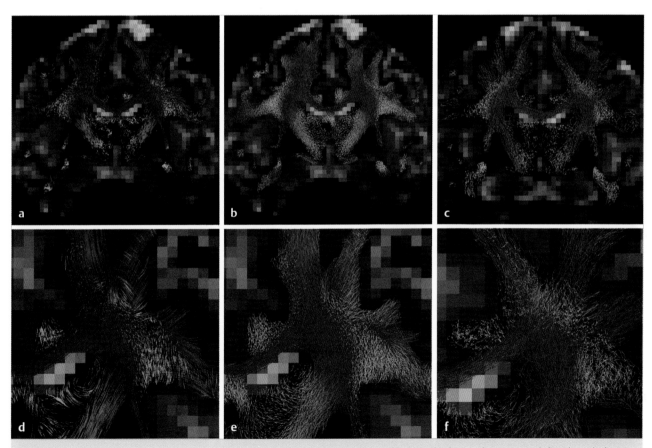

Fig. 9.10 Tractograms with the lowest angular error in region of interest-1 (ROI-1) (▶ Table 9.1). The figures show a coronal slice through the respective tractograms and a corresponding close-up view on the crossing between the corpus callosum (CC), corticospinal tract (CST), and superior longitudinal fasciculus (SLF) for deterministic CSD (**a,d**), probabilistic CSD (**b,e**), and global CSD tractography (**c,f**).

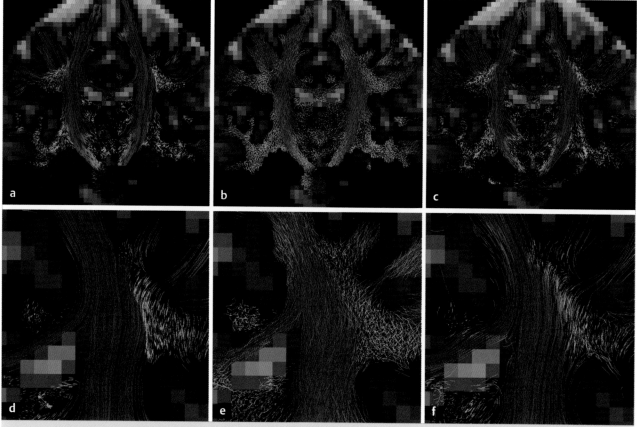

Fig. 9.11 Tractograms with the lowest angular error in region of interest-2 (ROI-2) (▶ Table 9.2). The figures show a coronal slice through the respective tractograms and a corresponding close-up view on the crossing between the corpus callosum (CC), corticospinal tract (CST), and superior longitudinal fasciculus (SLF) for deterministic Q-ball (**a,d**), global Q-ball (**b,e**), and probabilistic DT tractography (**c,f**).

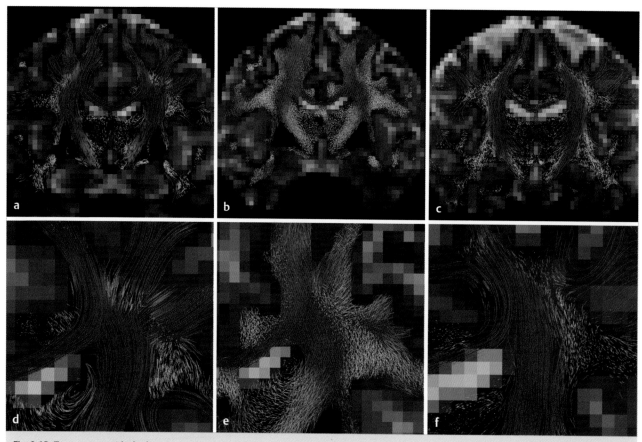

Fig. 9.12 Tractograms with the lowest angular error in region of interest-3 (ROI-3) (▶ Table 9.3). The figures show a coronal slice through the respective tractograms and a corresponding close-up view on the crossing between the corpus callosum (CC), corticospinal tract (CST), and superior longitudinal fasciculus (SLF) for deterministic Q-ball (**a,d**), global CSD (**b,e**) and probabilistic DT tractography (**c,f**).

Table 9.4 Best average local directional fiber plausibility (LDFP) results of region of interest-1 (ROI-1) and ROI-2

	Diffusion tensor (degrees)	Q-ball (degrees)	Constant solid angle (CSA) Q-ball (degrees)	Constrained spherical deconvolution (degrees)
Deterministic Streamline	23.6	16.49	44.77	8.64
Global Gibbs	25.05	20.89	14.66	9.88
Probabilistic Streamline	23.14	48.14	27.31	13.01

Note: Best average LDFP results of ROI-1 and ROI-2. Similar to the evaluation in the crossing region ROI-1 alone, the best average results over the two ROIs are obtained when using the CSD local model (dark blue cells).

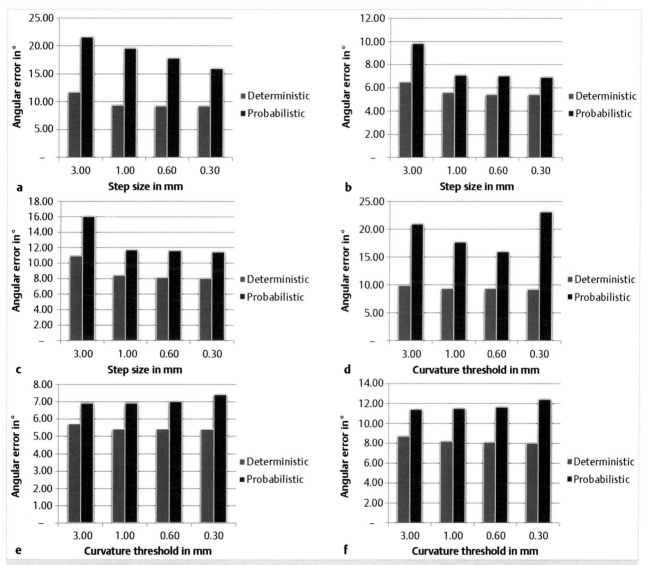

Fig. 9.13 The effect of the step size (a–c) and curvature threshold (d–f) parameters on the local directional fiber plausibility (LDFP). With shorter steps, the angular error decreased for all algorithms and in all regions of interest (ROIs). With a smaller curvature threshold, the error decreased for deterministic algorithms in all ROIs. For probabilistic algorithms, the results are more ROI-specific, and overall the angular error even increased with a smaller curvature threshold (c).

single-fiber results. ▶ Table 9.4 shows the angular errors of the pipelines that yielded the best averaged result of ROI-1 and ROI-2, which weights the results of crossing- and single-fiber voxels equally regardless of the number of voxels per region. Similar to the results in ROI-1, all algorithms performed best when using the CSD local model in this case.

The effect of different tractography parameters was analyzed separately for each ROI and deterministic, probabilistic, and global algorithm classes. In all ROIs, a decreasing step size led to a decreasing angular error (▶ Fig. 9.13a–c). Decreasing the minimum curvature threshold, which allows higher-fiber curvatures, has the same effect but on a smaller scale and only for deterministic algorithms. For probabilistic algorithms, the decreasing curvature threshold led to an increased angular error, both in single-fiber regions (ROI-2) and in the complete WM mask (ROI-3) (▶ Fig. 9.13e,f). In crossing-fiber regions the

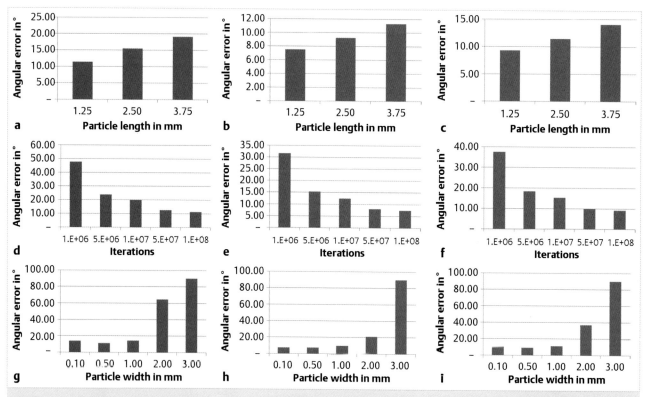

Fig. 9.14 The effect of the global tractography particle length, width, and number of iterations on the local directional fiber plausibility (LDFP). An increased particle length or width increased the angular error in all regions of interest (ROIs), whereas an increased number of iterations decreased the error.

error decreased at first but increased again for the smallest curvature threshold (► Fig. 9.13d).

The global Gibbs tractography results showed clear trends for all parameters consistent across all ROIs. With increasing particle length, the angular error increased (► Fig. 9.14a–c). A similar trend was observable for the increasing particle width, which resulted in a relatively constant angular error at lower values (≤ 1mm) and a strongly increasing error at higher values. Increasing the number of iterations resulted in a lower angular error (► Fig. 9.14d–i).

9.6 Conclusions

One of the main conclusions on fiber tractography that can be drawn is that currently no "perfect" fiber tractography algorithm exists, especially not under in vivo conditions. All methods show certain strengths and weaknesses that have to be carefully weighted before an algorithm is chosen for a specific task. Next we summarize the key issues, considering local signal modeling and fiber tracking.

9.6.1 Local Signal Modeling

Considering local modeling of the DWI-derived signal, the following can be concluded:

- In crossing-fiber situations, CSD outperforms all other models by far.
- In single-fiber situations, smoother models like DT and Q-ball, depending on the algorithm, perform best.

Nevertheless, the differences between the models are relatively small. Reasonable results can be obtained with all other evaluated combinations of models and algorithms except of the Q-ball probabilistic streamline tractography.

- The lowest average angular errors of ROIs-1 and -2 consistently point to CSD as being the most suitable local model for all algorithms.
- The combinations of tractography algorithms and local models that always yielded high angular errors are CSA Q-ball deterministic tractography and Q-ball probabilistic tractography. These combinations should be avoided.

Of the models investigated, CSD is always among the best-performing models and seems recommendable as the default method if one is unsure. Smooth models, such as Q-ball, show a particularly poor performance with probabilistic tractography, which needs sharp angular profiles to avoid an excessively arbitrary directional sampling. This is in concordance with earlier studies.[75,76,77,78]

In general the results strongly suggest that we need to move beyond DTI for meaningful fiber tractography, in particular for clinical applications of fiber tractography, where DTI is still the most commonly used method!

9.6.2 Fiber Tracking

Moving on to fiber tractography algorithms, one of the main issues with the state-of-the-art methods is the large number of fibers that end prematurely in the WM.[67,68] This is a general problem of purely DWI data-driven methods because it requires additional information not contained in DWI data sets. Tractography algorithms simply cannot know where fibers begin and end because DWI provides only localized directional information that ends at the voxel border. Algorithms such as the global Gibbs tractography or the online filtering tractography (OFT) try to mitigate this issue by including some kind of prior knowledge into the tracking process, which proved to be a successful approach, as also demonstrated by previous studies.[77] These attempts to guide the tractography process using prior information might be improved even further by additionally using techniques other than DWI, such as fMRI and imaging-based tissue classification. Besides forcing the exploitation of multimodality, which proved to be successful for many other tasks besides fiber tractography, a promising, purely DWI-based, approach is to include microstructural information into the tractography process, which rarely happens at the moment.[79,80] The choice of a suitable tractography algorithm, local modeling method, and corresponding parametrization has severe consequences for the validity of tasks such as connectomics, surgical planning, and tissue quantification that are based on tractography results. Surgery planning requires an unmitigated reconstruction of the tract of interest. An underestimation of such a tract can lead to decisions with potentially grave consequences for the patient.[81] The overestimation of the tract of interest on the other hand can lead to an incomplete resection of the tumor, which can significantly impair the survival rates after surgery.[82]

References

[1] Ciccarelli O, Catani M, Johansen-Berg H, Clark C, Thompson A. Diffusion-based tractography in neurological disorders: concepts, applications, and future developments. Lancet Neurol 2008; 7: 715–727

[2] Hüppi PS, Dubois J. Diffusion tensor imaging of brain development. Semin Fetal Neonatal Med 2006; 11: 489–497

[3] Johansen-Berg H, Behrens TE. Just pretty pictures? What diffusion tractography can add in clinical neuroscience. Curr Opin Neurol 2006; 19: 379–385

[4] Mori S, Itoh R, Zhang J et al. Diffusion tensor imaging of the developing mouse brain. Magn Reson Med 2001; 46: 18–23

[5] Sundgren PC, Dong Q, Gómez-Hassan D, Mukherji SK, Maly P, Welsh R. Diffusion tensor imaging of the brain: review of clinical applications. Neuroradiology 2004; 46: 339–350

[6] Yamada K, Sakai K, Akazawa K, Yuen S, Nishimura T. MR tractography: a review of its clinical applications. Magn Reson Med Sci 2009; 8: 165–174

[7] Jbabdi S, Lehman JF, Haber SN, Behrens TE. Human and monkey ventral prefrontal fibers use the same organizational principles to reach their targets: tracing versus tractography. J Neurosci 2013; 33: 3190–3201

[8] Mori S, van Zijl PC. Fiber tracking: principles and strategies—a technical review. NMR Biomed 2002; 15: 468–480

[9] Assaf Y, Pasternak O. Diffusion tensor imaging (DTI)-based white matter mapping in brain research: a review. J Mol Neurosci 2008; 34: 51–61

[10] Kinoshita M, Yamada K, Hashimoto N et al. Fiber-tracking does not accurately estimate size of fiber bundle in pathological condition: initial neurosurgical experience using neuronavigation and subcortical white matter stimulation. Neuroimage 2005; 25: 424–429

[11] Alexander DC, Barker GJ. Optimal imaging parameters for fiber-orientation estimation in diffusion MRI. Neuroimage 2005; 27: 357–367

[12] Caruyer E, Cheng J, Lenglet C, et al. Optimal design of multiple q-shells experiments for diffusion MRI. In: MICCAI Workshop on Computational Diffusion MRI. 2011

[13] Kamath A, Aganj I, Xu JG, et al. Generalized constant solid angle ODF and optimal acquisition protocol for fiber orientation mapping. In: MICCAI Workshop on Computational Diffusion MRI. Nice, France: 2012

[14] Alexander DC. Multiple-fiber reconstruction algorithms for diffusion MRI. Ann N Y Acad Sci 2005b; 1064: 113–133

[15] Rathi Y, Michailovich O, Shenton ME, Bouix S. Directional functions for orientation distribution estimation. Med Image Anal 2009; 13: 432–444

[16] Jbabdi S, Johansen-Berg H. Tractography: where do we go from here? Brain Connect 2011; 1: 169–183

[17] Stejskal EO, Tanner JE. Spin diffusion measurements: spin echoes in the presence of a time-dependent field gradient. J Chem Phys 1965; 42: 288–292

[18] Bihan D, Breton E. Imagerie de diffusion in vivo par résonance magnétique nucléaire. C R Acad Sci (Paris) 1985; 301: 1109–1112

[19] Callaghan P, MacGowan D, Packer K, Zelaya F. High-resolution q-space imaging in porous structures. J Magn Reson B 1990; 90: 177–182

[20] Callaghan PT, Eccles CD, Xia Y. NMR microscopy of dynamic displacements: k-space and q-space imaging. J Phys E Sci Instrum 1988; 21: 820

[21] Tuch D, Wiegell M, Reese T, et al. Measuring cortico-cortical connectivity matrices with diffusion spectrum imaging. In: Proceedings of International Society of Magnetic Resonance in Medicine. 2001:1

[22] Wedeen VJ, Hagmann P, Tseng W-YI, Reese TG, Weisskoff RM. Mapping complex tissue architecture with diffusion spectrum magnetic resonance imaging. Magn Reson Med 2005; 54: 1377–1386

[23] Kreher BW, Schneider JF, Mader I, Martin E, Hennig J, Il'yasov KA. Multitensor approach for analysis and tracking of complex fiber configurations. Magn Reson Med 2005; 54: 1216–1225

[24] Basser PJ, Mattiello J, LeBihan D. Estimation of the effective self-diffusion tensor from the NMR spin echo. J Magn Reson B 1994; 103: 247–254

[25] Tournier JD, Calamante F, Gadian DG, Connelly A. Direct estimation of the fiber orientation density function from diffusion-weighted MRI data using spherical deconvolution. Neuroimage 2004; 23: 1176–1185

[26] Chen Y, Guo W, Zeng Q, et al. Recovery of intra-voxel structure from hard DWI. In: IEEE International Symposium on Biomedical Imaging: From Nano to Macro. 2004:1028–1031

[27] Tuch DS, Reese TG, Wiegell MR, Makris N, Belliveau JW, Wedeen VJ. High angular resolution diffusion imaging reveals intravoxel white matter fiber heterogeneity. Magn Reson Med 2002; 48: 577–582

[28] Assaf Y, Basser PJ. Composite hindered and restricted model of diffusion (CHARMED) MR imaging of the human brain. Neuroimage 2005; 27: 48–58

[29] Panagiotaki E, Schneider T, Siow B, Hall MG, Lythgoe MF, Alexander DC. Compartment models of the diffusion MR signal in brain white matter: a taxonomy and comparison. Neuroimage 2012; 59: 2241–2254

[30] Zhang H, Hubbard PL, Parker GJ, Alexander DC. Axon diameter mapping in the presence of orientation dispersion with diffusion MRI. Neuroimage 2011a; 56: 1301–1315

[31] Zhang H, Schneider T, Wheeler-Kingshott CA, Alexander DC. NODDI: practical in vivo neurite orientation dispersion and density imaging of the human brain. Neuroimage 2012; 61: 1000–1016

[32] Tournier JD, Calamante F, Connelly A. Robust determination of the fibre orientation distribution in diffusion MRI: non-negativity constrained super-resolved spherical deconvolution. Neuroimage 2007; 35: 1459–1472

[33] Jansons KM, Alexander DC. Persistent Angular Structure: new insights from diffusion MRI data. Dummy version. Inf Process Med Imaging 2003; 18: 672–683

[34] Alexander DC. Maximum entropy spherical deconvolution for diffusion MRI. Inf Process Med Imaging 2005a; 19: 76–87

[35] Seunarine KK, Alexander DC. Linear persistent angular structure MRI and non-linear spherical deconvolution for diffusion MRI. Proc Internat Socr Magn Reson Med 2006; 14: 2726–2726

[36] Tuch DS. Q-ball imaging. Magn Reson Med 2004; 52: 1358–1372

[37] Descoteaux M, Angelino E, Fitzgibbons S, Deriche R. Regularized, fast, and robust analytical Q-ball imaging. Magn Reson Med 2007; 58: 497–510

[38] Aganj I, Lenglet C, Sapiro G. ODF reconstruction in q-ball imaging with solid angle consideration. In: IEEE International Symposium on Biomedical Imaging: From Nano to Macro. 2009:1398–1401

[39] Aganj I, Lenglet C, Sapiro G, Yacoub E, Ugurbil K, Harel N. Multiple Q-shell ODF reconstruction in Q-ball imaging. Med Image Comput Comput Assist Interv 2009b; 12: 423–431

[40] Basser PJ, Pajevic S, Pierpaoli C, Duda J, Aldroubi A. In vivo fiber tractography using DT-MRI data. Magn Reson Med 2000; 44: 625–632

[41] Batchelor PG, Calamante F, Tournier J-D, Atkinson D, Hill DL, Connelly A. Quantification of the shape of fiber tracts. Magn Reson Med 2006; 55: 894–903

[42] Conturo TE, Lori NF, Cull TS et al. Tracking neuronal fiber pathways in the living human brain. Proc Natl Acad Sci U S A 1999; 96: 10422–10427

[43] Jones DK, Simmons A, Williams SC, Horsfield MA. Non-invasive assessment of axonal fiber connectivity in the human brain via diffusion tensor MRI. Magn Reson Med 1999; 42: 37–41

[44] Mori S, Crain B, van Zijl P. 3D brain fiber reconstruction from diffusion MRI. In: Proceedings of International Conference on Functional Mapping of the Human Brain. 1998

[45] Mori S, Crain BJ, Chacko VP, van Zijl PC. Three-dimensional tracking of axonal projections in the brain by magnetic resonance imaging. Ann Neurol 1999; 45: 265–269

[46] Alexander DC, Seunarine KK. Mathematics of crossing fibers. In: Diffusion MRI: Theory, Methods, and Applications. New York, NY: Oxford University Press; 2011:451–464

[47] Behrens TE, Berg HJ, Jbabdi S, Rushworth MF, Woolrich MW. Probabilistic diffusion tractography with multiple fibre orientations: What can we gain? Neuroimage 2007; 34: 144–155

[48] Behrens TE, Woolrich MW, Jenkinson M et al. Characterization and propagation of uncertainty in diffusion-weighted MR imaging. Magn Reson Med 2003; 50: 1077–1088

[49] Björnemo M, Brun A, Kikinis R, Westin C-F. Regularized stochastic white matter tractography using diffusion tensor MRI. In: Medical Image Computing and Computer-Assisted Intervention. New York, NY: Springer; 2002:435–442

[50] Friman O, Farnebäck G, Westin CF. A Bayesian approach for stochastic white matter tractography. IEEE Trans Med Imaging 2006; 25: 965–978

[51] Parker GJ, Alexander DC. Probabilistic anatomical connectivity derived from the microscopic persistent angular structure of cerebral tissue. Philos Trans R Soc Lond B Biol Sci 2005; 360: 893–902

[52] Parker GJ, Haroon HA, Wheeler-Kingshott CA. A framework for a streamline-based probabilistic index of connectivity (PICo) using a structural interpretation of MRI diffusion measurements. J Magn Reson Imaging 2003; 18: 242–254

[53] Zhang F, Goodlett C, Hancock E, Gerig G. Probabilistic fiber tracking using particle filtering. In: Proceedings Medical Image Computing and Computer-Assisted Intervention. New York, NY; Springer; 2007:144–152

[54] Zhang M, Sakaie KE, Jones SE. Logical foundations and fast implementation of probabilistic tractography. IEEE Trans Med Imaging 2013; 32: 1397–1410

[55] Hagmann P, Jonasson L, Deffieux T, Meuli R, Thiran JP, Wedeen VJ. Fibertract segmentation in position orientation space from high angular resolution diffusion MRI. Neuroimage 2006; 32: 665–675

[56] Campbell JS, Siddiqi K, Rymar VV, Sadikot AF, Pike GB. Flow-based fiber tracking with diffusion tensor and q-ball data: validation and comparison to principal diffusion direction techniques. Neuroimage 2005; 27: 725–736

[57] Jbabdi S, Bellec P, Toro R, Daunizeau J, Pélégrini-Issac M, Benali H. Accurate anisotropic fast marching for diffusion-based geodesic tractography. Int J Biomed Imaging 2008; 2008: 320195

[58] Parker GJ, Wheeler-Kingshott CA, Barker GJ. Estimating distributed anatomical connectivity using fast marching methods and diffusion tensor imaging. IEEE Trans Med Imaging 2002; 21: 505–512

[59] Cheng P, Magnotta VA, Wu D et al. Evaluation of the GTRACT diffusion tensor tractography algorithm: a validation and reliability study. Neuroimage 2006; 31: 1075–1085

[60] Vorburger RS, Reischauer C, Boesiger P. BootGraph: Probabilistic fiber tractography using bootstrap algorithms and graph theory. Neuroimage 2013; 66: 426–435

[61] Hagmann P, Reese T, Tseng W, et al. Diffusion spectrum imaging tractography in complex cerebral white matter: an investigation of the centrum semiovale. International Society of Magnetic Resonance in Medicine. ISMRM Twelfth Scientific Meeting, Kyoto, Japan, 15-21 May 2004;12:623

[62] Tournier JD, Calamante F, Connelly A. MRtrix: Diffusion tractography in crossing fiber regions. Int J Imaging Syst Technol 2012; 22: 53–66

[63] Weinstein D, Kindlmann G, Lundberg E. Tensorlines: advection-diffusion based propagation through diffusion tensor fields. In: Proceedings of the Conference on Visualization'99: Celebrating Ten Years. IEEE Computer Society Press; 1999:249–253

[64] Lazar M, Weinstein DM, Tsuruda JS et al. White matter tractography using diffusion tensor deflection. Hum Brain Mapp 2003; 18: 306–321

[65] Poupon C, Roche A, Dubois J, Mangin JF, Poupon F. Real-time MR diffusion tensor and Q-ball imaging using Kalman filtering. Med Image Anal 2008b; 12: 527–534

[66] Malcolm JG, Shenton ME, Rathi Y. Neural tractography using an unscented Kalman filter. Inf Process Med Imaging 2009b; 21: 126–138

[67] Le Bihan D, Mangin J-F, Poupon C et al. Diffusion tensor imaging: concepts and applications. J Magn Reson Imaging 2001; 13: 534–546

[68] Mangin J-F, Fillard P, Cointepas Y, Le Bihan D, Frouin V, Poupon C. Toward global tractography. Neuroimage 2013; 80: 290–296

[69] Tschumperlé D, Deriche R. Orthonormal vector sets regularization with pde's and applications. Int J Comput Vis 2002; 50: 237–252

[70] Hagmann P, Thiran J-P, Jonasson L et al. DTI mapping of human brain connectivity: statistical fibre tracking and virtual dissection. Neuroimage 2003; 19: 545–554

[71] Aganj I, Lenglet C, Jahanshad N et al. A Hough transform global probabilistic approach to multiple-subject diffusion MRI tractography. Med Image Anal 2011; 15: 414–425

[72] Reisert M, Mader I, Anastasopoulos C, Weigel M, Schnell S, Kiselev V. Global fiber reconstruction becomes practical. Neuroimage 2011; 54: 955–962

[73] Van Essen DC, Ugurbil K, Auerbach E et al. WU-Minn HCP Consortium. The Human Connectome Project: a data acquisition perspective. Neuroimage 2012; 62: 2222–2231

[74] Caruyer E, Lenglet C, Sapiro G, Deriche R. Design of multishell sampling schemes with uniform coverage in diffusion MRI. Magn Reson Med 2013; 69: 1534–1540

[75] Côté MA, Girard G, Boré A, Garyfallidis E, Houde JC, Descoteaux M. Tractometer: towards validation of tractography pipelines. Med Image Anal 2013; 17: 844–857

[76] Farquharson S, Tournier J-D, Calamante F et al. White matter fiber tractography: why we need to move beyond DTI. J Neurosurg 2013; 118: 1367–1377

[77] Fillard P, Descoteaux M, Goh A et al. Quantitative evaluation of 10 tractography algorithms on a realistic diffusion MR phantom. Neuroimage 2011; 56: 220–234

[78] Nimsky C. Fiber tracking—we should move beyond diffusion tensor imaging. World Neurosurg 2014;82(1-2):3536

[79] Reisert M, Weigel M, Fieremans E, et al. Mesoft: mesoscopic structure and orientation with fiber tracking. International Society of Magnetic Resonance in Medicine. ISMRM Twenty-First Scientific Meeting, Salt Lake City, Utah, USA. 20-26 April 2013; 21

[80] Sherbondy AJ, Rowe MC, Alexander DC. Microtrack: an algorithm for concurrent projectome and microstructure estimation. In: Medical Image Computing and Computer-Assisted Intervention–MICCAI 2010. New York, NY: Springer; 2010:183–190

[81] Anderson AW, Gore JC. Analysis and correction of motion artifacts in diffusion weighted imaging. Magn Reson Med 1994; 32: 379–387

[82] Kang N, Zhang J, Carlson ES, Gembris D. White matter fiber tractography via anisotropic diffusion simulation in the human brain. IEEE Trans Med Imaging 2005; 24: 1127–1137

10 Functional MRI and Diffusion Tensor Imaging with Tractography

Anna Knobel and Robert J. Young

10.1 Introduction

Surgery is an effective and potentially curative treatment for many patients with brain tumors, with durable improvements in the length and quality of patient survival as well as the efficacy of adjuvant treatments after gross total resection.[1,2,3,4,5,6] Although surgery should maximize tumor resection, the overarching goal remains patient safety and avoiding inadvertent injury to eloquent brain that may cause profound neurologic deficits. Direct intraoperative mapping techniques remain the reference standards for mapping eloquent cortex and white matter. These are invasive, time-consuming techniques, however, which require a large craniotomy, exposure of the area of interest, and possibly an awake surgery with the risk of seizure or neurologic worsening.

Functional magnetic resonance imaging (fMRI) and diffusion tensor imaging (DTI) with tractography are complementary functional imaging techniques for the noninvasive evaluation and mapping of eloquent brain areas. Active clinical indications for fMRI and DTI are summarized in box Clinical applications of functional magnetic resonance imaging and diffusion tensor imaging (p. 123). Potential benefits include shortening the time of the operation spent mapping eloquent areas, maximizing resection of the tumor, and avoiding potentially devastating neurologic injuries. The two most common applications in brain tumor patients are for preoperative mapping of sensorimotor and language cortices and white matter tracts. This chapter reviews the basic principles of fMRI, DTI, and tractography with an emphasis on their applications, challenges, and limitations for clinical care.

> **Clinical applications of functional magnetic resonance imaging and diffusion tensor imaging**
>
> 1. To guide clinical decision making about whether to perform a resection and the planned extent of the resection, vs. a stereotactic biopsy or not to operate
> 2. To assist patient counseling about the feasibility, risks, and benefits of surgery
> 3. To determine the safest approach to reach the tumor
> 4. To guide intraoperative stimulation that is performed to confirm the imaging results rather than mapping de novo
> 5. To guide the procedure if intraoperative stimulation fails or the area in question is surgically inaccessible

10.2 fMRI

10.2.1 BOLD fMRI

Blood oxygenation level dependent (BOLD) fMRI indirectly measures changes in brain activation through the mechanism of neurovascular coupling. Increased neuronal activity leads to a predictable hemodynamic response where changes in the oxygenation state of hemoglobin can be measured as small alterations in the local magnetic environment. Oxyhemoglobin has diamagnetic properties with relatively small susceptibility and long T2* effects. In contrast, the four unpaired electrons of deoxyhemoglobin impart paramagnetic properties with relatively large susceptibility and short T2* effects. These local hemodynamic changes form the basis of BOLD imaging to estimate and localize areas of neuronal activation.

Local cortical activation initially consumes oxyhemoglobin, increasing the relative fraction of deoxyhemoglobin in blood and causing a tiny decrease in the BOLD signal that is difficult to detect.[7] The neuronal activity also causes rapid vasodilatation with increased cerebral blood flow (CBF), cerebral blood volume (CBV), and delivery of oxyhemoglobin. The increase in CBF and subsequent increase in oxyhemoglobin overshoot the increase in local cerebral metabolic rate of oxygen demand. Therefore, net increased BOLD signal is observed from the increased relative fraction of diamagnetic oxyhemoglobin, despite increased oxygen demand and extraction.[8] The net decrease in paramagnetic deoxyhemoglobin results in increased signal on the T2* images, which correlates to the site of the neuronal activity. The increased BOLD signal then decays and may undershoot as it returns to baseline. The magnitude of these BOLD changes is on the order of 2 to 4%.

Clinical BOLD fMRI is most commonly acquired with gradient echo (GE) echoplanar imaging (EPI), which permits whole brain coverage with high spatial resolution (< 3 mm) and high temporal resolution (2–3 s). Although the spatial resolution is adequate to localize activation signal to a gyrus, the functional data are routinely coregistered onto higher-resolution and higher-contrast anatomical images for interpretation. GE EPI is highly sensitive to changes in T2* signal resulting from increased magnetic susceptibility caused by deoxyhemoglobin. Contributions to T2* signal occur mostly from voxels containing the capillary and venous beds, however, indicating that mapping of the functional activity may be displaced toward the venous drainage and not at the actual site of cortical activation. fMRI may also be acquired with spin-echo (SE) EPI, which measures only the capillary BOLD signal. Despite a smaller measurable signal, and therefore lower contrast between active and rest phases, SE EPI generates smaller measureable signals and therefore lower contrast between active and rest phases. Despite these disadvantages, SE EPI has superior resolution to localize submm functional areas in eloquent cortex, and also performs better when susceptibility artifacts are prominent (e.g., due to prior surgery, metal, hemorrhage, air-bone interfaces).

Generation of activation maps requires several data analysis steps: preprocessing, regression, and inference. First, the raw images are preprocessed to temporally interpolate images obtained at different times, and spatially registered to correct for head motion. Spatial smoothing may be used to augment the signal-to-noise ratio, and spatial normalization to a standard

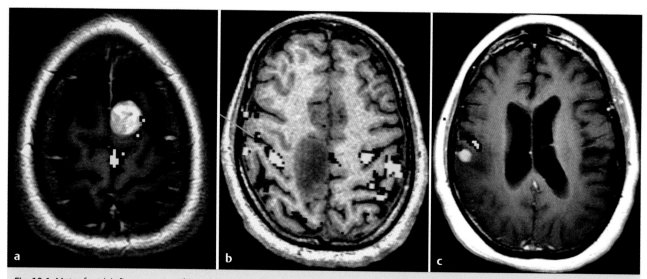

Fig. 10.1 Motor foot (**a**), finger tapping (**b**), and closed mouth tongue (**c**) blood oxygenation level-dependent functional magnetic resonance imaging scans overlaid on axial contrast T1-weighted images in three different patients. Patient in (**a**) has a meningioma superficial to the superior frontal gyrus, in (**b**) a low-grade astrocytoma in the posterior paramedian precentral gyrus and superior frontal gyrus (green line marks the central sulcus), and in (**c**) a primary central nervous system lymphoma in the postcentral gyrus. (Images courtesy of Nicole Petrovich Brennan, Memorial Sloan-Kettering Cancer Center.)

stereotactic space to enable group analyses. Second, the paradigm delivery is convolved with the hemodynamic response function estimate, and the subsequent general linear model fitted to generate a map of regression coefficients. Third, the regression coefficients are statistically translated into z scores or p-values to generate activation maps, which are color scaled to the magnitude above the statistical significance level.

10.2.2 Neurologic Planning with fMRI

fMRI has an important role in the neurosurgical planning and the treatment counseling of patients with brain tumors. Determining the location of eloquent brain and its relationship with the brain tumor allows the neurosurgeon to determine the safest approach for the resection, and to provide accurate assessments of the expected outcomes and risks involved. This information would not be available with more traditional, invasive intraoperative mapping techniques. Paradigms and their utilities are discussed in detail next.

Paradigm Design

Clinical fMRI is usually performed using block design paradigms, where stimulus presentations and/or active states are regularly alternated with rest states over a 3 to 4 min scan. Most default paradigms usually consist of 30 s active and 30 s rest states that are repeated four to six times. We perform 20 s active and 40 s rest states to permit more complete return of the hemodynamic response to baseline. The rest state may consist of no activity, or an activity similar to that in the active state minus the function being tested. Block design paradigms are more sensitive for detecting differences between active and rest states than event-related paradigms, which present a single event stimulus over the entire scan duration rather than multiple epochs of stimuli. The major disadvantage of the event-related paradigms is the long interstimulus interval (~ 20 s) that

often renders its use impractical. Paradigm selection is primarily determined by lesion location using information obtained by prior anatomical imaging, and must incorporate information about the patient's ability to perform the paradigms and preexisting neurologic deficits. Most brain tumor cases involve sensorimotor and language paradigms, although fMRI may also be used to localize auditory, visual, and memory areas.

Sensorimotor Paradigms

Sensorimotor paradigms are used to localize the primary motor cortex (M1) in the precentral gyrus and to identify the central sulcus. Paradigm selection is based on patient presentation and tumor location relative to the motor homunculus. From medial to lateral, the motor homunculus is organized with areas for legs, hands, fingers, lips, and tongue (► Fig. 10.1).

Foot motor paradigms include toe wiggling and foot dorsiflexion/plantarflexion (i.e., step on gas, lift up off gas). Somatomotor activation occurs in the paramedian precentral gyrus, paracentral lobule, and central sulcus. Visualization may be confounded by rich venous drainage from paramedian cortical veins into the superior sagittal sinus at this level. Somatosensory cortex, premotor, and cerebellar activation may also occur.

Hand motor paradigms usually consist of finger–thumb tapping or hand grasping. Due to the disproportionately large hand representation along the omega portion of the motor cortex, hand paradigms should be performed in all patients undergoing motor fMRI. Finger tapping results in activation in the omega portion of the primary somatomotor cortex as well as the supplementary motor area (SMA), sensory cortex, premotor cortex, and cerebellum.

Two common face motor paradigms are puckering or pouting for lips, and closed mouth tongue motions. Activation occurs in the lateral portion of the precentral gyrus assigned to the lower face, as well as in the sensory cortex, SMA, and premotor cortex.

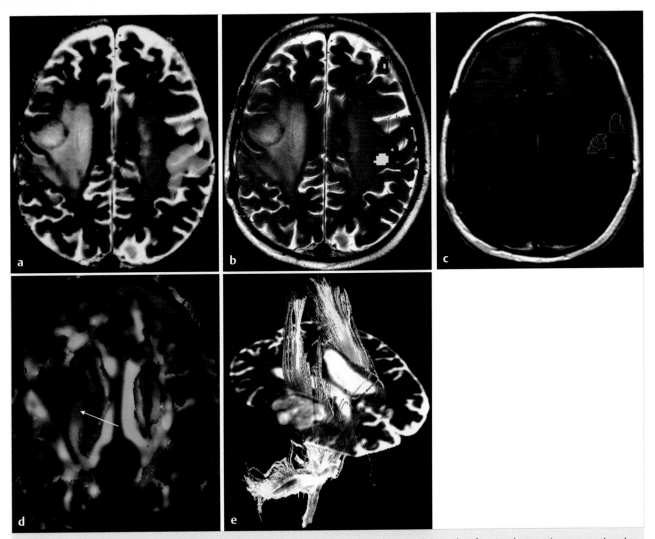

Fig. 10.2 Combined bilateral finger tapping and tongue motor paradigm. Blood oxygenation level-dependent functional magnetic resonance imaging from one patient overlaid on axial T2-weighted images (**a,b**) and contrast T1-weighted image (**c**) using three different postprocessing programs. The expansile nonenhancing tumor is localized to the lateral portion of the motor gyrus. Right activated voxels overlie the central sulcus in (**a**) and (**b**) due to bias of the signal generated by the hemodynamic response toward the venous drainage. Relatively less activation on the side of the recurrent glioblastoma (note much greater activation on the contralateral side) reflects a component of neurovascular decoupling. No activity is seen using the last technique in (**c**) despite adjusting the threshold, although localization of the normal contralateral motor cortex can be helpful in estimating the location of the motor cortex ipsilateral to the tumor. Axial directionally encoded color fractional anisotropy (FA) map (**d**) identifies the corticospinal tract along the posterior medial margin of the tumor (arrow) that is confirmed by corticospinal tractography (**e**). (Images a–c courtesy of Nicole Petrovich Brennan, Memorial Sloan-Kettering Cancer Center.)

Tongue motions activation occurs slightly more laterally in the primary sensorimotor cortex and is often associated with cerebellar activation.

Bilateral paradigms should be used to gain information from the (usually) normal contralateral side, which can aid localization inferences for the tumor side when suboptimal results occur. In addition, paradigms can be combined (e.g., hand and foot) in cooperative patients in order to save separate scan time for each paradigm (▶ Fig. 10.2). Because similar activation patterns are observed for similar motor paradigms, the exact paradigm chosen is usually not important.[9] Paradigms that require motor planning, such as sequential finger thumb tapping, occasionally result in exuberant activation of premotor, motor, and sensory areas that may obscure the localization of the primary motor cortex. In completely paralyzed patients, passive

movements may be performed to elicit BOLD motor activation. Active movements have been described as yielding more but not consistently better results.[10] Purely sensory paradigms (e.g., stroking the hand and/or foot) may also be performed to localize the primary somatosensory cortex (S1), in order to deduce the central sulcus and location of the primary somatomotor cortex (▶ Fig. 10.3 and ▶ Fig. 10.4).

Motor Mapping

The primary goal of motor fMRI is to localize the primary sensorimotor cortex by identifying the precentral or motor gyrus and the central sulcus. Activation occurs on the posterior cortex of the motor gyrus, or may occasionally follow the venous drainage and be displaced in a posterior direction onto the

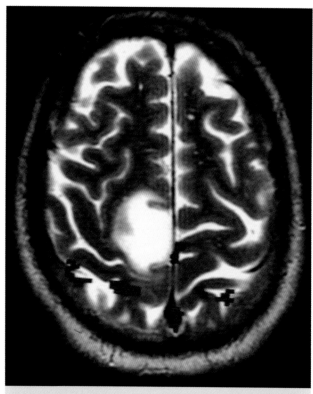

Fig. 10.3 Sensory leg stimulation. Blood oxygenation level dependent functional magnetic resonance imaging overlaid on an axial T2-weighted image. Activation is seen in the somatosensory cortex only. Despite the lack of activation, the foot motor is probably located at the posterior margin of the expansile hyperintense glioblastoma involving the paramedian precentral gyrus and the posterior superior frontal gyrus.

Table 10.1 Necessity for functional magnetic resonance imaging (fMRI) based on patient handedness, symptoms, and lesion location

Handedness	Lesion location	Aphasia	fMRI
Right	Right	Yes	Yes
	Left	Any	Yes
Left	Right	Any	Yes
	Left	Any	Yes
Ambidextrous	Right	Any	Yes
	Left	Any	Yes

central sulcus. The motor homunculus is organized, from medial to lateral, with cortical representations for the foot, leg, hand, trunk, face, and tongue. Many neurosurgeons consider the foot area to be the most important, with an inability to ambulate imposing greater morbidity than asymmetry of the face or an inability to use one hand. The foot motor area is also the most difficult portion of the homunculus to identify at intraoperative stimulation, due to its paramedian location deep to cortical veins converging on the superior sagittal sinus, and its deep extension down into the posterior interhemispheric fissure away from the brain surface.

Language Paradigms

Language paradigm selection has the additional complexity of patient handedness, diversity of primary and/or secondary language centers, and potential multilingualism. Formal evaluation of handedness using the Edinburgh inventory[11,12] should be performed if there is any doubt about hand dominance or ambidexterity. The implications of handedness on language lateralization are summarized in ▶ Table 10.1.

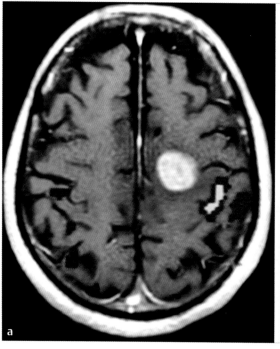
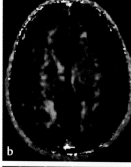
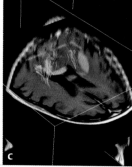

Fig. 10.4 Bilateral sensory motor hand stimulation paradigm. Blood oxygenation level-dependent functional magnetic resonance imaging overlaid on a contrast T1-weighted image (**a**) shows activation in motor and sensory gyri separate from the enhancing glioblastoma in the paramedian frontal lobe. Directionally encoded color fractional anisotropy map (**b**) demonstrates blue fibers along the posterior margin of the frontal lobe tumor. Tractography overlaid on three-dimensional contrast T1-weighted data (**c**) reveals posterior displacement of the left corticospinal tract, which is located along the posterior margin of the tumor.

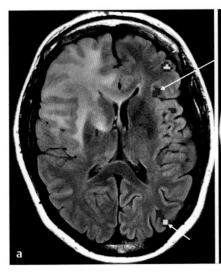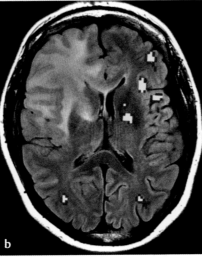

Fig. 10.5 Semantic fluency (a) and phonemic fluency (b) paradigms. Blood oxygenation level-dependent functional magnetic resonance imaging overlaid on axial fluid-attenuated inversion recovery images shows consistent activation in the Broca area (long arrow) and Wernicke area (short arrow) consistent with clear left language dominance. This left-handed patient had a large transcallosal low-grade astrocytoma centered in the right hemisphere.

The Broca and Wernicke areas are widely considered primary, essential language centers. In contradistinction to the motor cortex, no reliable anatomical landmarks are available to localize functional language areas. The Broca area is classically defined in the pars opercularis and pars triangularis of the inferior frontal gyrus (Brodmann area 44, 45). Damage may result in expressive language disorders such as dysarthria, nonfluent speech, semantic and phonemic paraphasias, and/or mutism. The Wernicke area is classically defined in the posterior superior temporal gyrus (Brodmann area 22), and/or in the middle temporal gyrus (Brodmann area 21), supramarginal gyrus (Brodmann area 40), and angular gyrus (Brodmann area 39). Damage may cause comprehension language disorders such as fluent aphasia, semantic and phonemic paraphasias, circumlocutions, and/or word-finding difficulties.

Speech paradigms may be performed silently (covertly) or vocalized (overtly). Silent language paradigms provide robust and reproducible language localization and lateralization that is comparable to vocalized language paradigms, although the magnitude of activation may be less.[13,14] Silent paradigms may also not correlate as well with sites of speech arrest at intraoperative stimulation as vocalized speech paradigms.[15] Language lateralization may be less robust with vocalized paradigms, however, due to confounding by increased bilateral motor activation.[14] We usually perform two to three speech paradigms in each patient, one of which will be vocalized with specific instructions to avoid head motion. Although uncommonly used, event-related designs may be applicable for vocalized speech paradigms intended to provide localization maps rather than lateralization.

Frontal language testing includes word-generation paradigms, verb-to-noun-generation paradigms, and object-naming paradigms. These require semantic processing to retrieve the concept from prior knowledge, phonological processing to retrieve a sound representation of the target, verbal working memory to store and manipulate the word-related data, and lexical search systems. The paradigms usually activate the Broca area, inferior frontal gyrus, and premotor frontal areas as well as the Wernicke area.[13,16] Common word-generation paradigms include phonemic fluency paradigms (e.g., name words that

begin with *R* or *M*, or generate an antonym to a presented word) and semantic fluency paradigms from a given lexical category (e.g., names of fruits and vegetables) (▶ Fig. 10.5). Word-generation paradigms may generate less activation than sentence-reading paradigms in patients with aphasia.[17] Object naming (e.g., name objects presented visually on a monitor or goggles) is a common paradigm to localize the inferior frontal and posterior parietal temporal speech and language regions, including the dorsolateral prefrontal cortex, inferior frontal gyrus, cingulate, SMA, premotor, and motor regions. Rest or control states may consist of rest or fixation on nonsense symbols. Occasionally, rest may involve reading or repeating matched control stimuli, which enable subtraction of semantic processing and phonological processing areas to better isolate working memory and lexical search areas in the inferior frontal gyrus.[18]

Posterior language testing includes forced choice reading and sentence completion paradigms (e.g., George cuts and washes other people's hair. He is a _____), semantic fluency paradigms (e.g., names of fruits or animals), and auditory response naming paradigms (e.g., What color is grass? What do you brush your hair with?). Sentence generation, processing, and semantic decision paradigms often lead to stronger activation in the Wernicke area than the single-word processing involved in word-generation and picture-naming paradigms.[19] The sentence and reading paradigms may also be more successful in eliciting language activation in aphasic patients.[17] In contrast to the sentence-reading paradigms that involve reproduction and production of only one appropriate word, success of the word-generation paradigms relies on the production of many words within the active state and may be suboptimal with production of only a few words. Rhyming paradigms may also be used. During the active state, the patient is shown pairs of words for 3 to 5 seconds and requested to press a button if the words rhyme. In the rest state, two rows of sticks are shown for 3 to 5 seconds and the patient is requested to press a button if the two rows match.

In severely aphasic patients unable to perform these paradigms, passive listening to vocalized speech or reading of visually presented words may evoke activation.[20] Activation in

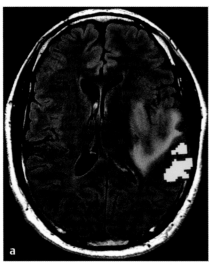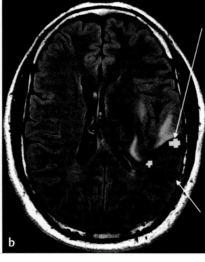

Fig. 10.6 Auditory response naming paradigm. Blood oxygenation level-dependent functional magnetic resonance imaging overlaid on axial fluid-attenuated inversion recovery images (**a,b**). The curvilinear activation of the Heschle gyrus or superior temporal gyrus (**b**) (long arrow) is located anterior to activation in the Wernicke area (short arrow). (Images courtesy of Nicole Petrovich Brennan, Memorial Sloan-Kettering Cancer Center.)

the Heschl gyrus or the primary auditory cortex in the posterior superior temporal lobe can help confirm localization of the Wernicke area, which is located just posterior to the Heschl gyrus (▶ Fig. 10.6). Tongue motor is often performed along with the language paradigms because injury to the inferior lateral motor gyrus can also result in speech arrest.

Language Mapping

The primary roles for preoperative fMRI are for lateralizing language dominance and localizing essential language areas. The Broca and Wernicke areas are considered essential for speech production and speech comprehension, respectively. Tumors in the frontal language areas may lead to nonfluent aphasia and normal speech comprehension, and tumors in the temporal language areas to fluent aphasia and difficulty with comprehension (e.g., picture naming). Clinical information is critical to tailor the fMRI examination and select appropriate paradigms.

Studies have shown favorable comparisons between preoperative language fMRI and invasive electrocorticography as well as intracarotid sodium amobarbital (Wada) procedures.[21–27] Intraoperative electrical stimulation is the gold standard for language mapping, but it is highly reliant on the brain exposed by the craniotomy, cognitive effects of anesthesia, number and quality of the neuropsychological paradigms, and cooperation of an awake patient. A meta-analysis of 442 patients reported by Dym et al[28] reported 80% concordance between fMRI and Wada testing in 91% of the studies they reviewed. In addition, fMRI showed 88% sensitivity for detecting left language dominance and 83% sensitivity for detecting non-left language dominance. High sensitivity and specificity for language localization were observed despite the wide range of paradigms, experimental procedures, data analysis, and interpretations across studies. Other investigators have confirmed consistently good concordance between fMRI and Wada testing, mostly in epilepsy patients.[24,25,29,30] The risks of Wada testing are not trivial—in a review of 677 patients, Loddenkemper et al[31] reported complications in 10.9%, including encephalopathy (by far the most common at 7.2%), seizure, stroke, and transient ischemic attack. At our institution (a National Cancer Institute–designated cancer center), Wada testing has been

supplanted by fMRI for language lateralization and localization. Although Wada testing allows language lateralization without localization, it remains the test of choice for memory lateralization and is considered superior for preoperative planning when memory is a primary concern, such as in patients with temporal lobe epilepsy.

Language fMRI performed in brain tumor patients has been described as successful on a technical basis in 100% and successful for localization and lateralization in 98%.[32] Language hemisphere dominance is typically described by calculating the laterality index from the number of voxels in the left hemisphere ($nV \times L$) and right hemisphere ($nV \times L$), where $LI = (nV \times L - nV \times R)/(nV \times L + nV \times R)$. This estimates the relative contributions to language activation from the left and right hemispheres and is therefore affected by the statistical threshold used to create the activation maps, although threshold-independent approaches have recently been advocated.[33] Evaluation of regional as well as hemispheric laterality indices may be useful to better elucidate interindividual spatial heterogeneity in language lateralization.[30,34] This is especially relevant for brain tumor patients, where large local changes in BOLD signal may result from tumor-related neurovascular decoupling, hemorrhage, and other sources of susceptibility artifact.[35]

In clinical practice, most patients show clear left language dominance with left hemisphere Broca area and Wernicke area confirmed across multiple paradigms. A right hemisphere Broca area analogue is often identified in strongly left hemisphere language dominant patients. This nondominant activation is associated with visual spatial processing and prosody functions related to the rhythm, tempo, emotion, pitch, and intonation of speech. Prosody deficits or aprosodia may present a severe handicap for some patients. True right hemisphere dominance manifest with the right Broca area and the right Wernicke area is unusual, even in left-handed individuals. The phonological processing recruited by word-generation paradigms may yield lateralization results that are superior to those elicited by semantic fluency, word-reading, and picture-naming paradigms.

Performance of multiple paradigms is recommended to improve the success and reproducibility of fMRI. Language paradigms may be biased toward the frontal or the temporal

Table 10.2 Common secondary language areas

Area	Brodmann area	Location	Function	Sample deficits
Middle frontal gyrus (dorsolateral prefrontal cortex, premotor area)	46	Superior to Broca area	Verbal working memory	Dysarthria, anomia
Supplementary motor area (SMA)	6	Superior frontal gyrus, with language SMA anterior to motor SMA	Complex coordinated movements, retrieval of motor memory	Transient speech paucity, mutism
Insula	13	Deep to sylvian fissure	Phonological and semantic processing, overt speech paradigms	Word finding difficulty, speech apraxia
Angular gyrus and supramarginal gyrus	39 and 40	Wrapped around posterior portion of sylvian fissure	Semantic processing, attention to phonological relations, working memory	Alexia, agraphia, semantic aphasia

language areas; however, they usually elicit activation in both areas (▶ Fig. 10.4). Benke et al[36] described superior agreement for frontal laterality indices, rather than temporal laterality indices between fMRI and Wada testing. Other groups have described higher laterality indices for the Broca area using word-generation and rhyming paradigms instead of sentence-completion or sentence-listening comprehension paradigms,[33, 37,38] and suggested that the expressive paradigms are sufficient for language lateralization and localization. Determining language lateralization in the receptive language areas with fMRI remains more problematic,[33] probably due to the wider distribution of language comprehension functions through the brain, as well as suboptimal receptive and semantic paradigm designs. The combined paradigm analysis is useful in identifying language areas involved in general language functions[19,26,27,39] and has been advocated as superior for language localization, rather than using a single paradigm, which may only identify language areas specific to the particular paradigm performed.[26]

Activation of secondary or supportive portions of the complex language neural network is nearly always present during fMRI. The locations, functions, and sequelae of damage to important secondary language areas[40–45] are summarized in ▶ Table 10.2. Similar to the primary areas, these secondary areas become relevant when located in close proximity to a tumor. For example, localization of the SMA when planning resection of a tumor in the superior frontal gyrus will help facilitate patient counseling. The SMA proper is responsible for planning motor movements and the pre-SMA for linguistic planning; injury to the SMA may cause SMA syndrome with profound but transient speech deficits or mutism. The middle frontal gyrus has a prominent role in phonological fluency and verbal working memory, in conjunction with the Broca area, premotor area, and SMA.

10.2.3 Challenges in fMRI

There are many potential challenges in fMRI that require attention to proper patient preparation, protocol optimization, and data processing standardization.

Patient Preparation

fMRI requires active patient effort to yield meaningful results. This contrasts most MRI sequences where patients are only required to remain motionless (or cooperate with breathing

instructions for nonneurologic protocols), and is superimposed upon the usual MRI constraints such as claustrophobia. Patients with brain tumors are often impaired, especially those who present with tumors located near eloquent brain areas. Paradigms must be selected for individual patients based on their clinical signs and symptoms, and location of the tumor on anatomical images. Results are often improved when the paradigms are rehearsed with the patient before entering the MRI suite. Monitoring BOLD signal on the scanner in real-time during paradigm delivery helps confirm that the patient is performing the specified paradigm.

Technical Considerations

fMRI requires balance between image signal and noise, and spatial and temporal resolution. Rapid imaging is necessary to capture the hemodynamic response, and $T2^*$ sensitive imaging to capture the 1 to 5% changes in $T2^*$ signal. Signal is affected by voxel volume, which is in turn affected by spatial resolution, which may be increased by decreasing the field of view and/or increasing the acquisition matrix size. Signal may also be increased by scanning at high field strengths of 3 T or more, permitting better resolution and better accuracy.[46] The increased field strength allows increased polarization of proton spins, and increased magnitude of BOLD changes. Most clinical studies include whole-brain scanning and are performed at spatial resolutions less than attained on routine anatomical images. This is acceptable because the activated voxels need only be mapped at the gyrus level and are routinely coregistered onto high-resolution anatomical images. The temporal resolution of fMRI is constrained by the evolution of the hemodynamic response caused by neuronal discharges, production, and diffusion of vascular agents to cause vasodilatation; fMRI therefore has less temporal resolution than electroencephalography (EEG) and magnetoencephalography (MEG) that directly measure electrical activity caused by neuronal discharges on the order of milliseconds rather than seconds.[47]

Neurovascular Decoupling

fMRI is dependent on neurovascular coupling, the relationship between neuronal activation, and changes in CBF, with the changes occurring primarily in the veins immediately removed from the local neuronal activity.[48] When neurons increase their firing rate, they release neurotransmitters that are removed by astrocytes. Vasodilators released by the astrocytes lead to increases in blood flow, and therefore increased concentration of oxygenated hemoglobin in the region of increased firing.

Intracranial pathologies may impede the normal hemodynamic response, such that an increase in neuronal firing will not cause a subsequent increase in blood flow or oxygenated hemoglobin. This phenomenon has been described in patients with arteriovenous malformations, high-grade gliomas, and high-grade vascular stenoses.[49,50,51] The marked tumor angiogenesis and neovascularity in high-grade gliomas such as glioblastoma may already be maximally dilated and unable to respond to the increased neuronal activity with any further dilatation. The functional activity may be undetectable due to physiological and/or technical noise despite optimal patient cooperation and technique. In these situations, where negative results are unreliable (i.e., is the expected function truly absent vs. just not measureable), evaluation of the normal contralateral side may be helpful (as for inferring the location of the motor cortex) or of other areas of activation (e.g., activation in the left Wernicke area should suggest left language dominance even if a frontal lobe tumor obscures the Broca area). The BOLD signal may also be affected by pharmacological agents—increased by caffeine and decreased by antihistamines.[52]

fMRI Postprocessing and Interpretation

fMRI postprocessing involves (1) image preprocessing to remove motion artifacts, align slices, and coregistration to anatomical images; and (2) statistical analysis of the changes in BOLD signal. Although the postprocessing efficacy may vary according to the manufacturer and vendor software, activation maps have been described as overlapping or partially overlapping in 100% of motor paradigms and 87% of language paradigms.[53] This suggests that reliable results may be obtained in the routine clinical setting with standard tools in the vast majority of cases, although advanced research tools such as Analysis of Functional NeuroImages (AFNI, http://afni.nimh.nih.gov/), Statistical Parametric Mapping (SPM, http://www.fil.ion.ucl.ac.uk/spm/), and FMRI of the Brain Software Library (FSL, http://fsl.fmrib.ox.ac.uk/fsl/) are often better for complex cases such as when severe motion artifact is present, when complex paradigm designs with unequal active/rest states are used, or when an independent component analysis is more useful than the standard *t*-test, general linear model, or cross-correlation methods.[54]

Statistical analysis relies on detection of local alterations in the BOLD signal when performing the paradigm as compared to baseline. The redundancy of the block paradigm design helps improve signal-to-noise to identify these small changes in BOLD signal. Unfortunately, since results are generated using a within-patient analysis each time, selection of appropriate *p*-values and display of the results vary according to patient and scan, limiting between-patient comparisons and group analysis. And despite the acceptance of certain eloquent areas as essential, such as the primary motor cortex, even relatively simple motor paradigms usually produce activation in other areas of the brain involved in motor planning and coordination such as the SMA, premotor area, and cerebellum. This is a common issue inherent in fMRI, which will often reveal the areas supportive of the function being tested—and potentially confound

localization of the essential areas.[47] Rather than identifying areas involved in generating a specific function, direct electrical stimulation reversibly interrupts function to predict the deficit that would result if that specific area of the brain were resected. Determining relevant thresholds and *p*-values and interpreting the functional maps thereby require an experienced operator to yield meaningful results.

Potential Effects of Brain Tumors on Language

Injury to the Broca area in the inferior frontal gyrus has classically been ascribed with severe expressive aphasia. This definition is controversial, with studies indicating that injury to the Broca area may occur without aphasia. There are three plausible explanations: (1) the Broca area is not involved in speech, (2) the Broca area is part of a wider network involved in speech, or (3) compensation by other language areas may take over the function of the Broca area. The considerable interindividual variability in the distribution of language function is compounded in tumor patients by potential displacement or infiltration by the tumor as well as potential brain plasticity or reorganization induced by the tumor. In particular, the brain's capacity to reorganize functional areas in the setting of long-standing and slow-growing tumors seems to play an important role in compensating for or avoiding speech deficits. Reorganization may involve shifting of the functional activity away from the peritumoral area to an adjacent ipsilateral area, or to the homologue in the contralateral hemisphere. In localizing 29 inferior frontal language sites in 16 patients with tumors in the Broca area, Lubrano et al[55] found that only 48% were present in the classic Broca area (Brodmann area 44, 45), consisting of 25% in patients with infiltrative grade II or III gliomas versus 100% in patients with well-circumscribed benign tumors. In addition to the classic Broca area, positive sites were identified in the premotor cortex and in the pars triangularis and pars orbitalis junction. These results suggest that well-circumscribed tumors may displace eloquent brain via simple mass effect, whereas infiltrative tumors may induce brain plasticity.

Despite the lack of standardization of multiple facets of the fMRI examination, fMRI has demonstrated its clinical utility across multiple studies for evaluating the feasibility, risk, and approach for potential surgery in brain tumor patients. Given the considerable normal and tumor-related variability in the language areas, however, further refinements in fMRI design, paradigms, postprocessing, and analysis will be necessary to continue to grow its applications in the neuro-oncological community.

10.2.4 Coding

Unique Current Procedural Terminology (CPT) codes are used by Medicare to identify specific diagnostic imaging procedures. The CPT system was developed and is updated annually by the American Medical Association (AMA). In early 2004, a collaboration between members of the American College of Radiology (ACR), American Society of Neuroradiology (ASNR), and the American Society of Functional Neuroradiology (ASFNR) aimed to develop CPT codes for fMRI. A single coordinated application was submitted by societies from Radiology and Neurology with support from Neurosurgery, and three category I (clinically

Table 10.3 Functional magnetic resonance imaging (fMRI) Current Procedural Terminology (CPT) codes

CPT code	Description [modifiers]	2013 Relative value units (RVUs)		
		Technical component	Professional component	Physician work
70554	fMRI by technician: not requiring physician or psychologist [Do not use with 96020] [Do not use 70554 or 70555 with 70551–70553 unless a separate brain MRI is performed]	11.70	3.02	2.11
70555	fMRI by physician or psychologist [Do not use 70555 unless 96020 is performed] [Do not use 70554 or 70555 with 70551–70553 unless a separate brain MRI is performed]	–	3.72	2.54
96020	Functional brain mapping: Neurofunctional test selection and administration during fMRI requiring physician or psychologist administration of entire neurofunctional test, with review and report of test results [Use with fMRI scan 70555] [Do not use with 96101–96103 or 96116–96120]	-	4.84	3.43

necessary) fMRI codes were approved for preoperative neurosurgical planning, effective January 1, 2007.

As summarized in ▶ Table 10.3, CPT code 70554 should be used when the fMRI is performed by a nonphysician or nonpsychologist. CPT code 70555 should be used to report the fMRI scan and CPT code 96020 to report the testing component when the fMRI is performed entirely by a physician or a psychologist. Each code has separate technical and professional components. The technical fee may vary based on the diagnosis-related group, Medicare physician fee schedule (MPFS), or carrier pricing, but usually increases from scanning in a hospital inpatient setting to a hospital outpatient setting and then an independent diagnostic imaging facility location. The professional fee is fixed by the MPFS and does not vary per setting. Any qualified physician or psychologist provider may administer the fMRI and use CPT codes 70555 and 96020. The 96020 code requires a report of clinical interactions with the patient to describe the time spent with the patient, the discussion with the patient, examinations performed, fMRI paradigms, and patient monitoring during the fMRI scan.

10.3 DTI and Tractography

10.3.1 Diffusion Tensor Imaging

The random or Brownian motion of unconstrained water molecules is described as isotropic. In contrast, the preferential motion of constrained water molecules in a particular direction is described as anisotropic. The water molecules in white matter tracts demonstrate anisotropic motion due to the constraints imposed by the myelin sheath of the axons. These local changes in anisotropy in the human brain form the basis of DTI.[56] By acquiring diffusion information in at least six directions, and usually many more on modern scanners, the directionality of diffusion can be described using an ellipsoid tensor. The major or principal eigenvector represents the main direction of diffusion, whereas the two minor eigenvectors describe the orthogonal directions in three-dimensional (3D) space. The corresponding major and minor eigenvalues in turn describe the magnitudes of the diffusion. The diffusion tensor allows the calculation of numerous scalar metrics. The most commonly applied is fractional anisotropy (FA), which is defined as follows:

$$FA = \frac{1}{\sqrt{2}} \sqrt{\frac{(\lambda_1 - \lambda_2)^2 + (\lambda_2 - \lambda_3)^2 + (\lambda_1 - \lambda_3)^2}{\lambda_1^2 + \lambda_2^2 + \lambda_3^2}} \qquad (10.1)$$

FA is a unitless metric that defines the shape of the tensor ellipsoid and varies from 0 (isotropy, or no net directionality) to 1 (anisotropy, or maximal directionality). Increased anisotropy is observed in highly organized white matter structures, and decreased anisotropy in gray matter structures. Anisotropy may also be decreased in areas of crossing fibers with net zero directionality despite complex fiber intersections. Tumors and peritumoral abnormalities may decrease anisotropy via one or more potential mechanisms, including displacement, edema, demyelination, axonal loss, tumor infiltration, and destruction.[57] As such, FA is a sensitive but nonspecific measure of white matter integrity and architecture. Additional descriptors of tensor shape include spherical, prolate (cylinder shaped), and oblate (disc shaped).

An FA map displays directional information where the brightness of each pixel corresponds to the degree of anisotropy. White matter structures with high directionality are shown as bright (maximum often seen in the highly directional corpus callosum fibers) and gray matter structures with low directionality are shown as dark. A directional encoded color FA map adds orientation data, where, by convention, red (x-axis) represents a left–right orientation, green (y-axis) represents an anterior–posterior orientation, and blue (z-axis) represents a superior–inferior orientation. These color FA maps facilitate the identification of specific white matter tracts, and, because they are calculated with minimal operator input (aside from selection of minimal and maximal FA thresholds), they may be considered to be more reliable representations of brain anisotropy and structure than tractography.

10.3.2 Tractography

Tractography is a unique tool in evaluating and localizing the eloquent white matter tracts adjacent to brain tumors, where the normal anatomy and anatomical references may be distorted by the tumor, edema, and/or infiltrating tumor. Tractography programs estimate and display the connectivity of the white matter tract fibers in 3D space. Many different tractography programs are currently being used in clinical and research settings—most are based on standard (deterministic) modeling and less commonly on probabilistic modeling.

Standard tractography generates connectivity maps by determining the principal direction for each voxel along a path. Tracking may be initiated by placing a seed region of interest (ROI) in a white matter tract of interest, then propagating the tract from voxel to voxel along the principal eigenvectors until termination criteria are met, when the FA is less than a predetermined threshold (e.g., < 0.15) or the turning angle is greater than a predetermined threshold (e.g., > 70 degrees). Many programs are based on the fiber assignment by continuous tracking (FACT) algorithm.[58,59] "Brute force" tracking, where every voxel is used as a seed to initiate propagations, may provide more robust tracts.[60] In this situation, tractography is performed first, and an ROI is only placed to display tracts that travel through the selected ROI. Standard tractography does well for uncomplicated tracts, such as the foot motor fibers of the corticospinal tract, which is a large tract that runs in a nearly straight vertical line from the brain to the spinal cord. For smaller or complex tracts that cross other paths or make acute turns, however, standard tractography often performs poorly. For example, the hand and face motor fibers of the corticospinal tract have a curved trajectory through intersecting superior longitudinal fasciculus tracts ("crossing fibers") that limit their reconstruction.

Rather than generating only a single projection for each voxel, probabilistic tractography performs a more complex analysis that calculates the probability density function of multiple tracts propagating in multiple directions for each voxel. The generated assignment probability enables the reconstruction of complex multiplanar tracts shown as the probability of connection between two seed ROIs.[61,62] Calculations of the uncertainty of the fiber trajectories may help resolve complex white matter voxels that contain crossing fibers, by Q-ball imaging reconstructions of the orientation distribution function (ODF), among other techniques.[63] In general, probabilistic tractography is capable of generating more tracts, particularly through areas of decreased FA, but these tracts may be weaker than those generated by standard tractography.

10.3.3 Neurosurgical Planning with DTI and Tractography

A deep brain tumor is more likely to lie in close proximity to eloquent white matter tract(s) rather than eloquent cortex. DTI mapping in these cases may supplement or supplant fMRI for imaging-based mapping of functional networks potentially at risk during surgery. Significant postoperative deficits may arise from purely white matter injuries,[64] which may be permanent. Visual inspection is often insufficient to discern tumor margins or identify specific white matter tracts, especially for primary glial tumors with infiltrative growth patterns into adjacent normal brain. The reference standard for white matter mapping remains intraoperative subcortical direct electrical stimulation. Stimulation is time consuming, technically challenging, and

may be associated with deficits in 20 to 80% of patients.[65,66] Although usually transient, with 77 to 94% returning to their baseline status by 3 months,[65,66,67,68] patients may experience significant morbidity.

By providing functional information about adjacent eloquent white matter tracts, DTI provides useful information for preoperative planning, including a prediction of the extent of resection.[69]

Stimulation is also highly dependent on close proximity to the target. This is not an issue for cortical stimulation along the surface of the brain. In contrast, white matter stimulation is usually limited to the exposed subcortical white matter. Stimulation may become more difficult or even impossible with minimally invasive surgeries or deep or otherwise inaccessible white matter tracts of interest. DTI allows the noninvasive evaluation of all white matter tracts in the brain, including the potentially normal contralateral tracts, which facilitate control comparisons within each patient. Even when the white matter is accessible, stimulation may occasionally fail. False-negative results (no response when the tract is stimulated) are difficult to interpret because it is unclear if the absence of response is due to (1) the tract is not actually present in the stimulated location, (2) the tract is present but not functional because of direct tumor effects (e.g., edema, demyelination, tumor infiltration), (3) the tract is present but suppressed (e.g., excessive anesthesia or sedation), or (4) the tract is present but insufficiently stimulated (i.e., maximum safe current intensity reached).

Motor Pathway Mapping

DTI and tractography decrease the time necessary for stimulation and localization and have been advocated as indispensable for resection of tumors in or near the corticospinal tract.[67,70] Reliable localization of the motor tracts facilitates the capacity of preoperative planning to define the feasibility of surgery, safety of margins, and opportunity for maximal resection[67] (▶ Fig. 10.7). Good correlations between pyramidal tractography and intraoperative subcortical electrical stimulation have been reported.[68,71,72]

The pyramidal tract is the major motor white matter tract in the brain, representing the direct activation pathway for voluntary muscle movement. The majority of the pyramidal tract fibers originate from Betz layer V cells in the precentral gyrus, with smaller contributions from the premotor region and supplemental motor area. Studies have also shown small contributions to the main (lateral) corticospinal tract from the primary sensory area (both precentral and postcentral gyri in 70%, only postcentral gyri in 7%) and the parietal lobe.[73] This introduces a potential source of error because candidate corticospinal tract fibers may be difficult to distinguish from somatosensory tract fibers, even after evaluation of the entire tract to the cortex. In clinical practice, we often consider only corticospinal tract fibers traveling from the primary motor cortex as essential; other contributions to motor function from the primary sensory area, SMA, premotor area, and insula involved in planning, control, and higher-level processing are not explicitly mapped. The corticospinal tract fibers usually decussate in the lower medulla and descend in the spinal cord ipsilateral and down to the level of the target muscle(s), where they synapse with motor nuclei of the spinal lower motor neurons.

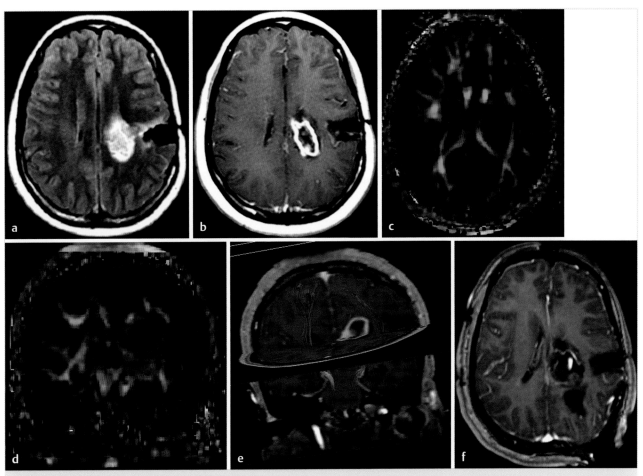

Fig. 10.7 Corticospinal tract mapping. Axial fluid-attenuated inversion recovery (FLAIR) (**a**) and contrast T1-weighted (**b**) images show a fluid-filled surgical cavity in the operculum and a heterogeneously enhancing FLAIR hyperintense recurrent oligodendroglioma in the lateral ventricle. Axial (**c**) and coronal (**d**) directionally encoded color fractional anisotropy maps overlaid on contrast T1-weighted images show craniocaudal blue motor fibers between the surgical cavity and the intraventricular tumor, which is confirmed by corticospinal tractography (**e**). Mass effect causes lateral deviation of the corticospinal tract. The shortest approach to the intraventricular tumor (through the original craniotomy and surgical cavity) was not taken. Intraoperative contrast T1-weighted image (**f**) shows a posterior lateral approach and gross total tumor resection.

At the primary motor cortex, the corticospinal tract has contributions, from medial to lateral, from the foot, hand, face, and tongue portions of the homunculus. Probabilistic tractography studies have shown rotation of these portions, such that the hand is located medial to the leg in the cerebral peduncle.[74] This weaving or crossing of the foot fibers from medial to lateral relative to the other portions of the corticospinal tract probably occurs at the level of the posterior limb of the internal capsule.[75] Recognition of this somatotopic organization of the corticospinal tract along its descent has implications for understanding potential deficits after injury.[76]

Even when using seed ROIs in the posterior limb of the internal capsule or brainstem, which should include all portions of the motor homunculus, standard tractography of the corticospinal tract often includes only the foot fibers. The foot fibers arising from the paramedian motor homunculus are a robust, large bundle that descends in a relatively vertical orientation. In contrast, fibers arising from the more lateral portions of the motor homunculus have medial inflections before descending, and face and tongue fibers from the far lateral portions must cross through the superior longitudinal fasciculus at the level of the corona radiata during their descent and are often truncated due

to crossing fiber errors.[71,77] These technical limitations of standard tractography can be overcome with probabilistic tractography techniques,[75] and likely also with other more advanced diffusion imaging techniques such as high angular resolution diffusion imaging. In practical terms, the standard tractography results are adequate for preoperative planning. Many neurosurgeons attribute much greater morbidity to an inability to ambulate than an inability to use a hand or asymmetry of the face. Therefore, medial cortical, subcortical, and deep white matter lesions in close proximity or involving the foot motor fibers of the corticospinal tract may be more difficult to resect than more lateral lesions.

Berman et al[78] found a mean distance between the site of the tractography-defined tract and the stimulation site of < 8.7 mm (while incorporating all potential sources of error, including from the neuronavigational system). Zolal et al[68] reported that stimulation elicited a motor response only when the distance between the DTI-determined tract and the tumor margin was ≤ 8 mm, with a steep nonlinear increase in the probability of eliciting a motor response when the distance was < 3 mm. Mikuni et al[79] reported positive motor-evoked potentials only when the distance was < 6 mm. Other groups have reported similar results, as well as the need for higher current intensities as the distance from the pyramidal tract is increased ≥ 1.5 to 1.9 mm.[80,81,82]

An important goal of motor DTI and tractography is to localize the corticospinal tract to a particular margin of the tumor. The neurosurgeon can then resect the rest of the tumor and approach this margin last, in order to attempt a complete resection if safe or leave a residual tumor if necessary based on white matter stimulation results. In a large study of 238 patients with brain tumors involving the pyramidal tract, who were randomized to either anatomical only ($n = 120$) or DTI ($n = 118$) neuronavigation groups, Wu et al[83] reported that the DTI group had a greater than 50% reduction in postoperative motor deterioration (15.3% vs. 32.8%, $p < 0.001$) and higher 6-month Karnofsky Performance Scale score (86 vs. 74). Patients with high-grade gliomas in the DTI group were also more likely to achieve gross total resection (74.4% vs. 33.3%, $p < 0.001$) and enjoy longer median survival (21.2 vs. 14 months, $p = 0.048$) with a 43% decrease in the risk of death. Other smaller nonrandomized studies have confirmed the benefits of DTI in accurately mapping the motor pathways to < 1 cm of the stimulation points, in order to maximize tumor resection and preserve motor function.[78,82,84,85,86,87]

Language Pathway Mapping

There is growing evidence that language function is distributed across large cortical and subcortical neural networks. The imaging representation of the language networks is further complicated by considerable variability in the localization, shape, and caliber of white matter tracts, as described by Bürgel et al.[88] The authors postulated that high interpatient variability of the language tracts reflects the late myelination of these long association fibers, in contrast to the motor corticospinal tract that undergoes early myelination and enjoys relatively low intersubject variability.

Five to six different perisylvian pathways have been implicated in language function, in addition to the classically recognized arcuate fasciculus pathway.[89] Saur et al[90] recently advocated a dual-stream architecture consisting of dorsal and ventral streams or pathways for language function. The dorsal or phonological stream is thought to be responsible for mapping sounds to articulatory and motor representations via the superior longitudinal fasciculus and arcuate fasciculus between the temporal lobe and the frontal lobe. These expressive language processing functions are considered strongly left-dominant. The ventral or semantic stream is thought to be responsible for the mapping sounds to linguistic processing centers via the uncinate fasciculus, extreme capsule, middle longitudinal fasciculus, inferior longitudinal fasciculus, and inferior fronto-occipital fasciculus. These receptive and semantic language processing functions are more bilateral in distribution.

While recognizing the complexity of the many association pathways involved in language function, and recent literature suggesting the absence of a direct link to language,[89] the arcuate fasciculus maintains prevailing importance for preoperative brain tumor planning. The arcuate fasciculus is the fourth part of the superior longitudinal fasciculus (SLF-IV). The SLF is the largest association fiber bundle in the brain, with connections between the parietal, occipital, temporal, and frontal lobe areas.

Table 10.4 Components of the superior longitudinal fasciculus (SLF)

SLF component	Connected areas	Direction	Connected areas
SLF-I	Superior parietal lobule, posterior parietal region	←→	Superior frontal gyrus, supplementary motor area (SMA)
SLF-II	Inferior parietal lobule, angular gyrus, lower bank of intraparietal sulcus	←→	Middle frontal gyrus, premotor cortex, SMA
SLF-III	Supramarginal gyrus, inferior parietal lobule, parietal operculum	←→	Inferior frontal gyrus, middle frontal gyrus, SMA
SLF-IV	Superior and middle temporal gyri	←→	Dorsolateral prefrontal area

The parts of the SLF are summarized in ▶ Table 10.4. Stimulation of the SLF may result in phonemic paraphasias or speech apraxias, whereas stimulation of the fronto-occipital fasciculus may result in semantic paraphasias.[91,92,93]

Conduction aphasia and impaired repetition have classically been ascribed to damage to the arcuate fasciculus and dissociation between the Wernicke and Broca areas (▶ Fig. 10.8). Various forms of conduction aphasia may occur with lesions along different segments of the arcuate fasciculus. Decreased FA and decreased white matter bundle size have been described for the anterior and posterior segments of the arcuate fasciculus in clinically evident Broca area–like conduction aphasia and Wernicke area–like conduction aphasia, respectively.[94] Conduction aphasia may also rarely occur with purely cortical lesions that appear to spare the arcuate fasciculus.[95] An essential role for the arcuate fasciculus is supported by a study by Hayashi et al,[96] which described increased visualization of the arcuate fasciculus after brain tumor resection that was correlated with improved postoperative language function ($p = 0.0039$). Intraoperative electrical stimulation of the arcuate fasciculus may induce articulatory, phonemic, and syntactic errors and less commonly semantic paraphasias. The arcuate fasciculus in verbal subjects shows asymmetrically increased size and fiber density,[97,98,99] which also support an important role of the arcuate fasciculus in the expressive language functions of the dorsal stream.

Tractography of the arcuate fasciculus will display fibers that ascend from the Wernicke area in the posterior perisylvian region and travel anteriorly along other superior longitudinal fasciculus components in the corona radiata toward the Broca area.[100] The anterior fibers often do not complete their travel to reach the Broca area, leading some investigators to postulate that the arcuate fasciculus instead connects the temporal language areas to motor and premotor relay areas and indirectly to the frontal language areas[101] (▶ Fig. 10.9). More recent work by Li et al[102] using probabilistic tractography showed complete arcuate fasciculus fibers connecting the Wernicke and Broca areas. The authors concluded that anterior truncations shown by standard tractography techniques were premature due to

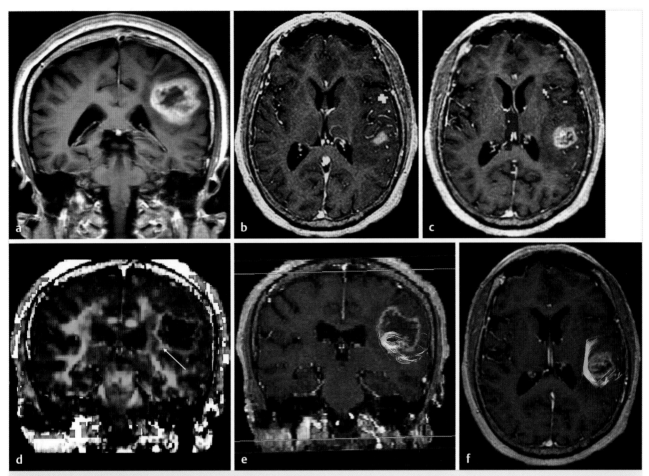

Fig. 10.8 Language functional magnetic resonance imaging. Contrast coronal T1-weighted image (**a**) reveals a large heterogeneously enhancing glioblastoma in the left parietal lobe. Word generation (**b**) and semantic fluency (**c**) tasks show activation in the Broca area without reliable localization of the Wernicke area. Coronal color-encoded directional fractional anisotropy map (**d**) suggests displacement of the green superior longitudinal fasciculus (SLF) fibers (arrow) to the inferior medial margin of the tumor (excluding green SLF-I at the superior medial margin). Tractography superimposed on axial (**e**) and coronal (**f**) images supports the proposed localization of the arcuate fasciculus.

technical issues innate to tractography when encountering crossing descending motor fibers, and that a full direct connection is present and usually visible with probabilistic tractography even in the presence of adjacent brain tumors.

10.3.4 Challenges in DTI and Tractography

Technical Considerations

There is currently little consensus on the optimal DTI acquisition, postprocessing, or analysis. DTI is vulnerable to the same artifacts common to other forms of single-shot echoplanar imaging, including signal degradation by susceptibility artifacts from the skull base and blood products, distortion by parallel imaging techniques, eddy currents, and rapid gradient changes. The quality of DTI and subsequent tractography is reliant upon signal-to-noise, which is, in turn, influenced primarily by the number of diffusion-weighting directions and the number of excitations. DTI requires ≥ 6 directions to calculate the diffusion ellipsoid. Increasing the number of directions is helpful to reduce the rotational variance of fractional anisotropy and increase the contrast-to-signal variance ratio, with relatively diminishing tensor benefits when acquiring ≥ 20 to 30 directions.[103,104] High-definition angular resolution diffusion techniques with acquisition of a very high number of directions (127–515) are capable of encoding multiple fiber orientations within each voxel to improve visualization of complex white matter architecture such as crossing fibers.[105,106] Recent advances[107,108] to reduce the scan times from > 60 min to a more reasonable 12 to 15 min may facilitate the entry of these techniques into clinical practice, despite requirements for a large number of encoding directions, higher b-values, and higher times to echo.

Seed Selection

Most tractography programs require the placement of a seed ROI to select the starting point for tracking. Additional ROIs used to refine the results fall into one of three categories: "and" to select only tracts traveling through both ROIs, "or" to select tracts traveling through either ROI, and "not" to exclude tracts traveling through the selected ROI. Seeds are usually placed manually, which requires a priori knowledge of white matter

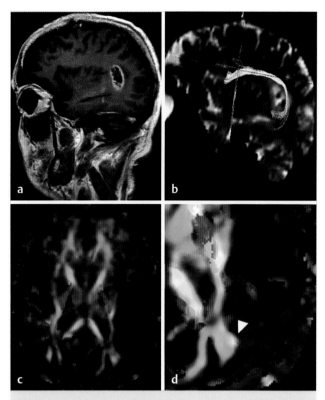

Fig. 10.9 Acute transient aphasia. Contrast sagittal T1-weighted image (**a**) shows a newly diagnosed glioblastoma with heterogeneously enhancing components in the posterior perisylvian tumor near the expected region of the Wernicke area. Tractography overlaid on sagittal b0 diffusion tensor imaging (DTI) (**b**) reveals the arcuate fasciculus tract along the posterior margin of the tumor. Axial directionally encoded color fractional anisotropy maps (**c,d** magnified) illustrate blue fibers running down around the posterior margin of the sylvian fissure, where blue (arrowhead, **d**) represents the descending portion of the superior longitudinal fasciculus. The arcuate fasciculus tract terminates anteriorly near the level of crossing motor fibers.

anatomy and entails unavoidable interobserver and intraobserver variability. Current research efforts into autosegmentation and seeding techniques should help reduce these potential sources of error.

The effects of distance provide cumulative opportunities for error, such that tracking accuracy decreases with increasing distance from the seed ROI. This effect is accompanied by decreasing fiber tract density with increasing distance from the seed ROI. Therefore, when seeding white matter tracts for preoperative planning, we advocate drawing the seed ROI(s) as close to the brain tumor as possible. The reconstructed tracts should be followed in both directions to assure that it conforms to expected anatomy and is representative of the tract of interest.

Tractography Failure

The most common effect of a brain tumor or peritumoral edema on DTI is decreased FA that may be quite dramatic. The usual consequence is failure of tractography, where few or no tracts are routed through the tumor or peritumoral region. These false-negative results, when the tract prematurely terminates despite preserved underlying function or successful subcortical stimulation, may occur with bland edema from a brain metastasis or infiltrating tumor and edema from an invasive glioma (▶ Fig. 10.10). False-positive results are also possible, when a tract is generated where none exists, or when the wrong tract is followed. Performing and interpreting tractography therefore requires a thorough knowledge of white matter anatomy, and the results should be rigorously tested against established techniques like stimulation prior to resection. Given wide subjective variabilities in postprocessing tractography, we advocate using the directionally encoded color FA maps to determine the location and relationship of the white matter tract relative to the tumor, and then using tractography to confirm the map results. We consider the color FA maps to be more reliable in these situations because the maps are calculated, and the results are less vulnerable to data manipulations.

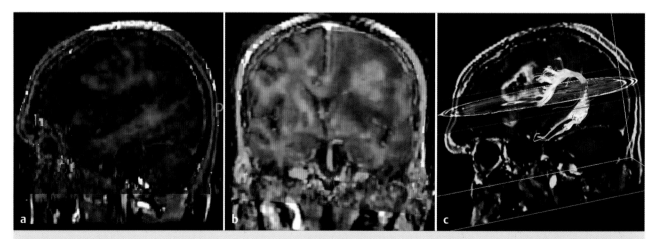

Fig. 10.10 Decreased anisotropy due to tumor and/or peritumoral abnormality. Sagittal (**a**) and coronal (**b**) directionally encoded fractional anisotropy maps overlaid on contrast T1-weighted images demonstrate an enhancing tumor in the frontal lobe along the anterior portion of the arcuate fasciculus, which stops at the posterior tumor margin and is displaced along the inferior lateral margin of the tumor. Oblique sagittal tractography (**c**) confirms lateral deviation of the anterior arcuate fibers.

Brain Shift

Brain shift is an unpredictable phenomenon where the brain changes position during surgery. The possible causes are numerous, including gravitation settling due to head position, craniotomy opening, dural opening, cerebrospinal fluid loss, edema, osmotic diuretics, surgical retraction, and tumor resection.[109] The direction of brain shift may be inward or outward depending on the complex relationship between the foregoing parameters. Although the magnitude of cortical brain shift has been described as reaching 2.4 cm,[110,111,112] the neurosurgeon may easily compensate for this by placing labels on the cortex and noting relationships with overlying veins and other anatomical markers. The magnitude of white matter brain shift has been described as reaching 11 mm for the corticospinal tract.[67,113,114] Although the mean shift was only 5.2 mm inward and 5.5 mm outward, when including both inward and outward possibilities, the total range of shift may be up to 20.7 mm.[114] White matter shift is potentially more problematic than gray matter shift because the localization of specific white matter tracts is often technically difficult due to the lack of anatomical landmarks, deep location, and unreliable negative stimulation results (e.g., Is the tract actually displaced away from the stimulation point? Is the tract present but nonfunctional? Is the tract present but the current is insufficient?). Because of its highly unpredictable nature, mathematical models perform quite poorly in attempting to compensate for brain shift. For these reasons, intraoperative MRI with DTI has been advocated by several groups as necessary to update the neuronavigational system during the surgery.[67,111,112,115] The costs of an intraoperative MRI scanner remain prohibitive for many institutions, however, limiting adoption of this promising technology.

10.4 Combining fMRI and DTI/ Tractography

fMRI and DTI are noninvasive; can be performed before surgery for preoperative planning purposes; can map the entire network involved in the function, including the contralateral brain; and are repeatable. They therefore facilitate preoperative planning in a manner that is not possible with intraoperative mapping techniques. Among the potential limitations of these imaging techniques, the primary limitation of fMRI is tumor-associated neurovascular decoupling and of DTI is tumor- or peritumoral-associated loss of anisotropy.

Modern postprocessing and neuronavigational systems enable integration of multiple data sources, such that the anatomical images can be merged with the BOLD activation maps, directionally encoded color FA maps, and tractography. Although Kleiser et al[116] described improved tractography results when using fMRI-driven seed ROIs, we have found that seeding from the ends of the tracts does not perform as well as seeding close to the tumor. Given that increased propagation from the seed ROI is associated with increases in error and decreases in tract volume, we advocate seeding adjacent to the tumor, which is also the area of greatest interest for the neurosurgeon.

Even when the data are integrated separately into a single navigable data set, fMRI and DTI can be valuable for preoperative planning. When pooling together 56 total patients

from several reports about the utility of fMRI and DTI, the neurosurgical approach was changed in 30.3% (range, 5–100%).[117,118,119] Proponents have suggested that the classical security margin around eloquent areas may be abandoned with the use of functional imaging techniques, allowing maximal resection of the entire tumor without increased permanent deficits.[120]

10.5 Conclusions

FMRI and DTI are considered complementary mapping methods and are not intended to completely replace intraoperative mapping. By providing information prior to surgery, invasive mapping may be performed in a targeted rather than a de novo manner to enable a smaller craniotomy and less time in the operating room. Given the different limitations of the noninvasive imaging mapping and of the invasive intraoperative mapping, the synergy of these complementary techniques will likely continue to evolve and remain invaluable in the evaluation of eloquent brain in brain tumor patients. Many neurosurgeons consider functional imaging the standard of care when treating patients with brain tumors near eloquent brain. Further advancements will require consensus on fMRI paradigms, and fMRI and DTI imaging protocols, data processing, and interpretation of results.

References

[1] Ammirati M, Vick N, Liao YL, Ciric I, Mikhael M. Effect of the extent of surgical resection on survival and quality of life in patients with supratentorial glioblastomas and anaplastic astrocytomas. Neurosurgery 1987; 21: 201–206

[2] Ushio Y, Kochi M, Hamada J, Kai Y, Nakamura H. Effect of surgical removal on survival and quality of life in patients with supratentorial glioblastoma. Neurol Med Chir (Tokyo) 2005; 45: 454–460, discussion 460–461

[3] Nomiya T, Nemoto K, Kumabe T, Takai Y, Yamada S. Prognostic significance of surgery and radiation therapy in cases of anaplastic astrocytoma: retrospective analysis of 170 cases. J Neurosurg 2007; 106: 575–581

[4] Burt M, Wronski M, Arbit E, Galicich JH Memorial Sloan-Kettering Cancer Center Thoracic Surgical Staff. Resection of brain metastases from non-small-cell lung carcinoma. Results of therapy. J Thorac Cardiovasc Surg 1992; 103: 399–410, discussion 410–411

[5] Wroński M, Arbit E, Burt M, Galicich JH. Survival after surgical treatment of brain metastases from lung cancer: a follow-up study of 231 patients treated between 1976 and 1991. J Neurosurg 1995; 83: 605–616

[6] Wroński M, Arbit E, Russo P, Galicich JH. Surgical resection of brain metastases from renal cell carcinoma in 50 patients. Urology 1996; 47: 187–193

[7] Detre JA, Wang J. Technical aspects and utility of fMRI using BOLD and ASL. Clin Neurophysiol 2002; 113: 621–634

[8] Heeger DJ, Ress D. What does fMRI tell us about neuronal activity? Nat Rev Neurosci 2002; 3: 142–151

[9] Johansen-Berg H, Dawes H, Guy C, Smith SM, Wade DT, Matthews PM. Correlation between motor improvements and altered fMRI activity after rehabilitative therapy. Brain 2002; 125: 2731–2742

[10] Kocak M, Ulmer JL, Sahin Ugurel M, Gaggl W, Prost RW. Motor homunculus: passive mapping in healthy volunteers by using functional MR imaging—initial results. Radiology 2009; 251: 485–492

[11] Fazio R, Coenen C, Denney RL. The original instructions for the Edinburgh Handedness Inventory are misunderstood by a majority of participants. Laterality 201 2; 17: 70–77

[12] Oldfield RC. The assessment and analysis of handedness: the Edinburgh inventory. Neuropsychologia 1971; 9: 97–113

[13] Palmer ED, Rosen HJ, Ojemann JG, Buckner RL, Kelley WM, Petersen SE. An event-related fMRI study of overt and covert word stem completion. Neuroimage 2001; 14: 182–193

[14] Partovi S, Konrad F, Karimi S et al. Effects of covert and overt paradigms in clinical language fMRI. Acad Radiol 2012; 19: 518–525

[15] Petrovich N, Holodny AI, Tabar V et al. Discordance between functional magnetic resonance imaging during silent speech tasks and intraoperative speech arrest. J Neurosurg 2005; 103: 267–274

[16] Lehéricy S, Cohen L, Bazin B et al. Functional MR evaluation of temporal and frontal language dominance compared with the Wada test. Neurology 2000; 54: 1625–1633

[17] Engström M, Karlsson M, Croné M et al. Clinical fMRI of language function in aphasic patients: reading paradigm successful, while word generation paradigm fails. Acta Radiol 2010; 51: 679–686

[18] Thompson-Schill SL, D'Esposito M, Kan IP. Effects of repetition and competition on activity in left prefrontal cortex during word generation. Neuron 1999; 23: 513–522

[19] Engström M, Ragnehed M, Lundberg P, Söderfeldt B. Paradigm design of sensory-motor and language tests in clinical fMRI. Neurophysiol Clin 2004; 34: 267–277

[20] Sunaert S. Presurgical planning for tumor resectioning. J Magn Reson Imaging 2006; 23: 887–905

[21] Binder JR, Swanson SJ, Hammeke TA et al. Determination of language dominance using functional MRI: a comparison with the Wada test. Neurology 1996; 46: 978–984

[22] FitzGerald DB, Cosgrove GR, Ronner S et al. Location of language in the cortex: a comparison between functional MR imaging and electrocortical stimulation. AJNR Am J Neuroradiol 1997; 18: 1529–1539

[23] Yetkin FZ, Swanson S, Fischer M et al. Functional MR of frontal lobe activation: comparison with Wada language results. AJNR Am J Neuroradiol 1998; 19: 1095–1098

[24] Baciu MV, Watson JM, Maccotta L et al. Evaluating functional MRI procedures for assessing hemispheric language dominance in neurosurgical patients. Neuroradiology 2005; 47: 835–844

[25] Woermann FG, Jokeit H, Luerding R et al. Language lateralization by Wada test and fMRI in 100 patients with epilepsy. Neurology 2003; 61: 699–701

[26] Giussani C, Roux FE, Ojemann J, Sganzerla EP, Pirillo D, Papagno C. Is preoperative functional magnetic resonance imaging reliable for language areas mapping in brain tumor surgery? Review of language functional magnetic resonance imaging and direct cortical stimulation correlation studies. Neurosurgery 2010; 66: 113–120

[27] Roux FE, Boulanouar K, Lotterie JA, Mejdoubi M, LeSage JP, Berry I. Language functional magnetic resonance imaging in preoperative assessment of language areas: correlation with direct cortical stimulation. Neurosurgery 2003; 52: 1335–1345, discussion 1345–1347

[28] Dym RJ, Burns J, Freeman K, Lipton ML. Is functional MR imaging assessment of hemispheric language dominance as good as the Wada test?: a meta-analysis. Radiology 2011; 261: 446–455

[29] Gaillard WD, Balsamo L, Xu B et al. Language dominance in partial epilepsy patients identified with an fMRI reading task. Neurology 2002; 59: 256–265

[30] Spreer J, Arnold S, Quiske A et al. Determination of hemisphere dominance for language: comparison of frontal and temporal fMRI activation with intracarotid amytal testing. Neuroradiology 2002; 44: 467–474

[31] Loddenkemper T, Morris HH, Möddel G. Complications during the Wada test. Epilepsy Behav 2008; 13: 551–553

[32] Stippich C, Rapps N, Dreyhaupt J et al. Localizing and lateralizing language in patients with brain tumors: feasibility of routine preoperative functional MR imaging in 81 consecutive patients. Radiology 2007; 243: 828–836

[33] Zacà D, Nickerson JP, Deib G, Pillai JJ. Effectiveness of four different clinical fMRI paradigms for preoperative regional determination of language lateralization in patients with brain tumors. Neuroradiology 2012; 54: 1015–1025

[34] Seghier ML, Kherif F, Josse G, Price CJ. Regional and hemispheric determinants of language laterality: implications for preoperative fMRI. Hum Brain Mapp 2011; 32: 1602–1614

[35] Holodny AI, Schulder M, Liu WC, Wolko J, Maldjian JA, Kalnin AJ. The effect of brain tumors on BOLD functional MR imaging activation in the adjacent motor cortex: implications for image-guided neurosurgery. AJNR Am J Neuroradiol 2000; 21: 1415–1422

[36] Benke T, Köylü B, Visani P et al. Language lateralization in temporal lobe epilepsy: a comparison between fMRI and the Wada Test. Epilepsia 2006; 47: 1308–1319

[37] Partovi S, Jacobi B, Rapps N et al. Clinical standardized fMRI reveals altered language lateralization in patients with brain tumor. AJNR Am J Neuroradiol 2012; 33: 2151–2157

[38] Sabbah P, Chassoux F, Leveque C et al. Functional MR imaging in assessment of language dominance in epileptic patients. Neuroimage 2003; 18: 460–467

[39] Ramsey NF, Sommer IE, Rutten GJ, Kahn RS. Combined analysis of language tasks in fMRI improves assessment of hemispheric dominance for language functions in individual subjects. Neuroimage 2001; 13: 719–733

[40] Sanai N, Mirzadeh Z, Berger MS. Functional outcome after language mapping for glioma resection. N Engl J Med 2008; 358: 18–27

[41] McDermott KB, Petersen SE, Watson JM, Ojemann JG. A procedure for identifying regions preferentially activated by attention to semantic and phonological relations using functional magnetic resonance imaging. Neuropsychologia 2003; 41: 293–303

[42] Banich MT, Milham MP, Jacobson BL et al. Attentional selection and the processing of task-irrelevant information: insights from fMRI examinations of the Stroop task. Prog Brain Res 2001; 134: 459–470

[43] Tanji J, Mushiake H. Comparison of neuronal activity in the supplementary motor area and primary motor cortex. Brain Res Cogn Brain Res 1996; 3: 143–150

[44] Majchrzak K, Bobek-Billewicz B, Tymowski M, Adamczyk P, Majchrzak H, Ladziński P. Surgical treatment of insular tumours with tractography, functional magnetic resonance imaging, transcranial electrical stimulation and direct subcortical stimulation support. Neurol Neurochir Pol 2011; 45: 351–362

[45] Smith EE, Jonides J, Marshuetz C, Koeppe RA. Components of verbal working memory: evidence from neuroimaging. Proc Natl Acad Sci U S A 1998; 95: 876–882

[46] Uğurbil K. The road to functional imaging and ultrahigh fields. Neuroimage 2012; 62: 726–735

[47] Korvenoja A, Kirveskari E, Aronen HJ et al. Sensorimotor cortex localization: comparison of magnetoencephalography, functional MR imaging, and intraoperative cortical mapping. Radiology 2006; 241: 213–222

[48] Hu X, Yacoub E. The story of the initial dip in fMRI. Neuroimage 2012; 62: 1103–1108

[49] Hou BL, Bradbury M, Peck KK, Petrovich NM, Gutin PH, Holodny AI. Effect of brain tumor neovasculature defined by rCBV on BOLD fMRI activation volume in the primary motor cortex. Neuroimage 2006; 32: 489–497

[50] Fujiwara N, Sakatani K, Katayama Y et al. Evoked-cerebral blood oxygenation changes in false-negative activations in BOLD contrast functional MRI of patients with brain tumors. Neuroimage 2004; 21: 1464–1471

[51] Wellmer J, Weber B, Urbach H, Reul J, Fernandez G, Elger CE. Cerebral lesions can impair fMRI-based language lateralization. Epilepsia 2009; 50: 2213–2224

[52] Laurienti PJ, Field AS, Burdette JH, Maldjian JA, Yen YF, Moody DM. Dietary caffeine consumption modulates fMRI measures. Neuroimage 2002; 17: 751–757

[53] González-Ortiz S, Oleaga L, Pujol T et al. Simple fMRI postprocessing suffices for normal clinical practice. AJNR Am J Neuroradiol 2013; 34: 1188–1193

[54] Pillai JJ. The significance of streamlined postprocessing approaches for clinical fMRI. AJNR Am J Neuroradiol 2013; 34: 1194–1196

[55] Lubrano V, Draper L, Roux FE. What makes surgical tumor resection feasible in Broca's area? Insights into intraoperative brain mapping. Neurosurgery 2010; 66: 868–875, discussion 875

[56] Mukherjee P, Berman JI, Chung SW, Hess CP, Henry RG. Diffusion tensor MR imaging and fiber tractography: theoretic underpinnings. AJNR Am J Neuroradiol 2008; 29: 632–641

[57] Jellison BJ, Field AS, Medow J, Lazar M, Salamat MS, Alexander AL. Diffusion tensor imaging of cerebral white matter: a pictorial review of physics, fiber tract anatomy, and tumor imaging patterns. AJNR Am J Neuroradiol 2004; 25: 356–369

[58] Mori S, Crain BJ, Chacko VP, van Zijl PC. Three-dimensional tracking of axonal projections in the brain by magnetic resonance imaging. Ann Neurol 1999; 45: 265–269

[59] Mori S, van Zijl PC. Fiber tracking: principles and strategies - a technical review. NMR Biomed 2002; 15: 468–480

[60] Jiang H, van Zijl PC, Kim J, Pearlson GD, Mori S. DtiStudio: resource program for diffusion tensor computation and fiber bundle tracking. Comput Methods Programs Biomed 2006; 81: 106–116

[61] Bürgel U, Mädler B, Honey CR, Thron A, Gilsbach J, Coenen VA. Fiber tracking with distinct software tools results in a clear diversity in anatomical fiber tract portrayal. Cent Eur Neurosurg 2009; 70: 27–35

[62] Kreher BHJ, Il'yasov K. DTI&FiberTools: a complete toolbox for DTI calculation, fiber tracking, and combined evaluation. In: Proceedings of ISMRM 14th International Scientific Meeting. Seattle, Washington; May 6–12, 2006

[63] Descoteaux M, Ang., elino E, Fitzgibbons S, Deriche R. Regularized, fast, and robust analytical Q-ball imaging. Magn Reson Med 2007; 58: 497–510

[64] Naeser MA, Alexander MP, Helm-Estabrooks N, Levine HL, Laughlin SA, Geschwind N. Aphasia with predominantly subcortical lesion sites:

description of three capsular/putaminal aphasia syndromes. Arch Neurol 1982; 39: 2–14

[65] Keles GE, Lundin DA, Lamborn KR, Chang EF, Ojemann G, Berger MS. Intraoperative subcortical stimulation mapping for hemispherical perirolandic gliomas located within or adjacent to the descending motor pathways: evaluation of morbidity and assessment of functional outcome in 294 patients. J Neurosurg 2004; 100: 369–375

[66] Duffau H, Capelle L, Denvil D et al. Usefulness of intraoperative electrical subcortical mapping during surgery for low-grade gliomas located within eloquent brain regions: functional results in a consecutive series of 103 patients. J Neurosurg 2003; 98: 764–778

[67] D'Andrea G, Angelini A, Romano A et al. Intraoperative DTI and brain mapping for surgery of neoplasm of the motor cortex and the corticospinal tract: our protocol and series in BrainSUITE. Neurosurg Rev 2012; 35: 401–412, discussion 412

[68] Zolal A, Hejčl A, Vachata P et al. The use of diffusion tensor images of the corticospinal tract in intrinsic brain tumor surgery: a comparison with direct subcortical stimulation. Neurosurgery 2012; 71: 331–340, discussion 340

[69] Castellano A, Bello L, Michelozzi C et al. Role of diffusion tensor magnetic resonance tractography in predicting the extent of resection in glioma surgery. Neuro-oncol 2012; 14: 192–202

[70] González-Darder JM, González-López P, Talamantes F et al. Multimodal navigation in the functional microsurgical resection of intrinsic brain tumors located in eloquent motor areas: role of tractography. Neurosurg Focus 2010; 28: E5

[71] Bello L, Castellano A, Fava E et al. Intraoperative use of diffusion tensor imaging fiber tractography and subcortical mapping for resection of gliomas: technical considerations. Neurosurg Focus 2010; 28: E6

[72] Coenen VA, Krings T, Weidemann J et al. Sequential visualization of brain and fiber tract deformation during intracranial surgery with three-dimensional ultrasound: an approach to evaluate the effect of brain shift. Neurosurgery 2005; 56 Suppl: 133–141, discussion 133–141

[73] Kumar A, Juhasz C, Asano E et al. Diffusion tensor imaging study of the cortical origin and course of the corticospinal tract in healthy children. AJNR Am J Neuroradiol 2009; 30: 1963–1970

[74] Kwon HG, Hong JH, Jang SH. Anatomic location and somatotopic arrangement of the corticospinal tract at the cerebral peduncle in the human brain. AJNR Am J Neuroradiol 2011; 32: 2116–2119

[75] Pan C, Peck KK, Young RJ, Holodny AI. Somatotopic organization of motor pathways in the internal capsule: a probabilistic diffusion tractography study. AJNR Am J Neuroradiol 2012; 33: 1274–1280

[76] Lee JS, Han MK, Kim SH, Kwon OK, Kim JH. Fiber tracking by diffusion tensor imaging in corticospinal tract stroke: Topographical correlation with clinical symptoms. Neuroimage 2005; 26: 771–776

[77] Jones DK. Determining and visualizing uncertainty in estimates of fiber orientation from diffusion tensor MRI. Magn Reson Med 2003; 49: 7–12

[78] Berman JI, Berger MS, Chung SW, Nagarajan SS, Henry RG. Accuracy of diffusion tensor magnetic resonance imaging tractography assessed using intraoperative subcortical stimulation mapping and magnetic source imaging. J Neurosurg 2007; 107: 488–494

[79] Mikuni N, Okada T, Nishida N et al. Comparison between motor evoked potential recording and fiber tracking for estimating pyramidal tracts near brain tumors. J Neurosurg 2007; 106: 128–133

[80] Maesawa S, Fujii M, Nakahara N, Watanabe T, Wakabayashi T, Yoshida J. Intraoperative tractography and motor evoked potential (MEP) monitoring in surgery for gliomas around the corticospinal tract. World Neurosurg 2010; 74: 153–161

[81] Prabhu SS, Gasco J, Tummala S, Weinberg JS, Rao G. Intraoperative magnetic resonance imaging-guided tractography with integrated monopolar subcortical functional mapping for resection of brain tumors. Clinical article. J Neurosurg 2011; 114: 719–726

[82] Vassal F, Schneider F, Nuti C. Intraoperative use of diffusion tensor imaging-based tractography for resection of gliomas located near the pyramidal tract: comparison with subcortical stimulation mapping and contribution to surgical outcomes. Br J Neurosurg 2013; 27: 668–675

[83] Wu JS, Zhou LF, Tang WJ et al. Clinical evaluation and follow-up outcome of diffusion tensor imaging-based functional neuronavigation: a prospective, controlled study in patients with gliomas involving pyramidal tracts. Neurosurgery 2007; 61: 935–948, discussion 948–949

[84] Ohue S, Kohno S, Inoue A et al. Accuracy of diffusion tensor magnetic resonance imaging-based tractography for surgery of gliomas near the pyramidal tract: a significant correlation between subcortical electrical stimulation and postoperative tractography. Neurosurgery 2012; 70: 283–293, discussion 294

[85] Okada T, Mikuni N, Miki Y et al. Corticospinal tract localization: integration of diffusion-tensor tractography at 3-T MR imaging with intraoperative white matter stimulation mapping–preliminary results. Radiology 2006; 240: 849–857

[86] Mikuni N, Okada T, Enatsu R et al. Clinical significance of preoperative fibre-tracking to preserve the affected pyramidal tracts during resection of brain tumours in patients with preoperative motor weakness. J Neurol Neurosurg Psychiatry 2007; 78: 716–721

[87] Roessler K, Donat M, Lanzenberger R et al. Evaluation of preoperative high magnetic field motor functional MRI (3 Tesla) in glioma patients by navigated electrocortical stimulation and postoperative outcome. J Neurol Neurosurg Psychiatry 2005; 76: 1152–1157

[88] Bürgel U, Amunts K, Hoemke L, Mohlberg H, Gilsbach JM, Zilles K. White matter fiber tracts of the human brain: three-dimensional mapping at microscopic resolution, topography and intersubject variability. Neuroimage 2006; 29: 1092–1105

[89] Dick AS, Tremblay P. Beyond the arcuate fasciculus: consensus and controversy in the connectional anatomy of language. Brain 2012; 135: 3529–3550

[90] Saur D, Kreher BW, Schnell S et al. Ventral and dorsal pathways for language. Proc Natl Acad Sci U S A 2008; 105: 18035–18040

[91] Duffau H, Capelle L, Sichez N et al. Intraoperative mapping of the subcortical language pathways using direct stimulations. An anatomo-functional study. Brain 2002; 125: 199–214

[92] Duffau H, Gatignol P, Denvil D, Lopes M, Capelle L. The articulatory loop: study of the subcortical connectivity by electrostimulation. Neuroreport 2003; 14: 2005–2008

[93] Duffau H, Gatignol P, Mandonnet E, Peruzzi P, Tzourio-Mazoyer N, Capelle L. New insights into the anatomo-functional connectivity of the semantic system: a study using cortico-subcortical electrostimulations. Brain 2005; 128: 797–810

[94] Song X, Dornbos D, III, Lai Z et al. Diffusion tensor imaging and diffusion tensor imaging-fibre tractograph depict the mechanisms of Broca-like and Wernicke-like conduction aphasia. Neurol Res 2011; 33: 529–535

[95] Quigg M, Geldmacher DS, Elias WJ. Conduction aphasia as a function of the dominant posterior perisylvian cortex. Report of two cases. J Neurosurg 2006; 104: 845–848

[96] Hayashi Y, Kinoshita M, Nakada M, Hamada J. Correlation between language function and the left arcuate fasciculus detected by diffusion tensor imaging tractography after brain tumor surgery. J Neurosurg 2012; 117: 839–843

[97] Nucifora PGPVR, Verma R, Melhem ER, Gur RE, Gur RC. Leftward asymmetry in relative fiber density of the arcuate fasciculus. Neuroreport 2005; 16: 791–794

[98] Vernooij MW, Smits M, Wielopolski PA, Houston GC, Krestin GP, van der Lugt A. Fiber density asymmetry of the arcuate fasciculus in relation to functional hemispheric language lateralization in both right- and left-handed healthy subjects: a combined fMRI and DTI study. Neuroimage 2007; 35: 1064–1076

[99] Wan CY, Marchina S, Norton A, Schlaug G. Atypical hemispheric asymmetry in the arcuate fasciculus of completely nonverbal children with autism. Ann N Y Acad Sci 2012; 1252: 332–337

[100] Bernal B, Altman N. The connectivity of the superior longitudinal fasciculus: a tractography DTI study. Magn Reson Imaging 2010; 28: 217–225

[101] Bernal B, Ardila A. The role of the arcuate fasciculus in conduction aphasia. Brain 2009; 132: 2309–2316

[102] Li Z, Peck KK, Petrovich Brennan N et al. Diffusion tensor tractography of the arcuate fasciculus in patients with brain tumors: comparison between deterministic and probabilistic models J Biomed Sci Engineering 2013; 6: 192–200

[103] Giannelli M, Cosottini M, Michelassi MC et al. Dependence of brain DTI maps of fractional anisotropy and mean diffusivity on the number of diffusion weighting directions. J Appl Clin Med Phys 2010; 11: 2927

[104] Lebel C, Benner T, Beaulieu C. Six is enough? Comparison of diffusion parameters measured using six or more diffusion-encoding gradient directions with deterministic tractography. Magn Reson Med 2012; 68: 474–483

[105] Gorczewski K, Mang S, Klose U. Reproducibility and consistency of evaluation techniques for HARDI data. MAGMA 2009; 22: 63–70

[106] Wedeen VJ, Wang RP, Schmahmann JD et al. Diffusion spectrum magnetic resonance imaging (DSI) tractography of crossing fibers. Neuroimage 2008; 41: 1267–1277

[107] Cho KH, Yeh CH, Chao YP, Wang JJ, Chen JH, Lin CP. Potential in reducing scan times of HARDI by accurate correction of the cross-term in a hemispherical encoding scheme. J Magn Reson Imaging 2009; 29: 1386–1394

[108] Khare K, Hardy CJ, King KF, Turski PA, Marinelli L. Accelerated MR imaging using compressive sensing with no free parameters. Magn Reson Med 2012; 68: 1450–1457

[109] Nimsky C. Intraoperative acquisition of fMRI and DTI. Neurosurg Clin N Am 2011; 22: 269–277, ix

[110] Mandelstam SA. Challenges of the anatomy and diffusion tensor tractography of the Meyer loop. AJNR Am J Neuroradiol 2012; 33: 1204–1210

[111] Nimsky C, Ganslandt O, Buchfelder M, Fahlbusch R. Intraoperative visualization for resection of gliomas: the role of functional neuronavigation and intraoperative 1.5 T MRI. Neurol Res 2006; 28: 482–487

[112] Nimsky C, Ganslandt O, Cerny S, Hastreiter P, Greiner G, Fahlbusch R. Quantification of, visualization of, and compensation for brain shift using intraoperative magnetic resonance imaging. Neurosurgery 2000; 47: 1070–1079, discussion 1079–1080

[113] Nimsky C, Ganslandt O, Merhof D, Sorensen AG, Fahlbusch R. Intraoperative visualization of the pyramidal tract by diffusion-tensor-imaging-based fiber tracking. Neuroimage 2006; 30: 1219–1229

[114] Romano A, D'Andrea G, Calabria LF et al. Pre- and intraoperative tractographic evaluation of corticospinal tract shift. Neurosurgery 2011; 69: 696–704, discussion 704–705

[115] Nimsky C, Grummich P, Sorensen AG, Fahlbusch R, Ganslandt O. Visualization of the pyramidal tract in glioma surgery by integrating diffusion tensor imaging in functional neuronavigation. Zentralbl Neurochir 2005; 66: 133–141

[116] Kleiser R, Staempfli P, Valavanis A, Boesiger P, Kollias S. Impact of fMRI-guided advanced DTI fiber tracking techniques on their clinical applications in patients with brain tumors. Neuroradiology 2010; 52: 37–46

[117] Buchmann N, Gempt J, Stoffel M, Foerschler A, Meyer B, Ringel F. Utility of diffusion tensor-imaged (DTI) motor fiber tracking for the resection of intracranial tumors near the corticospinal tract. Acta Neurochir (Wien) 2011; 153: 68–74, discussion 74

[118] Rasmussen IA, Jr, Lindseth F, Rygh OM et al. Functional neuronavigation combined with intra-operative 3D ultrasound: initial experiences during surgical resections close to eloquent brain areas and future directions in automatic brain shift compensation of preoperative data. Acta Neurochir (Wien) 2007; 149: 365–378

[119] Romano A, Ferrante M, Cipriani V et al. Role of magnetic resonance tractography in the preoperative planning and intraoperative assessment of patients with intra-axial brain tumours. Radiol Med (Torino) 2007; 112: 906–920

[120] Gil-Robles S, Duffau H. Surgical management of World Health Organization Grade II gliomas in eloquent areas: the necessity of preserving a margin around functional structures. Neurosurg Focus 2010; 28: E8

11 Metabolic Imaging: MR Spectroscopy

Isabella M. Björkman-Burtscher and Pia C. Sundgren

11.1 Introduction

Magnetic resonance spectroscopy (MRS) allows noninvasive detection and measurement of clinically relevant metabolites in the brain and has the potential to play an important role in the diagnostic workup of brain lesions in children and adults. In recent years MRS has also shown to provide additional information for treatment planning and monitoring treatment response, particularly in patients with brain tumors. This chapter presents the methodological concept of performing and evaluating MRS in the context of brain tumors as well as the limitations of the technique. The chapter is focused on the use of MRS as a complement to conventional MR imaging (MRI) in daily clinical practice and not as a scientific research tool.

11.2 Metabolites

A large number of reviews and original articles elucidate the function and physical properties of metabolites detected with MRS.[1] ▶ Table 11.1 summarizes the major neurometabolites of interest for clinical brain tumor evaluation (*N*-acetyl aspartate [NAA], choline [Cho], creatine [Cr], myoinositol, lactate, and lipids). The chapter discusses a variety of resonances, which, due to their low concentration in normal brain tissue, broad resonance frequencies, or spectral overlaps, are usually more difficult to detect or quantify unless they are clearly increased (e.g., glutamine [Gln] and glutamate [Glu], and a variety of amino acids).

11.3 Methodology

11.3.1 Data Acquisition

MRS physics have been described extensively in several text-books,[2] and only some basics need to be discussed here for the understanding of methodological challenges related to the clinical interpretation of data acquired. MRS can be performed using several nuclei (C13, F19, Na23, P31), however the hydrogen nucleus (H1) is by far the most used in clinical MRS. H1 has a high abundance within multiple neurometabolites and most clinical scanners mainly operate at its resonance frequency. This allows the combination of MRS with morphological MRI and other functional MR techniques in the clinical setting, which is a prerequisite for successful clinical MRS examinations.

Based on morphological reference images (▶ Fig. 11.1) a volume of interest is chosen for the MRS examination. A single voxel (single voxel spectroscopy [SVS]) with a usual voxel size of 3 to 8 cm³ is preferably used to characterize the metabolic profile of a rather homogeneous solid or cystic part in a tumor (▶ Fig. 11.1b,c), whereas multiple smaller voxels (multivoxel MRS or chemical shift imaging [CSI]) in one or several slices (single-slice two-dimensional chemical shift imaging [2D CSI]; multislice three-dimensional CSI [3D CSI]) are used to characterize the metabolic profile over different parts of a heterogeneous tumor and/or surrounding tissue (▶ Fig. 11.1d–f). In this context it is important to emphasize the need to review conventional MR images prior to voxel/region of interest (ROI) positioning to define the area of the lesion that is most

Table 11.1 Magnetic resonance spectroscopy (MRS) metabolites: neurometabolites in clinical brain tumor evaluation

Metabolite	Main components contributing to the signal	Resonance frequency	Main functions	Main occurrence
NAA	*N*-acetylaspartate (NAA), *N*-acetylaspartylglutamate (NAAG)	2.02 parts per million (ppm)	Marker for neuronal integrity and function, osmolyte, metabolic precursor	Neurons
Cr	Creatine (Cr), phosphocreatine (PCr)	3.02 ppm	Marker of energy metabolism	All types of cells
Cho	Choline (Cho), phosphorylcholine (PC), glycerophosphorylcholine (GPC)	3.2 ppm	Marker for cell membrane turnover	All types of cells
mI	Myoinositol	3.56 ppm	Glial marker, osmolyte	Glia cells/myelin breakdown product
Lac	Lactate (Lac)	Doublet peak at 1.33 ppm	Very low detectable concentrations in normal tissue	Pathologically altered cells and cerebrospinal fluid
Lip	Lipids	0.9–1.3 ppm	Membrane marker	All types of cells

Note: Although NAA, Cr, and Cho are seen in both short (20–35 ms), intermediate (144 ms), and long (288 ms) TE (echo time) spectra, mI is seen only in short TE spectra. Lactate and lipid concentrations are low or not detectable in normal brain tissue unless the latter appear due to contamination artifacts from the scalp due to inappropriate voxel positioning.

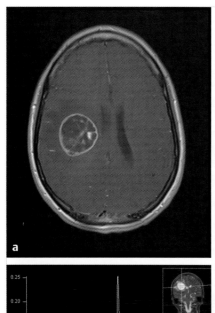

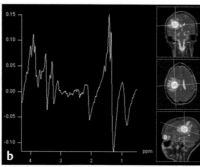

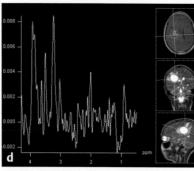

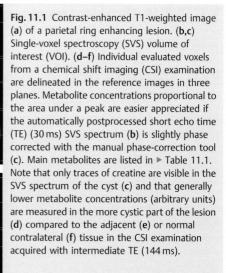

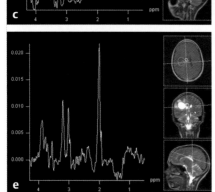

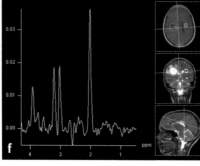

Fig. 11.1 Contrast-enhanced T1-weighted image (a) of a parietal ring enhancing lesion. (b,c) Single-voxel spectroscopy (SVS) volume of interest (VOI). (d–f) Individual evaluated voxels from a chemical shift imaging (CSI) examination are delineated in the reference images in three planes. Metabolite concentrations proportional to the area under a peak are easier appreciated if the automatically postprocessed short echo time (TE) (30 ms) SVS spectrum (b) is slightly phase corrected with the manual phase-correction tool (c). Main metabolites are listed in ▶ Table 11.1. Note that only traces of creatine are visible in the SVS spectrum of the cyst (c) and that generally lower metabolite concentrations (arbitrary units) are measured in the more cystic part of the lesion (d) compared to the adjacent (e) or normal contralateral (f) tissue in the CSI examination acquired with intermediate TE (144 ms).

interesting for MRS and relevant for the clinical question to be answered. The defined area might not necessarily coincide with the area technically most accessible for MRS. Compared to the wide variety of available sequences and parameters in MRI the choice of MRS sequences can be standardized regarding sequence type and acquisition parameters in a very robust way to allow for comparable data not only within one patient but within larger clinical populations (▶ Table 11.2). Short echo times allow for evaluation of metabolites with short relaxation times (e.g., myoinositol). Intermediate echo times are used to more clearly depict lactate because the resonance inverts in the spectrum and points below the baseline, and to assure lesser relaxation effects on the main metabolites NAA, Cho, and Cr compared to long echo times. Use of the latter usually generates spectra of high quality, however, including a more limited number of metabolites compared to short echo time spectra.

11.3.2 Data Postprocessing

Acquired MRS raw data need to be postprocessed with software provided by the manufacturers or with postprocessing tools such as LCModel (LCMODEL, Inc. Oakville, Ontario, Canada).[3] For clinical examination in brain tumor patients, automated postprocessing with manufacturer-provided software is mainly sufficient and limited to a few steps: water reference processing, filtering, zero filling, Fourier transformation, frequency shift correction, baseline correction, phase correction, and curve fitting. Of these mainly phase correction might need some manual adjustment as illustrated in ▶ Fig. 11.1b. Generated spectra may be saved in Picture Archiving and Communication System (PACS) systems or made available for interpretation by other means. Using curve fitting tools the generated spectra may also include information on, for example,

Table 11.2 Clinical magnetic resonance spectroscopy (MRS) sequences, single-voxel spectroscopy (SVS), and chemical shift imaging (CSI) with parameter suggestions

MRS technique	SVS	CSI
Voxel size[a]	3–8 cm³	1–1.5 cm³
Number of acquired spectra	1	4–100 depending on region of interest size
Repetition time (TR) (ms)	1,500–2,000	
Echo time (TE) (ms)	Short (20–35) Intermediate (135–144)[b] Long (270–288)[b]	
Number of excitations	96–128	1–2
Acquisition method[c]	PRESS or STEAM	

[a]The voxel size in SVS is determined by the width of the slice selection pulses and in CSI by the field of view (e.g., 16 × 16 cm) and the number of phase-encoding steps (e.g., 16 × 16) in combination with the slice thickness (e.g., 1.5 cm). The number of acquired spectra in CSI depends on the size of the region of interest (ROI; 2 × 2 to 10 × 10 cm) in combination with the voxel size above.

[b]Echo time (TE) of 135 or 270 ms is usually used on 1.5 T systems and 144 and 288 ms on 3 T systems.

[c]Although stimulated echo acquisition mode (STEAM) earlier was often preferred, especially for SVS because it allowed for more precise slice selection and usage of shorter TE, point resolved spectroscopy (PRESS) is now the clinical method of choice because earlier technical problems have been overcome, and the method allows for twice the signal-to-noise ratio compared to STEAM.

semiquantitative metabolite concentrations in arbitrary units, resonance position, and resonance assignment. Using automated curve fitting, the reader of the spectrum should make sure that, first, the fitted baseline coincides with the actual spectral baseline—because metabolites will otherwise be over- or underestimated—and that, second, the metabolite assignments are correct and there has been no frequency shift of metabolites. Voxel position should be illustrated to the reader of the spectrum with reference images (▶ Fig. 11.1b–f). The area under a peak of the MR spectrum equals the signal intensity of the resonance and is proportional to the concentration of the metabolite within the voxel because it is a function of the number of nuclei contributing to the signal. However, besides the number of contributing nuclei the detected signal is influenced by many factors, such as J-coupling, relaxation times and thus pulse sequences and acquisition parameters, as well as spectral quality and artifacts. Strict rules need to be applied for spectral quality if absolute metabolite concentrations are calculated with methods employing referencing to internal signals (mainly brain water signal from the same voxel) or external signals (phantom). Furthermore, tissue inhomogeneity within the voxel—not only due to partial volume effects of, for example, cerebrospinal fluid (CSF), but also tumor inhomogeneities—needs to be taken into account. A more robust and clinically often more feasible method of data interpretation is a semiquantitative approach with calculation or visual appreciation of metabolite ratios. Either ratios normalizing the individual metabolites to the creatine signal (e.g., NAA:Cr) are used or the metabolites are directly compared to each other (e.g., NAA:Cho). This also allows the use of spectra with lower spectral quality for clinical

evaluation (▶ Fig. 11.2). When looking at an isolated voxel metabolite ratio, such as Cho:NAA, the problem arises of not knowing whether the abnormality causing an observed spectral change is in the numerator or in the denominator. Therefore, in multivoxel MRS, further tissue characterization might be achieved when the tumor signals are expressed in the contralateral normal brain tissue metabolite signals (e.g., tumor Cho to Cho from normal-appearing contralateral brain tissue). A drawback of this method, however, is the risk that general signal decrease due to edema, tissue necrosis, or artifacts might lead to an underestimation of a possible peak increase compared to the other metabolites in the same voxel.

11.3.3 Data Interpretation

Radiologists are trained to take confounding artifacts into account when interpreting MR images, and the awareness of interpretation pitfalls related to image artifacts is usually high. Artifacts affecting MR spectra are generally less well known but are well described and illustrated by Kreis.[4] As a first step in the clinical interpretation the spectral quality should be evaluated. Subsequently, voxel position should be related to morphological findings to establish the clinical question to be answered with the spectra from each voxel. Spectra acquired from outside the periphery or the center of a lesion need to be looked upon in different ways: while the tumor center primarily might be of interest for tumor differential diagnosis or grading, tumor periphery and surrounding tissue are often evaluated for tumor infiltration or as reference areas. When evaluating the spectral patterns the reader needs to keep in mind spectral changes in metabolite concentrations related to age, which is primarily of interest in neonates and infants, who show increasing NAA concentrations parallel to decreasing choline concentrations with increasing age. The following spectral changes are common in brain tumor MRS (▶ Fig. 11.3): (1) decrease of NAA as a marker for a decreased number of neurons or neuronal function per volume as seen not only in the tumor itself but also in the surrounding edema; (2) increase of choline as a marker of increased cell membrane turnover, which might reflect tumor growth, tumor necrosis, or gliosis; (3) increase of lactate and or lipids mainly as a marker of tumor necrosis, which is not only related to treatment response but is also a natural feature in viable tumor with energy requirements exceeding energy supply; and (4) decrease of all metabolites as a marker of general cell destruction and general decrease of molecules contributing to the spectrum.

11.4 Limitations

Despite MRS being used in the workup of brain tumors there are still several important limitations associated with the clinical use of proton MRS for brain tumor imaging. MRS data processing is time consuming and user dependent, or it might require third party postprocessing tools. Regardless of which technique is used the size of the MRS voxel is limited, thus the total tumor volume might not be evaluated and heterogeneous parts of a tumor might contribute to a single spectrum leading to partial volume effects, which are difficult to interpret. The location of the lesion and components like calcification and hemorrhage might cause artifacts and provide limited spectral quality. Further, there is no obvious single spectral pattern that

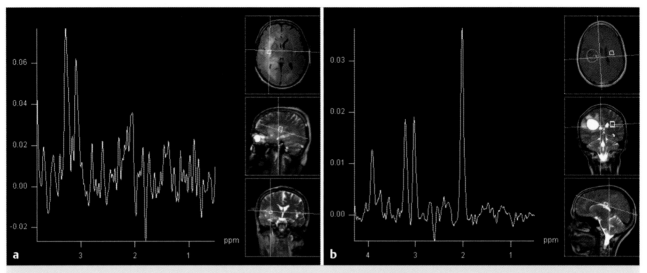

Fig. 11.2 Suboptimal quality spectrum representing tumor in a patient with low-grade astrocytoma (**a**). Although the spectral quality is suboptimal the change of metabolite ratios from *N*-acetylaspartate (NAA) > choline (Cho) in normal tissue (**b**) to Cho > NAA in this tumor spectrum (**a**) is easily appreciated visually without sophisticated quantitative evaluation.

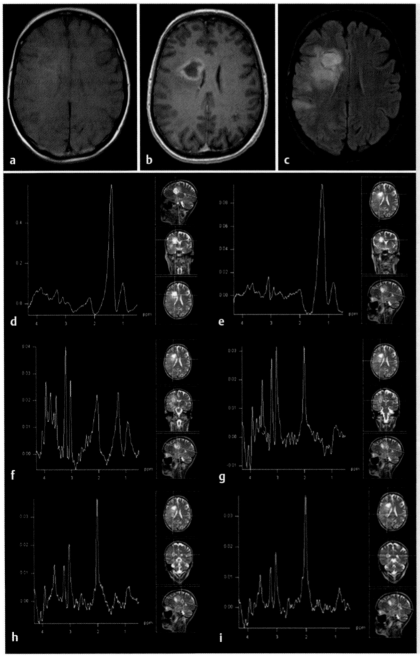

Fig. 11.3 T1 (**a**) and contrast-enhanced T1 (**b**) and fluid-attenuated inversion recovery (FLAIR) (**c**) images of a glioblastoma multiforme with surrounding edema. Short TE (echo time) (30 ms) single voxel spectroscopy (SVS) (**d**) and chemical shift imaging (CSI) (**e**) spectra from the cystic part of the lesion show high concentrations of lipids and lactate. The CSI measurement covers several further areas within the tumor and surrounding tissue. To the spectrum from the narrow contrast-enhancing rim of the lesion (**f**) contribute, due to partial volume effects from adjacent tissue, the contrast-enhancing tumor portion, the tumor cyst/necrosis, and surrounding less infiltrated tissue with elevated choline, lactate, and lipids and decreased NAA. Decreased NAA is found in adjacent tissue with edema (**g**), whereas spectra from areas without T2 signal increase (**h**) and from the contralateral side (**i**) are normal.

correlates with tumor histopathology, and nonspecific spectral findings as described earlier are common. Still, despite a considerable volume of research in the field, no consensus exists regarding the use of normalized versus nonnormalized ratios or quantitative data, the specificity and sensitivity of the method, or the true value of the method in clinical decision making. The ultimate clinically oriented scientific paper on the use of MRS in brain tumor diagnosis is yet to be written.

11.5 Clinical Applications

Despite some controversy the clinical potential for MRS in brain tumor workup is well documented. MRS has been shown to be a valuable additional tool along with conventional imaging and other advanced MR techniques for grading brain tumors, differentiating brain lesions, and differentiating recurrent tumor and radiation injury. MRS has also demonstrated its value as an imaging-guiding tool for surgical brain biopsy. The focus here is on the metabolic changes relevant for tumor grading, tumor characterization prior to treatment, and differentiation of radiation injury and necrosis from recurrent tumor. Furthermore spectral patterns of primary pediatric and adult intracranial tumors and secondary tumors are presented, and the findings in some common differential diagnoses are described.

11.5.1 Tumor Grading

Conventional MRI is limited in its ability to reliably grade gliomas. Contrast enhancement on postcontrast T1-weighted images is one of the most common methods for assessing glioma grade. However, malignancy often extends beyond contrast enhancement, and some tumors graded as World Health Organization (WHO) grade III or IV might not always present with contrast enhancement as well as low grade tumors might.[5] Some studies suggest that the choline signal in gliomas and peritumoral regions is able to distinguish regions with tumor infiltration from nontumor tissue, but it may not be a surrogate marker for the pathological grade of a tumor.[6,7,8] A common MRS finding in malignant gliomas is increased choline and decreased NAA and creatine concentrations compared with normal brain tissue. It is clear that the contrast enhancement does not necessarily correspond to the regions of high choline concentration because elevated choline levels have been found beyond the contrast-enhancing tumor area or, in cases of no enhancement, in areas with hyperintense signal on T2-weighted and fluid-attenuation inversion recovery (FLAIR) images representing tumor.[7,9,10,11] Indication of malignant transformation and early progression of initial low-grade gliomas is the increase in the creatine concentration and progressive decrease in NAA and myoinositol concentrations and increased choline concentration.[12] Significantly increased Cho:Cr and Cho:NAA ratios are usually seen in high-grade tumors compared to less increased Cho:Cr or decreased NAA:Cr in low-grade tumors compared to normal brain tissue. ▸ Fig. 11.4 illustrates a WHO grade III oligodendroglioma with highly increased Cho and decreased NAA. In comparison a WHO grade IV glioblastoma multiforme demonstrates almost

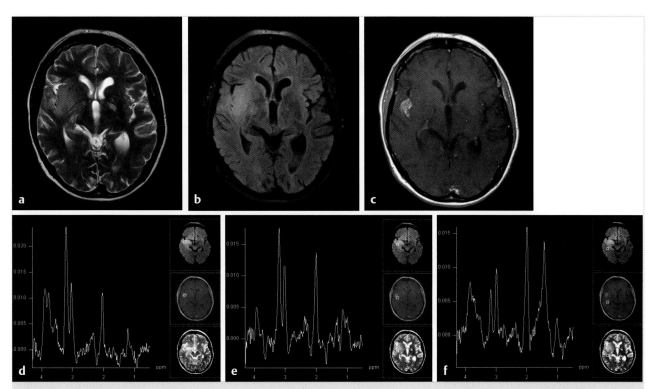

Fig. 11.4 T2 (**a**), fluid-attenuated inversion recovery (FLAIR) (**b**), and contrast-enhanced T1-weighted magnetic resonance (MR) (**c**) images of an oligodendroglioma World Health Organization (WHO) grade III. The spectrum (echo time [TE] 144 ms) (**d**) from the contrast-enhancing area demonstrates significantly elevated choline (Cho) and decreased N-acetylaspartate (NAA) resulting in high Cho:NAA and low NAA to creatine (NAA:Cr) ratios. Cho:NAA ratios decrease with increasing distance from the contrast-enhancing area (**e,f**). Spectral patterns with significantly elevated Cho over NAA are consistent with higher-grade tumor; however, differentiation between grade III and grade IV tumors might be difficult.

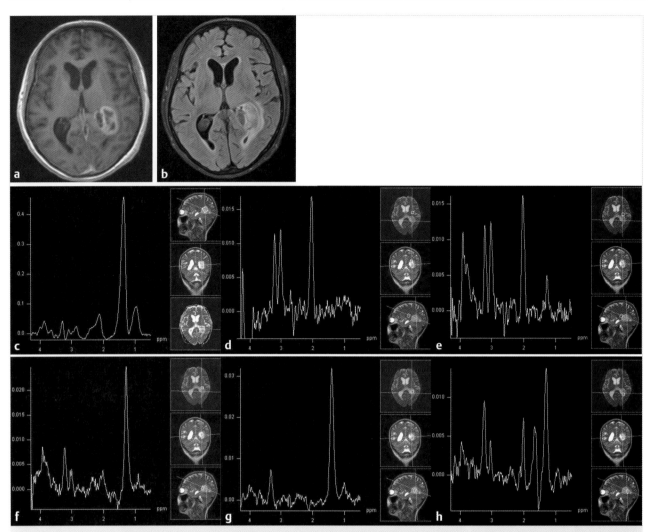

Fig. 11.5 Contrast-enhanced T1-weighted (**a**) and fluid-attenuated inversion recovery (FLAIR) (**b**) images of a glioblastoma multiforme (World Health Organization grade IV). In (**c**) the single-voxel spectroscopy (SVS) volume of interest (VOI) and in (**d–h**) individual evaluated voxels from a chemical shift imaging (CSI) examination are delineated in the reference images in three planes. The short echo time (TE) (30 ms) SVS spectrum (**c**) is unspecific for necrosis with a dominating lactate resonance (1.33 ppm) and a broad lipid peak to the right and underlying lactate. Compared to a normal intermediate TE (144 ms), spectral pattern for basal ganglia in (**d**) the spectrum from tissue directly adjacent to the contrast-enhancing lesion (**e**) shows a slight decrease of N-acetylaspartate (NAA) (a neuron marker) and a slight increase of lactate. Spectra from the lesion center (**f,g**) show generally decreased metabolites and a marked increase of the Cho:NAA ratio and of lactate. The contrast-enhancing periphery of the lesion is characterized by a less pronounced increase of the Cho:NAA ratio (**h**), which is not an indicator for lower malignancy but of partial volume effects from adjacent, more normal tissue.

complete absence of NAA in the contrast-enhancing periphery of the necrotic tumor and elevated Cho (▶ Fig. 11.5f,g).

Several MRS studies have demonstrated significantly higher Cho:Cr and Cho:NAA ratios in high-grade than in low-grade glioma ($p < 0.001$),[13,14] whereas the NAA:Cr ratios were significantly lower in high-grade than in low-grade glioma ($p < 0.001$).[13] Using a threshold for Cho:Cr of 2.04 resulted in sensitivity, specificity, positive predicted value (PPV), and negative predicted value (NPV) of 84%, 83.33%, 91.3% and 71.43%, respectively.[13] A threshold value of 2.2 for the Cho:NAA ratio resulted in sensitivity, specificity, PPV, and NPV of 88%, 66.67%, 84.62%, and 72.73%, respectively.[13] The presence of lipid or lactate on MRS is highly suggestive of higher-grade malignant gliomas mainly seen in grade IV gliomas but not correlated to the degree of tumor infiltration.[8,9] Paradoxically malignant MR spectra can be present in pilocytic astrocytoma because lactate is frequently elevated in this type of tumor.[15] Other metabolites like glycine (Gly) and myoinositol (Myo) might be present in high-grade or low-grade tumors, respectively. A recent study demonstrated that glycine levels were significantly elevated in glioblastoma multiforme (GBM), low-grade astrocytoma, and metastases and significantly higher in GBM than low-grade astrocytomas.[16] The same study demonstrated that the myo-inositol levels were elevated in low-grade astrocytoma and metastases and reduced in meningioma and GBM.[16] In addition they found that the Gly:Myo ratio did distinguish GBM from metastases and low-grade astrocytomas, suggesting that Gly might be a useful biomarker for tumor characterization.[16]

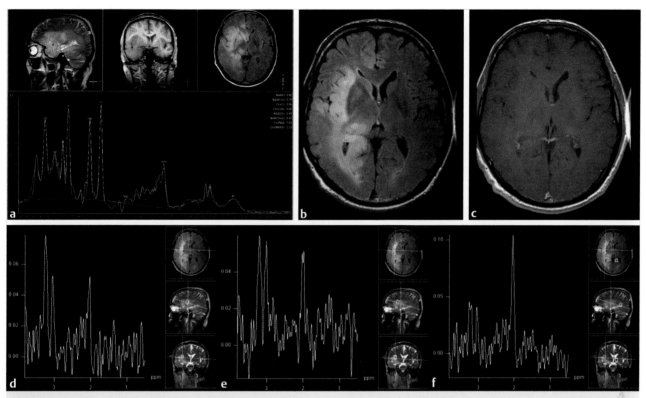

Fig. 11.6 A lesion initially diagnosed as encephalitis after stereotactic biopsy showed in a preoperative single-voxel spectroscopy (SVS) (echo time [TE] 30 ms) spectrum a marked decrease of *N*-acetylaspartate (NAA) and elevated myoinositol (**a**) suggestive for low-grade astrocytoma. Follow-up magnetic resonance imaging (MRI) showed decreased edema but otherwise stable disease on fluid-attenuated inversion recovery (FLAIR) (**b**) and contrast-enhanced T1 (**c**) images but chemical shift imaging (CSI) (TE 288 ms) revealed in some areas an increase in the ratio of choline to NAA (Cho: NAA) (**d**), again suggestive of tumor. In the other areas magnetic resonance spectroscopy (MRS) was consistent with unspecific edema (**e**). Normal contralateral MRS (**f**). A second stereotactic biopsy was consistent with World Health Organization grade II astrocytoma.

11.5.2 Imaging-Guided Surgical Brain Biopsy

Due to the tissue heterogeneity often present in brain tumors, especially in gliomas, and the diffuse infiltrative growth without a delineable central tumor portion in many low-grade tumors, sampling error associated with surgical biopsy might occur. Conventional MRI is limited in its ability to guide biopsy sites to the most aggressive, or for the pathologist most interesting, portion of the tumor, especially in brain tumors without contrast enhancement. ▶ Fig. 11.6a–f illustrates a case with MRS findings consistent with low-grade astrocytoma with decreased NAA, increased myoinositol, and no marked increase in Cho or decrease in Cr (▶ Fig. 11.6a). Initial stereotactic biopsy suggested encephalitis. Follow-up MRS showed a marked increase of Cho:NAA (▶ Fig. 11.6) in some parts of the lesion, although no contrast enhancement was present. Other parts revealed decreased NAA with a Cho:NAA ratio of approximately 1 consistent with edema (▶ Fig. 11.6e). A repeated stereotactic biopsy from the relevant area revealed astrocytoma WHO grade II.

MRS performed for the purpose of image-guided biopsy is preferably using 2D or 3D CSI methods with robust long echo time (TE), point resolved spectroscopy (PRESS) sequences if large tumor/lesion areas need to be evaluated or single-voxel spectroscopy (SVS) short TE sequences if different focal areas at some distance from each other need to be evaluated. Areas characterized with MRS as appropriate regions for biopsy need to be carefully evaluated on MRI to exclude confounding factors, such as extensive edema or areas of hemorrhage that might cause artifacts. Especially areas of suspected high cellularity might be confirmed with MRS demonstrated by a significant increase in Cho and low or no NAA.[17] However, by MRS defined areas of interest for surgical intervention are not always accessible for stereotactic biopsy or open surgery as they might represent eloquent brain areas with a high risk of postoperative sequel.

11.5.3 Monitoring Brain Tumor Treatment

One of the major concerns in the follow-up of brain tumor treatment is the difficulty of differentiating between radiation injury and recurrent tumor when new contrast-enhancing lesions are presenting at the vicinity of a previously treated brain tumor (▶ Fig. 11.7). These lesions are in regions that have been subjected to radiation, with or without chemotherapy, and often adjacent to surgical resection. In most cases there are no specific conventional MRI characteristics that enable discrimination between tumor recurrence, tumor progression, pseudoprogression, and inflammatory or necrotic changes that can result from radiation therapy, all potentially presenting

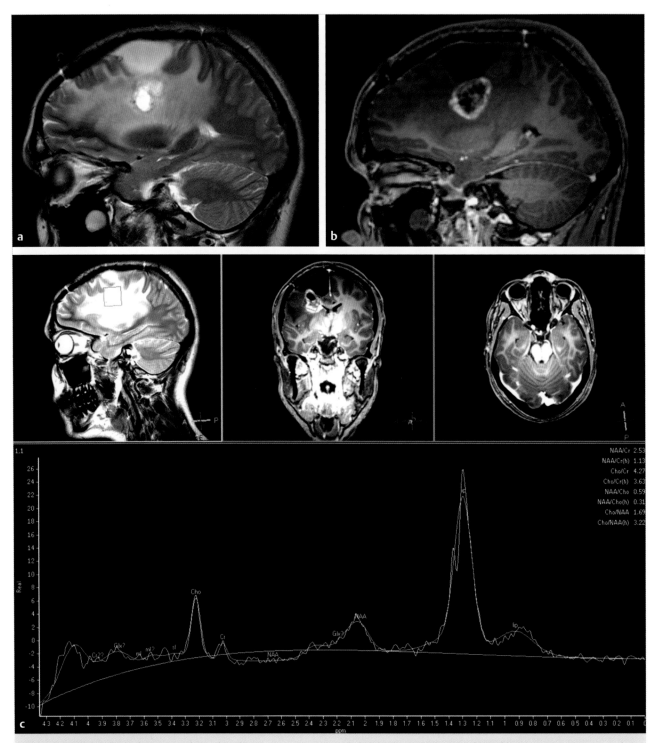

Fig. 11.7 Sagittal T2 (a) and contrast-enhanced T1 (b) images in a patient with anaplastic astrocytoma World Health Organization (WHO) grade III showing progression with increased contrast enhancement and necrosis after radiation therapy. Long echo time (TE 288 ms) single-voxel spectroscopy (SVS) shows a clearly increased choline to creatine (Cho:Cr) ratio and increased lipids and lactate (c). Although spectral quality is suboptimal the spectrum supports the clinical and morphological suspicion of tumor progression and increased malignancy. Tumor resection reveals high-grade glioma WHO grade IV.

with contrast enhancement.[18] Unfortunately, in many of the new enhancing regions, both tumor cells and radiation injury are present, and the spectral patterns in such cases are less definitive than in pure tumor or pure radiation necrosis.[19] When performing MRS as part of the workup of suspected

radiation injury versus recurrent or progressive tumor 2D-CSI MRS is preferred to SVS. With 2D CSI, the coverage of contrast-enhancing tissue, surrounding tissue, and normal-appearing white matter in the contralateral hemisphere is allowed. This enables sampling of multiple regions, which may be necessary to discern the subtle differences between tumor recurrence and radiation injury and for the identification of areas of both tumor and inflammatory changes in the same enhancing lesion.[20]

A previous 2D-CSI MRS study using a cutoff value of 1.8 for either the Cho:NAA ratio or the Cho:Cr ratio as a marker for tumor recurrence reported a 97% success rate to retrospectively differentiate recurrent tumor from radiation injury.[21] These findings are in agreement with those in a previous multivoxel MRS study that correlated spectroscopy findings with histological specimens.[22] The odds of a lesion being pure tumor compared to pure necrosis are higher with a Cho:Cr ratio > 1.79 or a lipid (Lip) and lactate (Lac):Cho ratio < 0.75, and the odds of biopsy-proven pure necrosis were higher when having either a Cho:normalized Cr (nCr) value < 0.89 or a Cho:normalized Cho (nCho) value < 0.66.[22] A multivoxel 3D proton MRS study demonstrated significantly higher Cho:NAA and Cho:Cr ratios in recurrent tumor than in radiation injury, whereas the NAA:Cr ratios were lower in recurrent tumor than in radiation injury. When using receiver operating characteristic analysis, the resulting sensitivity, specificity, and diagnostic accuracy of 3D MR spectroscopy were 94.1%, 100%, and 96.2%, respectively, based on the cutoff values of 1.71 for Cho:Cr or 1.71 for Cho:NAA or both as tumor criteria.[23] In a recent study comparing MRS with ^{18}F fluorodeoxyglucose positron-emission tomography (FDG-PET), MRS demonstrated a PPV and NPV of 100%, whereas for FDG-PET, PPV and NPV were 66.6% and 60%, concluding that MRS and MR perfusion are superior to FDG-PET in discriminating tumor recurrence, grade increase, and radiation injury or radiation necrosis.[24] In another study the investigators found significantly higher Lac:Cho ratios in the radiation necrosis group compared with the recurrent tumor group.[25] There are, however, also other imaging techniques used in the workup of this patient group. For example, a recent study indicates that pentavalent technetium-99 m dimercaptosuccinic acid brain single photon emission computed tomography (SPECT) is more accurate compared with ^{1}H-MRS for the detection of tumor residual tissues or recurrence in glioma patients with previous radiotherapy.[26] Clinical course, MR findings including MRS, and techniques other than MR need to be interpreted together to assure as accurate treatment monitoring as possible. Slight depression of NAA and variable changes in Cho and Cr are spectroscopic changes that occur in radiation injury.[27,28,29] In addition, radiation necrosis may show a broad peak between 0 and 2 ppm reflecting cellular debris containing fatty acids, lactate, and amino acids. A complete radiation necrosis cannot be differentiated from a tumor necrosis by either imaging or spectroscopy. Both will present with a cystic necrosis on MRI and flat spectra or spectra with nonspecific elevation of lactate and or lipids.

The degree of metabolic changes most likely depends on the radiation dose. Frequent reported findings are a decrease in NAA or a reduction in the NAA:Cr ratio and an increase in the Cho:Cr ratio after radiation therapy, proportional to the radiation dose.[27–33] Another ratio that has been used in the attempt to diagnose radiation necrosis is the Cho:Lip or Lac ratio. One study showed that the positive predictive value of a Cho:Lip or Lac ratio < 0.3 and the positive predictive value of a Cho:Cr < 2.48 for diagnosing radiation necrosis were 100% and 71.4%, respectively.[34] The authors concluded that it is possible to statistically differentiate radiation necrosis from metastatic

brain tumor but not from glioblastoma by using the Cho:Cr ratio or the Cho:Lip or Lac ratio.[34] A more relevant diagnostic dilemma is the differentiation between recurrent brain tumor and radiation injury as presented earlier.

11.5.4 Meningioma and Hemangiopericytoma

Although often easily diagnosed with computed tomography (CT) or conventional MRI, meningiomas are well evaluated with MRS because they often present as large and homogeneous tumors that allow for good tumor tissue representation in MR spectra. Meningiomas are characterized by high choline levels and the absence of NAA, except for rare cases of infiltrative growth or—probably more common—partial volume effects from adjacent tissue or artifacts (▶ Fig. 11.8). Alanine might be seen as an inverted doublet in 144 TE spectra.[35] On rare occasion grading of meningioma might be of interest prior to surgery. A recent SVS ^{1}H-MRS study on 100 intracranial meningiomas performed before their surgical resection showed no significant differences regarding mobile lipids, lactate, alanine, NAA, and choline-containing compounds between different grades of meningioma.[36] However, absolute choline concentration has been demonstrated to be significantly higher in malignant compared with benign meningiomas.[37] Decreased NAA and lower NAA:Cho ratios have been demonstrated in the perilesional edema in the vicinity of meningiomas and might, according to Chernov et al, suggest a more aggressive tumor pattern.[38] Depending on location, hemangiopericytoma is, based on common imaging features, a differential diagnosis to meningioma. In general, these tumors can be difficult to analyze with spectroscopy because of artifacts due to hemorrhagic components commonly seen in this tumor. A recent study has suggested relative ratios of myoinositol, glucose, and glutathione with respect to glutamate being higher in hemangiopericytoma compared to meningioma; whereas the relative ratios of creatine, glutamine, alanine, glycine, and choline-containing compounds with respect to glutamate are lower in hemangiopericytoma compared to meningioma.[39] Myoinositol has earlier been described to be elevated in hemangiopericytoma.[40] However, it is too early to draw any conclusions as to whether MRS can be helpful in clinical differentiation of the two entities.

11.5.5 Pediatric Cerebellar Brain Tumors

Spectral pattern overlaps are common in pediatric brain tumors and their differential diagnoses in adults (▶ Fig. 11.9). Studies evaluating the use of MRS to differentiate the most common primary cerebellar pediatric brain tumors—astrocytoma, ependymoma, and medulloblastoma—are mainly based on complex evaluation methods combining absolute MRS metabolite quantification, other MR techniques, and statistical methods such as linear discriminant analysis, principal component analysis, and cross-validation methods.[41,42] In the study presented by Davies et al[42] medulloblastomas were characterized by high taurine, phosphocholine, and glutamate and low glutamine; ependymomas were differentiated by high myoinositol and glycerophosphocholine; and astrocytomas presented with low creatine and

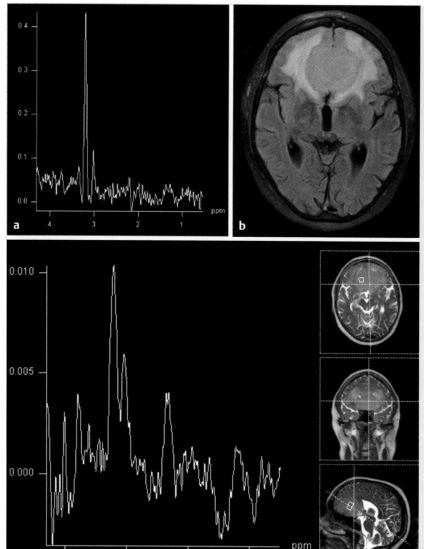

Fig. 11.8 The normal spectral appearance (echo time [TE] 288 ms) of a meningioma with clearly increased choline (Cho) and absence of N-acetylaspartate (NAA) (**a**) is not seen in all meningiomas. T1 contrast-enhanced magnetic resonance imaging (MRI) of an olfactory bulb meningioma (**b**). Chemical shift imaging (CSI) magnetic resonance spectroscopy (MRS) (TE 144 ms) from the lesion shows increased Cho (3.2 ppm) and increased creatine (Cr) (3 ppm) and an unassigned resonance to the right of Cr as well as minor concentrations of lactate—inverted at TE 144 ms (**c**).

high NAA. Schneider et al[41] showed that linear discriminant analysis using diffusion-weighted imaging (DWI) and MRS using water as internal reference discriminates the most frequent posterior fossa tumors in children, whereas tumors could not be discriminated with the use of metabolite ratios or apparent diffusion coefficient (ADC) values alone, nor could they be differentiated using creatine as an internal reference even in combination with ADC values. MRS has also been used in attempts to differentiate between pediatric low- and high-grade astrocytomas. A recent study has shown that a decrease of NAA and an increase of Cho concentrations were more pronounced in WHO grade III than in WHO grade II astrocytomas and that the best discriminator to differentiate low- from high-grade gliomas was the NAA:Cho ratio.[43] The same group showed that choline as a single parameter cannot be considered as reliable in the differential diagnosis of low-grade astrocytomas in children.[44] The use of clinical MRS in pediatric tumors, especially in the posterior fossa, warrants confirmation by larger studies.

11.5.6 Lymphoma

The high cellularity and the limited infiltrative growth beyond the MR-visible borders of the tumor give lymphomas an intermediate status between gliomas and metastases regarding MRS interpretation (▶ Fig. 11.10). Their generally high Cho:Cr ratios within the lesion compares to both differential diagnoses,[45] whereas their noninfiltrative CSI pattern in surrounding tissue[45,46] more closely resembles metastases.

11.5.7 Metastases

Considering the possible spectral changes related to tumor growth described earlier, it should be possible to differentiate metastases from high-grade glial tumors due to their primarily noninfiltrative growth not yielding high choline levels in their vicinity and the absence of NAA within metastases. Areas of high T2 signal surrounding contrast-enhancing lesions are often referred to as perilesional or peritumoral edema. Although true

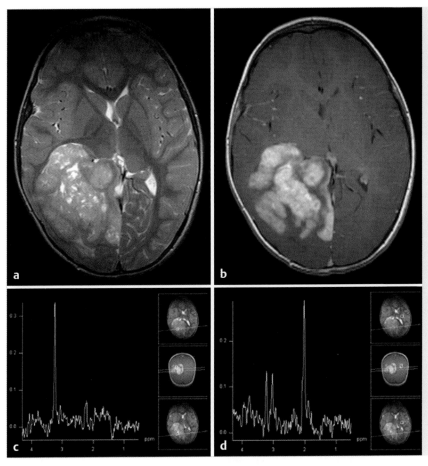

Fig. 11.9 T2 (**a**) and contrast-enhanced T1 (**b**) axial images of a supratentorial ependymoma in a 5-year-old girl. The center of the tumor (**c**) exhibits excessive choline (Cho) (3.2 ppm) and no clearly detectable signal of creatine (Cr) (3.02 ppm) and *N*-acetylaspartate (NAA) (2 ppm). The spectrum is not specific for ependymoma but represents a common finding in pediatric differential diagnoses such as meningioma, medulloblastoma, and high-grade glioma but is unlikely for low-grade astrocytoma. Contralateral normal long echo time (TE 288 ms) spectrum (**d**).

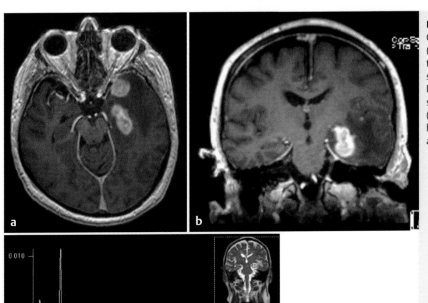

Fig. 11.10 Right temporal lymphoma. Contrast-enhanced T1 axial (**a**) and coronal (**b**) magnetic resonance imaging. The location of the lesion is not in favor for magnetic resonance spectroscopy due to its proximity to areas with large susceptibility differences. However, despite suboptimal quality, (**c**) chemical shift imaging (CSI) (echo time [TE] 288 ms) reveals clearly a high choline to *N*-acetylaspartate (Cho:NAA) ratio and but no marked increase of lactate or lipids.

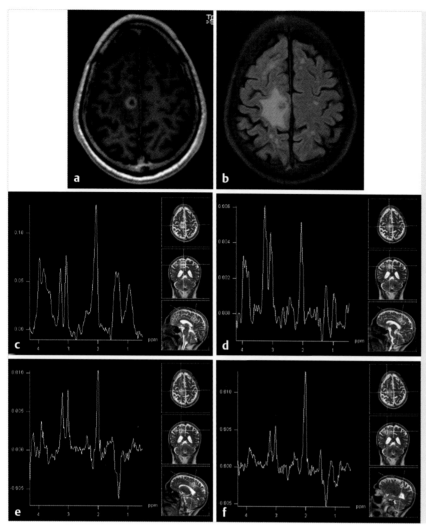

Fig. 11.11 The size of the small ring-enhancing lung adenocarcinoma metastasis (**a**) surrounded by edema (**b**) in the right central region does not allow acquisition of magnetic resonance (MR) spectra, only representing the center or the contrast-enhancing rim with conventional magnetic resonance spectroscopy (MRS) techniques. Therefore single-voxel spectroscopy (SVS) (echo time [TE] 30 ms) (**c**) and chemical shift imaging (CSI) (TE 144 ms) (**d**) spectra represent a mixture of tissues from the lesion complicating differential diagnosis. Absence of high choline (Cho) and N-acetylaspartate (NAA: Cho) > 1 suggests absence of infiltration to tissue surrounding the contrast-enhancing rim (**e,f**) and therefore metastasis.

for metastases, in high-grade gliomas these areas frequently represent tumor infiltration (see ▶ Fig. 11.3 and ▶ Fig. 11.5). Because NAA, a marker of neuronal function and neuronal density per volume, should decrease in areas of edema as well as in areas of tumor, NAA can be expected to play a minor role in the differentiation of the two tumor entities regarding infiltrative growth. In 1996 Siejens et al[47] showed that metastases do not contain NAA. Within the metastatic lesion Bendini et al[46] showed in general high concentrations of lipids and a variable Cho:Cr ratio, whereas tumor infiltration characterized by high Cho levels was absent from perilesional areas of edema. Similar results are demonstrated by Server et al,[48] reporting significant differences in the Cho:Cr, Cho:NAA, and NAA:Cr ratios between high-grade gliomas and metastases in areas outside the contrast-enhancing tumor regions. Because the peritumoral area is of great interest in the differential diagnosis of metastases from high-grade gliomas the use of multivoxel techniques covering larger areas within and in the vicinity of the tumors is important. Furthermore, careful positioning of the region of interest in areas suspected for possible infiltration is a prerequisite

for detection of infiltrative growth (▶ Fig. 11.11). To position the CSI volume through the center of a cystic lesion neglecting off-center areas of suspected infiltration might lead to spectra not representative for the true tumor growth pattern.

11.5.8 Differential Diagnosis From Nonneoplastic Lesions

MRS can add information to the clinical workup of suspected brain tumors. The chapter now focuses on metabolic patterns that can be expected in the common differential diagnoses encephalitis, cerebritis, and abscesses. Encephalitis and cerebritis lead to local diffuse tissue injury, cell proliferation, and tissue repair. Depending on cause and severity of the changes, including ongoing repair mechanisms, imaging findings can range from subtle to tissue necrosis or abscess formation. As with variable MRI findings, MRS presents with a variety of spectral patterns in these lesions. In cases of less severe changes lacking obvious necrosis and contrast enhancement, differentiation of

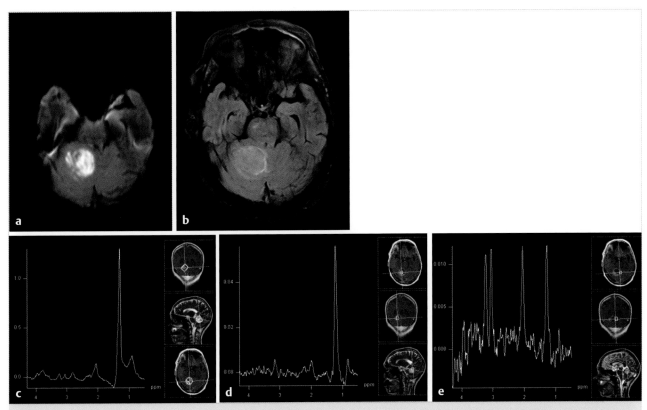

Fig. 11.12 Diffusion-weighted imaging (DWI) (**a**) with restricted diffusion and fluid-attenuated inversion recovery (FLAIR) (**b**) in a patient with a treated abscess. Single-voxel spectroscopy (SVS) (echo time [TE] 30 ms) (**c**) and chemical shift imaging (CSI) (TE 144 ms) (**d**) show unspecific spectra with high lipids. The voxel directly adjacent to the lesion (**e**) demonstrates a typical spectrum for edema and contamination from the cystic part of the lesion.

low-grade gliomas from encephalitis and early cerebritis might be difficult for both conventional MR and MRS. Sequential examinations showing spectral normalization corresponding to treatment response might be of value in unclear cases of diffuse nonenhancing lesions. When a bacterial infection has led to abscess formation the lesion may be difficult to distinguish from other ring-enhancing lesions on MRI, although DWI, with its ability to detect the restricted diffusion in the abscess cavity, is of substantial help. MRS has proven to be valuable in the detection of spectral patterns specific to bacterial abscesses with the occurrence of acetate, succinate, and different amino acids, such as valine, alanine, and leucine, and in spectra representing the cystic area of lesions.[49,50,51] A change of spectral patterns under antibiotic treatment of abscesses resulting in uncharacteristic spectra revealing lipids or lactate needs to be considered when one is interpreting spectra of treated abscesses[50,51] (▶ Fig. 11.12). Evaluation of the cystic part of the lesion might be compromised by hemorrhage (▶ Fig. 11.13) or the occurrence of abnormal resonances, such as sialic acids (2 ppm) in some adenocarcinoma metastases.[17] Differential diagnostics do not usually benefit from spectra representing the contrast-enhancing ring of the lesions because partial volume effects from the cystic compartment and especially surrounding

tissue increase the spectral overlap with other ring-enhancing lesions. In tissue outside the contrast enhancement neither metastases nor abscesses should show an increase of the Cho: NAA ratio above levels expected for tissue edema.

11.6 Conclusions

This has chapter focused on the use of MRS as a complement to conventional MRI in daily clinical practice and demonstrated the possible clinical use of MRS despite limitations related to technical challenges such as spatial resolution and data post-processing and often nonspecific spectral patterns. In the hands of skilled MR spectroscopists and neuroradiologists, and if performed and interpreted in conjunction with other functional or MRI techniques, MRS may provide additional biochemical information and thus support a suspected diagnosis of brain tumor, help to differentiate between brain lesions, depict therapy-related changes, and help to direct stereotactic biopsy. However, the well-known spectral pattern of tumors with mainly variable levels of decreased NAA and increased Cho, lactate, or lipids leaves a wide range of spectral overlaps between a variety of different diagnoses within tumor biology.

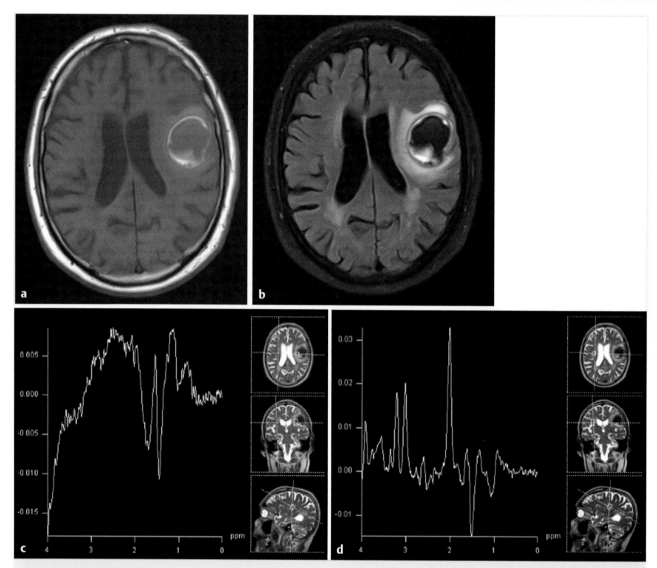

Fig. 11.13 (a,b) Hemorrhagic components in a cystic malignant melanoma metastasis cause local inhomogeneities in the magnetic field leading to artefacts in the chemical shift imaging (CSI) spectrum (echo time [TE] 30 ms) of the lesion (c) compared to the spectrum from the normal contralateral side (d).

References

[1] Govindaraju V, Young K, Maudsley AA. Proton NMR chemical shifts and coupling constants for brain metabolites. NMR Biomed 2000; 13: 129–153

[2] Barker PB, Bizzi A, De Stefano N, et al. Clinical MR Spectroscopy: Techniques and Applications. Cambridge: Cambridge University Press; 2009

[3] Provencher SW. Estimation of metabolite concentrations from localized in vivo proton NMR spectra. Magn Reson Med 1993; 30: 672–679

[4] Kreis R. Issues of spectral quality in clinical 1H-magnetic resonance spectroscopy and a gallery of artifacts. NMR Biomed 2004; 17: 361–381

[5] Louis DN, Ohgaki H, Wiestler OD, Cavenee WK, eds. WHO classification of tumours of the central nervous system. Lyon, France: IARC; 2007

[6] Nelson SJ. Multivoxel magnetic resonance spectroscopy of brain tumors. Mol Cancer Ther 2003; 2: 497–507

[7] McKnight TR, von dem Bussche MH, Vigneron DB et al. Histopathological validation of a three-dimensional magnetic resonance spectroscopy index as a predictor of tumor presence. J Neurosurg 2002; 97: 794–802

[8] Croteau D, Scarpace L, Hearshen D et al. Correlation between magnetic resonance spectroscopy imaging and image-guided biopsies: semiquantitative and qualitative histopathological analyses of patients with untreated glioma. Neurosurgery 2001; 49: 823–829

[9] Li X, Lu Y, Pirzkall A, McKnight T, Nelson SJ. Analysis of the spatial characteristics of metabolic abnormalities in newly diagnosed glioma patients. J Magn Reson Imaging 2002; 16: 229–237

[10] Vigneron D, Bollen A, McDermott M et al. Three-dimensional magnetic resonance spectroscopic imaging of histologically confirmed brain tumors. Magn Reson Imaging 2001; 19: 89–101

[11] Pirzkall A, Li X, Oh J et al. 3D MRSI for resected high-grade gliomas before RT: tumor extent according to metabolic activity in relation to MRI. Int J Radiat Oncol Biol Phys 2004; 59: 126–137

[12] Bulik M, Jancalek R, Vanicek J, Skoch A, Mechl M. Potential of MR spectroscopy for assessment of glioma grading. Clin Neurol Neurosurg 2013; 115: 146–153

[13] Zeng Q, Liu H, Zhang K, Li C, Zhou G. Noninvasive evaluation of cerebral glioma grade by using multivoxel 3D proton MR spectroscopy. Magn Reson Imaging 2011; 29: 25–31

[14] Zou QG, Xu HB, Liu F, Guo W, Kong XC, Wu Y. In the assessment of supratentorial glioma grade: the combined role of multivoxel proton MR spectroscopy and diffusion tensor imaging. Clin Radiol 2011; 66: 953–960

[15] Hwang JH, Egnaczyk GF, Ballard E, Dunn RS, Holland SK, Ball WS, Jr. Proton MR spectroscopic characteristics of pediatric pilocytic astrocytomas. AJNR Am J Neuroradiol 1998; 19: 535–540

[16] Righi V, Andronesi OC, Mintzopoulos D, Black PM, Tzika AA. High-resolution magic angle spinning magnetic resonance spectroscopy detects glycine as a biomarker in brain tumors. Int J Oncol 2010; 36: 301–306

[17] Burtscher IM, Skagerberg G, Geijer B, Englund E, Ståhlberg F, Holtås S. Proton MR spectroscopy and preoperative diagnostic accuracy: an evaluation of intracranial mass lesions characterized by stereotactic biopsy findings. AJNR Am J Neuroradiol 2000; 21: 84–93

[18] Bonavita S, Di Salle F, Tedeschi G. Proton MRS in neurological disorders. Eur J Radiol 1999; 30: 125–131

[19] Rock JP, Scarpace L, Hearshen D et al. Associations among magnetic resonance spectroscopy, apparent diffusion coefficients, and image-guided histo-pathology with special attention to radiation necrosis. Neurosurgery 2004; 54: 1111–1117, discussion 1117–1119

[20] Sundgren PC. MR spectroscopy in radiation injury. AJNR Am J Neuroradiol 2009; 30: 1469–1476

[21] Weybright P, Sundgren PC, Maly P et al. Differentiation between brain tumor recurrence and radiation injury using MR spectroscopy. AJR Am J Roentgenol 2005; 185: 1471–1476

[22] Rock JP, Hearshen D, Scarpace L et al. Correlations between magnetic resonance spectroscopy and image-guided histopathology, with special attention to radiation necrosis. Neurosurgery 2002; 51: 912–919, discussion 919–920

[23] Zeng QS, Li CF, Zhang K, Liu H, Kang XS, Zhen JH. Multivoxel 3D proton MR spectroscopy in the distinction of recurrent glioma from radiation injury. J Neurooncol 2007; 84: 63–69

[24] Prat R, Galeano I, Lucas A et al. Relative value of magnetic resonance spectros-copy, magnetic resonance perfusion, and 2-(18F) fluoro-2-deoxy-D-glucose positron emission tomography for detection of recurrence or grade increase in gliomas. J Clin Neurosci 2010; 17: 50–53

[25] Nakajima T, Kumabe T, Kanamori M et al. Differential diagnosis between radiation necrosis and glioma progression using sequential proton magnetic resonance spectroscopy and methionine positron emission tomography. Neurol Med Chir (Tokyo) 2009; 49: 394–401

[26] Amin A, Moustafa H, Ahmed E, El-Toukhy M. Glioma residual or recurrence ver-sus radiation necrosis: accuracy of pentavalent technetium-99m-dimercaptosuc-cinic acid [Tc-99 m (V) DMSA] brain SPECT compared to proton magnetic reso-nance spectroscopy (1H-MRS): initial results. J Neurooncol 2012; 106: 579–587

[27] Schlemmer HP, Bachert P, Henze M et al. Differentiation of radiation necrosis from tumor progression using proton magnetic resonance spectroscopy. Neuroradiology 2002; 44: 216–222

[28] Chong VF, Rumpel H, Fan YF, Mukherji SK. Temporal lobe changes following radiation therapy: imaging and proton MR spectroscopic findings. Eur Radiol 2001; 11: 317–324

[29] Schlemmer HP, Bachert P, Herfarth KK, Zuna I, Debus J, van Kaick G. Proton MR spectroscopic evaluation of suspicious brain lesions after stereotactic radiotherapy. AJNR Am J Neuroradiol 2001; 22: 1316–1324

[30] Chan YL, Roebuck DJ, Yuen MP et al. Long-term cerebral metabolite changes on proton magnetic resonance spectroscopy in patients cured of acute lym-phoblastic leukemia with previous intrathecal methotrexate and cranial irradiation prophylaxis. Int J Radiat Oncol Biol Phys 2001; 50: 759–763

[31] Rutkowski T, Tarnawski R, Sokol M, Maciejewski B. 1H-MR spectroscopy of normal brain tissue before and after postoperative radiotherapy because of primary brain tumors. Int J Radiat Oncol Biol Phys 2003; 56: 1381–1389

[32] Sundgren PC, Nagesh V, Elias A et al. Metabolic alterations: a biomarker for radiation-induced normal brain injury-an MR spectroscopy study. J Magn Reson Imaging 2009; 29: 291–297

[33] Sundgren PC, Cao Y. Brain irradiation: effects on normal brain parenchyma and radiation injury. Neuroimaging Clin N Am 2009; 19: 657–668

[34] Kimura T, Sako K, Gotoh T, Tanaka K, Tanaka T. In vivo single-voxel proton MR spectroscopy in brain lesions with ring-like enhancement. NMR Biomed 2001; 14: 339–349

[35] Cho YD, Choi GH, Lee SP, Kim JK. (1)H-MRS metabolic patterns for distinguishing between meningiomas and other brain tumors. Magn Reson Imaging 2003; 21: 663–672

[36] Chernov MF, Kasuya H, Nakaya K et al. 1H-MRS of intracranial meningiomas: what it can add to known clinical and MRI predictors of the histopathological and biological characteristics of the tumor? Clin Neurol Neurosurg 2011; 113: 202–212

[37] Yue Q, Isobe T, Shibata Y, Kawamura H, Anno I, Matsumura A. Usefulness of quantitative proton MR spectroscopy in the differentiation of benign and malignant meningioma. Sheng Wu Yi Xue Gong Cheng Xue Za Zhi 2011; 28: 1103–1109

[38] Chernov MF, Nakaya K, Kasuya H et al. Metabolic alterations in the peritu-moral brain in cases of meningiomas: 1H-MRS study. J Neurol Sci 2009; 284: 168–174

[39] Righi V, Tugnoli V, Mucci A, Bacci A, Bonora S, Schenetti L. MRS study of meningeal hemangiopericytoma and edema: a comparison with meningo-thelial meningioma. Oncol Rep 2012; 28: 1461–1467

[40] Barba I, Moreno A, Martinez-Pérez I et al. Magnetic resonance spectroscopy of brain hemangiopericytomas: high myoinositol concentrations and discrimination from meningiomas. J Neurosurg 2001; 94: 55–60

[41] Schneider JF, Confort-Gouny S, Viola A et al. Multiparametric differentiation of posterior fossa tumors in children using diffusion-weighted imaging and short echo-time 1H-MR spectroscopy. J Magn Reson Imaging 2007; 26: 1390–1398

[42] Davies NP, Wilson M, Harris LM et al. Identification and characterisation of childhood cerebellar tumours by in vivo proton MRS. NMR Biomed 2008; 21: 908–918

[43] Porto L, Kieslich M, Franz K et al. MR spectroscopy differentiation between high and low grade astrocytomas: a comparison between paediatric and adult tumours. Eur J Paediatr Neurol 2011; 15: 214–221

[44] Porto L, Kieslich M, Franz K, Lehrbecher T, Pilatus U, Hattingen E. Proton magnetic resonance spectroscopic imaging in pediatric low-grade gliomas. Brain Tumor Pathol 2010; 27: 65–70

[45] Tang YZ, Booth TC, Bhogal P, Malhotra A, Wilhelm T. Imaging of primary central nervous system lymphoma. Clin Radiol 2011; 66: 768–777

[46] Bendini M, Marton E, Feletti A et al. Primary and metastatic intraaxial brain tumors: prospective comparison of multivoxel 2D chemical-shift imaging (CSI) proton MR spectroscopy, perfusion MRI, and histopatholog-ical findings in a group of 159 patients. Acta Neurochir (Wien) 2011; 153: 403–412

[47] Sijens PE, Levendag PC, Vecht CJ, van Dijk P, Oudkerk M. 1 H MR spectroscopy detection of lipids and lactate in metastatic brain tumors. NMR Biomed 1996; 9: 65–71

[48] Server A, Josefsen R, Kulle B et al. Proton magnetic resonance spectroscopy in the distinction of high-grade cerebral gliomas from single metastatic brain tumors. Acta Radiol 2010; 51: 316–325

[49] Foerster BR, Thurnher MM, Malani PN, Petrou M, Carets-Zumelzu F, Sundgren PC. Intracranial infections: clinical and imaging characteristics. Acta Radiol 2007; 48: 875–893

[50] Lai PH, Ho JT, Chen WL et al. Brain abscess and necrotic brain tumor: discrim-ination with proton MR spectroscopy and diffusion-weighted imaging. AJNR Am J Neuroradiol 2002; 23: 1369–1377

[51] Burtscher IM, Holtås S. In vivo proton MR spectroscopy of untreated and treated brain abscesses. AJNR Am J Neuroradiol 1999; 20: 1049–1053

12 Molecular Imaging: PET and SPECT

Asim K. Bag and Samuel Almodóvar

12.1 Introduction

In the last decade there has been great interest in the clinical application of molecular imaging of tumors following the success of positron-emission tomography (PET) using ^{18}F-fluorodeoxyglucose (FDG) in clinical oncology. Although FDG is extensively and successfully used in different cancers, its sensitivity and specificity are not optimal for all cancer types. FDG evaluates only glucose metabolism of tissue. Numberous PET tracers have been developed to investigate other aspects of tumor physiology in addition to glucose metabolism and are very helpful in detecting tumors, identifying tumor grades and prognosis, guiding and monitoring treatment, and differentiating tumor recurrence from treatment related changes. Many of these radiotracers are at various stages of translation to clinical practice in the United States and have already been in clinical practice in other countries.

In addition to development of newer radiotracers, there has also been tremendous improvement of the molecular (single photon emission computed tomography [SPECT] and PET) imaging instrumentation and reconstruction algorithms allowing imaging with spatial resolution of as little as 3 mm in clinical PET systems.[1] There has been remarkable improvement in temporal resolution as well, allowing dynamic PET acquisition. A PET magnetic resonance imaging (MRI) system has been introduced for clinical use and has tremendous potential in oncological imaging.[2]

12.2 Molecular Imaging: Concepts

Molecular imaging has been defined as "visualization, characterization, and measurement of biological processes at the molecular and cellular levels in human and other living systems."[3] Imaging techniques available for this purpose include nuclear medicine techniques, advanced functional MRI techniques, optical imaging, ultrasonography, and other nanoimaging technologies. The goals of molecular imaging include improved understanding of tumor biology (cancer development, progression, angiogenesis, metastasis, etc.), visualization and noninvasive quantification of different cellular receptors that are typically activated/suppressed in the process of tumorigenesis, studying pharmacokinetics and pharmacodynamics of novel anticancer drugs, and noninvasive quantification of response to predict outcomes in response to such novel therapies.[4] Molecular imaging thus differs greatly from the conventional anatomical imaging that is still predominantly used to characterize structural abnormalities, which often correspond to the end result of molecular processes at the cellular and subcellular levels.

12.3 Molecular Imaging: Need in Brain Tumors

MRI is the workhorse in neuro-oncology. In the last 2 decades, there has been significant improvement of MRI instrumentation and development and validation of several MRI-based estimations of tumor physiology, such as diffusion imaging, perfusion imaging, and MR spectroscopy. Even with the availability of these advanced MRI techniques, there are several unmet clinical needs, particularly in detection of actual tumor margin and treatment monitoring. The limitations of MRI become prominent following the clinical availability of increasingly popular antiangiogenic drugs for brain tumor therapy. Antitumor drugs are being developed that target different molecular/genetic events of gliomas, which necessitates accurate and precise molecular imaging technology.

12.4 Molecular Imaging: Instrumentation

12.4.1 SPECT

Brain SPECT has been pursued since the early 1960s. Brain SPECT allows three-dimensional (3D) acquisition of functional information with high sensitivity and specificity. When compared with PET, SPECT provides lower sensitivity, poorer resolution, and lower potential for quantification, and it is uncommonly used in the practice of neuro-oncology. SPECT, however, remains more widely available and is less expensive than PET.

Unlike computed tomography (CT), the source of radioactivity is the patient. The patient is injected with radioactive material that selectively binds to the area of interest and acts as a source of radiation, which is captured using detectors. SPECT systems use collimators to allow only photons approaching at certain angles to reach the detectors from the body part being imaged. To maximize resolution, collimators must be kept as close as possible to the patient. In brain imaging, this means that the collimator must clear the bed and the shoulders of the patient. Head holders are used for brain SPECT and provide comfort while limiting patient motion.

Information from the captured photons is used to reconstruct images using different computational algorithms. Filtered back projection (FBP) with various filters or iterative reconstruction is routinely used to reconstruct images in SPECT. Iterative reconstruction has advantages over FBP in that it allows better control of noise, scatter, attenuation, and other factors affecting image quality. SPECT images can be fused to a separately acquired CT scan or can be obtained in dedicated SPECT/CT scanners.[5]

12.4.2 PET CT

PET imaging relies on the nature of the positron and positron decay. The positron is the antimatter counterpart to the electron and therefore has the same mass as the electron but the opposite charge.[6] Positron decay can be explained with the equation:

$$(P+) \rightarrow N + (\beta+) + \nu + E$$

where, (P+) is a proton, N is a neutron, (β+) is a positron, ν is a neutrino, and E is excess energy released. Positrons are emitted from the atomic nucleus, and as they pass through matter they travel a short distance and interact with an electron via annihilation. From this interaction, two photons are emitted, each with an energy of 511 keV, in opposite directions of each other. Simultaneous emission of annihilation photons traveling 180 degrees from each other forms the basis of PET imaging, through coincidence detection and coincidence imaging.[6] The detector in a conventional PET scanners consists of a ring of scintillation crystals in a 360 degree array. The basic principle of coincidence imaging is that two photons detected in close temporal proximity by two opposed detectors in the ring are likely to be from a single annihilation event. When simultaneous detection of two photons is registered at opposite directions of each other within the ring, it can be assumed that the annihilation event took place somewhere on a line (line of response [LOR]) between the two detectors.[6] When LORs are combined, they represent all of the coincidence events for a given acquisition, which can be depicted as a sinogram. An extremely fast and accurate electronic circuit is required to identify whether two detected photons are the result of a single coincidence event and to analyze the sonogram for quick image reconstruction.

Events detected by PET scanners can be true, scattered, or random events, all of which may be recorded as coincidence events, provided that both annihilation photons are actually detected by opposite detectors within the coincidence window. However, only true coincidence events provide the desired information needed for accurate images of the distribution of the positron emitting radiopharmaceutical for clinical imaging. Because coincidence imaging requires registration of two photons produced during a single annihilation reaction, attenuation of photons at the time of traveling toward detectors markedly impact the final raw data set. Attenuation correction is, therefore, an extremely important step in PET imaging.[6,7]

Attenuation correction can be performed by either calculated or measured methods. The calculated method is no longer used in current systems. On current hybrid PET/CT scanners, a low-dose CT scan is obtained prior to positron-emission imaging, which yields information used to create an attenuation map for attenuation correction of the PET raw data set. Positioning for the low-dose CT scan needs to be the same as for the positron-emission imaging. It is important to account for factors that may alter the attenuation map because these can introduce alterations in the data that can translate into artifacts in the final corrected images. In addition to attenuation correction, CT is also used for accurate anatomical localization of increased tracer accumulation in tissues.[7]

Images on a PET scanner can be acquired by using either two-dimensional (2D) or 3D techniques. Two-dimensional imaging uses an axial collimator made of thin septa of lead or tungsten placed between detectors, such that coincidence events are accepted by only adjacent detectors in a ring. This allows for a defined plane or slice and eliminates out-of-plane scatter. Two-dimensional imaging is usually performed when imaging small structures or limited fields of view, such as in brain imaging. Two-dimensional acquisitions provide better image quality, although sensitivity is reduced secondary to collimation.[7]

Three-dimensional acquisition is volume based and allows for imaging of larger structures or fields of view. When compared with 2D techniques, 3D has higher sensitivity because it allows registration of more coincidence photons, but image quality is reduced as a result of a larger amount of scatter. Three-dimensional imaging is commonly used when imaging small fields of view and areas of low scatter, such as imaging of the brain. Final image processing will require converting the emission data into an image format, either by FBP or using iterative reconstruction.[7]

PET allows semiquantification of the activity accumulated in tissue at a particular location. This measure is called standardized uptake value (SUV), and it is defined as the image-based concentration of the positron emitter in tissue, divided by the injected dose and multiplied by a calibration factor. Usually the maximal activity is determined from the pixel with highest concentration of the radiopharmaceutical. Semiquantitative determination of tracer accumulation in lesions allows a more objective tool to assess tumor physiology as well as a tool to follow lesions over time and to monitor therapy effects.

12.4.3 PET-MRI

A PET-MRI system has been introduced for clinical use. There are two main imaging approaches in PET-MRI, based on either sequential or simultaneous acquisition of the PET and the MRI data. A sequential system is simple sequential acquisition of PET and MRI data that are later fused through coregistration. Performing simultaneous PET and MRI acquisition poses multiple technical challenges but provides advantages over the sequentially acquired studies, including optimal image registration, correction of the PET data for motion during the scan, and MR-guided PET image reconstruction. Simultaneously acquired studies have markedly improved spatial resolution and allow a unique opportunity for studying transient phenomena with both modalities, a unique advantage of this approach.[8]

12.5 Molecular Imaging: Glioma

12.5.1 Imaging of Tumor Physiology

Evaluation of Tumor Proliferation

Uncontrolled cellular proliferation is the key pathophysiologic abnormality of cancer. The rate of cell division is an important characteristic of malignancies, particularly in glioblastoma multiforme (GBM). Even though the percentage of cellular proliferation has not been included in the diagnostic criteria of higher grade gliomas in the most recent World Health Organization (WHO) definition, the percentage of tumor cells in the active cell cycle (as identified by the MIB-1 score) is an important biomarker of tumor physiology for high-grade gliomas and correlates well with tumor cell density, histopathological grade of the tumor, and, most importantly, survival time.[9] The ability to assess the cell proliferation rate of tumors by noninvasive imaging markers can improve diagnosis, grading, and staging of cancers as well as being useful for longitudinal follow-up and prediction of tumor response to anticancer drugs.[10] The most commonly used PET tracer for evaluation of tumor proliferation is: (3'-[18]fluoro-3'-deoxy-L-thymidine [FLT]).

DNA replication is the key prerequisite for cell division. Thymidine is one of the four nucleosides required for DNA synthesis, which can be synthesized de novo within the cell by thymidylate synthase or can be obtained through phosphorylation of thymine deoxyriboside (TdR) by thymidine kinase (TK) through the so-called salvage pathway. Expression of DNA synthesis enzymes is a highly regulated process and depends on the cellular cycle. The expression of TK1 increases as much as 10 to 20 times the baseline in G1/S phase transition, remains high in S, G2, and M phases, and then rapidly declines as the cell approaches the G0 to G1 phase.[10] TK2, another isoform of TK, is constitutively expressed, and expression of TK2 is not dependent on cell cycle phase.[10]

FLT is a thymidine nucleoside analogue that was originally developed as an anticancer and antiretroviral agent. Due to the high incidence of side effects, it has never been approved for clinical use. However, experience from clinical trials forms the background of using the compound as a PET tracer. The principle mechanism of FLT PET is uptake of FLT by proliferating tumor cells, mostly in the S phase.[11] Inside the cell, FLT is phosphorylated by TK1 to an intermediary metabolite that is resistant to degradation and phosphorylated, as a result of which FLT is trapped inside proliferating cells.[10] The rate-limiting step in FLT accumulation is phosphorylation by TK1; therefore, the intracellular level of phosphorylated FLT indirectly reflects TK1 activity that has also been shown to strongly correlate with thymidine incorporation into DNA.[12,13] Over time, there is a very slow efflux of FLT due to dephosphorylation, allowing a significant period of relatively stable tracer retention inside cells for imaging.

The injected does of FLT is based on body weight, and the usual dose is 2.7 MBq/kg with a maximum dose of 185 MBq. There are two different approaches to analyze FLT PET imaging. The first is the standard SUV-based method as used in FDG PET. The other method uses dynamic imaging sequence and kinetic modeling of tracer uptake. This approach is unique in the sense that it can quantify FLT uptake and retention over time and estimate the rates of underlying biological processes.

Evaluation of Tumor Metabolism

Living cells require a relentless supply of essential nutrients. Transmembrane transport and biosynthesis generate and maintain an internal pool of these essential molecules for internal metabolism. Transports of nutrient molecules are tightly regulated and largely depend on the demand of the cell at a given time. Therefore, imaging strategies that can noninvasively image the nutrient uptake can provide insight about the real-time metabolism of the cell.

Glucose Metabolism

Malignant tumors have higher rates of glucose usage and glycolysis. Based on this knowledge, FDG has been developed and is being successfully used to evaluate numerous cancer types. FDG differs from glucose only for the replacement of a hydroxyl group with radioactive fluorine. FDG actively enters cells via the same group of carrier-mediated active transport molecules (glucose transporter 1 [GLUT1]) as for glucose. Similar to glucose ^{18}FDG undergoes phosphorylation within the cell by hexokinase to FDG-6-phosphate, which cannot be metabolized rapidly. Essentially FDG-6-phosphate is trapped inside cells. Therefore imaging with FDG allows noninvasive assessment of the rate of glucose uptake/ requirement of a cell.

There is upregulation of expression of GLUT1 as well as hexokinase in tumor cells because tumor cells use a large amount of glucose as the only energy source. As a result, uptake of FDG is increased in tumor cells. Normal neurons in brain also depend heavily on glucose as a source of energy to maintain high energy-consuming synaptic activity. Expectedly there is also high FDG uptake in normal brain, particularly in the neuron-rich gray matter. This explains significantly lower tumor-to-background contrast, even in high grade central nervous system (CNS) tumors and limits the use of FDG in evaluation of brain tumors.

Several processes determine FDG uptake in tumor cells. The most important factor is the intact blood supply for delivery of the tracer into tumor cells. The number of tumor cells and degree of cellular proliferation also increase uptake of FDG. Uptake of FDG in the hypoxic area of a tumor depends on a complex interaction between the tumor microenvironment and the blood supply. In hypoxic areas there is less delivery of FDG; however, uptake of FDG in tumor cell is very high due to hypoxia-inducible factor 1-alpha (HIP1-α) further upregulation of GLUT1 and hexokinase.[14] A necrotic area of a tumor does not uptake FDG for obvious reasons. Steroid use may also interfere with FDG uptake in tumor cells.[15]

There are several limitations of FDG in evaluation of brain tumors. First, the sensitivity of detection of low-grade gliomas using FDG PET is low due to the relatively small differences in the rates of glucose usage in tumor cells and normal brain cells.[16] Increased FDG uptake is not specific for tumor cells. Inflammatory cells, particularly macrophages, also intensely uptake FDG, even inside a tumor.[17] As a result, high FDG uptake by a lesion is not tumor specific, and FDG PET has demonstrated low sensitivity in differentiation treatment effects from recurrent glioblastoma.[18,19] Finally, it is difficult to precisely delineate the tumor margin if the tumor is located close to the basal ganglia or close to the cortex because of high FDG uptake in normal gray matter.[20]

Amino Acid Metabolism

Due to the inherent limitations of FDG PET, the use of alternative tracers has been proposed for evaluation of metabolism of brain tumors. In this regard, imaging with radiolabeled amino acid is a brilliant concept. Amino acid imaging allows excellent contrast between tumor and background normal brain because there is very limited uptake of amino acids by normal brain tissue. This allows easy tumor detection and better delineation of tumor margin in comparison to FDG. Amino acids are transported inside the cell by specific transporter systems and are essential cellular nutrients, particularly in rapidly dividing cells.[21] Amino acid uptake depends on the flux of amino acids to the tissue, expression of amino acid transporters, and rate of amino acid metabolism. In animal models increased amino acid uptake has been linked to upregulation of amino acid transport in the supporting vasculature of the tumor regardless of the phase of the cell cycle and even in the absence of increased vascular permeability.[22,23] These results indicate that tumor uptake of amino acids does not depend on breakdown of the blood–brain barrier.[24]

L-(methyl-^{11}c) Methionine (Met)

Met has been most extensively studied in evaluation of brain tumors, and in many European countries this is the most popular amino acid PET tracer routinely used for brain tumor evaluation. High uptake of Met is related to increased amino acid transport mediated by L-type amino acid transporter and has been shown to correlate with in vitro cell proliferation, Ki 67 nuclear antigen expression, and microvessel density in primary brain tumors, suggesting that this could be a biomarker for tumor proliferation as well as angiogenesis.[20] Unlike FDG, Met is accumulated mostly in viable cancer cells with minimum uptake in macrophages and other nonspecific cellular components of the tumor.[17] Significant uptake is seen in low-grade tumor as well, although the uptake in low-grade tumors is lower in comparison to high-grade tumors. The major limitation of this tracer is very short half-life (only 20 minutes).

2-[18F]-fluoroethyl)-L-Tyrosine (FET)

FLT is a fluoro-alkylated analogue of another essential amino acid, L-tyrosine. During the last 2 decades more and more studies have been performed with FET PET, mainly because of the longer half-life of ^{18}F (t1/2 = 110 min) in comparison to the shorter half-life (t1/2 = 20 min) of ^{11}C, allowing imaging even without an on-site cyclotron. It does not accumulate in normal brain tissue, but uptake is higher in tumor tissue. Multiple studies[28,29,30] have demonstrated that FET PET is better than FDG PET in showing markedly elevated uptake in both high- and low-grade gliomas. It has been shown that diagnostic performance of FET PET as a tumor marker in gliomas and metastatic brain tumors is similar to that of Met PET, with a sensitivity of 91% and s specificity of 100%.[28]

3,4-dihydroxy-6-[[18F]-fluoro-L-phenylalanine (FDOPA)

Although the mother compound of FDOPA is not an amino acid, it is a product of an essential amino acid, L-tyrosine, and is considered as amino acid analogue. Tumor-to-background contrast is very good because of elevated amino acid transport in malignant brain tumors.

Oxidative Metabolism

Acetate is one of the most common building blocks for biosynthesis in the living organisms. In tumor cells, most of the acetate is converted into fatty acid synthetase and is predominantly incorporated into intracellular phosphatidylcholine membranes. Due to this feature, ^{11}C acetate (ACE) can serve as a PET tracer.

Evaluation of Angiogenesis and Invasion

Tumor neovascularization, the formation of new blood vessels from preexisting vasculature, plays a vital role in tumor growth and is recognized as a key event in the natural progression of gliomas.[29] Tumor neovascularization is an extremely complex tumor physiology and is the end result of the interaction of hundreds of pro- and antiangiogenic molecules. At least five different mechanisms have been described in GBM, of which angiogenesis is the predominant mechanism.[30]

Activated endothelial cells expresses $\alpha_v\beta_3$, a dimeric transmembrane integrin that interacts with extracellular matrix protein and regulates migration of endothelial cells through the extracellular matrix during neoangiogenesis.[31] Additionally, $\alpha_v\beta_3$ and different other integrins are also expressed by glioma cells that function at almost every step of tumorigenesis, including development and progression of gliomas,[32] tumor cell

migration, and invasion.[33,34,35] $\alpha_v\beta_3$ binds to arginine-glycine-aspartic acid (RGD) containing motif of the interstitial matrix proteins such as vitronectin, fibronectin, and thrombospondin.[36,37] Based on this observation, both linear and cyclic RGD compounds have been introduced for imaging and have been shown to have high binding affinity and selectivity to the $\alpha_{v\beta3}$ integrin. Numerous chemical modifications have been suggested for better pharmacokinetic profiles of the RGD-containing molecules. Similarly, several different radionuclides have been also been used to tag these molecules in order to optimize imaging properties. The most commonly used radionuclide is 18-Fluoride. It is not known yet proved whether RGD imaging actually images $\alpha_v\beta_3$ expression by the endothelial cells or by the glioma cells. Using a human glioma cell line in mouse models Battle et al have demonstrated that $^{18}Fluciclatide$ (a PET imaging agent with an RGD sequence) can detect changes in tumor uptake of this PET tracer after acute antiangiogenic therapy.[38]

Vascular Endothelial Growth Factor

Vascular endothelial growth factor (VEGF) is one of the key regulators in glioma angiogenesis. Among the *VEGF* gene family, VEGF-A is a homodimeric glycoprotein that has seven different isoforms with varying numbers of amino acid length.[39] All isoforms of VEGF-A bind to both the VEGF receptors family: VEGFR1 and VEGFR2. Binding to VEGFR2 plays an orchestrating role in angiogenesis.[39] PET imaging probes that specifically bind to the VEGF or VEGFR2 can provide a tumorwide angiogenesis profile that can serve as a more precise assessment of tumor angiogenesis and can be used to assess the effects of antiangiogenic therapy. It has been shown that there is rapid, prominent, and specific uptake of a new ^{64}Cu labeled DOTA-VEGF121 (VEGF-A isoform with 121 amino acids) PET probe in the U87MG cell line with high expression of VEGFR2 in comparison to the same U87MG cell line with low VEGFR2 expression.[40,41] It has also been shown that this particular PET tracer is able to demonstrate the dynamic expression profile of VEGFR2 expression at different stages of tumor.[40]

Evaluation of Hypoxia

FMISO

In GBM, tumor cell growth outstrips the vascular development. As a result, oxygen delivery is decreased beyond its diffusion distance, and there is hypoxia in the tumor microenvironment.[42] Hypoxia is a predominant feature of the microenvironment of higher-grade gliomas, particularly in GBM. It has been well established that hypoxia is associated with tumor growth, progression, angiogenesis, invasion, increased cancer stem cell population, genomic instability, resistance of conventional therapies, recurrence, and decreased patient survival.[43,44] Hypoxia-inducible factors (HIFs) is the master regulator of the aforementioned tumor biology acting as a transcription factor and activating hundreds of downstream genes.[45] Active research has been ongoing for accurate imaging of hypoxia using immunohistochemistry, MRI, PET, and SPECT. Several PET and SPECT tracers have been investigated to quantify tumor hypoxia.

Nitroimidazole Agents

3-[18]Fluoro-1-(20-nitro-10-imidazolyl)-2-propanol (FMISO)

FMISO is the most extensively investigated and validated PET radiotracer for hypoxia imaging to date.[46] FMISO is a nitroimidazole compound that undergoes reduction into a reactive intermediary metabolite within a living cell. Uptake of [18]FMISO is inversely proportional to O_2 level, its delivery to the tumor core is not dependent on tumor perfusion, and the molecule diffuses freely into all cells. In normoxic cells (where electron transport is occurring), the NO_2 subunit of FMISO takes an electron to form a radical anion reduction product, then rapidly transfers the electron to O_2 and returns to its original structure. However, in hypoxic cells the molecule undergoes further reduction, forms covalent bonds to intracellular macromolecules, and is thereby trapped inside the cell.[42,47] It is not retained in necrotic tissue because there is no electron transport.[47] Several studies have proved that uptake of FMISO directly correlates with tissue oxygenation level.[48,49,50] Binding of FMISO to tissue is dependent on the level of hypoxia, and oxygen levels of 3 to 10 mm Hg lead to FMSIO binding.[51,52] More hypoxic tissue binds FMISO more avidly. Because there is no uptake of FMISO in normoxic brain cells, FMISO PET allows excellent contrast between the tumor and normal brain.[42]

There is a longer waiting period (90–140 min) between injection and the start of the scan for FMISO in comparison to FDG because of slower clearance kinetics, low uptake in hypoxic cells, and the absence of any active transport system for FMISO.[53] The usual injection dose is 3.7 MBq/kg with a maximum dose of 260 MBq.[42] Typically, image analysis is performed after coregistration of the PET data with contrast-enhanced 3D MRI to delineate tumor margins and to identify the regions of interest. Typically, the degree of radiotracer uptake of tumor is compared with the venous blood sample after decay time correction. FMISO image data are divided with the blood radiotracer level to generate the pixel-by-pixel tissue/blood (T/B) level map.[54] T/B > 1.2 is considered significant hypoxia and is usually used to generate a hypoxic volume map.

Imaging in very early stage, FMISO distribution reflects tumor blood flow, whereas later on this mostly accumulates in hypoxic cells with a very high tumor-to-background ratio. The metabolites of FMISO rapidly clear from plasma, allowing no need of normalization for delivery. FMISO has no protein binding, and relatively early imaging is possible. Additionally FMISO has been validated in numerous animal models and human disease conditions, and its signal is independent of other tumor-related factors, such as regional glucose consumption, glutathione level, and local pH.

Other Nitroimidazole Agents

Several other nitroimidazole compounds have been developed for hypoxia imaging, including 18F-labeled fluoroerythronitroimidazole ([18]FETNIM),[44,52,53] 1-α-D-(5-Deoxy-5-[18F]fluoroarabinofuranosyl)-2-nitroimidazole (^{18}F-FAZA),[44,54] 18F-2-(2-Nitroimidazol-1H-yl)-(3,3,3-trifluoropropyl) acetamide (^{18}F-EF3), and 18F-labeled 2-(2-nitro-(1)H-imidazol-1-yl)-N-(2,2,3,3,3-pentafluoropropyl)-acetamide (EF5) ^{18}F-EF5[55,56,57,58] compounds, with variable potential.

Non-Nitroimidazole Agent

CU ATSM

[60,62,64]Cu-diacetyl-bis(N4-methylthiosemicarbazone)

Cu-ATSM has a low molecular weight and a high cell membrane permeability (because this is a lipophilic compound), allowing rapid diffusion of this molecule to tissue from the bloodstream. The compound can be tagged to any of the radioactive copper isotopes, but the most suitable is [64]Cu. Cu-ATSM is a promising new hypoxia-imaging agent for delineating the extent of hypoxia within tumors. Cu-ATSM is retained within hypoxic cells at a higher level compared to FMISO. Cu-ATSM enters and exits normoxic cells metabolically unchanged. In hypoxic cells Cu-ATSM undergoes change of its three-dimensional structure secondary to a hypoxia-induced altered redox environment.[62] Unlike FMISO, Cu-ATSM is able to image acute as well as chronic tumoral hypoxia. Uptake of Cu-ATSM is relatively high in GBM, and there is correlation between T/B ratio and HIF-1α expression.[53]

Evaluation of Cell Membrane Proliferation

Choline is an essential phospholipid, an indispensable cell membrane constituent. Increased cellular proliferation entails high choline uptake. Choline is then phosphorylated by choline kinases and ultimately is incorporated in phospholipids. In tumor tissues, there is increased uptake of choline. This finding corresponds to the increased choline peak in magnetic resonance spectroscopy in brain tumors. Increased ^{18}F choline (Cho) has been seen in gliomas, including oligodendrogliomas.[63,64] Increased Cho uptake has been associated with tumor aggressiveness and resistance to chemotherapy. Cho PET has also been shown useful to monitor antiangiogenic therapy.[64]

Similar to amino acid PET, Cho PET cannot reliably differentiate between high- and low-grade tumors and also cannot differentiae from inflammatory conditions because inflammatory cells also take up Cho.[65,66] Additionally, uptake of Cho is highly affected by blood–brain barrier disruption in gliomas.

Evaluation of Epidermal Growth Factor Receptor Expression

Epidermal growth factor receptor (EGFR) has been associated with multiple solid tumors, including GBM. EGFR is a member of the structurally related ErbB family of receptor tyrosine kinase. Activation of EGFR contributes to several tumorigenic mechanisms. Overexpression of EGFR acts as a prognostic indicator in GBM, predicting poor survival and more advanced disease stage.[39] Currently, many molecular antibodies have been developed that block the binding of EGFR to the extracellular ligand-binding domain of the receptor and inhibit tyrosine kinase. This family of molecules has shown promise for the treatment of cancer, with expression of EGFR as a therapeutic option as well as for PET imaging.

Cetuximab is the first monoclonal antibody targeted against EGFR. A new molecular imaging probe, ^{64}Cu-DOTA-cetuximab, has been used as a PET probe to image EGFR expression in GBM xenografts[67] with good correlation with tumor EGR expression identified by western blot analysis.

Evaluation of Apoptosis

Apoptosis is the energy-dependent, organized self-disassembly of unneeded or senescent cells. When triggered by appropriate internal/external signals, these cells undergo programmed cytoplasmic shrinkage, membrane disruption, and budding off of intracellular contents packaged into small membrane-bound packets. The packets are taken up by phagocytes and surrounding cells without mounting any inflammatory response. Initiation of apoptotic cell death leads to activation of a family of cysteine proteases (caspases) that act as the central regulator of apoptosis processes. Antitumor therapy induces apoptosis. Estimation of rate and extent of apoptosis after treatment can provide a great insight about the efficacy of treatment.

Annexin V, a member of the calcium and phospholipid binding family of annexin proteins that has very high affinity toward phosphatidylserine residues, has been extensively studied as a PET imaging probe.[68,69,70] ML10, a member of the Aposense family of biomarkers for apoptosis, has been proposed as another PET tracer for apoptosis imaging, with ^{18}F being the radionuclide with selective binding to the apoptotic cells and favorable biodistribution.[71,72]

12.5.2 Clinical Utility of Molecular Imaging in Gliomas

Tumor Detection

FDG uptake within high-grade gliomas is less than or similar to that in normal gray matter, allowing very poor tumor-to-background ratio.[73] The sensitivity of detection is further compromised by variable FDG uptake within a single tumor that has both high and low areas of uptake very close to each other.[73] Imaging of newly diagnosed gliomas with FDG is, therefore, very problematic and "comment about tumor grade must be applied with caution."[73] Tumor-to-white matter ratio of > 1.5 and tumor-to-gray matter ratio of > 0.6 of FDG can distinguish between high- and low-grade tumors.[74] Delayed imaging can improve the tumor-to-background contrast because normal cells excrete FDG more rapidly than do tumor cells.

Because of higher contrast than FDG, Met PET can detect both low- and high-grade gliomas. The reported sensitivity of Met PET in detection of primary brain tumor ranges from 76 to 95%. This variability is largely because of different study designs and a different percentage of tumors evaluated in different studies. There has also been evidence of uptake of Met PET in nontumorous pathologies such as around abscess, hematoma, and acute infarcts.[20] Despite the possibilities of a false-positive test, the specificity of Met PET for detection of primary brain tumor is high at 87 to 100%. The accuracy of Met PET in detection of tumor can be improved with a tumor to background ratio calculation, with a ratio of > 1.5 generally being indicative of tumor.[20]

Tumor-to-background contrast is also much better with FLT imaging in comparison with FDG because there is no appreciable uptake of FLT by normal brain tissue.[75] Sensitivity of detection of tumor is lower with FLT, particularly of low-grade tumors, in comparison with Met.[76] FLT is also a poorer agent to identify low-grade gliomas in comparison with FDG and FDOPA.[77]

Prognosis and Grading

FDG uptake within gliomas has a positive correlation with histological grade, cell density, and poor survival.[74] Interval increased FDG uptake of a previously low-grade tumor with low-FDG uptake establishes diagnosis of transformation to a higher grade.[78] However, because of the high uptake of normal brain tissue, detection of tumor can be difficult. FDG uptake in low-grade gliomas is similar to the uptake in normal white matter, whereas uptake in high-grade gliomas can be equal to, less than, or higher than uptake in normal gray matter, thus decreasing the sensitivity of lesion detection. High-grade gliomas (WHO grade III and IV) show high uptake that is often heterogeneous because of the necrosis (▶ Fig. 12.1). Low-grade tumors, such as pilocytic astrocytomas, have low FDG uptake.

Unlike FDG, FLT can cross an intact blood–brain barrier, though very slowly.[79] For this reason and because of the very slow proliferation of neurons and astrocytes, normal background brain activity is very low, allowing a nice contrast

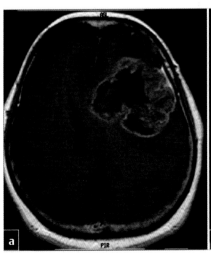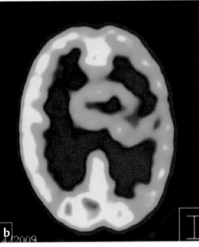

Fig. 12.1 Glioblastoma multiforme. Postcontrast T1-weighted image (**a**) demonstrates a heterogeneous ring-enhancing lesion in the left frontal lobe with mass effect that crossed the midline through the genu of the corpus callosum (not shown). On the axial ^{18}F-fluorodeoxyglucose (FDG) image (**b**), there is heterogeneous uptake of FDG at the periphery of the tumor with no uptake at the central areas of necrosis. (Image courtesy of Juan Manuel Isusi, MD, Department of Radiology, Universidad Nacional Autonoma de Mexico [UNAM], Mexico.)

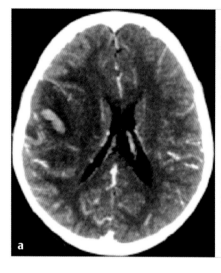 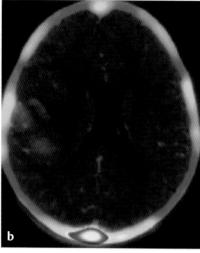

Fig. 12.2 Grade III astrocytoma. Postcontrast computed tomography (CT) (**a**) demonstrates a large, isodense mass with a focal are of enhancement in the left frontoparietal region with mass effect over the ventricle. 3′-¹⁸fluoro-3′-deoxy-L-thymidine (FLT) positron-emission tomography image overlaid on a postcontrast CT image (**b**) demonstrated increased FLT uptake in the entire tumor. Of note, very low background normal brain activity allowing nice delineation of tumor margin. (Image courtesy of Juan Manuel Isusi, MD, Department of Radiology, Universidad Nacional Autonoma de Mexico [UNAM], Mexico.)

between rapidly proliferating tumor and background brain activity.[76] Tumor accumulation of the tracer can be very fast, reaching the maximum level within 5 to 10 minutes of injection and remaining high thereafter.[75] There is a minimal decrease of tracer level over time.[75] FLT is taken up by all high-grade gliomas (▶ Fig. 12.2). In contrast, there is no appreciable uptake of FLT in low-grade gliomas. High FLT uptake by the tumor is a strong predictor of tumor proliferation (ki-67 index or MIB 1 score), tumor progression and overall survival. SUV_{max} strongly correlates with ki-67 index.[75]

Met PET uptake has been shown to be an independent significant prognostic factor in cerebral gliomas in comparison to FDG.[80] A higher tumor-to-background ratio has been shown to be associated with poor survival. There is significant correlation between Met uptake and Ki-67 expression. Relatively higher methionine uptake is seen in oligodendrogliomas compared to astrocytomas of a similar grade.[81] It has been shown that both high- and low-grade brain tumors are well visualized with FDOPA.[82] The sensitivity to identify tumors was substantially higher with FDOPA in comparison to FDG, especially for evaluating low-grade brain tumors.[82] FDOPA has high sensitivity (96%) and specificity (100%) for diagnosing brain tumor; however, FDOPA cannot reliably differentiate low grade from high grade.[82]

It has also been proved that ACE PET is a useful imaging biomarker of gliomas; however, the role of ACE PET in differentiating high- from low-grade gliomas is not clear.[83,84]

Multiple studies have shown that severity of hypoxic burden of the tumor after surgical intervention significantly impacts the overall and progression-free survival for GBM.[54,85]

Tumor Extent Delineation

It has been well established that conventional MRI underestimates the exact extent of the tumor. In fact, even with advanced MRI techniques it is not possible to determine the exact tumor margin. As stated earlier, FDG PET is poor in delineating exact tumor margin secondary to high normal background activity. It has been shown that the tumor margin identified by Met PET is different from that of MRI and FDG PET in most cases. In a small sample of GBM patients, it has been shown that the extent of tumor as delineated by Met PET is larger than the area of

contrast enhancement but smaller than the area of abnormal T2 signal.[86] It has also been shown that there is tumor recurrence in patients with areas of high Met uptake after resection of gadolinium-enhanced areas clearly suggestive of tumor extension beyond the gadolinium-enhanced areas.[86] FLT PET can also correctly identify extent of tumor beyond the enhancing margin of the tumor.[76]

Treatment Guidance

Biopsy Guidance

To avoid understaging of tumor, biopsies should always be performed for the most aggressive region of the tumor. However, because of the heterogeneous nature of gliomas, it is often difficult to identify the most anaplastic area of the tumor from conventional MRI. Perfusion MRI can correctly demonstrate the most vascular area of the tumor. For obvious reasons, as stated earlier, FDG cannot be reliably used to guide biopsy. In a study with FLT PET in combination with multiple advanced MRI techniques, it has been shown that areas of high vascularity correspond to the areas of high proliferation as detected by FLT PET.[87] FLT uptake rate (K1) is also correlated well with the MIB-1 labeling index in biopsy samples.[88] Amino acid imaging has also been used in targeting the biopsy site. It has been shown that incorporation of Met PET in biopsy planning reduced the number of required attempts,[89] and the biopsy yield using Met PET is superior to that with FDG.[90]

Guide to Resection

In a large study of 63 low-grade gliomas and 40 high-grade gliomas Pirotte et al demonstrated that imaging guidance with PET generated independent and complementary information that helped to define tumor extent and plan tumor resection better than MRI alone.[91] FDG uptake of high-grade tumors in this study demonstrated less tumor volume compared to gadolinium-enhanced MRI.

Radiation Planning

Computerized treatment planning using multimodality anatomical–physiological imaging techniques in combination with sophisticated radiation dose delivery systems (intensity-modulated radiation therapy [IMRT]) that deliver the maximum intended dose to the tumor with little or no dose to the adjacent normal tissue are gradually becoming the standard of care in radiation oncology.[92,93] Dose painting allows radiation oncologists to deliver different radiation doses to different areas of tumor. This powerful technique warrants the use of molecular imaging to identify areas of tumor that should be treated with a higher radiation dose. Because hypoxia incurs treatment resistance (to radiation therapy, as well as chemotherapy) and worse outcome, there is a recent emphasis on integrating hypoxia imaging in the planning of radiation therapy. Hypoxia imaging with FMISO,[94] FAZA,[95] and Cu-ATSM[96] has been investigated for guiding IMRT as a means to overcome hypoxia-induced radioresistance with varying success. Currently this hybrid imaging technology for radiation planning has not been standardized, and it is not established which hypoxic imaging agent should be used for which subtype of tumor. The role of hypoxia imaging is currently being actively investigated in a phase 2 multicenter study sponsored by the American College of Radiology Imaging Network (ACRIN 6684).

Even though FDG PET is increasingly being used for planning radiation treatment in other body parts (head and neck cancer and lung cancers), it is not used to plan radiation treatment in brain tumors in clinical practice due to the high intensity of FDG uptake in normal brain tissue.[97] In fact, Douglas et al demonstrated no improvement in overall survival and progression-free survival in a study of 40 patients with radiation dose escalation based on FDG PET imaging.[98] In a study with 16 gliomas, Li et al demonstrated that a Cho-PET combination with contrast-enhanced MRI is useful in determining as well as delineating a radiotherapeutic target volume and making decisions in selecting treatment regimens after tumor resection and before radiation treatment.[99] Similarly Grosu et al demonstrated that Met PET is very helpful in identifying residual tumor in operated gliomas for delineating gross tumor volume. The authors demonstrated that in 79% of their patient population ($n = 39$) regions with high Met uptake were larger than the contrast-enhanced MRI.[100]

Monitoring Treatment Response and Follow-Up

The assessment of response to treatment is key in routine patient care in neuro-oncology. Traditionally, patients are followed up with MRI. However, imaging findings are not specific and certainly are not reflective of actual tumor activity. Detection of nonresponse to treatment can be delayed secondary to nonspecific imaging appearances on MRI. It is may be difficult to differentiate tumor recurrence from treatment effects using MRI because both of these pathologies share similar imaging findings. Advanced MRI techniques, such as perfusion and diffusion imaging and MR spectroscopy, can differentiate between these two processes; however, they are not 100% specific. PET imaging can be complementary to MRI in differentiating between the two.

FLT is a promising PET tracer for treatment monitoring. FLT PET is a better technique to monitor testament of high grade brain tumors in comparison to 18FDG and MRI.[101] An early drop of SUV value during treatment that remains low thereafter is a predictor of long-term survival. An SUV value returning to pretreatment level after an initial drop predicts poor survival.[13] Dynamic FLT PET imaging early in the treatment is a powerful method for evaluating the efficacy of the therapeutic regimen.[102] It is also possible to differentiate short-term survivors from long-term survivors using dynamic FLT imaging.[102]

Imaging with amino acid PET imaging demonstrated more promising results. Popperl et al demonstrated tumor$_{max}$ to background ratio of 2.4 or higher can differentiate tumor recurrence from treatment-related effect with sensitivity of 82% and specificity of 100%.[103] Increased Met uptake by a tumor between two follow-up scans is consistent with tumor progression or recurrence. It has been shown that Met uptake > 14.6% in between two follow-up scans can distinguish tumor progression from stable disease with sensitivity of 90% and specificity of 92.3%.[104] Using FET PET, Mehrkens et al demonstrated a positive predictive value of 84% in predicting glioma recurrence in glioma patients treated with multimodality treatment, although the positive predictive value is not high enough to replace biopsy.[105]

Assessment of Radiation Necrosis and Recurrence

Differentiation between radiation necrosis and tumor recurrence is an extremely important aspect of high-grade glioma management because these two entities require entirely different treatment. Differentiation between these two pathologies is not *always* possible using MRI because radiation necrosis and tumor recurrence may share similar imaging appearances. Even with advanced MRI techniques, it is not always possible to differentiate between these two entities, and a re-biopsy is often required. There is a dire need for a sensitive and specific noninvasive imaging technique to differentiate these two entities.

Using FDG to differentiate tumor recurrence and treatment effect is problematic. In cases with predominant tumor recurrence there is high FDG uptake (▶ Fig. 12.3). Conversely, there is low FDG uptake in cases with predominant radiation necrosis (▶ Fig. 12.4). However, this simple approach is inefficient in cases with mixed tumor and treatment effect. Also, it is important to know the timing of the PET study in reference to radiation therapy and type and amount of radiation delivered because FDG uptake is dependent on all of these variables. For this reason, there is a wide range of sensitivity (81–86%) and specificity (40–94%) in distinguishing radiation necrosis from tumor recurrence.[19] An SUV-based approach is not reliable because the use of FDG is widely variable across different tumor types. Relative tumor uptake (in comparison with the contralateral hemisphere) is also not a useful approach. This is because an area of treated brain has a wide range of background metabolic activity (lower than normal brain). Recurring tumor can similarly have a wide variation of metabolic activity that is also lower in comparison to the normal brain. Delayed imaging with FDG PET has been suggested for better performance given the faster excretion of FDG from the necrotic tissue in comparison with proliferating tumors, but this has not been validated with a large study.[78] However, interval increase in FDG uptake in a previously diagnosed low-grade glioma with low FDG uptake is diagnostic of tumor progression/anaplastic transformation.[106] In the absence of differentiation to higher

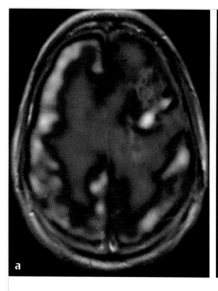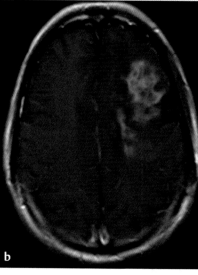

Fig. 12.3 Tumor recurrence. A 63-year-old patient with a World Health Organization (WHO) grade III oligodendroglioma, status postresection and chemoradiation therapy. (a) ^{18}F-fluorodeoxyglucose (FDG) positron-emission tomography image overlaid on a postcontrast T1-weighted sequence demonstrates diminished FDG uptake in most of the left frontal lobe in contrast to the normal FDG uptake in the right frontal lobe, with a focal area of increased uptake in the posteromedial aspect of the enhancement, suggestive of tumor recurrence (proved by biopsy). (b) Postcontrast T1-weighted image demonstrates heterogeneous enhancement of the left frontal lobe. Of note, there is no difference in the enhancement pattern in the areas of recurrence with high FDG uptake (posterior aspect of the lesion) compared to the areas of treatment-related changes with low FDG uptake (anterior aspect of the lesion). (Image courtesy of Anson Thaggard, MD, University of Mississippi, Jackson, MS.)

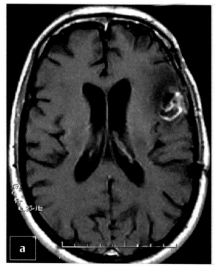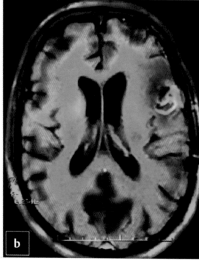

Fig. 12.4 Treatment effects. A 45-year-old man with previously treated glioblastoma multiforme developed new enhancement approximately 1 year after completion of radiation therapy. Postcontrast (a) image demonstrates heterogeneous enhancement in the left frontal lobe. ^{18}F-fluorodeoxyglucose (FDG) positron-emission tomography image overlaid on a postcontrast T1-weighted image (b) demonstrates diminished FDG uptake in the left frontal lobe compared to the rest of the brain, suggestive of treatment-related changes rather than tumor recurrence. (Proved on biopsy). (Image courtesy of Juan Manuel Isusi, MD, Department of Radiology, Universidad Nacional Autonoma de Mexico [UNAM], Mexico.)

grade, FDG is not sensitive in identifying recurrent low-grade tumors.

FLT can be used to differentiate treatment-related changes from tumor recurrence. FLT influx rate and phosphorylation rate can differentiate tumor recurrence form treatment-related effect, whereas simple SUV cannot.[107] FLT influx rate and phosphorylation rate can be estimated from compartmental modeling of dynamic FLT PET imaging.[107] Using the kinetic analysis of FLT PET in previously treated recurrent gliomas, it is possible to differentiate patients with predominant treatment-related changes from tumor-predominant patients.[108]

Met PET is also a promising PET tracer in differentiating treatment-related changes from tumor recurrence. Ogawa et al demonstrated increased Met uptake in all of 10 patients with tumor recurrence, whereas none of the radiation necrosis patients showed increased Met uptake.[109] In another study, Sonoda et al demonstrated positive Met PET in all five cases of

tumor recurrence, whereas only one of the seven patients with radiation necrosis showed high Met uptake.[110] Increased Met uptake can also be seen before any change on conventional MRI and even before onset of clinical symptoms.[111] Some investigators have used a semiquantitative approach to differentiate between tumor recurrence and radiation necrosis using Met PET with a better predictive value. Tumor-to-background ratio of > 1.5 to 2 is usually indicative of viable tumor. In cases with borderline tumor-to-background ratio, Crippa et al suggested repeating the Met PET scan after steroid administration to reduce the perfusion.[20] Recurrence of low-grade gliomas from radiation necrosis may not be possible using Met PET because there is overlap of the degree of low Met uptake in low-grade tumor and radiation necrosis.

In a rat model of radiation necrosis, it has been shown that the FET uptake profile in radiation necrosis is much better in comparison with FDG and Cho PET, suggesting a promising role of FET PET in the evaluation of radiation necrosis.[112] Focal increased FET uptake can be seen in recurrent gliomas in comparison with homogeneous low-level uptake in radiation necrosis, and FET PET can distinguish radiation necrosis from tumor recurrence with 100% accuracy.[78] In fact FET PET is more sensitive (100%) and specific (92%) in differentiating radiation necrosis from tumor recurrence in comparison with MRI, which showed sensitivity of 93.5% and specificity of only 50%.[113]

FDOPA, an amino acid analogue, has also been shown to be useful in differentiating tumor recurrence from radiation necrosis.[82] Tumor to striatum ratio of 0.75 or more is suggestive of tumor recurrence and can differentiate tumor recurrence from radiation necrosis with a sensitivity of 98% and an accuracy of 95%.[78]

12.5.3 Molecular Imaging in Gliomas: Current Recommendation

Unlike rest of the body parts, FDG PET is not a useful PET imaging agent for evaluation of brain tumors. Met PET and FET PET appear to be the best-performing imaging biomarkers in gliomas. However, these radiotracers also have limitations. Currently there is no PET tracer available that is highly sensitive and specific with high diagnostic accuracy for major brain tumor types that can be reliably used to monitor treatment and that can confidently diagnose tumor recurrence in the least possible time.

Careful analysis demonstrates that a combination of FDG PET and Met PET could be considered a gold standard in glioma evaluation.[28] However, FET PET has been shown to be an equally effective, if not better, radiotracer that is more widely available, and the combination of FET and FDG PET may eventually replace the FDG PET and Met PET combination as the optimal gold standard.[28] With the availability of PET MRI systems for clinical use, it is possible that multitracer imaging in combination with advanced MRI techniques will soon become a reality for evaluation of gliomas.

12.6 Molecular Imaging: Nonglial Brain Tumors

12.6.1 Brain Metastasis

Brain metastases occur in 20 to 40% of systemic cancers and constitute approximately half of all brain tumors.[114] CT and MRI remain the primary modalities for evaluation of brain metastases. On FDG, depending on the source of the tumor, it can be either hypermetabolic or hypometabolic compared to the normal brain (▶ Fig. 12.5 and ▶ Fig. 12.6).

12.6.2 Primary CNS Lymphoma

Primary CNS lymphoma (PCNSL) is a highly malignant tumor with high cellularity and is highly active metabolically. As expected, FDG uptake of PCNSL is very high, even higher than that for high-grade gliomas.[117] It has been shown that PCNSL has the maximum FDG uptake in comparison to high-grade gliomas, and metastasis with an SUV_{max} of > 15 is highly suggestive of PCNSL.[118] Differentiating PCNSL from CNS toxoplasmosis

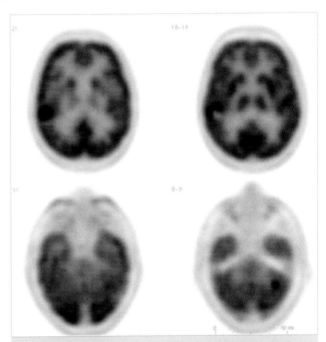

Fig. 12.5 Hypermetabolic lung cancer metastases to brain. Multiple axial ^{18}F-fluorodeoxyglucose positron-emission tomography images through the brain demonstrate multiple hypermetabolic lesions in the brain (right parietotemporal region, left frontal region, and left cerebellum) consistent with hypermetabolic metastasis.

is a very important clinical question in immunocompromised patients and often cannot be confidently diagnosed with conventional MRI. FDG can differentiate between these two entities. There is a high SUV ratio (ratio of SUV_{max} within PCNSL in comparison to the contralateral hemisphere) in PCNSL in comparison to toxoplasmosis, with no overlap of values.[119] This result has been validated in multiple studies.[115,116] SPECT imaging with ^{201}Tl can also be used to differentiate between PCNSL and CNS toxoplasmosis in immunocompromised patients with very high sensitivity and specificity.[120]

12.6.3 Meningioma

In meningiomas, FDG uptake is variable and may be related to aggressiveness and the probability of recurrence.[121] FDG uptake was also shown to be higher in meningiomas with higher cellularity, a higher proliferation index, and a higher grade (WHO grade II and III) in comparison to meningiomas with low cellularity, a low proliferation index, and a lower grade (WHO grade I).[122] In evaluation of meningioma with Met PET and FDG PET, it has been shown that the Met uptake, not FDG uptake, is significantly correlated with tumor proliferation (Ki-67 index).[123]

12.6.4 Pituitary Tumor

Pituitary adenoma is the most common tumor arising from the pituitary gland. MRI evaluation of pituitary tumors is the current standard practice. However, up to 80% of pituitary adenomas showed high uptake on FDG scans[124] (▶ Fig. 12.7), and SUV_{max} has been shown to correlate well with the size of the tumor.[124] Although clinically occult pituitary adenomas can also

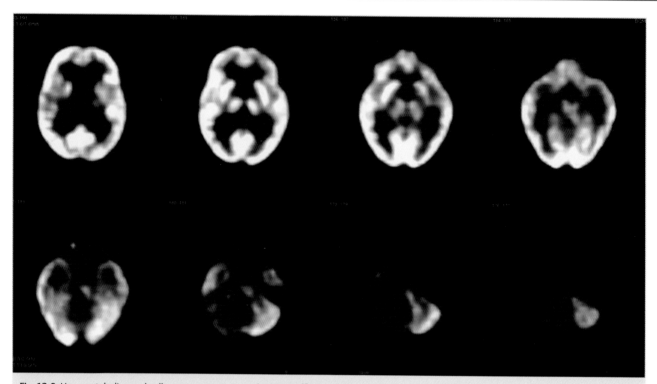

Fig. 12.6 Hypometabolic renal cell cancer metastasis. Multiple axial ^{18}F-fluorodeoxyglucose positron-emission tomography images through the brain demonstrate a large focal hypometabolic right cerebellar mass (compared to the contralateral cerebellar hemisphere). Heterogeneous ring enhancement was seen on postcontrast magnetic resonance imaging (not included).

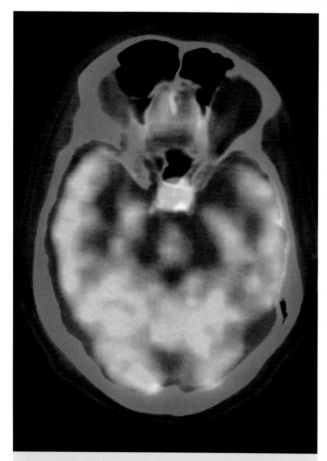

Fig. 12.7 Pituitary macroadenoma. Seizure workup with ^{18}F-fluoro-deoxyglucose (FDG) in a 48-year-old man. Incidental high FDG uptake is seen at the sella, which was very suggestive of pituitary macro-adenoma on magnetic resonance imaging (not removed, the patient was asymptomatic without any hormonal abnormality).

be incidentally detected on FDG scans, SUV_{max} of 4.1 or higher is usually suggestive of pathological uptake and warrants further diagnostic evaluation.[125]

References

[1] Rahmim A, Zaidi H. PET versus SPECT: strengths, limitations and challenges. Nucl Med Commun 2008; 29: 193–207

[2] von Schulthess GK, Kuhn FP, Kaufmann P, Veit-Haibach P. Clinical positron emission tomography/magnetic resonance imaging applications. Semin Nucl Med 2013; 43: 3–10

[3] Mankoff DA. A definition of molecular imaging. J Nucl Med 2007; 48: 18N–21N, 21N

[4] Schöder H, Ong SC. Fundamentals of molecular imaging: rationale and applications with relevance for radiation oncology. Semin Nucl Med 2008; 38: 119–128

[5] Accorsi R. Brain single-photon emission CT physics principles. AJNR Am J Neuroradiol 2008; 29: 1247–1256

[6] Turkington TG. Introduction to PET instrumentation. J Nucl Med Technol 2001; 29: 4–11

[7] Mettler FAGM. Essentials of Nuclear Medicine Imaging. 6th ed. Philadelphia, PA: Elsevier; 2012

[8] Vaska P, Cao T. The state of instrumentation for combined positron emission tomography and magnetic resonance imaging. Semin Nucl Med 2013; 43: 11–18

[9] Kiss R, Dewitte O, Decaestecker C et al. The combined determination of proliferative activity and cell density in the prognosis of adult patients with supratentorial high-grade astrocytic tumors. Am J Clin Pathol 1997; 107: 321–331

[10] Bading JR, Shields AF. Imaging of cell proliferation: status and prospects. J Nucl Med 2008; 49 Suppl 2: 64S–80S

[11] Zhang CC, Yan Z, Li W et al. [(18)F]FLT-PET imaging does not always "light up" proliferating tumor cells. Clin Cancer Res 2012; 18: 1303–1312

[12] Salskov A, Tammisetti VS, Grierson J, Vesselle H. FLT: measuring tumor cell proliferation in vivo with positron emission tomography and 3-deoxy-3-[18F]fluorothymidine. Semin Nucl Med 2007; 37: 429–439

[13] Herholz K, Langen KJ, Schiepers C, Mountz JM. Brain tumors. Semin Nucl Med 2012; 42: 356–370

[14] Marín-Hernández A, Gallardo-Pérez JC, Ralph SJ, Rodríguez-Enríquez S, Moreno-Sánchez R. HIF-1alpha modulates energy metabolism in cancer cells by inducing over-expression of specific glycolytic isoforms. Mini Rev Med Chem 2009; 9: 1084–1101

[15] Roelcke U, Blasberg RG, von Ammon K et al. Dexamethasone treatment and plasma glucose levels: relevance for fluorine-18-fluorodeoxyglucose uptake measurements in gliomas. J Nucl Med 1998; 39: 879–884

[16] Bénard F, Romsa J, Hustinx R. Imaging gliomas with positron emission tomography and single-photon emission computed tomography. Semin Nucl Med 2003; 33: 148–162

[17] Kubota R, Kubota K, Yamada S et al. Methionine uptake by tumor tissue: a microautoradiographic comparison with FDG. J Nucl Med 1995; 36: 484–492

[18] Chao ST, Suh JH, Raja S, Lee SY, Barnett G. The sensitivity and specificity of FDG PET in distinguishing recurrent brain tumor from radionecrosis in patients treated with stereotactic radiosurgery. Int J Cancer 2001; 96: 191–197

[19] Langleben DD, Segall GM. PET in differentiation of recurrent brain tumor from radiation injury. J Nucl Med 2000; 41: 1861–1867

[20] Crippa F, Alessi A, Serafini GL. PET with radiolabeled aminoacid. Q J Nucl Med Mol Imaging 2012; 56: 151–162

[21] Isselbacher KJ. Sugar and amino acid transport by cells in culture—differences between normal and malignant cells. N Engl J Med 1972; 286: 929–933

[22] Sasajima T, Miyagawa T, Oku T, Gelovani JG, Finn R, Blasberg R. Proliferation-dependent changes in amino acid transport and glucose metabolism in glioma cell lines. Eur J Nucl Med Mol Imaging 2004; 31: 1244–1256

[23] Miyagawa T, Oku T, Uehara H et al. "Facilitated" amino acid transport is upregulated in brain tumors. J Cereb Blood Flow Metab 1998; 18: 500–509

[24] Roelcke U, Radü EW, von Ammon K, Hausmann O, Maguire RP, Leenders KL. Alteration of blood-brain barrier in human brain tumors: comparison of [18F]fluorodeoxyglucose, [11C]methionine and rubidium-82 using PET. J Neurol Sci 1995; 132: 20–27

[25] Plotkin M, Blechschmidt C, Auf G, et al. Comparison of F-18 FET-PET with F-18 FDG-PET for biopsy planning of non-contrast-enhancing gliomas. Eur Radiol. 2010;20(10):2496–2502

[26] Pauleit D, Stoffels G, Bachofner A, et al. Comparison of (18)F-FET and (18)F-FDG PET in brain tumors. Nucl Med Biol. 2009;36(7):779–787

[27] Lau EW, Drummond KJ, Ware RE, et al. Comparative PET study using F-18 FET and F-18 FDG for the evaluation of patients with suspected brain tumour. J Clin Neurosci. 2010;17(1):43–49

[28] Gulyás B, Halldin C. New PET radiopharmaceuticals beyond FDG for brain tumor imaging. Q J Nucl Med Mol Imaging 2012; 56: 173–190

[29] Fischer I, Gagner JP, Law M, Newcomb EW, Zagzag D. Angiogenesis in gliomas: biology and molecular pathophysiology. Brain Pathol 2005; 15: 297–310

[30] Hardee ME, Zagzag D. Mechanisms of glioma-associated neovascularization. Am J Pathol 2012; 181: 1126–1141

[31] Eliceiri BP, Cheresh DA. The role of alphav integrins during angiogenesis. Mol Med 1998; 4: 741–750

[32] Gingras MC, Roussel E, Bruner JM, Branch CD, Moser RP. Comparison of cell adhesion molecule expression between glioblastoma multiforme and autologous normal brain tissue. J Neuroimmunol 1995; 57: 143–153

[33] Tysnes BB, Larsen LF, Ness GO et al. Stimulation of glioma-cell migration by laminin and inhibition by anti-alpha3 and anti-beta1 integrin antibodies. Int J Cancer 1996; 67: 777–784

[34] Kawataki T, Yamane T, Naganuma H et al. Laminin isoforms and their integrin receptors in glioma cell migration and invasiveness: Evidence for a role of alpha5-laminin(s) and alpha3beta1 integrin. Exp Cell Res 2007; 313: 3819–3831

[35] Gritsenko PG, Ilina O, Friedl P. Interstitial guidance of cancer invasion. J Pathol 2012; 226: 185–199

[36] Ruoslahti E, Pierschbacher MD. New perspectives in cell adhesion: RGD and integrins. Science 1987; 238: 491–497

[37] Xiong JP, Stehle T, Zhang R et al. Crystal structure of the extracellular segment of integrin alpha Vbeta3 in complex with an Arg-Gly-Asp ligand. Science 2002; 296: 151–155

[38] Battle MR, Goggi JL, Allen L, Barnett J, Morrison MS. Monitoring tumor response to antiangiogenic sunitinib therapy with 18F-fluciclatide, an 18F-labeled αV beta3-integrin and αV beta5-integrin imaging agent. J Nucl Med 2011; 52: 424–430

[39] Chen K, Chen X. Positron emission tomography imaging of cancer biology: current status and future prospects. Semin Oncol 2011; 38: 70–86

[40] Cai W, Rao J, Gambhir SS, Chen X. How molecular imaging is speeding up antiangiogenic drug development. Mol Cancer Ther 2006; 5: 2624–2633

[41] Chen K, Cai W, Li ZB, Wang H, Chen X. Quantitative PET imaging of VEGF receptor expression. Mol Imaging Biol 2009; 11: 15–22

[42] Swanson KR, Chakraborty G, Wang CH et al. Complementary but distinct roles for MRI and 18F-fluoromisonidazole PET in the assessment of human glioblastomas. J Nucl Med 2009; 50: 36–44

[43] Bar EE. Glioblastoma, cancer stem cells and hypoxia. Brain Pathol 2011; 21: 119–129

[44] Jensen RL. Brain tumor hypoxia: tumorigenesis, angiogenesis, imaging, pseudoprogression, and as a therapeutic target. J Neurooncol 2009; 92: 317–335

[45] Yang L, Lin C, Wang L, Guo H, Wang X. Hypoxia and hypoxia-inducible factors in glioblastoma multiforme progression and therapeutic implications. Exp Cell Res 2012; 318: 2417–2426

[46] Vallabhajosula S, Solnes L, Vallabhajosula B. A broad overview of positron emission tomography radiopharmaceuticals and clinical applications: what is new? Semin Nucl Med 2011; 41: 246–264

[47] Imam SK. Review of positron emission tomography tracers for imaging of tumor hypoxia. Cancer Biother Radiopharm 2010; 25: 365–374

[48] Koh WJ, Rasey JS, Evans ML et al. Imaging of hypoxia in human tumors with [F-18]fluoromisonidazole. Int J Radiat Oncol Biol Phys 1992; 22: 199–212

[49] Rasey JS, Koh WJ, Evans ML et al. Quantifying regional hypoxia in human tumors with positron emission tomography of [18F]fluoromisonidazole: a pretherapy study of 37 patients. Int J Radiat Oncol Biol Phys 1996; 36: 417–428

[50] Troost EG, Laverman P, Kaanders JH et al. Imaging hypoxia after oxygenation-modification: comparing [18F]FMISO autoradiography with pimonidazole immunohistochemistry in human xenograft tumors. Radiother Oncol 2006; 80: 157–164

[51] Rasey JS, Nelson NJ, Chin L, Evans ML, Grunbaum Z. Characteristics of the binding of labeled fluoromisonidazole in cells in vitro. Radiat Res 1990; 122: 301–308

[52] Gross MW, Karbach U, Groebe K, Franko AJ, Mueller-Klieser W. Calibration of misonidazole labeling by simultaneous measurement of oxygen tension and labeling density in multicellular spheroids. Int J Cancer 1995; 61: 567–573

[53] Tateishi K, Tateishi U, Sato M et al. Application of 62Cu-diacetyl-bis (N4-methylthiosemicarbazone) PET imaging to predict highly malignant tumor grades and hypoxia-inducible factor-1α expression in patients with glioma. AJNR Am J Neuroradiol 2013; 34: 92–99

[54] Spence AM, Muzi M, Swanson KR et al. Regional hypoxia in glioblastoma multiforme quantified with [18F]fluoromisonidazole positron emission tomography before radiotherapy: correlation with time to progression and survival. Clin Cancer Res 2008; 14: 2623–2630

[55] Yang DJ, Wallace S, Cherif A et al. Development of F-18-labeled fluoroerythro-nitroimidazole as a PET agent for imaging tumor hypoxia. Radiology 1995; 194: 795–800

[56] Grönroos T, Bentzen L, Marjamäki P et al. Comparison of the biodistribution of two hypoxia markers [18F]FETNIM and [18F]FMISO in an experimental mammary carcinoma. Eur J Nucl Med Mol Imaging 2004; 31: 513–520

[57] Reischl G, Dorow DS, Cullinane C et al. Imaging of tumor hypoxia with [124I] IAZA in comparison with [18F]FMISO and [18F]FAZA—first small animal PET results. J Pharm Pharm Sci 2007; 10: 203–211

[58] Mahy P, Geets X, Lonneux M et al. Determination of tumour hypoxia with [18F]EF3 in patients with head and neck tumours: a phase I study to assess the tracer pharmacokinetics, biodistribution and metabolism. Eur J Nucl Med Mol Imaging 2008; 35: 1282–1289

[59] Dubois L, Landuyt W, Cloetens L et al. [18F]EF3 is not superior to [18F]FMISO for PET-based hypoxia evaluation as measured in a rat rhabdomyosarcoma tumour model. Eur J Nucl Med Mol Imaging 2009; 36: 209–218

[60] Komar G, Seppänen M, Eskola O et al. 18F-EF5: a new PET tracer for imaging hypoxia in head and neck cancer. J Nucl Med 2008; 49: 1944–1951

[61] Evans SM, Judy KD, Dunphy I et al. Hypoxia is important in the biology and aggression of human glial brain tumors. Clin Cancer Res 2004; 10: 8177–8184

[62] Mendichovszky I, Jackson A. Imaging hypoxia in gliomas. Br J Radiol 2011; 84: S145–S158

[63] Wyss MT, Spaeth N, Biollaz G et al. Uptake of 18F-Fluorocholine, 18F-FET, and 18F-FDG in C6 gliomas and correlation with 131I-SIP(L19), a marker of angiogenesis. J Nucl Med 2007; 48: 608–614

[64] Vanpouille C, Le Jeune N, Kryza D et al. Influence of multidrug resistance on (18)F-FCH cellular uptake in a glioblastoma model. Eur J Nucl Med Mol Imaging 2009; 36: 1256–1264

[65] Utriainen M, Komu M, Vuorinen V et al. Evaluation of brain tumor metabolism with [11C]choline PET and 1H-MRS. J Neurooncol 2003; 62: 329–338

[66] Huang Z, Zuo C, Guan Y et al. Misdiagnoses of 11C-choline combined with 18F-FDG PET imaging in brain tumours. Nucl Med Commun 2008; 29: 354–358

[67] Cai W, Chen K, He L, Cao Q, Koong A, Chen X. Quantitative PET of EGFR expression in xenograft-bearing mice using 64Cu-labeled cetuximab, a chimeric anti-EGFR monoclonal antibody. Eur J Nucl Med Mol Imaging 2007; 34: 850–858

[68] Blankenberg FG. Recent advances in the imaging of programmed cell death. Curr Pharm Des 2004; 10: 1457–1467

[69] Koopman G, Reutelingsperger CP, Kuijten GA, Keehnen RM, Pals ST, van Oers MH. Annexin V for flow cytometric detection of phosphatidylserine expression on B cells undergoing apoptosis. Blood 1994; 84: 1415–1420

[70] Boersma HH, Kietselaer BL, Stolk LM et al. Past, present, and future of annexin A5: from protein discovery to clinical applications. J Nucl Med 2005; 46: 2035–2050

[71] Cohen A, Shirvan A, Levin G, Grimberg H, Reshef A, Ziv I. From the Gla domain to a novel small-molecule detector of apoptosis. Cell Res 2009; 19: 625–637

[72] Höglund J, Shirvan A, Antoni G et al. 18F-ML-10, a PET tracer for apoptosis: first human study. J Nucl Med 2011; 52: 720–725

[73] Heiss WD, Raab P, Lanfermann H. Multimodality assessment of brain tumors and tumor recurrence. J Nucl Med 2011; 52: 1585–1600

[74] Delbeke D, Meyerowitz C, Lapidus RL et al. Optimal cutoff levels of F-18 fluorodeoxyglucose uptake in the differentiation of low-grade from high-grade brain tumors with PET. Radiology 1995; 195: 47–52

[75] Chen W, Cloughesy T, Kamdar N et al. Imaging proliferation in brain tumors with 18F-FLT PET: comparison with 18F-FDG. J Nucl Med 2005; 46: 945–952

[76] Jacobs AH, Thomas A, Kracht LW et al. 18F-fluoro-L-thymidine and 11C-methylmethionine as markers of increased transport and proliferation in brain tumors. J Nucl Med 2005; 46: 1948–1958

[77] Tripathi M, Sharma R, D'Souza M et al. Comparative evaluation of F-18 FDOPA, F-18 FDG, and F-18 FLT-PET/CT for metabolic imaging of low grade gliomas. Clin Nucl Med 2009; 34: 878–883

[78] Chen W. Clinical applications of PET in brain tumors. J Nucl Med 2007; 48: 1468–1481

[79] Stahle L, Borg N. Transport of alovudine (3-fluorothymidine) into the brain and the cerebrospinal fluid of the rat, studied by microdialysis. Life Sci 2000; 66: 1805–1816

[80] Kim S, Chung JK, Im SH et al. 11C-methionine PET as a prognostic marker in patients with glioma: comparison with 18F-FDG PET. Eur J Nucl Med Mol Imaging 2005; 32: 52–59

[81] Kracht LW, Miletic H, Busch S et al. Delineation of brain tumor extent with [11C]L-methionine positron emission tomography: local comparison with stereotactic histopathology. Clin Cancer Res 2004; 10: 7163–7170

[82] Chen W, Silverman DH, Delaloye S et al. 18F-FDOPA PET imaging of brain tumors: comparison study with 18F-FDG PET and evaluation of diagnostic accuracy. J Nucl Med 2006; 47: 904–911

[83] Liu RS, Chang CP, Chu LS et al. PET imaging of brain astrocytoma with 1–11C-acetate. Eur J Nucl Med Mol Imaging 2006; 33: 420–427

[84] Tsuchida T, Takeuchi H, Okazawa H, Tsujikawa T, Fujibayashi Y. Grading of brain glioma with 1–11C-acetate PET: comparison with 18F-FDG PET. Nucl Med Biol 2008; 35: 171–176

[85] Cher LM, Murone C, Lawrentschuk N et al. Correlation of hypoxic cell fraction and angiogenesis with glucose metabolic rate in gliomas using 18F-fluoromisonidazole, 18F-FDG PET, and immunohistochemical studies. J Nucl Med 2006; 47: 410–418

[86] Miwa K, Shinoda J, Yano H et al. Discrepancy between lesion distributions on methionine PET and MR images in patients with glioblastoma multiforme: insight from a PET and MR fusion image study. J Neurol Neurosurg Psychiatry 2004; 75: 1457–1462

[87] Weber MA, Henze M, Tüttenberg J et al. Biopsy targeting gliomas: do functional imaging techniques identify similar target areas? Invest Radiol 2010; 45: 755–768

[88] Price SJ, Fryer TD, Cleij MC et al. Imaging regional variation of cellular proliferation in gliomas using 3-deoxy-3-[18F]fluorothymidine positron-emission tomography: an image-guided biopsy study. Clin Radiol 2009; 64: 52–63

[89] Pirotte B, Goldman S, Salzberg S et al. Combined positron emission tomography and magnetic resonance imaging for the planning of stereotactic brain biopsies in children: experience in 9 cases. Pediatr Neurosurg 2003; 38: 146–155

[90] Pirotte B, Goldman S, Massager N et al. Comparison of 18F-FDG and 11C-methionine for PET-guided stereotactic brain biopsy of gliomas. J Nucl Med 2004; 45: 1293–1298

[91] Pirotte B, Goldman S, Dewitte O et al. Integrated positron emission tomography and magnetic resonance imaging-guided resection of brain tumors: a report of 103 consecutive procedures. J Neurosurg 2006; 104: 238–253

[92] Scripes PG, Yaparpalvi R. Technical aspects of positron emission tomography/computed tomography in radiotherapy treatment planning. Semin Nucl Med 2012; 42: 283–288

[93] Brunetti J, Caggiano A, Rosenbluth B, Vialotti C. Technical aspects of positron emission tomography/computed tomography fusion planning. Semin Nucl Med 2008; 38: 129–136

[94] Hendrickson K, Phillips M, Smith W, Peterson L, Krohn K, Rajendran J. Hypoxia imaging with [F-18] FMISO-PET in head and neck cancer: potential for guiding intensity modulated radiation therapy in overcoming hypoxia-induced treatment resistance. Radiother Oncol 2011; 101: 369–375

[95] Grosu AL, Souvatzoglou M, Röper B et al. Hypoxia imaging with FAZA-PET and theoretical considerations with regard to dose painting for individualization of radiotherapy in patients with head and neck cancer. Int J Radiat Oncol Biol Phys 2007; 69: 541–551

[96] Chao KS, Bosch WR, Mutic S et al. A novel approach to overcome hypoxic tumor resistance: Cu-ATSM-guided intensity-modulated radiation therapy. Int J Radiat Oncol Biol Phys 2001; 49: 1171–1182

[97] Gross MW, Weber WA, Feldmann HJ, Bartenstein P, Schwaiger M, Molls M. The value of F-18-fluorodeoxyglucose PET for the 3-D radiation treatment planning of malignant gliomas. Int J Radiat Oncol Biol Phys 1998; 41: 989–995

[98] Douglas JG, Stelzer KJ, Mankoff DA et al. [F-18]-fluorodeoxyglucose positron emission tomography for targeting radiation dose escalation for patients with glioblastoma multiforme: clinical outcomes and patterns of failure. Int J Radiat Oncol Biol Phys 2006; 64: 886–891

[99] Li FM, Nie Q, Wang RM et al. 11C-CHO PET in optimization of target volume delineation and treatment regimens in postoperative radiotherapy for brain gliomas. Nucl Med Biol 2012; 39: 437–442

[100] Grosu AL, Weber WA, Riedel E et al. L-(methyl-11C) methionine positron emission tomography for target delineation in resected high-grade gliomas before radiotherapy. Int J Radiat Oncol Biol Phys 2005; 63: 64–74

[101] Chen W, Delaloye S, Silverman DH et al. Predicting treatment response of malignant gliomas to bevacizumab and irinotecan by imaging proliferation with [18F] fluorothymidine positron emission tomography: a pilot study. J Clin Oncol 2007; 25: 4714–4721

[102] Wardak M, Schiepers C, Dahlbom M et al. Discriminant analysis of 18F-fluorothymidine kinetic parameters to predict survival in patients with recurrent high-grade glioma. Clin Cancer Res 2011; 17: 6553–6562

[103] Pöpperl G, Götz C, Rachinger W et al. Serial O-(2-[(18)F]fluoroethyl)-L:-tyrosine PET for monitoring the effects of intracavitary radioimmunotherapy in patients with malignant glioma. Eur J Nucl Med Mol Imaging 2006; 33: 792–800

[104] Ullrich RT, Kracht L, Brunn A et al. Methyl-L-11C-methionine PET as a diagnostic marker for malignant progression in patients with glioma. J Nucl Med 2009; 50: 1962–1968

[105] Mehrkens JH, Pöpperl G, Rachinger W et al. The positive predictive value of O-(2-[18F]fluoroethyl)-L-tyrosine (FET) PET in the diagnosis of a glioma recurrence after multimodal treatment. J Neurooncol 2008; 88: 27–35

[106] De Witte O, Levivier M, Violon P et al. Prognostic value positron emission tomography with [18F]fluoro-2-deoxy-D-glucose in the low-grade glioma. Neurosurgery 1996; 39: 470–476, discussion 476–477

[107] Spence AM, Muzi M, Link JM et al. NCI-sponsored trial for the evaluation of safety and preliminary efficacy of 3-deoxy-3-[18F]fluorothymidine (FLT) as a marker of proliferation in patients with recurrent gliomas: preliminary efficacy studies. Mol Imaging Biol 2009; 11: 343–355

[108] Schiepers C, Chen W, Dahlbom M, Cloughesy T, Hoh CK, Huang SC. 18F-fluorothymidine kinetics of malignant brain tumors. Eur J Nucl Med Mol Imaging 2007; 34: 1003–1011

[109] Ogawa T, Kanno I, Shishido F et al. Clinical value of PET with 18F-fluorodeoxyglucose and L-methyl-11C-methionine for diagnosis of recurrent brain tumor and radiation injury. Acta Radiol 1991; 32: 197–202

[110] Sonoda Y, Kumabe T, Takahashi T, Shirane R, Yoshimoto T. Clinical usefulness of 11C-MET PET and 201Tl SPECT for differentiation of recurrent glioma from radiation necrosis. Neurol Med Chir (Tokyo) 1998; 38: 342–347, discussion 347–348

[111] Nariai T, Tanaka Y, Wakimoto H et al. Usefulness of L-[methyl-11C] methionine-positron emission tomography as a biological monitoring tool in the treatment of glioma. J Neurosurg 2005; 103: 498–507

[112] Spaeth N, Wyss MT, Weber B et al. Uptake of 18F-fluorocholine, 18F-fluoroethyl-L-tyrosine, and 18F-FDG in acute cerebral radiation injury in the rat: implications for separation of radiation necrosis from tumor recurrence. J Nucl Med 2004; 45: 1931–1938

[113] Rachinger W, Goetz C, Pöpperl G et al. Positron emission tomography with O-(2-[18F]fluoroethyl)-l-tyrosine versus magnetic resonance imaging in the diagnosis of recurrent gliomas. Neurosurgery 2005; 57: 505–511, discussion 505–511

[114] Jeong HJ, Chung JK, Kim YK et al. Usefulness of whole-body (18)F-FDG PET in patients with suspected metastatic brain tumors. J Nucl Med 2002; 43: 1432–1437

[115] Westwood TD, Hogan C, Julyan PJ, et al. Utility of FDG-PETCT and magnetic resonance spectroscopy in differentiating between cerebral lymphoma and non-malignant CNS lesions in HIV-infected patients. Eur J Radiol. 2013;82(8): e374–379

[116] Lewitschnig S, Gedela K, Toby M, et al. 18F-FDG PET/CT in HIV-related central nervous system pathology. Eur J Nucl Med Mol Imaging. 2013;40(9):1420–1427

[117] Makino K, Hirai T, Nakamura H et al. Does adding FDG-PET to MRI improve the differentiation between primary cerebral lymphoma and glioblastoma? Observer performance study. Ann Nucl Med 2011; 25: 432–438

[118] Kosaka N, Tsuchida T, Uematsu H, Kimura H, Okazawa H, Itoh H. 18F-FDG PET of common enhancing malignant brain tumors. AJR Am J Roentgenol 2008; 190: W365–9

[119] Sathekge M, Goethals I, Maes A, van de Wiele C. Positron emission tomography in patients suffering from HIV-1 infection. Eur J Nucl Med Mol Imaging 2009; 36: 1176–1184

[120] De La Peña RC, Ketonen L, Villanueva-Meyer J. Imaging of brain tumors in AIDS patients by means of dual-isotope thallium-201 and technetium-99 m sestamibi single-photon emission tomography. Eur J Nucl Med 1998; 25: 1404–1411

[121] Di Chiro G, Hatazawa J, Katz DA, Rizzoli HV, De Michele DJ. Glucose utilization by intracranial tumors as an index of tumor aggressivity and probability of recurrence: a PET study. Radiology 1987; 164: 521–526

[122] Lippitz B, Cremerius U, Mayfrank L et al. PET-study of intracranial meningiomas: correlation with histopathology, cellularity and proliferation rate. Acta Neurochir Suppl (Wien) 1996; 65: 108–111

[123] Iuchi T, Iwadate Y, Namba H et al. Glucose and methionine uptake and proliferative activity in meningiomas. Neurol Res 1999; 21: 640–644

[124] Seok H, Lee EY, Choe EY et al. Analysis of 18F-fluorodeoxyglucose positron emission tomography findings in patients with pituitary lesions. Korean J Intern Med 2013; 28: 81–88

[125] Hyun SH, Choi JY, Lee KH, Choe YS, Kim BT. Incidental focal 18F-FDG uptake in the pituitary gland: clinical significance and differential diagnostic criteria. J Nucl Med 2011; 52: 547–550

13 It's Not Just the Tumor: Treatment Effects

Brent Griffith and Rajan Jain

13.1 Introduction

Imaging plays a major role in monitoring brain tumor patients; however, assessment of treatment response is currently limited to sequential measurements of only the contrast-enhancing component of the lesion using either Macdonald criteria or Response Evaluation Criteria in Solid Tumors (RECIST).[1] These methods use changes in the size of the contrast enhancement as a biomarker for treatment response or failure. However, because these methods rely on direct correlation between changes in enhancement and disease response or progression, they may not completely assess the nonenhancing component of the tumor. More importantly, these imaging biomarkers may not provide an accurate assessment of the tumor physiology, vascularity, and metabolism.

Brain tumor enhancement, or lack thereof, is affected by the presence and integrity of the blood–brain barrier (BBB). Therefore, any factors affecting the BBB will also affect the enhancement pattern on imaging. And, although changes in enhancement pattern can result from disease response or progression, a number of additional factors, particularly those related to the therapy, can affect enhancement patterns as well. For example, processes such as postictal changes, postoperative infarcts, or treatment-related inflammatory processes can disrupt the BBB, resulting in increased enhancement, thus mimicking disease progression and referred to as pseudoprogression. In addition, other factors, such as steroid treatment and antiangiogenic agents, can actually improve the integrity of the BBB, leading to decreased enhancement without much cytotoxic effect and hence mimicking treatment response, also referred to as pseudoresponse.[1,2] The Response Assessment in Neuro-Oncology (RANO) Working Group recently updated the criteria and included assessment of the nonenhancing part of the tumor based on T2 fluid-attenuated inversion recovery (T2/FLAIR) imaging to counter the issue of pseudoresponse following treatment with antiangiogenic agents.[3]

Other common adverse treatment effects seen in busy neuro-oncology centers are related to radiation therapy, with delayed radiation necrosis being a common nemesis. Differentiating radiation necrosis from tumor progression is usually not possible based solely on morphological magnetic resonance imaging (MRI) features.[4]

13.2 Clinical Implications

Accurately identifying treatment effects is especially challenging for brain tumors due to the rapidly changing and evolving field of combination therapy regimens, which is a consequence of the disease's poor overall prognosis. In 2005 a study by Stupp et al found a small advantage in progression-free survival (PFS), as well as a significant benefit in 2-year overall survival with the use of temozolomide plus radiation therapy.[5] This has since become the standard of care following tumor resection.[6] In 2009 the U.S. Food and Drug Administration approved the use of bevacizumab, an antiangiogenic agent, for the treatment of recurrent gliomas.[7] Although new treatments offer hope for improving the overall dismal prognosis, they also lead to new imaging patterns, which can create confusion in differentiating treatment response or failure from treatment effects. Imaging biomarkers that provide early indication of treatment failure and timely opportunity to select an alternative treatment, or those that correctly diagnose treatment effects and prevent premature discontinuation of an effective treatment, are therefore of very active clinical interest. In particular, many studies rely on PFS and radiographic response (RR) to determine the effectiveness of a given therapy. However, because these methods have traditionally relied on changes in enhancement as the major differentiating factor, incorrectly categorizing these changes can lead to falsely high response or failure rates for a particular therapy.[8] Functional imaging modalities can provide additional information that may help differentiate treatment effects from true tumor progression and are discussed in this chapter.

13.3 Radiation Therapy–Induced Treatment Effects and Toxicity

Radiation therapy combined with chemotherapy is the standard of care following resection of high-grade gliomas. In patients undergoing treatment for malignant gliomas, radiation therapy is typically administered over a span of 6 to 7 weeks, usually consisting of fractionated focal irradiation at a dose of 2 Gy per fraction for a total dose of 60 Gy.[5,9] Although this therapy regimen has led to improved overall patient survival, delivering high doses of radiation can lead to a number of treatment-related effects, which can confound the overall clinical and imaging picture. Understanding the presentation of these changes from both a clinical and an imaging standpoint is, therefore, essential to ensure proper patient management.

The incidence and severity of radiation-induced effects depend on a number of factors, including patient factors, such as overall patient health; factors related to the treatment regimen, such as the use of concomitant chemotherapy; or factors related to the radiation therapy itself, such as the amount and type of radiation being administered.[10] In addition, recent studies have identified tumor-specific factors that also may influence the frequency of certain radiation-related effects. A study by Brandes et al in 2008 found that the incidence of pseudoprogression, a well-known cause of postradiation changes mimicking tumor progression, is significantly correlated with methylation of O^6-methylguanine-DNA methyltransferase, a DNA repair enzyme, and in fact may be associated with survival benefit.[11]

Classically, the effects of radiation on the central nervous system have been divided into three categories: acute, early delayed or subacute, and late effects.[12,13]

Acute effects of radiation therapy occur either during or within days to weeks following therapy.[10,12,13] Symptoms, which are generally mild and typically reversible, can include fatigue, dizziness, and signs of elevated intracranial pressure.[12,13]

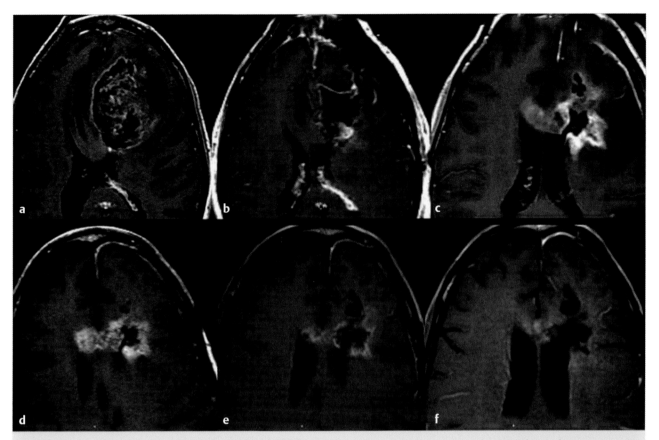

Fig. 13.1 Pseudoprogression. Preoperative (**a**) contrast-enhanced T1-weighted axial magnetic resonance imaging (MRI) shows a large heterogeneously enhancing high-grade glioma in the left frontal region with associated mass effect. (**b**) Immediate postoperative baseline MRI shows mild residual enhancement along the posterior margin of the surgical cavity. (**c**) Follow-up MRI 10 weeks after temozolomide and radiation therapy shows increase in size of the enhancing lesion. (**d–f**) Sequential follow-up MRI studies done over the next 8 months show decrease in the enhancing area without any change in the chemotherapy, suggesting the initial increase in enhancement after chemoradiation therapy was pseudoprogression and not true tumor progression.

Subacute or early delayed effects of radiation therapy generally occur a few weeks to several months following radiation treatment.[10,12] Symptoms during this period, which are also typically reversible, include generalized weakness and somnolence and are thought to relate to transient demyelination.[13] During this subacute phase of radiation injury the relatively new phenomenon known as pseudoprogression may arise. *Pseudoprogression* refers to a treatment-related increase in enhancing lesion size and/or edema without actual increase in tumor burden. This is confirmed on follow-up imaging demonstrating either regression or lack of progression of the imaging abnormalities without any change in therapy regimen (► Fig. 13.1). Although a number of factors can lead to increased enhancement or edema following treatment, including postictal changes, postoperative infarcts, and changes in steroid dose, radiation injury has also been identified as a causative factor. Pseudoprogression is believed to occur more frequently in patients undergoing combination therapy with radiation and temozolomide, although it is also seen in patients treated only with radiation.[14] Pseudoprogression typically occurs in the 2 to 6 month period following chemoradiation, with a median occurrence time of 3 months.[15] The reported incidence of pseudoprogression ranges from 15 to 30%.[12] Pseudoprogression can have important implications in patient treatment. First, mischaracterization of recurrent tumor as pseudoprogression or vice versa can either delay necessary changes in therapy or result in continuation of an ineffective treatment.[3] Second, pseudoprogression may have important implications for patient prognosis and has been, in fact, associated with improved survival.[11]

Late effects of radiation classically relate to delayed radiation necrosis. These effects generally occur between 3 and 12 months following radiation therapy, although they can be seen up to decades following completion of treatment.[12,16] Radiation necrosis is reported to occur in approximately 3 to 24% of adults undergoing standard radiation therapy.[14] Clinical symptoms related to these late effects of therapy, including focal neurological deficits, seizures, and cognitive dysfunction, as well as symptoms related to swelling, mass effect, and increased intracranial pressure, are typically more severe than those seen early on and are often irreversible.[13,17] In addition, because the clinical presentation of radiation necrosis is difficult to distinguish from tumor progression, decisions regarding patient management are often complicated.

13.3.1 Pathophysiology of Radiation-Induced Central Nervous System Injury

The exact pathophysiological mechanisms leading to radiation damage are still under investigation. However, understanding the changes occurring within the local tissues following radiation therapy is important when attempting to differentiate tumor recurrence from treatment effects based on imaging analysis. The ability of normal brain parenchyma to withstand radiation damage is dependent on a number of factors, including total dose administered, length of exposure, volume of tissue irradiated, as well as other concomitant therapies.[13] Although the pathophysiology leading to radiation-induced brain injury is likely a complex process involving a number of causes, two primary factors have classically been described: injury to the glial cells and injury to the endothelial cells of the cerebral vasculature.[13,18,19]

Studies have shown that oligodendrocytes are radiosensitive, with cell death occurring soon after radiation exposure.[20] In addition, radiation leads to loss of O-2A progenitor cells, which are the source of new oligodendrocytes. Given the radiosensitivity of oligodendrocytes and their precursors, they have long been suspected as a potential etiology for radiation injury. Supporting this is the fact that oligodendrocytes are responsible for the production of myelin, and demyelination is one of the histological changes seen following early delayed radiation injury.[21] However, although radiation effects on oligodendrocytes and their precursors may explain the transient demyelination observed in the early stages of radiation injury, the time course of these changes does not explain the radiation necrosis seen in the later stages.[13,22]

In addition to radiation's effect on oligodendrocytes and their precursors, the early effects of radiation also result in damage and breakdown of the BBB, likely resulting from loosened endothelial tight junctions, vascular leakage, and endothelial cell death.[23,24] Although this initial effect on the BBB is transient, the endothelial cells have already suffered significant chromosomal damage that leads to declining cell numbers.[23] Eventually, once the number of functioning endothelial cells falls below a certain threshold, the integrity of the BBB is severely inhibited, leading to an increase in vascular permeability.[18,23] Such damage to the vasculature subsequently leads to thickening of the vessel walls and hyalinization, as well as fibrinoid necrosis with resultant thrombosis and infarction, finally leading to coagulative necrosis within the perivascular parenchyma.[25]

In addition to the direct deleterious effects of radiation on the vasculature and glial cells, secondary injury due to production of reactive oxygen species and the production of other inflammatory mediators by increased numbers of reactive cells at the site of tissue injury have also been implicated as causes of late effects of radiation therapy.[13]

Pseudoprogression

Although the exact mechanism for pseudoprogression is not known, it likely relates to the changes seen in the BBB during the early subacute phase of radiation injury. These changes result in a combination of increased inflammation, edema, and abnormal vessel permeability in the local tissues following treatment, which in turn allows the movement of fluid into the interstitial space, resulting in brain edema.[11] This alteration in capillary permeability, while enhancing the effect of chemotherapy by allowing maximized uptake of the drug, also leads to increased contrast enhancement.[11] This increased

enhancement and edema results in an overall imaging appearance that mimics tumor progression while actually likely reflecting treatment effect, thus the name *pseudoprogression*.

13.3.2 Radiation Toxicity: Role of Imaging

Acute Radiation Injury

The typical imaging appearance of acute radiation injury on standard MRI is focal edema, which presents as increased T2/FLAIR signal abnormality.[12] A 2009 study by Cao et al found that both vascular volume and BBB permeability showed an initial increase during the course of radiation therapy followed by a gradual decrease after radiation therapy completion.[26] The study also found that areas of the brain receiving the highest doses of radiation showed the most rapid and significant changes.[26] The changes in vascular volume were felt to be secondary to vessel dilation in response to radiation with the increased BBB permeability resulting from endothelial cell death and apoptosis.[26] An earlier study by Cao et al also found that, although increased gadolinium diethylenctriamine penta-acetic acid (Gd-DTPA) uptake was observed in the nonenhancing tumor region following radiation therapy, a similar phenomenon was not seen in the remaining brain during the course of radiation therapy, suggesting a selective effect of radiation on the blood–tumor barrier over the BBB.[24]

Subacute Radiation Injury (Pseudoprogression)

Unfortunately, the morphological features identified in pseudoprogression, including increased enhancement and/or edema, are similar to those seen with early tumor progression. As a result, differentiating the two using morphological MRI is not possible. A study by Young et al assessing the use of conventional MRI in diagnosing pseudoprogression found it to be of limited utility.[27] However, although the study failed to find a sign with sufficient negative predictive value to confidently diagnose pseudoprogression, it did find that subependymal spread of an enhancing lesion was a useful marker for early progression.[27] Similarly, a recent study by Agarwal et al evaluating 20 morphological features in an attempt to differentiate pseudoprogression from early tumor progression found that the only statistically significant findings were larger size of the T2/FLAIR signal abnormality and larger size of the enhancing component, both of which favored early tumor progression.[28] Although the presence of ependymal enhancement, poorly defined margin of the enhancing component, and corpus callosum involvement were all found more often in early tumor progression, the findings were not statistically significant.[28] Despite these findings, currently the only method to definitively diagnose pseudoprogression is based retrospectively on serial follow-up imaging.

Functional Imaging Techniques: Perfusion Imaging

Contrast enhancement in pseudoprogression, a result of increased vessel permeability and disruption of the BBB, is

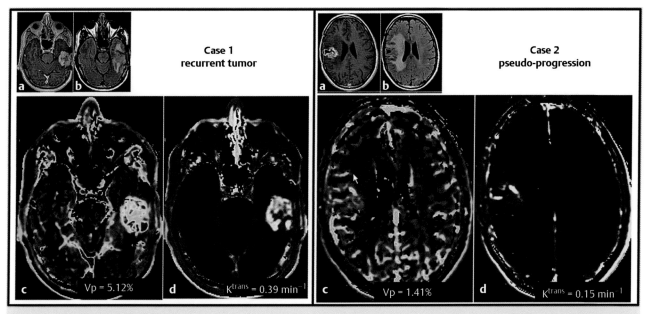

Fig. 13.2 Postcontrast T1-weighted (a) and fluid-attenuated inversion recovery (FLAIR) (b) axial images in two different patients with high-grade gliomas treated with surgery and chemoradiation therapy demonstrate recurrent progressive enhancing lesions within 3 months. Dynamic contrast-enhanced magnetic resonance imaging (DCE-MRI) showing a much higher fractional plasma volume (Vp) and K^{trans} in case 1 (Case 1; c and d) consistent with recurrent tumor and much lower values of these parameters in case 2 (Case 2; c and d) consistent with pseudoprogression.

indistinguishable on MRI from that produced by the process of angiogenesis in progressive tumor, thus precluding their differentiation. However, by assessing changes occurring on the microvasculature level, perfusion imaging allows quantification of certain parameters, including tumor blood volume and vascular permeability, thus providing a potential tool for discriminating between the two processes. Whereas many studies have assessed the performance of perfusion imaging in differentiating radiation necrosis and recurrent progressive tumor, fewer have assessed pseudoprogression. However, radiation necrosis and pseudo-progression have different pathophysiologic mechanisms, but they share a number of similarities, resulting in similar imaging features.[29] In particular, enhancing lesions related to pseudoprogression should demonstrate lower blood volume and permeability when compared to recurrent tumor (▸ Fig. 13.2), reflecting the absence of angiogenesis, as well as lower-grade leakiness due to radiation-induced BBB disruption rather than the marked leakiness associated with angiogenesis and tumor vasculature in recurrent tumor.[29]

A study by Mangla et al confirmed these findings, demonstrating that relative cerebral blood volume (rCBV) at 1 month was able to distinguish pseudoprogression from recurrent progressive disease with a sensitivity of 77% and specificity of 86%.[30] Similarly, a study by Young et al found that pseudoprogression demonstrated a lower median rCBV and lower permeability (measured by percent signal recovery) when compared to disease progression.[29] Gahramanov et al also found lower rCBV in cases of pseudoprogression and, in addition, found that ferumoxytol, a blood pool agent, offered a potentially simpler model for blood volume assessment by not requiring correction for leakage of contrast.[31]

Given the complicated multicompartment physiological models required to quantitatively assess tumor blood volume

and permeability, which potentially limit its clinical applicability, model-free "semiquantitative" indices have also been used in the past to assess tissue perfusion.[32] These semiquantitative methods, in addition to assessing the shape of the uptake and washout of the contrast agent, also offer a variety of non-model-based semiquantitative indices, which provide a more objective means of assessment. These indices include maximum slope of enhancement in the initial vascular phase (MSIVP), which assesses change of signal intensity per second; normalized slope of the delayed equilibrium phase (nSDEP), which is the slope of the fitted linear curve to the final 25% of samples; as well as the initial area under the time–intensity curve (IAUC) at 60 and 120 seconds (IAUC$_{60}$ and IAUC$_{120}$).[32] Using these semiquantitative indices, Jain et al found that pseudoprogression demonstrated a lower mean MSIVP, lower nIAUC$_{60}$, and higher nSDEP compared to early tumor progression (▸ Fig. 13.3).[32]

Functional Imaging Techniques: Diffusion-Weighted Imaging

Diffusion-weighted imaging (DWI) is performed as part of routine serial imaging in brain tumor patients and is sensitive to the microscopic movement of water molecules. Along with the apparent diffusion coefficient (ADC), DWI can help provide information about tumor cellularity, which is not available on conventional MRI. Because increased tumor cellularity leads to a decrease in the volume of the extracellular space, it can be inferred that lower ADC values (more restricted diffusion) may relate to higher cellularity, indicating higher-grade tumor or tumor recurrence, whereas higher ADC values (less restricted diffusion) may relate to low cellularity indicating lower-grade tumor or treatment effects.

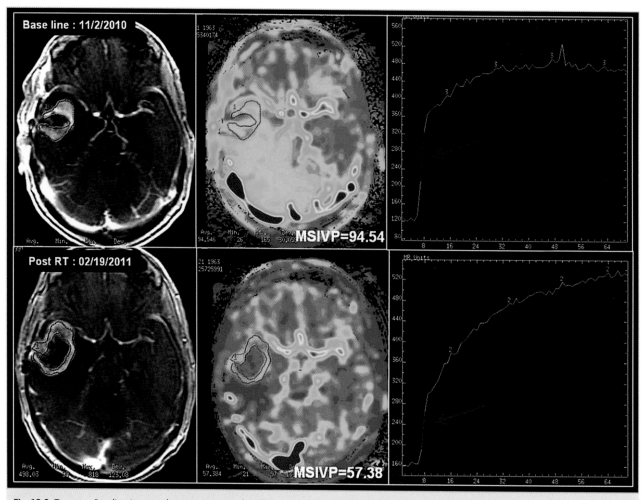

Fig. 13.3 Top row: Baseline images demonstrate an enhancing tumor with maximum slope of enhancement in the initial vascular phase (MSIVP) of 94.54. Bottom row: Post-radiation therapy images demonstrate interval decrease in the MSIVP to 57.38 suggesting response to therapy.

There is not a lot of literature regarding the use of DWI in differentiating pseudoprogression from true progression. A study by Lee et al assessed the pattern of high signal intensity on DWI, as well as mean ADC values, within an enlarging or newly enhancing lesion on first follow-up MRI. The study found that enhancing lesions representing true progression mostly showed homogeneous or multifocal high signal intensity on DWI, whereas lesions representing pseudoprogression mostly demonstrated either high signal intensity at the rim of the lesion or no high signal intensity.[33] The study also found that quantitative analysis of the mean ADC value within the enhancing lesion was able to differentiate true progression from pseudoprogression with a sensitivity, specificity, and accuracy of 80%, 83.3%, and 81.2%, respectively, when a threshold vale of $1,200 \times 10^{-6}$ mm^2/s was used, with the true progression group mostly having values lower than the threshold and the pseudoprogression group mostly having values above the threshold.[33]

Diffusion tensor imaging (DTI) has also been evaluated as a means of differentiating pseudoprogression from true progression. DTI, which uses diffusion-sensitization gradients applied in multiple directions to probe the directionality of water, has been used to demonstrate alteration of white matter tracts by tumor, differentiate high-grade gliomas, and evaluate the extent of cellular infiltration. Quantitative indices in DTI can help discriminate myelin loss and axonal injury and has been used to assess white matter injury in children and adults. However, a study by Agarwal et al found that DTI metrics were not helpful in differentiating between the two groups.[28]

Late Radiation Effects (Delayed Radiation Necrosis)

Radiation necrosis, one of the late effects of radiation injury, most commonly occurs at the site of maximum radiation dose, which is usually in the vicinity of the original tumor and surrounding the surgical cavity.[4] The most common MRI manifestation of radiation necrosis is that of an enhancing mass with central necrosis, the enhancement resulting from BBB breakdown secondary to endothelial cell damage.[4] This typically demonstrates a T2 hypointense solid component with increased signal within the central necrotic component.[4] Kumar et al went on to describe a variety of spatial and temporal MRI patterns that may be seen in radiation necrosis, including (1) development of enhancement within a previously nonenhancing tumor; (2) development of an enhancing focus away from the original site of the primary glioma; (3) development of an enhancing focus within the periventricular white matter, which is among the areas most susceptible to radiation necrosis; and (4) development of a new enhancing lesion exhibiting a soap bubble or Swiss cheese pattern.[4] Kumar et al also found that, because radiation necrosis was a dynamic process, the outcome was not always the same. In particular, they noted that, whereas lesion growth with cytotoxic edema and mass effect is commonly seen, some lesions eventually stabilize and others will actually regress.[4] Unfortunately, differentiating radiation necrosis from recurrent tumor on standard morphological imaging is quite difficult given their many similar characteristics, including proximity to the original tumor site, contrast enhancement, growth over time, edema, and mass effect.[4,34]

Functional Imaging Techniques: Perfusion Imaging

As gliomas grow, there is increased reliance on the process of angiogenesis—promoted by proangiogenic factors such as vascular endothelial growth factor (VEGF)—to provide the nutrients and oxygen required for continued survival and growth.[35] This growth and the subsequent tumor heterogeneity complicate tumor assessment by morphological imaging. However, the abnormal vasculature and resultant altered hemodynamic parameters offer potential functional imaging markers for differentiating recurrent tumor from treatment effects. Prior studies using a variety of dynamic contrast-enhanced perfusion techniques to assess tumor hemodynamics and treatment response have identified a number of perfusion parameters that correlate with tumor grade, aggressiveness, and prognosis.[25]

Using changes in the vasculature and resulting change in hemodynamics, both MR and CT techniques have been developed to help differentiate delayed radiation necrosis from tumor progression. The most commonly used parameter, rCBV, is obtained by comparing a measurement in a particular area of interest, typically at the site of suspected recurrence, and comparing that against a region of normal-appearing white matter in the contralateral hemisphere.[2] Studies have found that an elevated rCBV raises concern for progression of disease, whereas a reduced rCBV is typically indicative of treatment effects and radiation necrosis.[36,37,38] MRI estimation of vascular leakiness (K^{trans}) also offers a means of differentiating radiation necrosis from tumor progression, as blood vessels within previously irradiated tissues, unlike in recurrent tumor, maintain an intact BBB and therefore demonstrate a lower K^{trans} (▶ Fig. 13.4).[25] Also, as with pseudoprogression, semi-quantitative indices can be used to differentiate radiation necrosis and recurrent progressive tumor, with recurrent tumor showing higher MSIVP (▶ Fig. 13.5), nMSIVP, $nIAUC_{60}$, and $nIAUC_{120}$.[32]

Computed tomographic (CT) perfusion is another tool used to assess brain tumor response to treatment by assessing CBV and permeability surface area-product (PS). Although CT perfusion allows both CBV and PS to be obtained in the same examination, the drawback is additional radiation exposure as well as requiring an additional examination—because contrast-enhanced MRI and MR perfusion have become the standard of care in brain tumor follow-up. As with MR perfusion imaging, differentiating recurrent tumor from posttreatment change based on blood volume relies on the differences in vascularity

between the two entities. Although recurrent tumors have high blood volume due to increased tumor vascularity and angiogenesis, posttreatment radiation change will have low blood volume due to damaged blood vessels and hypoperfusion.[18] A 2007 study by Jain et al found that recurrent tumors showed higher nCBV and normalized cerebral blood flow, as well as lower normalized mean transit time when compared to radiation necrosis (▶ Fig. 13.6).[39] A later study by the same group also found that PS estimates increased the accuracy of perfusion CT in differentiating recurrent tumor and posttreatment radiation necrosis.[18]

Functional Imaging Techniques: Proton Magnetic Resonance Spectroscopy (^{1}H-MRS)

Proton MR spectroscopic (MRS) imaging has shown promise in differentiating recurrent progressive tumor and radiation necrosis by characterizing the chemical makeup of targeted regions of interest. It is hypothesized that by detecting early changes in metabolic activity, MRS may be able to predict structural degradation in cerebral tissue following radiation therapy.[12] Spectral patterns in radiation necrosis have been shown to demonstrate decreased N-acetylaspartate (NAA) and variable changes in choline (Cho) and creatine (Cr).[25] In addition, radiation necrosis may show a broad peak corresponding to cellular debris containing fatty acids, lactate (Lac), and amino acids.[25]

A study by Rock et al found that using spectral data for Cho, Cr, NAA, and lipid-lactate (Lip-Lac) allowed for reliable clinical differentiation among spectroscopically normal tissue and pure tumor, mixed tumor and necrosis, and pure necrosis. The study found that elevated (> 1.79) Cho: normal Cr (nCr) ratio or decreased (< 0.75) Lip-Lac: normal Cho (nCho) ratio suggested pure tumor rather than pure necrosis (▶ Fig. 13.7). Similarly, areas demonstrating decreased (< 0.66) Cho:nCho ratio or decreased (< 0.89) Cho:nCr ratio suggested pure necrosis.[21] However, the results were less definitive in tissues composed of varying degrees of mixed tumor and necrosis. In addition, the timing of MRS measurements in relation to treatment must be considered because normal brain tissue can demonstrate an increase in Cho:Cr in the short term (▶ Fig. 13.8).[25]

Functional Imaging Techniques: Diffusion-Weighted Imaging

Although attempts have been made to use ADC values to differentiate radiation necrosis from recurrent tumor, there is disagreement in the literature regarding which has higher ADC values. Although a study by Asao et al found the maximal ADC values in radiation necrosis to be significantly higher than those in tumor recurrence, Sundgren et al found that ADC values in contrast-enhancing lesions were significantly higher for the recurrence group than for the radiation injury group.[40,41]

As with pseudo-progression, DTI has also been used to differentiate radiation necrosis and recurrent tumor. A study by Sundgren et al in 2006 found that both the principal eigenvalue ($\lambda_{\square}$) and the mean of eigenvalues perpendicular to the principle eigenvalue ($\lambda_{\square}$) were significantly higher in contrast-enhancing lesions in the recurrence group than in those in the radiation injury group.[41]

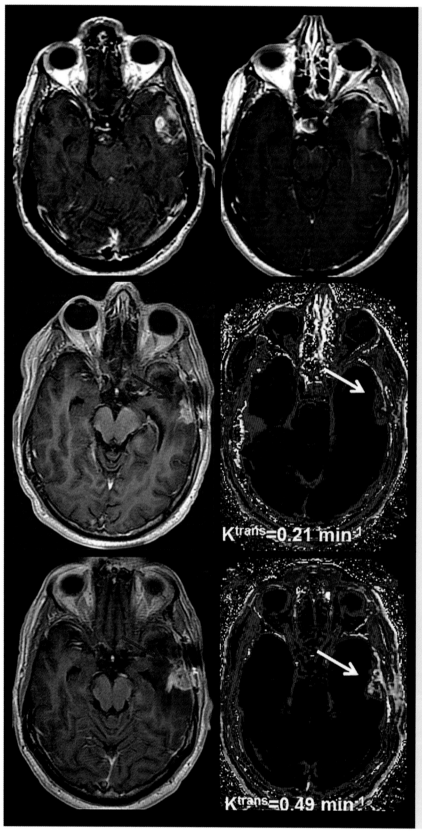

Fig. 13.4 Top row: Preoperative (left) contrast enhanced T1-weighted axial magnetic resonance imaging (MRI) shows a heterogeneously enhancing grade III glioma (red arrow) in the left temporal lobe; (right) immediate postoperative baseline MRI shows mild residual enhancement (red arrow) along the margin of the surgical cavity. Second row: 7-month follow-up imaging showed a progressively increasing lesion on postcontrast T1-weighted images with K^{trans} 0.21 min^{-1} on dynamic contrast-enhanced (DCE) MRI. Third row: Follow-up imaging 1 month later showed increased size of the enhancing lesion with increased K^{trans} on DCET1 consistent with recurrent tumor, which was proven on histopathology.

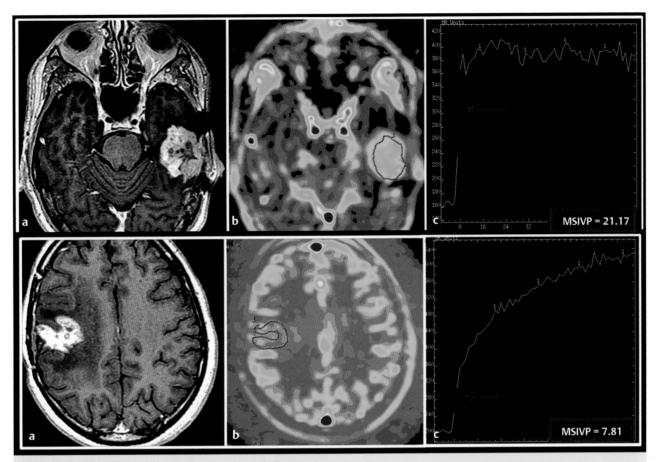

Fig. 13.5 Top row: (**a**) Magnetic resonance imaging (MRI) following resection, chemotherapy, and external beam radiation therapy of astrocytoma showed recurrent enhancing lesion in the left temporal region within the radiation field. (**b**) Maximum slope of enhancement in the initial vascular phase (MSIVP) parametric map and (**c**) graph of MSIVP showed high MSIVP (red arrow) suggesting recurrent/progressive tumor, which was confirmed by histopathology. Bottom row: (**a**) MRI following chemotherapy and external beam radiotherapy (EBR) of glioblastoma multiforme showed recurrent enhancing lesion in the right parietal region. (**b**) MSIVP parametric map and (**c**) graph of MSIVP showed low MSIVP (blue arrow) suggesting treatment-induced necrosis, which was confirmed by histopathology. (Used with permission from Narang J, Jain R, Arbab AS, et al. Differentiating treatment-induced necrosis from recurrent/progressive brain tumor using nonmodel-based semiquantitative indices derived from dynamic contrast-enhanced T1-weighted MR perfusion Neuro-oncology 2011;13(9):1043.)

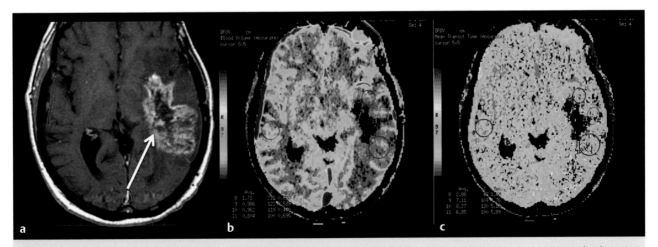

Fig. 13.6 Left temporal-parietal glioma with biopsy-proven radiation necrosis 4.5 years following radiation therapy. Postcontrast T1-weighted imaging (**a**) showing "Swiss-cheese" pattern of enhancement (arrow). Perfusion computed tomography: cerebral blood volume (CBV) (**b**) and mean transit time (MTT) (**c**) maps showing low normalized CBV and higher normalized MTT suggestive of radiation necrosis.

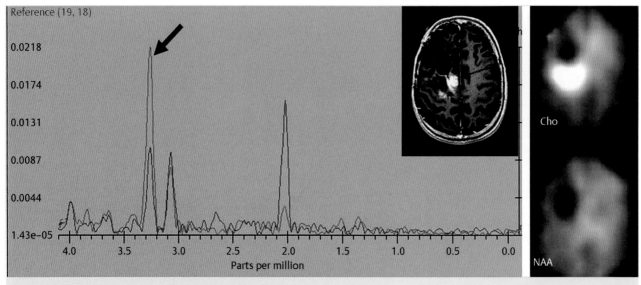

Fig. 13.7 Magnetic resonance spectroscopy (blue line) of a recurrent enhancing lesion (inset, red arrow) in a patient with previously treated high-grade glioma demonstrates increased choline (Cho) (black arrow) with decreased N-acetylaspartate (NAA) (green arrow) suggestive of recurrent tumor. Spectrum from the contralateral normal-appearing white matter (red line) showing normal levels of the metabolites. Corresponding metabolite maps are shown. (Used with permission from Jain R, Narang J, Sundgren PM, et al. Treatment induced necrosis versus recurrent/progressing brain tumor: going beyond the boundaries of conventional morphologic imaging. J Neurooncol 2010;100(1):23.)

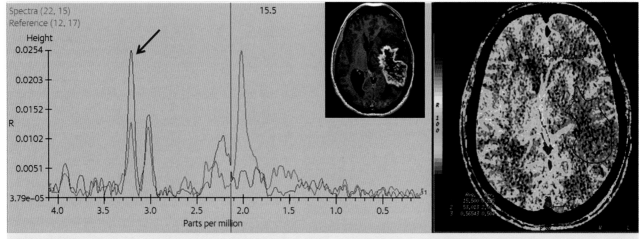

Fig. 13.8 Magnetic resonance spectroscopy (red line) from a recurrent enhancing lesion (inset) shows increased choline:creatine (Cho:Cr) (red arrow) with decrease in the N-acetylaspartate (NAA) suggestive of recurrent tumor. Spectrum from the contralateral normal-appearing white matter (blue line) shows normal levels of the metabolites. However, the perfusion computed tomography blood volume map showed reduced blood volume in the lesion, suggesting predominant treatment effects. Histopathology revealed pure radiation necrosis with no viable tumor cells confirming that the Cho:Cr ratio was probably increased due to active demyelination rather than tumor. (Used with permission from Jain R, Narang J, Sundgren PM, et al. Treatment induced necrosis versus recurrent/progressing brain tumor: going beyond the boundaries of conventional morphologic imaging. J Neurooncol 2010;100(1):23.)

Functional Imaging Techniques: Positron-Emission Tomography Imaging

Evaluating the metabolic properties of a recurrent enhancing lesion using either fluorodeoxyglucose (^{18}F) positron-emission tomography (FDG-PET), ^{11}C-methionine PET, other amino acid analogue tracers, or ^{201}Tl single photon emission computed tomography (SPECT), have also been used to differentiate recurrent progressive tumor from radiation necrosis. These techniques are based on the principle that active tumor should

demonstrate increased metabolism and therefore increased radiotracer uptake, whereas radiation necrosis should demonstrate decreased metabolism (► Fig. 13.9).[25]

One of the difficulties encountered in FDG-PET imaging is the variability of metabolic activity within the adjacent normal brain, which often demonstrates decreased metabolism when compared to normal untreated brain.[42] Thus, when differentiating recurrent tumor from radiation necrosis using FDG-PET, it is important to compare the metabolism of the enhancing lesion to the background activity in the adjacent brain tissue

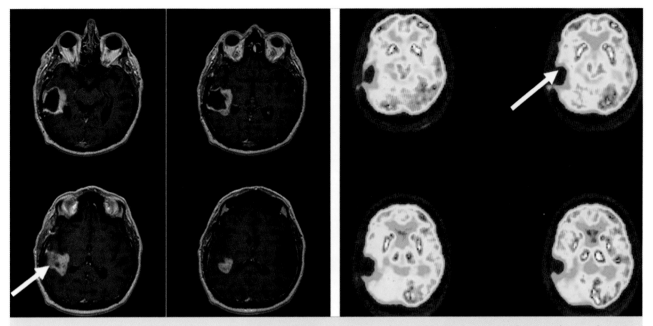

Fig. 13.9 (a) Postcontrast T1-weighted magnetic resonance images show a recurrent enhancing lesion in a patient with previously treated tumor. (b) Fluorodeoxyglucose (^{18}F) positron-emission tomography (FDG-PET) scan shows reduced tracer uptake (arrow) suggestive of hypometabolism. Histopathology revealed radiation necrosis. (Used with permission from Jain R, Narang J, Sundgren PM, et al. Treatment induced necrosis versus recurrent/progressing brain tumor: going beyond the boundaries of conventional morphologic imaging. J Neurooncol 2010;100(1):25.)

rather than to normal, untreated brain parenchyma. A study by Wang et al found [18]FDG-PET to have a sensitivity of 96% and specificity of 77% for distinguishing recurrent tumor from radiation necrosis. In that study, lesions were considered suspicious for recurrent tumor if they demonstrated uptake higher than expected background activity in the adjacent brain tissue or demonstrated uptake in areas showing contrast enhancement.[43]

Additional difficulties in using [18]FDG-PET to differentiate recurrent disease and treatment effects include increased metabolism within nonneoplastic processes, such as abscesses, as well as variable FDG uptake depending on timing of the scan following radiation therapy.[42] Although the optimal timing for performing [18]FDG-PET following radiation therapy is not defined, it is generally recommended that it not be performed until at least 6 weeks following therapy.[42]

Beyond [18]FDG imaging, which evaluates glucose metabolism, a number of additional molecular imaging tracers have also been developed to evaluate different features of tumor physiology, including cellular proliferation, metabolism (glucose, amino acid, oxidative), and hypoxia, among others. These techniques, including their use in differentiating tumor from treatment effects, are discussed in detail in Chapter 12 (Molecular Imaging: PET and SPECT).

13.3.3 Pseudoresponse

Pseudoresponse refers to improvement in the size of the enhancing tumor and/or edema in patients undergoing treatment for brain tumor in the absence of true antitumor effect. The phenomenon occurs when the BBB, which is quite leaky in higher-grade brain tumors, effectively normalizes following particular treatments. The entity has long been known to occur following treatment with corticosteroids, which act to stabilize

the BBB, thereby decreasing tumoral enhancement and surrounding edema. However, the introduction of treatments specifically targeting the VEGF signaling pathway has brought this entity to the forefront of early tumor response assessment.

Two such treatments include bevacizumab, a monoclonal antibody that binds to vascular endothelial growth factor-A (VEGF-A) blocking its interaction with receptors on endothelial cell surfaces, and cediranib, a VEGF receptor tyrosine kinase inhibitor.[25] Both drugs target VEGF-induced angiogenesis and, like corticosteroids, can lead to a rapid reduction in contrast enhancement and surrounding edema.[44] A phase 1 study evaluating bevacizumab in combination with irinotecan found a response rate of 57% with 6-month PFS of 46%.[45] This was markedly better than the response rates of less than 10% and 6-month PFS rates of 15% seen with traditional chemotherapies.[14] These changes were also observed with cediranib, which demonstrated rapid normalization of the BBB following a single dose.[44] However, although these treatments demonstrate improvement in both response rate and 6-month PFS, their effect on overall survival has been minimal,[44] suggesting that measuring response solely based on contrast enhancement and traditional methods overestimated the efficacy of these regimens.

Pathophysiology of Pseudoresponse

The dichotomous response to therapy with anti-VEGF treatment, marked by significant early response to therapy but only modest effect on overall survival, suggests that the early imaging changes correspond to stabilization of the BBB and not a true antitumor effect. This is supported by the rebound enhancement and edema noted in patients requiring drug holidays, as well as subsequent improvement following reinitiation of therapy.[2]

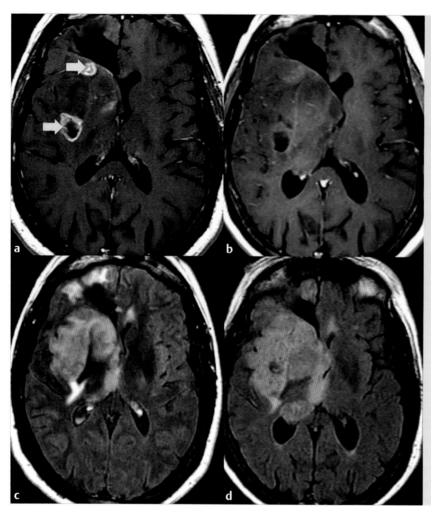

Fig. 13.10 Baseline (**a**) contrast-enhanced T1-weighted and (**c**) T2-weighted fluid-attenuated inversion recovery (FLAIR) axial magnetic resonance imaging (MRI) in a patient with high-grade recurrent glioma shows multiple enhancing areas in the right cerebral hemisphere with surrounding FLAIR signal abnormality. Follow-up imaging 6 weeks after treatment with an antiangiogenic agent (bevacizumab) shows complete response (CR) with resolution of all enhancing areas on the contrast-enhanced T1-weighted MRI (**b**). However, (**d**) the nonenhancing FLAIR signal abnormality and mass effect demonstrates interval increase. This phenomenon has been labeled pseudoresponse.

The hypothesized reasoning behind this response dichotomy is that, although antiangiogenic agents effectively control local response to tumor growth, as evidenced by the decreased enhancement and peritumoral edema, they fail to stop the spread of diffuse infiltrating tumor.[46,47] By inhibiting angiogenesis through blockage of VEGF receptor interactions, antiangiogenic agents lead to decreased microvascular density and vascular permeability, effectively inhibiting local tumor growth.[48] Batchelor et al showed that a single dose of cediranib led to improved tumor enhancement and reduced BBB permeability (measured by K^{trans}) within 24 hours.[44]

However, despite blockage of neoangiogenesis, a subset of glioma cells may actually co-opt existing host vessels to facilitate continued growth.[49] This model is supported by murine models and rat studies, which found that treatment with a VEGF receptor antibody actually promoted tumor growth along preexisting cerebral blood vessels with satellite tumor formation.[50,51] Thus, while resulting in an initial reduction in tumor contrast enhancement, anti-VEGF therapy may also lead to the invasive growth of nonenhancing tumor through vessel co-option.[52]

Role of Imaging in Identifying Pseudoresponse

Following treatment with antiangiogenic therapies, it is common to see a rapid reduction in the degree of contrast enhancement and edema due to inhibition of neoangiogenesis and decreased vascular permeability. However, despite this apparent improvement, there is a concomitant increase in the size of the non-enhancing lesion, which is seen as increased nonenhancing T2 or FLAIR-weighted signal abnormality (▶ Fig. 13.10).

However, although certain imaging findings such as mass effect, cortical ribbon infiltration, and location outside of the radiation field can suggest tumor infiltration, differentiating changes in signal due to tumor progression from other causes such as radiation effect, decreased steroid dose, demyelination, ischemic change, seizures, or other treatment-related effects can remain challenging.[3] In addition, quantifying the change in T2/FLAIR signal due to tumor progression can be difficult as well.[3]

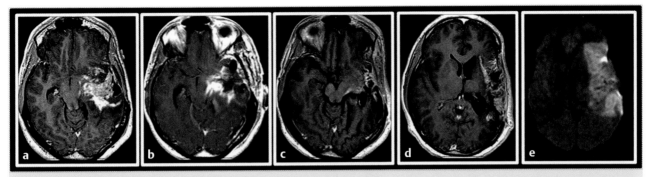

Fig. 13.11 Postoperative infarct with pseudoprogression. Preoperative (**a**) contrast-enhanced T1-weighted axial magnetic resonance imaging (MRI) shows a large heterogeneously enhancing glioma in the left temporal lobe. (**b**) Immediate postoperative baseline MRI shows residual enhancement along the medial margin of the surgical cavity. Follow-up MRI 6 weeks following surgery demonstrates decreased enhancement at the primary tumor site (**c**), but increasing enhancement superior to the resection cavity (**d**), which correlated with an area of large infarct (**e**) on the immediate postoperative MRI scan.

Diffusion-Weighted Imaging

DWI, which is routinely obtained in follow-up imaging of brain tumor patients, is an important supplement to routine MR sequences due to its ability to provide information about tumor cellularity based on assessment of water diffusivity.[48] DWI and calculation of the ADC have been used to distinguish normal white matter from necrosis, cyst formation, edema, and solid enhancing tumor.[48]

Jain et al evaluated the use of DWI as a follow-up tool for recurrent malignant gliomas treated with bevacizumab.[48] The study hypothesized that, due to the antiangiogenic properties of bevacizumab, progressors would show higher volumes of infiltrative nonenhancing lesion with decreased ADC values due to increasing tumor cell density. The study found that both progressors and nonprogressors had an initial decrease in volume of the contrast-enhancing lesion, supporting the limited role of contrast-enhancing lesion size in evaluating response in patients treated with antiangiogenic agents.[48] Additionally, nonprogressors showed no significant change in ADC values, whereas progressors demonstrated a progressive negative change in ADC in both the contrast-enhancing lesion and the non-enhancing lesion, suggesting restricted diffusion due to increased tumor cell density and treatment failure.[48] These findings supported the potential role of ADC values as an early predictor of treatment failure.[48]

Functional diffusion mapping (fDM) was developed as a means of assessing localized differences in diffusion by measuring changes in ADC (ΔADC) in the same patient over time. By assessing localized differences in diffusion, this technique prevents potentially obscuring relevant changes in ADC values within certain tumor segments due to averaging of all values.

The fDM technique has been used to predict the effect of chemotherapy and radiation therapy within both the contrast-enhancing tumor bed and regions of FLAIR signal abnormality.[53] Moffat et al found that areas demonstrating interval increase in ADC correlated with regions of treatment-induced cell death, while regions demonstrating decreased ADC correlated with foci of tumor undergoing rapid cellular proliferation.[54] More recently, Ellingson et al found that graded fDMs, which allow visualization and quantification of more subtle differences in ADC, were more predictive of overall survival than traditional fDMs.[53]

13.3.4 Other Treatment Effects

In addition to the problems related to radiation therapy and antiangiogenic agents, a number of other treatment methods can also complicate the imaging picture. Surgery can lead to development of enhancement at the resection margins between 48 and 72 hours.[3] As a result, the RANO Working Group recommends obtaining a baseline MRI within 24 to 48 hours following surgery.[3] They also recommend the inclusion of DWI in the immediate postoperative period to help differentiate enhancement due to recurrent tumor from sequelae of postoperative ischemia/infarct (▶ Fig. 13.11).[3] ▶ Fig. 13.12 demonstrates a flexible algorithm for imaging of brain tumor patients following treatment that incorporates the use of both conventional and functional imaging.

In addition, a number of locally administered therapies, including chemotherapy wafers, directly administered immunotoxins or gene therapies, immunotherapies, and focal irradiation with brachytherapy can further complicate the post-treatment evaluation of brain tumors.

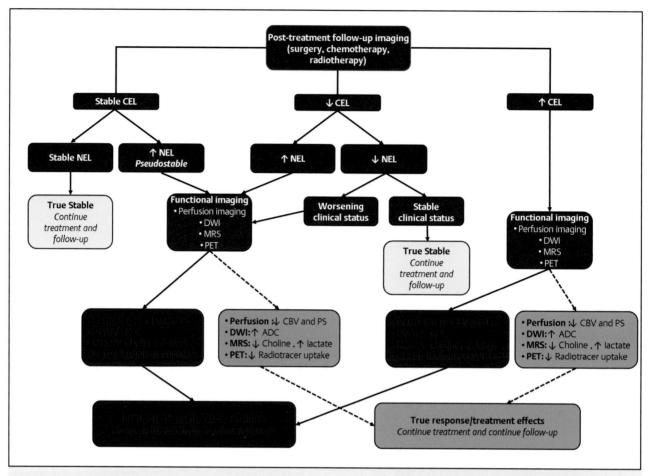

Fig. 13.12 Brain tumor posttreatment follow-up algorithm. (Abbreviations: ADC, apparent diffusion coefficient; CBV, cerebral blood volume; CEL, contrast-enhancing lesion; DWI, diffusion-weighted imaging; MRS, magnetic resonance spectroscopy; NNA, N-acetylaspartate; NEL, nonenhancing lesion; PET, positron emission tomography; PS, permeability surface area product.) (Adapted with permission from Jain R, Narang J, Sundgren PM, et al. Treatment induced necrosis versus recurrent/progressing brain tumor: going beyond the boundaries of conventional morphologic imaging. J Neurooncol 2010;100 (1):23.)

References

[1] Vogelbaum MA, Jost S, Aghi MK et al. Application of novel response/progression measures for surgically delivered therapies for gliomas: Response Assessment in Neuro-Oncology (RANO) Working Group. Neurosurgery 2012; 70: 234–243, discussion 243–244

[2] Clarke JL, Chang S. Pseudoprogression and pseudoresponse: challenges in brain tumor imaging. Curr Neurol Neurosci Rep 2009; 9: 241–246

[3] Wen PY, Macdonald DR, Reardon DA et al. Updated response assessment criteria for high-grade gliomas: response assessment in neuro-oncology working group. J Clin Oncol 2010; 28: 1963–1972

[4] Kumar AJ, Leeds NE, Fuller GN et al. Malignant gliomas: MR imaging spectrum of radiation therapy- and chemotherapy-induced necrosis of the brain after treatment. Radiology 2000; 217: 377–384

[5] Stupp R, Mason WP, van den Bent MJ et al. European Organisation for Research and Treatment of Cancer Brain Tumor and Radiotherapy Groups, National Cancer Institute of Canada Clinical Trials Group. Radiotherapy plus concomitant and adjuvant temozolomide for glioblastoma. N Engl J Med 2005; 352: 987–996

[6] Hygino da Cruz LC, Jr, Rodriguez I, Domingues RC, Gasparetto EL, Sorensen AG. Pseudoprogression and pseudoresponse: imaging challenges in the assessment of posttreatment glioma. AJNR Am J Neuroradiol 2011; 32: 1978–1985

[7] FDA Approval for Bevacizumab. http://www.cancer.gov/cancertopics/druginfo/fda-bevacizumab. Accessed March 4, 2013

[8] Lutz K, Radbruch A, Wiestler B, Bäumer P, Wick W, Bendszus M. Neuroradiological response criteria for high-grade gliomas. Clin Neuroradiol 2011; 21: 199–205

[9] Buatti J, Ryken TC, Smith MC et al. Radiation therapy of pathologically confirmed newly diagnosed glioblastoma in adults. J Neurooncol 2008; 89: 313–337

[10] Rabin BM, Meyer JR, Berlin JW, Marymount MH, Palka PS, Russell EJ. Radiation-induced changes in the central nervous system and head and neck. Radiographics 1996; 16: 1055–1072

[11] Brandes AA, Franceschi E, Tosoni A et al. MGMT promoter methylation status can predict the incidence and outcome of pseudoprogression after concomitant radiochemotherapy in newly diagnosed glioblastoma patients. J Clin Oncol 2008; 26: 2192–2197

[12] Sundgren PC, Cao Y. Brain irradiation: effects on normal brain parenchyma and radiation injury. Neuroimaging Clin N Am 2009; 19: 657–668

[13] Kim JH, Brown SL, Jenrow KA, Ryu S. Mechanisms of radiation-induced brain toxicity and implications for future clinical trials. J Neurooncol 2008; 87: 279–286

[14] Brandsma D, Stalpers L, Taal W, Sminia P, van den Bent MJ. Clinical features, mechanisms, and management of pseudoprogression in malignant gliomas. Lancet Oncol 2008; 9: 453–461

[15] Fatterpekar GM, Galheigo D, Narayana A, Johnson G, Knopp E. Treatment-related change versus tumor recurrence in high-grade gliomas: a diagnostic conundrum—use of dynamic susceptibility contrast-enhanced (DSC) perfusion MRI. AJR Am J Roentgenol 2012; 198: 19–26

[16] Giglio P, Gilbert MR. Cerebral radiation necrosis. Neurologist 2003; 9: 180–188

[17] Shah AH, Snelling B, Bregy A et al. Discriminating radiation necrosis from tumor progression in gliomas: a systematic review what is the best imaging modality? J Neurooncol 2013; 112: 141–152

[18] Jain R, Narang J, Schultz L et al. Permeability estimates in histopathology-proved treatment-induced necrosis using perfusion CT: can these add to other perfusion parameters in differentiating from recurrent/progressive tumors? AJNR Am J Neuroradiol 2011; 32: 658–663

[19] Hopewell JW. Radiation injury to the central nervous system. Med Pediatr Oncol 1998 Suppl 1: 1–9

[20] Vrdoljak E, Bill CA, Stephens LC, van der Kogel AJ, Ang KK, Tofilon PJ. Radiation-induced apoptosis of oligodendrocytes in vitro. Int J Radiat Biol 1992; 62: 475–480

[21] Rock JP, Hearshen D, Scarpace L et al. Correlations between magnetic resonance spectroscopy and image-guided histopathology, with special attention to radiation necrosis. Neurosurgery 2002; 51: 912–919, discussion 919–920

[22] New P. Radiation injury to the nervous system. Curr Opin Neurol 2001; 14: 725–734

[23] Remler MP, Marcussen WH, Tiller-Borsich J. The late effects of radiation on the blood brain barrier. Int J Radiat Oncol Biol Phys 1986; 12: 1965–1969

[24] Cao Y, Tsien CI, Shen Z et al. Use of magnetic resonance imaging to assess blood-brain/blood-glioma barrier opening during conformal radiotherapy. J Clin Oncol 2005; 23: 4127–4136

[25] Jain R, Narang J, Sundgren PM et al. Treatment induced necrosis versus recurrent/progressing brain tumor: going beyond the boundaries of conventional morphologic imaging. J Neurooncol 2010; 100: 17–29

[26] Cao Y, Tsien CI, Sundgren PC et al. Dynamic contrast-enhanced magnetic resonance imaging as a biomarker for prediction of radiation-induced neurocognitive dysfunction. Clin Cancer Res 2009; 15: 1747–1754

[27] Young RJ, Gupta A, Shah AD et al. Potential utility of conventional MRI signs in diagnosing pseudoprogression in glioblastoma. Neurology 2011; 76: 1918–1924

[28] Agarwal A, Kumar S, Narang J et al. Morphologic MRI features, diffusion tensor imaging and radiation dosimetric analysis to differentiate pseudoprogression from early tumor progression. J Neurooncol 2013; 112: 413–420

[29] Young RJ, Gupta A, Shah AD et al. MRI perfusion in determining pseudoprogression in patients with glioblastoma. Clin Imaging 2013; 37: 41–49

[30] Mangla R, Singh G, Ziegelitz D et al. Changes in relative cerebral blood volume 1 month after radiation-temozolomide therapy can help predict overall survival in patients with glioblastoma. Radiology 2010; 256: 575–584

[31] Gahramanov S, Muldoon LL, Varallyay CG et al. Pseudoprogression of glioblastoma after chemo- and radiation therapy: diagnosis by using dynamic susceptibility-weighted contrast-enhanced perfusion MR imaging with ferumoxytol versus gadoteridol and correlation with survival. Radiology 2013; 266: 842–852

[32] Narang J, Jain R, Arbab AS et al. Differentiating treatment-induced necrosis from recurrent/progressive brain tumor using nonmodel-based semiquantitative indices derived from dynamic contrast-enhanced T1-weighted MR perfusion. Neuro-oncol 2011; 13: 1037–1046

[33] Lee WJ, Choi SH, Park CK et al. Diffusion-weighted MR imaging for the differentiation of true progression from pseudoprogression following concomitant radiotherapy with temozolomide in patients with newly diagnosed high-grade gliomas. Acad Radiol 2012; 19: 1353–1361

[34] Rogers LR, Gutierrez J, Scarpace L et al. Morphologic magnetic resonance imaging features of therapy-induced cerebral necrosis. J Neurooncol 2011; 101: 25–32

[35] Jain R, Griffith B, Narang J et al. Blood-brain-barrier imaging in brain tumors: Concepts and methods. Neurographics 2012; 2: 48–59

[36] Cha S, Lupo JM, Chen MH et al. Differentiation of glioblastoma multiforme and single brain metastasis by peak height and percentage of signal intensity recovery derived from dynamic susceptibility-weighted contrast-enhanced perfusion MR imaging. AJNR Am J Neuroradiol 2007; 28: 1078–1084

[37] Hu LS, Baxter LC, Smith KA et al. Relative cerebral blood volume values to differentiate high-grade glioma recurrence from posttreatment radiation effect: direct correlation between image-guided tissue histopathology and localized dynamic susceptibility-weighted contrast-enhanced perfusion MR imaging measurements. AJNR Am J Neuroradiol 2009; 30: 552–558

[38] Barajas RF, Chang JS, Sneed PK, Segal MR, McDermott MW, Cha S. Distinguishing recurrent intra-axial metastatic tumor from radiation necrosis following gamma knife radiosurgery using dynamic susceptibility-weighted contrast-enhanced perfusion MR imaging. AJNR Am J Neuroradiol 2009; 30: 367–372

[39] Jain R, Scarpace L, Ellika S et al. First-pass perfusion computed tomography: initial experience in differentiating recurrent brain tumors from radiation effects and radiation necrosis. Neurosurgery 2007; 61: 778–786, discussion 786–787

[40] Asao C, Korogi Y, Kitajima M et al. Diffusion-weighted imaging of radiation-induced brain injury for differentiation from tumor recurrence. AJNR Am J Neuroradiol 2005; 26: 1455–1460

[41] Sundgren PC, Fan X, Weybright P et al. Differentiation of recurrent brain tumor versus radiation injury using diffusion tensor imaging in patients with new contrast-enhancing lesions. Magn Reson Imaging 2006; 24: 1131–1142

[42] Chen W. Clinical applications of PET in brain tumors. J Nucl Med 2007; 48: 1468–1481

[43] Wang SX, Boethius J, Ericson K. FDG-PET on irradiated brain tumor: ten years' summary. Acta Radiol 2006; 47: 85–90

[44] Batchelor TT, Sorensen AG, di Tomaso E et al. AZD2171, a pan-VEGF receptor tyrosine kinase inhibitor, normalizes tumor vasculature and alleviates edema in glioblastoma patients. Cancer Cell 2007; 11: 83–95

[45] Vredenburgh JJ, Desjardins A, Herndon JE, II et al. Bevacizumab plus irinotecan in recurrent glioblastoma multiforme. J Clin Oncol 2007; 25: 4722–4729

[46] Norden AD, Young GS, Setayesh K et al. Bevacizumab for recurrent malignant gliomas: efficacy, toxicity, and patterns of recurrence. Neurology 2008; 70: 779–787

[47] Narayana A, Kelly P, Golfinos J et al. Antiangiogenic therapy using bevacizumab in recurrent high-grade glioma: impact on local control and patient survival. J Neurosurg 2009; 110: 173–180

[48] Jain R, Scarpace LM, Ellika S et al. Imaging response criteria for recurrent gliomas treated with bevacizumab: role of diffusion weighted imaging as an imaging biomarker. J Neurooncol 2010; 96: 423–431

[49] Holash J, Maisonpierre PC, Compton D et al. Vessel cooption, regression, and growth in tumors mediated by angiopoietins and VEGF. Science 1999; 284: 1994–1998

[50] Kunkel P, Ulbricht U, Bohlen P et al. Inhibition of glioma angiogenesis and growth in vivo by systemic treatment with a monoclonal antibody against vascular endothelial growth factor receptor-2. Cancer Res 2001; 61: 6624–6628

[51] Rubenstein JL, Kim J, Ozawa T et al. Anti-VEGF antibody treatment of glioblastoma prolongs survival but results in increased vascular cooption. Neoplasia 2000; 2: 306–314

[52] Bergers G, Hanahan D. Modes of resistance to anti-angiogenic therapy. Nat Rev Cancer 2008; 8: 592–603

[53] Ellingson BM, Cloughesy TF, Lai A et al. Graded functional diffusion map-defined characteristics of apparent diffusion coefficients predict overall survival in recurrent glioblastoma treated with bevacizumab. Neuro-oncol 2011; 13: 1151–1161

[54] Moffat BA, Chenevert TL, Meyer CR et al. The functional diffusion map: an imaging biomarker for the early prediction of cancer treatment outcome. Neoplasia 2006; 8: 259–267

14 It's Not Just the Tumor: CNS Paraneoplastic Syndromes and Cerebrovascular Complications of Cancers

Prashant Nagpal and Rajan Jain

14.1 Introduction

A variety of neurologic complications and syndromes can be seen in patients with cancer. Other than direct tumor infiltration and/or metastatic spread, neurologic symptoms may arise in cancer patients due to a paraneoplastic cause or stroke and cerebrovascular complications, which in turn may be due to direct tumor-related causes or the side effects of tumor therapy. Stroke and cerebrovascular complications may be responsible for significant morbidity and mortality in patients with cancer and are the second most common pathology of the nervous system, seen in around 15% of cases in various autopsy series.[1,2]

Paraneoplastic syndromes are the remote effects of the primary tumor and encompass various disorders unrelated to direct tumor invasion of the nervous system or resulting from the indirect effects of the cancer and its therapies, such as infections, coagulopathy, metabolic disturbance, or other side effects of treatment.[3,4] The term *paraneoplastic* was first introduced by Guichard and Vignon in a patient with uterine cancer presenting with multiple cranial and radicular neuropathies.[5] However, the first report of involvement of the peripheral nervous system in a patient with known malignancy dates back to late 19th century.[6] The pathogenesis of these syndromes is poorly understood; however, most studies have shown them to be due to immune response to the underlying malignancy. Knowledge of these entities in patients with cancer is crucial because their pathogenesis in this subgroup differs from that in the general population; hence their correct identification may be necessary for appropriate treatment to be initiated. The clinical manifestations of these neurologic complications may in fact precede the detection of primary tumor in a significant proportion of cases. Hence recognition of these syndromes is even more important because they provide a window for early detection of cancer and can impact patient management and survival.

Neuroimaging plays a crucial role in evaluation of cancer patients. In cases with extra central nervous system (CNS) malignancy presenting with neurologic symptoms, neuroimaging is used primarily to rule out the metastatic spread of disease. A computed tomographic (CT) scan is usually the first imaging test performed in these patients, and magnetic resonance imaging (MRI) is then performed for further evaluation and better characterization of the disease. Angiography or venography is performed in patients suspected to have stroke and cerebrovascular complications and can be noninvasive with the use of CT or magnetic resonance angiography (MRA) or venography techniques. Catheter angiography (digital subtraction angiography) is usually reserved for patients who need more detailed examination of the vasculature or patients needing endovascular therapeutic intervention.

This chapter describes various CNS paraneoplastic syndromes and cerebrovascular complications commonly seen in cancer patients with an emphasis on early diagnosis based on characteristic imaging features.

14.2 CNS Paraneoplastic Syndromes

14.2.1 Cerebellar Degeneration

Paraneoplastic cerebellar degeneration (PCD) is a well known entity associated commonly with small cell lung cancer, gynecological and breast cancers, as well as Hodgkin lymphoma.[7] This disorder is usually associated with the presence of anti-Yo, anti-Hu, or anti-Tr antibodies in the cerebrospinal fluid (CSF). The loss of Purkinje cells in the cerebellum is the pathognomonic finding on histology. Though the clinical manifestations (ataxia, diplopia, and dysarthria) are disabling, neuroimaging in the early stage of disease is usually unremarkable. Abnormal enlargement of the cerebellar hemisphere and corticomeningeal enhancement have been shown in some instances,[8] and a few case reports have shown fluid-attenuated inversion recovery (FLAIR) signal abnormalities in patients with fulminant cerebellar degeneration. Functional imaging techniques like positron-emission tomographic (PET) scan can help in earlier diagnosis of this entity. In the initial phase a fluorodeoxyglucose (FDG)-PET scan shows increased tracer uptake within the cerebellum, even in patients with a normal-appearing MRI scan. However, in the later stages, CT and MRI scans show diffuse cerebellar atrophy (most marked in midline), and PET scans demonstrate decreased tracer uptake.[9]

14.2.2 Limbic Encephalitis

Paraneoplastic limbic encephalitis (PLE) is the inflammatory disorder confined to the limbic system due to autoimmune response to cancer cells. The malignancies commonly associated with this are small cell lung cancer, testicular germ cell neoplasms, thymoma, teratoma, and Hodgkin lymphoma.[10] Unlike most other CNS paraneoplastic disorders, the imaging studies are abnormal in the majority of patients with PLE. MRI usually shows bilateral but asymmetric increased T2 and FLAIR signal in the amygdala region and hippocampal formation of mesial temporal lobes (▸ Fig. 14.1). Involvement of the unilateral temporal lobe can be seen as well and additionally the altered signal may also extend into other limbic structures like the insular cortex.[11] Contrast enhancement is rare and, if present, is usually minimal. Diffusion-weighted and high-resolution FLAIR sequences are shown to be better than conventional spin-echo sequences for earlier diagnosis of the condition.[12] Involvement of brain cortex prior to involvement of the temporal lobe in these patients has also been reported (▸ Fig. 14.2).[13] A case series on PLE showed bilateral temporal lobe involvement in around 70% of cases, with extra temporal cortical signal abnormality in 37% and abnormal contrast enhancement in 21% of patients.[14] With time, the T2 hyperintense signal decreases and focal, temporal, or generalized cerebral atrophy ensues. An

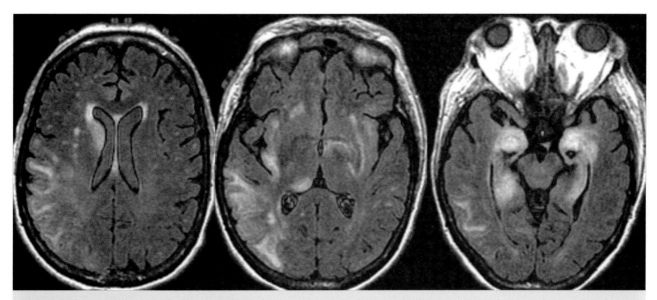

Fig. 14.1 Limbic encephalitis. Axial fluid-attenuated inversion recovery magnetic resonance imaging in a patient with memory loss and altered mental status, showing involvement of the bilateral mesial temporal lobes and asymmetric involvement of the bilateral insular cortices as well as the right cerebral cortex. During further workup, he was diagnosed with small cell lung cancer and had anti-Hu antibodies.

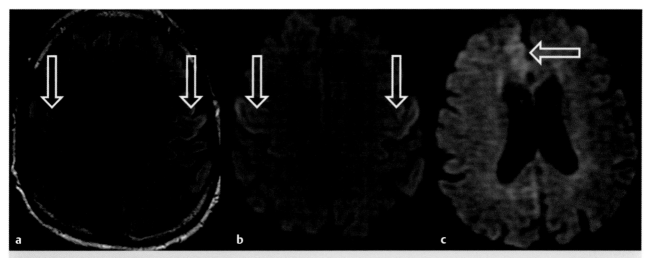

Fig. 14.2 Limbic encephalitis. (**a**) Axial fluid-attenuated inversion recovery and (**b**) diffusion-weighted imaging (DWI) in a patient with known pancreatic adenocarcinoma and seizure showing subtle increased signal within bilateral precentral cortex (arrows). (**c**) Axial DWI in another patient with lung cancer showing only involvement of the right cingulate gyrus and medial frontal lobe.

FDG-PET scan shows hypermetabolism in the affected areas. MRI signal abnormality in these patients does not vary with levels of oncoantibodies associated with limbic encephalitis. However, the tracer uptake on FDG-PET is shown to increase simultaneously with increase in the level of oncoantibodies. Hence the tracer uptake in these patients may also help to assess response to the treatment.[15]

The temporal lobe may be affected by various other pathologies with overlapping clinical manifestations; imaging plays an important role in diagnosis and differentiation of these disorders. Infectious encephalitis (e.g., herpes), non-PLE mesial temporal sclerosis, and gliomatosis cerebri are other disorders that may have imaging similar to this. Differentiation of limbic encephalitis from herpes encephalitis is the primary consideration. PLE tends to have multifocal brain involvement, lesser local

mass effect, and a lesser degree of contrast enhancement on MRI scans. The presence of associated antibodies and a history of cancer (if already diagnosed) may further add to the diagnosis of PLE.[11]

14.2.3 Brainstem Encephalitis

Paraneoplastic brainstem encephalitis is often seen along with the presence of other paraneoplastic syndromes like limbic encephalitis, cerebellar degeneration, or multifocal encephalomyelitis.[16] It is seen in patients with small-cell carcinoma of the lung, testicular tumors, breast cancer, hypernephroma, or prostate cancer and is commonly associated with the presence of anti-Hu, anti-NMDAR, or anti-Ma2 antibodies in serum or CSF.[17,18] MRI may show T2/FLAIR hyperintensity in the

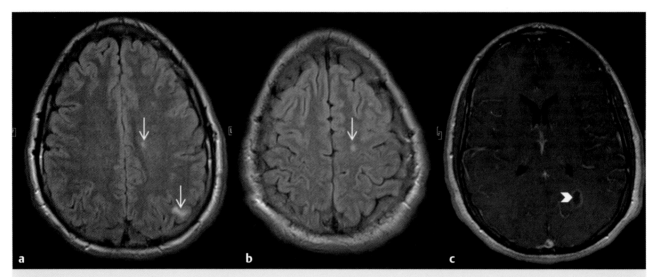

Fig. 14.3 Paraneoplastic encephalitis. (**a, b**) Axial fluid-attenuated inversion recovery magnetic resonance imaging in a patient with behavioral disturbances and positive anti-NMDA (*N*-methyl-D-aspartate) receptor antibodies in the serum and cerebrospinal fluid showing multiple subcortical white matter lesions on the left side (arrows). (**c**) One of the deep white matter lesions also shows peripheral enhancement (arrowhead) on postcontrast T1-weighted image. (Courtesy of Suyash Mohan, MD, University of Pennsylvania.)

midbrain tectum, periaqueductal gray matter, substantia nigra, pons, medulla, and superior/middle cerebellar peduncles. Contrast enhancement is usually not seen, but nodular enhancement along the structures just described has also been reported.[19,20] Though uncommon, involvement of the cortex or the juxtacortical white matter (► Fig. 14.3) along with involvement of brainstem may be seen in patients with onconeural antibodies. The radiological differential diagnosis of paraneoplastic brainstem encephalitis includes infectious encephalitis, vasculitis, demyelination, or low-grade glial neoplasm.

14.2.4 Striatal Encephalitis or Chorea

Paraneoplastic striatal encephalitis is most often seen in patients with small cell lung cancer and thymoma and is commonly associated with presence of anti-CV2/CRMP-5 antibodies.[21] MRI in these patients is often abnormal and may show T2/FLAIR signal abnormality in bilateral caudate nuclei and putamen. The signal abnormality may also extend into the adjacent white matter. There is usually no contrast enhancement or restricted diffusion (increased signal) on diffusion-weighted imaging (DWI).[17] Basal ganglia signal changes are seen to resolve with clinical improvement of the patient condition. With this imaging appearance, the radiological differential diagnosis of paraneoplastic striatal encephalitis includes viral encephalitis, sporadic Creutzfeldt-Jakob disease (CJD), acute disseminated encephalomyelitis (ADEM), anoxic brain injury, and various metabolic conditions. Absence of restricted diffusion and extension of signal abnormality into the adjacent white matter help to distinguish paraneoplastic striatal encephalitis from prion disease. On MRI scans the presence of signal abnormalities associated with other paraneoplastic CNS disorders

may also help to distinguish paraneoplastic striatal encephalitis from other radiological differentials.

14.2.5 Paraneoplastic Myelitis

Paraneoplastic myelitis is a severely disabling disorder of the spinal cord and is associated with various cancers (lung, breast, kidney, and ovary) in the literature.[22,23] Symmetric, longitudinally extensive tract or gray matter-specific T2/FLAIR hyperintensity, which may enhance on contrast administration, has been described in these patients on spine MRI.[20]

14.2.6 Hypertrophic Polyneuropathy

Hypertrophic polyneuropathy is a rare paraneoplastic neurologic disorder that is characterized by thickening and necrosis of the involved nerve roots. It has been reported with lung tumor, carcinoid, melanoma, lymphoproliferative malignancies, and malignant thymoma.[24,25,26,27] Characteristically, inflammatory and malignant cells are absent within the involved nerves, distinguishing it from inflammatory demyelinating polyneuropathy or a metastatic disease, which are common causes of neuropathy. Although there is no classical onconeural antibody associated with hypertrophic polyneuropathy, various nonspecific antibodies may be seen in patients with paraneoplastic neuropathy. There may be involvement of single or multiple nerve roots, and there is varying involvement of sensory and motor nerve fibers. Selective involvement of multiple cauda equina nerve roots has been reported.[26,27,28] On MRI scan, hypertrophic polyneuropathy is characterized by thickening of the involved nerve roots, which enhance on contrast administration (► Fig. 14.4). Hypertrophy and enhancement of these nerve roots have been reported to resolve following resection of the primary tumor.[29]

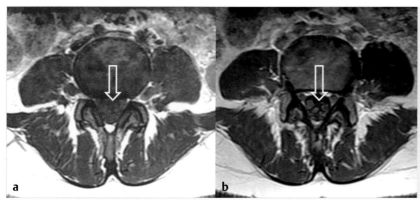

Fig. 14.4 Paraneoplastic hypertrophic polyneuropathy. (**a**) Pre- and (**b**) postcontrast enhanced T1 axial magnetic resonance images showing marked thickening and enhancement (arrows) of the cauda equina nerve roots in a patient with known malignant thymoma. Cerebrospinal fluid was negative for any malignant cells.

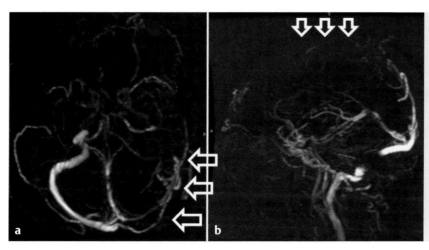

Fig. 14.5 Dural venous thrombosis. Three-dimensional phase contrast magnetic resonance venogram, reformatted maximum intensity projection (**a**) caudal and (**b**) sagittal view showing nonvisualization of the right transverse and sigmoid sinus (arrows in **a**) and the superior sagittal sinus (arrows in **b**) consistent with venous sinus thrombosis in a patient with breast carcinoma.

14.3 Tumor-Related Stroke and Cerebrovascular Complications

14.3.1 Cerebral Venous Thrombosis

Cerebral venous thrombosis (CVT) may occur due to a hypercoagulable state in cancer patients or it may be because of direct invasion of the dural venous sinuses by primary brain neoplasm or metastatic deposits in meninges/calvarium.[29] Patients with CVT may present with headache, convulsions, focal neurologic deficits, or coma. The presence of thrombosis of vessels of extra-CNS organ systems may be a useful clue to diagnosis.

Noncontrast CT (NCCT) is usually the first imaging investigation in these patients and may show a hyperdense thrombus within the dural venous sinus or the cortical vein. Further, there may be infarction (hemorrhagic or nonhemorrhagic) within the brain parenchyma that does not conform to any arterial territory. On contrast administration, there may be enhancement of the margins of the dural venous sinus (known as the empty-delta sign) due to collateral veins within the walls of the dural venous sinus and prominent tentorial enhancement due to retrograde venous congestion.[30] However, conventional CT findings may be insignificant in a third of these patients. With advances in CT technology, CT venography can be quickly obtained in these patients and with faster scans and isotropic acquisition; three-dimensional reformats can be obtained from

the data. CT venography is not limited by flow artifacts as in MRI, is faster to obtain, and may be obtained in the setting of the initial CT study if the clinical suspicion is high. CT venography has been shown to be equally as good as MR venography in these patients in various studies.[31,32,33]

MRI is better for detection of parenchymal changes in these patients. On conventional fast spin-echo sequences, thrombosed venous sinuses are seen as loss of normal flow voids. In the very early stage (< 5 days), the thrombosed sinus appears isointense on T1-weighted MRI and hypointense on T2-weighted MRI and hence may be missed on conventional MRI. However, MR venography overcomes this and shows nonvisualization of thrombosed sinus (▶ Fig. 14.5). MRI is also better for delineation of parenchymal changes (edema, hemorrhagic, or nonhemorrhagic infarct) of the CVT.[34] DWI is a relatively new tool in imaging of patients with CVT. On DWI, the brain parenchyma shows heterogeneous signal with increased or normal apparent diffusion coefficient (ADC). These signal changes signify the presence of a combination of vasogenic and cytotoxic edema. The combination of these MRI sequences is usually helpful in diagnosis of cerebral venous sinus thrombosis. But in equivocal cases or in patients with isolated cortical venous thrombosis, conventional catheter angiography may be required. The direct sign of cerebral sinus thrombosis is nonvisualization of the venous sinus. The other indirect signs, which may point to the occlusion of the cerebral venous system, are dilatation of collateral veins with a corkscrew appearance, delayed venous emptying, and dilation of collateral circulation.[35] Another

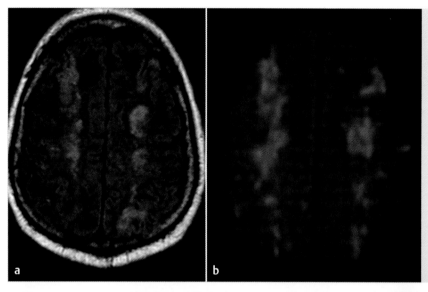

Fig. 14.6 Hypereosinophilic syndrome (HES). Axial (**a**) fluid-attenuated inversion recovery and (**b**) diffusion-weighted imaging in a patient with hypereosinophilia who presented with stroke, showing multiple acute infarcts in both cerebral hemispheres.

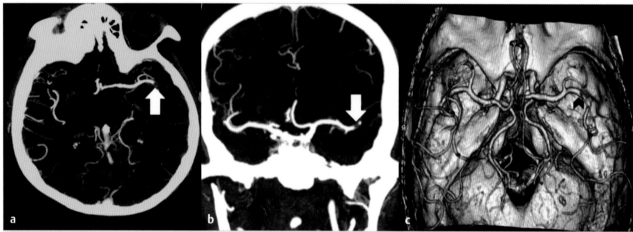

Fig. 14.7 Nonbacterial thrombotic endocarditis (NBTE). (**a**) Axial, (**b**) coronal maximum intensity projection, and (**c**) three-dimensional surface shaded volume rendered computed tomographic angiogram images in a patient with renal cell carcinoma shows a well-defined intraluminal filling defect in the distal M1 segment of the left middle cerebral artery (arrows) with resultant paucity of its distal branches. Echocardiogram (not shown) in this patient showed multiple small vegetations on cardiac valves suggesting NBTE.

possible mechanism of cerebral sinus thrombosis in patients with tumor is by direct invasion or compression of the venous structures by parenchymal, dural, or calvarial metastases. CT and MRI both may show the enhancing mass responsible for venous thrombosis. However, these imaging modalities may not be able to distinguish bland and tumor thrombus. There may be enhancement of tumor thrombus, but the same may also be seen in the subacute stage of bland thrombus.

14.3.2 Ischemic Stroke and Arterial Compromise

The occlusion of the arterial system too can be either due to systemic hypercoagulable stage in cancer patients or due to compression/invasion of the arterial structures by the mass. The arterial occlusion may also be caused by abnormal activation of the coagulation system in cancer patients due to disseminated intravascular coagulation (DIC) or due to nonbacterial thrombotic endocarditis (NBTE) in which sterile platelet-fibrin vegetations on the cardiac valves may embolize to cerebral

circulation and hence lead to stroke in these patients. NBTE should be considered in all cancer patients with acute embolic stroke and especially in patients with multiterritorial or multiple organ system emboli.[36] Echocardiography is useful in patients suspected with NBTE to look for vegetations. Ischemic stroke may also be seen in patients with hypereosinophilia syndrome (HES). An increased number of circulating eosinophils causes damage to the cardiac endocardium and myocardium, which may then embolize to cause stroke in these patients. In the early stage, HES infarcts classically involve the arterial watershed zones, whereas in later stages large infarcts often involve the cortex and subcortical region (▶ Fig. 14.6).[37,38] Depending on the involved arterial territory, patients may present with neurologic deficits. In the hyperacute stage, the NCCT may be normal in patients with acute embolic stroke. Later, there is hypodensity in the involved territorial distribution with edema and loss of gray–white matter interface. Using multidetector CT scanners, CT angiography can be done in the same setting with the initial CT, and the exact site of arterial block can be determined (▶ Fig. 14.7).[39] MRI along with MRA is more

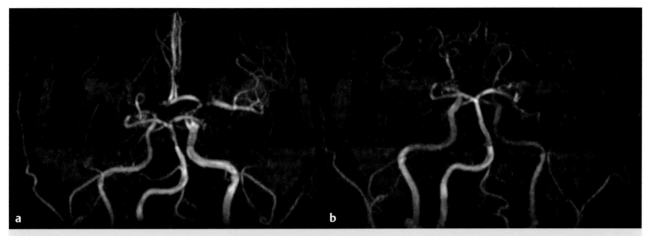

Fig. 14.8 Paraneoplastic vasculitis. (**a**) Maximum intensity projection magnetic resonance angiography (MRA) image in a patient with thymic carcinoma showing marked irregularity and narrowing of bilateral supraclinoid internal carotid arteries, worse on the right side. The patient did not respond to treatment and (**b**) MRA done 1 month later shows worsening of the narrowing of the left internal carotid artery.

sensitive for detection of acute stroke. DWI is especially useful for early detection of ischemic stroke in these patients.

Tumors adjacent to the intracranial arterial structures occasionally lead to stroke by encasement, compression, infiltration, or displacement of these vessels. Some of the tumors that have caused arterial compromise via these mechanisms are craniopharyngioma, suprasellar germinoma, hypothalamic tumors, pituitary adenoma with apoplexy, and astrocytoma.[40,41] Hence stroke in cancer patients can be caused by a varied pathogenesis, but careful clinical assessment, imaging studies, assessment of coagulation profile, and echocardiography are the most useful modalities to identify the cause of stroke.

14.3.3 Paraneoplastic Vasculitis

Vasculitis in a patient with cancer may occur as an immune-mediated process and usually involves the small- or medium-sized vessels. Paraneoplastic vasculitis is usually associated with hematological malignancies but may also occur in a few solid tumors, such as small-cell lung cancer, and renal and gastrointestinal neoplasias. Clinically, these patients present with acute/subacute encephalopathy rather than focal neurologic deficits. MRI findings are nonspecific and may show the presence of infarcts in both cerebral hemispheres. Vascular luminal compromise is seen on angiography (▶ Fig. 14.8). The role of imaging is to rule out cerebral metastases, carcinomatous meningitis, and other common entities that may present with acute/subacute encephalopathy. A biopsy will show the presence of lymphocytic vascular damage along with infarcts, which is highly suggestive of the disorder.

14.3.4 Neoplastic Aneurysms and Tumor Emboli

Neoplastic aneurysm is a rare entity described in patients with lung cancer, cardiac myxoma, or choriocarcinoma.[42,43,44] The neoplastic aneurysm is usually seen in small peripheral arteries due to infiltration of the vessel wall by the tumor cells and resultant weakening of the internal elastic lamina. Neoplastic

aneurysms can be very small and may mimic systemic necrotizing vasculitis on imaging studies. CT and MRI play a primary role in diagnosis of parenchymal/subarachnoid hemorrhage due to these aneurysms. However, these small peripheral aneurysms are best diagnosed by conventional catheter angiography.[45] These are seen as small, irregular, fusiform outpouching from the walls of distal arteries.

Tumor fragments may also embolize to the cerebral circulation and cause cerebral ischemia. Tumor itself or thrombus overlying the tumor may detach and enter the systemic circulation with involvement of cerebral circulation in approximately 50% of cases with tumor emboli.[46] These tumor emboli have been reported mostly in patients with cardiac myxoma or in patients with lung cancer during surgical resection.[47,48,49] Due to the dominant flow vessel, these tumor emboli usually involve the middle cerebral artery territory (▶ Fig. 14.9). They may further progress to formation of discrete parenchymal metastatic masses or may lead to neoplastic aneurysm.[39]

14.3.5 Hemorrhagic Stroke

Hemorrhage within the tumor mass is the most common cause of hemorrhagic stroke in patients with solid brain tumors. It is more commonly seen in metastatic deposits than in primary brain neoplasms.[50] The pathological mechanism of hemorrhage within brain tumors is increase in morphologically abnormal intratumoral vessels along with tumor necrosis. Metastases of primary tumors from various organ systems like thyroid, liver, kidney, and lung have increased propensity to undergo hemorrhagic transformation. Various primary neoplasms like pituitary adenoma, glioma, meningioma, and primitive neuroectodermal tumors have also been associated with intratumoral hemorrhage (▶ Fig. 14.10).[51] Hemorrhagic transformation of the mass may cause worsening of the preexisting symptoms, or it may be responsible for presenting symptoms. Imaging is particularly challenging in patients with a previously undiagnosed mass or a single metastasis/tumor. A few of the imaging features that may point toward hemorrhagic transformation of mass rather than benign parenchymal bleed are atypical

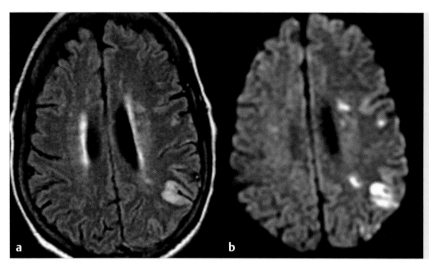

Fig. 14.9 Tumor emboli. Axial (**a**) fluid-attenuated inversion recovery and (**b**) diffusion-weighted imaging in a patient with metastatic breast carcinoma who presented with stroke, showing multiple acute infarcts in the left cerebral hemisphere (middle cerebral artery territory).

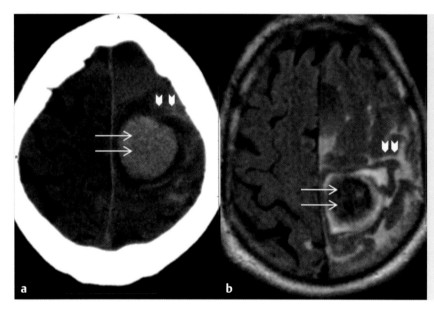

Fig. 14.10 Tumor-related hemorrhagic stroke. Axial (**a**) noncontrast computed tomography and (**b**) fluid-attenuated inversion recovery magnetic resonance images show hemorrhage within a meningioma (arrows) with surrounding edema and subarachnoid hemorrhage (arrowheads) within adjacent sulci. The patient presented with sudden-onset severe headache due to intratumoral and subarachnoid hemorrhage.

location, multiplicity, disproportionate vasogenic edema, early enhancement, changes in signal/attenuation of the previously known mass, and the absence of a complete well-defined hemosiderin rim on follow-up scan. Depending on the location of the tumor, the intratumoral bleed can extend into the surrounding structures, and an associated subarachnoid, subdural, epidural, or intraventricular bleed may occur.[52] When a tumor causes recurrent subarachnoid hemorrhage, there can be hemosiderin deposition in the leptomeninges and along the subpial tissue of brain, spinal cord, and cranial nerves, which leads to superficial siderosis.[53] The presence of intratumoral bleed or superficial siderosis may sometimes point to the aggressive nature of a benign-appearing mass.

14.3.6 Primary Angiitis of the Central Nervous System

Primary angiitis of the CNS (PACNS) is an isolated CNS vasculitis and is associated with various etiologies (autoimmune, infective, drugs, or malignancy).[54,55,56] Among the malignancies, PACNS is associated mostly with Hodgkin and non-Hodgkin

lymphoma. It typically causes granulomatous inflammation of the medium to small arteries of the brain and spinal cord. Involvement of small veins and venules is atypical but has been reported. The common presenting symptoms of PACNS are headache and encephalopathy. The most important differential of PACNS is reversible cerebral vasoconstriction syndrome (RCVS), which is also characterized by acute-onset severe recurrent headache, usually with neurologic deficits.[57] MRI is helpful in diagnosing this disorder, and biopsy establishes the definitive diagnosis. On MRI, there are foci of T2-weighted hyperintensity involving both the gray and white matter, which represent a combination of inflammation, ischemia, and infarction. The inflammation of the perforating arteries and the perivascular tissues is seen as linear enhancing areas within the white matter and brainstem on gadolinium administration (▶ Fig. 14.11). Less commonly, these patients may present with parenchymal hemorrhage or with focal neurologic deficit mimicking a mass lesion.[58] MRA in these patients shows short segment (< 0.5 cm) stenosis, arterial occlusion, and aneurysms, usually seen in the anterior circulation, and involve the proximal part of the vessels.[59] Such MRI findings have angiographic correlates in

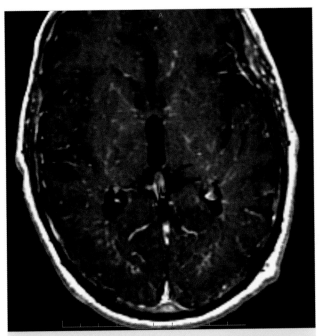

Fig. 14.11 Primary angiitis of the central nervous system (PACNS). Axial postcontrast T1-weighted magnetic resonance imaging in a patient with renal transplant and lymphoma, showing multiple enhancing foci in white matter almost in a perivascular configuration. Biopsy showed PACNS and granulomatous perivascular infiltrates.

approximately 40 to 50% of cases. There are areas of focal luminal narrowing on angiography, which most commonly involve the middle cerebral artery and its branches. Digital subtraction angiography (DSA) provides more information regarding the true extent of disease and better explains symptoms that cannot be attributed to abnormalities on MRI.[60]

14.4 Stroke and Cerebrovascular Complications Related to Tumor Therapy

14.4.1 Radiation-Induced Stroke and Cerebrovascular Complications

In the last few decades, treatment of various brain neoplasms has been revolutionized by the use of radiotherapy and chemotherapy. Radiotherapy-induced neurologic complications may be classified as acute (during radiation of up to 2 weeks), early-delayed (up to 6 months postirradiation), and late-delayed (more than 6 months to several years postirradiation).[61,62]

Acute Encephalopathy

Acute encephalopathy usually occurs within 2 weeks of onset of radiotherapy and is seen in patients receiving high-dose radiation. Its incidence has decreased due to the use of low-dose (< 3 Gy) radiation. In patients with multiple metastases or a large posterior fossa tumor, the encephalopathy is exceptionally severe. Pathologically, it is linked to the disruption of the blood–brain barrier by the radiation and is seen as increased edema on imaging.

Early-Delayed Complications

Early-delayed complications occur within 2 weeks to 4 months of the onset of radiotherapy. Early-delayed complications of brain tumors include somnolence syndrome, severe leukoencephalopathy with cognitive dysfunction, and pseudobulbar syndrome. In spinal cord tumors the presence of the Lhermitte sign (electric shock–like sensation on neck flexion) is considered a classic symptom of radiation-induced early-delayed complications. In the majority of patients radiological imaging is normal; however, increased edema or the presence of a new area of contrast enhancement is seen in approximately 15% of patients. MRI of the spine is usually normal in patients with the Lhermitte phenomenon.

Delayed Complications

Delayed complications occur 4 months after the onset of radiotherapy and have been reported as late as 30 years after the last cycle of radiotherapy. Radionecrosis and leukoencephalopathy are the major delayed complications of radiation therapy. Other delayed radiation complications include radiogenic tumors, vascular abnormalities, and endocrinopathies.

Radiation Necrosis

The latency period for radiation necrosis is between 1 and 2 years. Patients may present with new-onset focal neurologic deficits, or the necrosis may mimic tumor recurrence clinically. It classically occurs in the white matter with sparing of the cortex. Because radiation necrosis may show contrast enhancement, the role of morphological imaging in distinguishing recurrent tumor from radiation necrosis is limited. Various functional imaging techniques like PET may distinguish hypometabolic radiation necrosis from hypermetabolic recurrent tumor.

Radiation-Induced Leukoencephalopathy

Radiation-induced leukoencephalopathy is the most common neurologic complication of radiation in long-term survivors. Clinically, patients present with cognitive decline and dementia-like symptoms. Although it is a diagnosis of exclusion, and other causes of dementia need to be ruled out, MRI can show T2/FLAIR hyperintensity in the periventricular white matter along with prominence of cerebral sulci and the ventricular system.

Vascular Complications

Radiation therapy has adverse effects on both medium and large vessels of the CNS. The latency for its effect on medium-sized vessels is approximately 7 years, whereas the latency period for large vessels is 20 years. But in patients who receive/undergo interstitial radiotherapy the incubation period can be substantially less. These vascular effects can adversely affect the quality of life in long-term survivors. Accelerated carotid atherosclerosis is one of the most common effects of radiation on CNS vasculature and can lead to transient ischemic attack or stroke. Other factors that may exacerbate atherosclerosis in these patients are hypertension, diabetes, hypercholesterolemia, and obesity.[63] Rarely, radiation may cause excessive thinning or complete

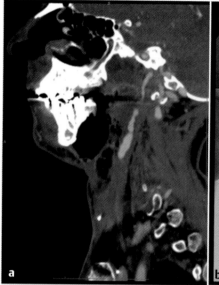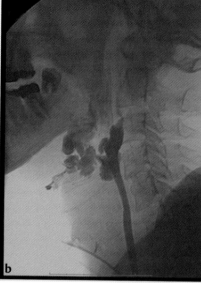

Fig. 14.12 Postradiotherapy carotid blowout. (a) Sagittal computed tomographic angiography in a patient who had a history of radiotherapy for head and neck cancer shows marked irregularity and narrowing of the luminal outline of the internal carotid artery (ICA) with surrounding air density and soft tissue heterogeneity. (b) Conventional contrast angiography done 1 day later shows complete blowout of the anterior margin of the ICA with active contrast extravasation.

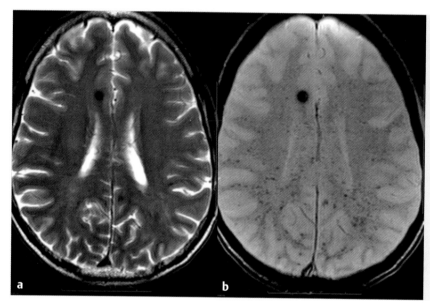

Fig. 14.13 Postradiotherapy cavernoma. (a) Axial T2-weighted and (b) gradient echo image showing multiple small hypointense foci in bilateral cerebral hemispheres, which show prominent blooming suggesting cavernoma. The patient had a history of whole-brain radiotherapy in childhood for medulloblastoma.

necrosis of the carotid wall, and the patient may present with carotid "blow-out" syndrome (▶ Fig. 14.12).[64] Moyamoya pattern vasculopathy may be seen, especially in children. Other CNS vascular malformations, such as telangiectasias, cavernomas, and aneurysms, may also appear as delayed manifestations of radiotherapy (▶ Fig. 14.13). Because the latency period for such vascular malformations is longer, they are seen most often in patients who receive radiotherapy early in life. These malformations have been reported in both the brain and the spinal cord.[62,65]

14.4.2 Chemotherapy-Induced Stroke and Cerebrovascular Complications

A multimodal treatment approach has led to increased use of chemotherapy for both CNS and extra-CNS malignancies. Various vascular and nonvascular complications can occur due to chemotherapeutic drugs. Although the occurrence of stroke due to chemotherapeutic drugs is rare, it can be caused by other factors. The use of anti-VEGF (bevacizumab) is associated with arterial infarcts and cerebral hemorrhage. In patients on L-asparaginase therapy, there is depletion of fibrinolytic factors, which may lead to venous sinus thrombosis. Antithrombin concentrate has shown promise in prevention of thrombosis due to L-asparaginase therapy. L-asparaginase also depletes various coagulation factors and may cause cerebral hemorrhage.[66,67]

Reversible posterior leukoencephalopathy syndrome (PRES) is a well-known CNS complication of various chemotherapeutic drugs like cisplatin, cytarabine, and methotrexate. The exact pathogenesis of PRES is unknown. Vasogenic edema is the most accepted cause of reversible posterior leukoencephalopathy. On CT, there is symmetric subcortical hypodensity in bilateral cerebral hemispheres. These changes are most commonly seen in the parieto-occipital region. On MRI, there is symmetric T2/FLAIR subcortical hyperintensity in the involved areas. The presence of restricted diffusion is atypical but can still be

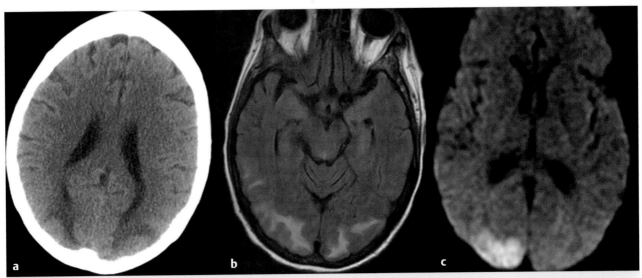

Fig. 14.14 Posterior reversible encephalopathy syndrome (PRES). Axial (**a**) noncontrast computed tomography, (**b**) fluid-attenuated inversion recovery, and (**c**) diffusion-weighted magnetic resonance imaging in a patient with lymphoma on treatment shows white matter signal abnormality in parieto-occipital white matter with restricted diffusion within the cortex.

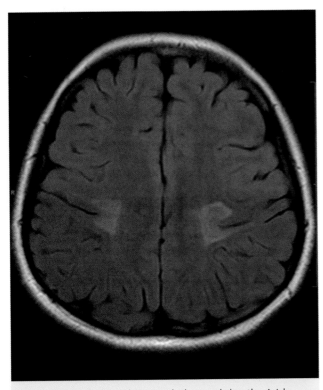

Fig. 14.15 Intrathecal methotrexate leukoencephalopathy. Axial fluid-attenuated inversion recovery magnetic resonance imaging in a patient with acute lymphoblastic leukemia on intrathecal methotrexate therapy shows symmetrical white matter signal abnormality in bilateral frontoparietal white matter.

observed in the involved areas (▶ Fig. 14.14). The presence of restricted diffusion represents infarction or tissue injury and hence may predict poor outcome.[68]

Certain chemotherapeutic drugs like methotrexate are given specifically for CNS neoplasms because they can be delivered/ administered intrathecally and they cross the blood–brain barrier when administered at high dosage intravenously. Methotrexate is associated with toxic leukoencephalopathy, which may present clinically with strokelike episodes. Toxic leukoencephalopathy usually presents within 2 weeks of intrathecal methotrexate administration. On MRI, areas of T2/FLAIR hyperintensity are seen in deep or periventricular white matter (▶ Fig. 14.15). These areas represent cytotoxic edema and hence show restricted diffusion on DWI. White matter signal abnormalities may reverse completely or progress to gliosis/ encephalomalacia.[62]

14.5 Conclusions

The role of imaging in patients with neurologic complications of cancer is manifold. The primary goal is to rule out the presence of any structural lesion, such as neoplastic disease, traumatic or spontaneous intracranial hemorrhage, extra-axial collections, or ischemic disease, which may be responsible for the patient's symptoms. Second, imaging may also help to identify and characterize abnormalities in brain signal intensity and seek any alternative cause of encephalopathy responsible for subacute presentation of the patient. The recognition of cerebrovascular complications due to tumor is important because they can be life threatening, and any delay in treatment can significantly increase patient morbidity and mortality. A majority of patients present with paraneoplastic CNS syndromes prior to the diagnosis of cancer; hence, imaging also plays an important role in early diagnosis of the primary cancer.[69]

Various imaging modalities like ultrasonography, CT, and MRI may aid in early diagnosis of malignancy and may point to the appropriate site for tissue diagnosis. The role of FDG-PET in these patients is well established because it may detect the tumor in patients even when conventional imaging results are normal. FDG-PET tracer may also correlate with the disease activity, and it may also help in guiding biopsies for histological diagnosis, especially when tumor is not visualized on conventional imaging.[70] With rapid advances in CT, MRI, and PET, the role of imaging in evaluation of cancer patients presenting with neurologic symptoms continues to evolve.

References

[1] DeAngelis LM, Posner JB. Neurologic Complications of Cancer. 2nd ed. New York, NY: Oxford University Press; 2008

[2] Graus F, Rogers LR, Posner JB. Cerebrovascular complications in patients with cancer. Medicine (Baltimore) 1985; 64: 16–35

[3] Posner JB, Furneaux HM. Paraneoplastic syndromes. Res Publ Assoc Res Nerv Ment Dis 1990; 68: 187–219

[4] Darnell RB, Posner JB. Paraneoplastic syndromes involving the nervous system. N Engl J Med 2003; 349: 1543–1554

[5] Guichard MMA, Vignon G. La polyradiculonévrite cancéreuse métastatique; paralysies multiples des nerfs craniens et rachidiens par généralisation microscopique d'un épithélioma du colutérin. J Med Lyon 1949; ; 30: 197–207

[6] Auche M. Des nevrites peripheriques chez les cancereux. Rev Med. 1890; 10: 785–807

[7] Dalmau J, Rosenfeld MR. Paraneoplastic syndromes of the CNS. Lancet Neurol 2008; 7: 327–340

[8] de Andrés C, Esquivel A, de Villoria JG, Graus F, Sánchez-Ramón S. Unusual magnetic resonance imaging and cerebrospinal fluid findings in paraneoplastic cerebellar degeneration: a sequential study. J Neurol Neurosurg Psychiatry 2006; 77: 562–563

[9] Choi KD, Kim JS, Park SH, Kim YK, Kim SE, Smitt PS. Cerebellar hypermetabolism in paraneoplastic cerebellar degeneration. J Neurol Neurosurg Psychiatry 2006; 77: 525–528

[10] Gultekin SH, Rosenfeld MR, Voltz R, Eichen J, Posner JB, Dalmau J. Paraneoplastic limbic encephalitis: neurologic symptoms, immunological findings and tumour association in 50 patients. Brain 2000; 123: 1481–1494

[11] Lacomis D, Khoshbin S, Schick RM. MR imaging of paraneoplastic limbic encephalitis. J Comput Assist Tomogr 1990; 14: 115–117

[12] Thuerl C, Müller K, Laubenberger J, Volk B, Langer M. MR imaging of autopsy-proved paraneoplastic limbic encephalitis in non-Hodgkin lymphoma. AJNR Am J Neuroradiol 2003; 24: 507–511

[13] Brierley JB, Corsellis JA, Hierons R, Nevin S. Subacute encephalitis of later adult life mainly affecting the limbic areas. Brain 1960; 83: 57–368

[14] Lawn ND, Westmoreland BF, Kiely MJ, Lennon VA, Vernino S. Clinical, magnetic resonance imaging, and electroencephalographic findings in paraneoplastic limbic encephalitis. Mayo Clin Proc 2003; 78: 1363–1368

[15] Scheid R, Lincke T, Voltz R, von Cramon DY, Sabri O. Serial 18F-fluoro-2-deoxy-D-glucose positron emission tomography and magnetic resonance imaging of paraneoplastic limbic encephalitis. Arch Neurol 2004; 61: 1785–1789

[16] Dalmau J, Graus F, Rosenblum MK, Posner JB. Anti-Hu—associated paraneoplastic encephalomyelitis/sensory neuronopathy. A clinical study of 71 patients. Medicine (Baltimore) 1992; 71: 59–72

[17] Saiz A, Bruna J, Stourac P et al. Anti-Hu-associated brainstem encephalitis. J Neurol Neurosurg Psychiatry 2009; 80: 404–407

[18] Voltz R, Gultekin SH, Rosenfeld MR et al. A serologic marker of paraneoplastic limbic and brain-stem encephalitis in patients with testicular cancer. N Engl J Med 1999; 340: 1788–1795

[19] Dalmau J, Graus F, Villarejo A et al. Clinical analysis of anti-Ma2-associated encephalitis. Brain 2004; 127: 1831–1844

[20] Saket RR, Geschwind MD, Josephson SA, Douglas VC, Hess CP. Autoimmune-mediated encephalopathy: classification, evaluation, and MR imaging patterns of disease. Neurographics 2011; 1: 2–16

[21] Honnorat J, Cartalat-Carel S, Ricard D et al. Onco-neural antibodies and tumour type determine survival and neurologic symptoms in paraneoplastic neurologic syndromes with Hu or CV2/CRMP5 antibodies. J Neurol Neurosurg Psychiatry 2009; 80: 412–416

[22] Taraszewska A, Piekarska A, Kwiatkowski M, Wierzba-Bobrowicz T, Czorniuk-Sliwa A. A case of the subacute brainstem encephalitis. Folia Neuropathol 1998; 36: 217–220

[23] Flanagan EP, McKeon A, Lennon VA et al. Paraneoplastic isolated myelopathy: clinical course and neuroimaging clues. Neurology 2011; 76: 2089–2095

[24] Kidher ES, Briceno N, Taghi A, Chukwuemeka A. An interesting collection of paraneoplastic syndromes in a patient with a malignant thymoma. BMJ Case Rep 2012 Jul 3; 2012

[25] Flanagan EP, Sandroni P, Pittock SJ, Inwards DJ, Jones LK, Jr. Paraneoplastic lower motor neuronopathy associated with Hodgkin lymphoma. Muscle Nerve 2012; 46: 823–827

[26] Burton M, Anslow P, Gray W, Donaghy M. Selective hypertrophy of the cauda equina nerve roots. J Neurol 2002; 249: 337–340

[27] Kumar N, Dyck PJ. Hypertrophy of the nerve roots of the cauda equina as a paraneoplastic manifestation of lymphoma. Arch Neurol 2005; 62: 1776–1777

[28] Lins H, Kanakis D, Dietzmann K, Wallesch CW, Mawrin C. Paraneoplastic necrotizing myelopathy with hypertrophy of the cauda equina. J Neurol 2003; 250: 1388–1389

[29] Raizer JJ, DeAngelis LM. Cerebral sinus thrombosis diagnosed by MRI and MR venography in cancer patients. Neurology 2000; 54: 1222–1226

[30] Inhaul KM, Maser F. Cerebral venous and sinus thrombosis - an update. Eur J Neurol 1994; 1: 109–126

[31] Ozsvath RR, Casey SO, Lustrin ES, Alberico RA, Hassankhani A, Patel M. Cerebral venography: comparison of CT and MR projection venography. AJR Am J Roentgenol 1997; 169: 1699–1707

[32] Rizzo L, Crasto SG, Rudà R et al. Cerebral venous thrombosis: role of CT, MRI and MRA in the emergency setting. Radiol Med (Torino) 2010; 115: 313–325

[33] Khandelwal N, Agarwal A, Kochhar R et al. Comparison of CT venography with MR venography in cerebral sinovenous thrombosis. AJR Am J Roentgenol 2006; 187: 1637–1643

[34] Wasay M, Azeemuddin M. Neuroimaging of cerebral venous thrombosis. J Neuroimaging 2005; 15: 118–128

[35] Perkin GD. Cerebral venous thrombosis: developments in imaging and treatment. J Neurol Neurosurg Psychiatry 1995; 59: 1–3

[36] Terashi H, Uchiyama S, Iwata M. Stroke in cancer patients [in Japanese]. Brain Nerve 2008; 60: 143–147

[37] Lee EJ, Lee YJ, Lee SR, Park DW, Kim HY. Hypereosinophilia with multiple thromboembolic cerebral infarcts and focal intracerebral hemorrhage. Korean J Radiol 2009; 10: 511–514

[38] Sethi HS, Schmidley JW. Cerebral infarcts in the setting of eosinophilia: three cases and a discussion. Arch Neurol 2010; 67: 1275–1277

[39] Rogers LR. Cerebrovascular complications in patients with cancer. Semin Neurol 2010; 30: 311–319

[40] Mori K, Takeuchi J, Ishikawa M, Handa H, Toyama M, Yamaki T. Occlusive arteriopathy and brain tumor. J Neurosurg 1978; 49: 22–35

[41] Aoki N, Sakai T, Oikawa A, Takizawa T, Koike M. Dissection of the middle cerebral artery caused by invasion of malignant glioma presenting as acute onset of hemiplegia. Acta Neurochir (Wien) 1999; 141: 1005–1008

[42] Gliemroth J, Nowak G, Kehler U, Arnold H, Gaebel C. Neoplastic cerebral aneurysm from metastatic lung adenocarcinoma associated with cerebral thrombosis and recurrent subarachnoid haemorrhage. J Neurol Neurosurg Psychiatry 1999; 66: 246–247

[43] Tamulevičiūtė E, Taeshineetanakul P, Terbrugge K, Krings T. Myxomatous aneurysms: a case report and literature review. Interv Neuroradiol 2011; 17: 188–194

[44] Chang IB, Cho BM, Park SH, Yoon DY, Oh SM. Metastatic choriocarcinoma with multiple neoplastic intracranial microaneurysms: case report. J Neurosurg 2008; 108: 1014–1017

[45] Iihara K, Kikuchi H, Nagata I. Left atrial myxoma with cerebral oncotic aneurysms with special reference to the importance of serial angiography [in Japanese]. No Shinkei Geka 1991; 19: 857–860

[46] Branch CL, Jr, Laster DW, Kelly DL, Jr. Left atrial myxoma with cerebral emboli. Neurosurgery 1985; 16: 675–680

[47] Taccone FS, Jeangette SM, Blecic SA. First-ever stroke as initial presentation of systemic cancer. J Stroke Cerebrovasc Dis 2008; 17: 169–174

[48] Lee SJ, Kim JH, Na CY, Oh SS. Eleven years' experience with Korean cardiac myxoma patients: focus on embolic complications. Cerebrovasc Dis 2012; 33: 471–479

[49] Uner A, Dogan M, Sal E, Peker E. Stroke and recurrent peripheral embolism in left atrial myxoma. Acta Cardiol 2010; 65: 101–103

[50] Kondziolka D, Bernstein M, Resch L et al. Significance of hemorrhage into brain tumors: clinicopathological study. J Neurosurg 1987; 67: 852–857

[51] Lieu AS, Hwang SL, Howng SL, Chai CY. Brain tumors with hemorrhage. J Formos Med Assoc 1999; 98: 365–367

[52] Lee CS, Huh JS, Sim KB, Kim YW. Cerebellar pilocytic astrocytoma presenting with intratumor bleeding, subarachnoid hemorrhage, and subdural hematoma. Childs Nerv Syst 2009; 25: 125–128

[53] Konya D, Peker S, Ozgen S, Kurtkaya O, Necmettin Pamir M. Superficial siderosis due to papillary glioneuronal tumor. J Clin Neurosci 2006; 13: 950–952

[54] Zuber M, Blustajn J, Arquizan C, Trystram D, Mas JL, Meder JF. Angiitis of the central nervous system. J Neuroradiol 1999; 26: 101–117

[55] Volcy M, Toro ME, Uribe CS, Toro G. Primary angiitis of the central nervous system: report of five biopsy-confirmed cases from Colombia. J Neurol Sci 2004; 227: 85–89

[56] Birnbaum J, Hellmann DB. Primary angiitis of the central nervous system. Arch Neurol 2009; 66: 704–709

[57] Hajj-Ali RA, Calabrese LH. Central nervous system vasculitis. Curr Opin Rheumatol 2009; 21: 10–18

[58] Greenan TJ, Grossman RI, Goldberg HI. Cerebral vasculitis: MR imaging and angiographic correlation. Radiology 1992; 182: 65–72

[59] Aviv RI, Benseler SM, Silverman ED et al. MR imaging and angiography of primary CNS vasculitis of childhood. AJNR Am J Neuroradiol 2006; 27: 192–199

[60] Pomper MG, Miller TJ, Stone JH, Tidmore WC, Hellmann DB. CNS vasculitis in autoimmune disease: MR imaging findings and correlation with angiography. AJNR Am J Neuroradiol 1999; 20: 75–85

[61] Keime-Guibert F, Napolitano M, Delattre JY. Neurologic complications of radiotherapy and chemotherapy. J Neurol 1998; 245: 695–708

[62] Rollins N, Winick N, Bash R, Booth T. Acute methotrexate neurotoxicity: findings on diffusion-weighted imaging and correlation with clinical outcome. AJNR Am J Neuroradiol 2004; 25: 1688–1695

[63] Abayomi OK. Neck irradiation, carotid injury and its consequences. Oral Oncol 2004; 40: 872–878

[64] Chang FC, Lirng JF, Luo CB et al. Carotid blowout syndrome in patients with head-and-neck cancers: reconstructive management by self-expandable stent-grafts. AJNR Am J Neuroradiol 2007; 28: 181–188

[65] Greene-Schloesser D, Robbins ME, Peiffer AM, Shaw EG, Wheeler KT, Chan MD. Radiation-induced brain injury: A review. Front Oncol 2012; 2: 73

[66] Soussain C, Ricard D, Fike JR, Mazeron JJ, Psimaras D, Delattre JY. CNS complications of radiotherapy and chemotherapy. Lancet 2009; 374: 1639–1651

[67] Imamura T, Morimoto A, Kato R et al. Cerebral thrombotic complications in adolescent leukemia/lymphoma patients treated with L-asparaginase-containing chemotherapy. Leuk Lymphoma 2005; 46: 729–735

[68] Bartynski WS. Posterior reversible encephalopathy syndrome, part 1: fundamental imaging and clinical features. AJNR Am J Neuroradiol 2008; 29: 1036–1042

[69] Dalmau J, Gonzalez RG, Lerwill MF. Case records of the Massachusetts General Hospital. Case 4-2007. A 56-year-old woman with rapidly progressive vertigo and ataxia. N Engl J Med 2007; 356: 612–620

[70] Kostakoglu L, Agress H, Jr, Goldsmith SJ. Clinical role of FDG PET in evaluation of cancer patients. Radiographics 2003; 23: 315–340, quiz 533

15 Image-Guided Neurosurgery: Intraoperative MRI

Ian Y. Lee

15.1 Introduction

Since the development and introduction of intraoperative magnetic resonance imaging (iMRI) in the late 1990s, applications for neurosurgical interventions have become increasingly widespread as more and more centers across the world adopt this technology. Following is a brief outline of the historical development of iMRI and a description of current applications.

15.2 Historical Background

The historical development and use of iMRI applications evolved out of the adoption of neuronavigational systems. With the development of frame-based and frameless applications, neurosurgeons were able to target deep intracranial lesions with previously unattainable accuracy.[1-10] The availability of neuronavigation greatly aided in localization of lesions as well as surgical planning, allowing for a minimally invasive approach toward intracranial surgery. However, the accuracy of neuronavigation was dependent on a preoperative scan. Once the cranial vault was accessed, and as an operation progressed, numerous factors (egress of cerebrospinal fluid, resection of tissue, local tissue swelling) could result in a shift of up to 5 mm, potentially compromising the accuracy of any navigation system.[6]

The next step in attempting to improve accuracy during an operation was to develop real-time intraoperative imaging to provide updated information with which to guide a procedure. Intraoperative ultrasonography was one such development; however, use was limited because it was unable to interface with other simultaneously available navigational modalities.[11] Computed tomography was also explored in the 1980s, but was never widely adopted due largely to the perception of an unfavorable cost-to-benefit ratio.[12,13,14,15] With the multiplanar capability and image quality of MRI, development of an iMRI was the next logical progression.

The earliest experience of development and application was described by Peter Black and his colleagues at Brigham and Women's Hospital in conjunction with General Electric Medical Systems.[16,17] The first of its kind, the Magnetic Resonance Therapy Unit at Brigham and Women's Hospital represented a major collaboration and nearly a decade of work through the 1980s. This initial application used an open low-field scanner built within the operative suite, a so-called double doughnut configuration. The 0.15 T magnet configuration provided a spherical imaging volume of 30 cm in diameter and allowed a 56-cm space between two magnets where a surgeon and assistant could stand or sit to operate. The surgical field would remain within the scanner, which would allow for image acquisition during the procedure. A requisite for this configuration would be MRI-compatible instruments, which had to be developed independently. In addition, an integrated navigational system was also developed and could be updated with each scan that was done during the procedure. Although use of this early iMRI added increased operating time due to the additional time required to position a patient properly, there were no adverse events reported in this initial experience. Interventions that

were described included stereotactic biopsies and cyst drainages, as well as craniotomies for tumor resection.

The experience published at Brigham and Women's Hospital illustrated that iMRI could prove a powerful tool in the hands of a neurosurgeon. However, such a system would pose great costs in terms of both installation and maintenance. Other magnet configurations were also developed, including a high-field-strength cylindrical superconducting short-bore system, and a biplanar open MRI design.[18] Rudolph Fahlbusch and colleagues at Erlangen developed a side-opening high-field system where the operative table would rotate into a 1.5 T close-bored magnet.[19] Moshe Hadani and his colleagues in conjunction with Medtronic Navigation (Louisville, CO) introduced the PoleStar N-10 iMRI, which offered an open-configuration 0.12 T portable magnet.[20] This particular system had a much smaller footprint and could be stored within a small area in the operating room and brought into the surgical field. In addition, its small footprint meant that the system could be installed in a conventional operating room.

The open-configuration iMRI systems were limited by low-field magnets, and over time could not produce the same high-quality image resolution as the 1.5 T and 3 T scanners that were being introduced for diagnostic purposes. As a result, efforts to introduce iMRI systems using closed high-field scanners continued apace. One such configuration involved using a separate conventional operating room connected via a transport corridor to a room containing the scanner.[21] This design had some advantages. It allowed the institution to use a commercially available scanner instead of an iMRI-specific scanner. In addition, the use of a conventional operating room also allowed for standard surgical instruments. The twin room configuration also meant the MRI was available for conventional studies when not being used during surgery. The cumulative result was a more cost-effective approach than some of the dedicated intraoperative units in use elsewhere. Another configuration involves the use of an intraoperative rail-mounted system that brings the scanner to the patient. The 1.5 T magnet is stored in a separate room that is shielded from the operating room via sliding radiofrequency- and sound-shielded doors. This configuration also allows the magnet to be used while not in use in the operating room. The operating suite features an MR-compatible operating room table and an MR-compatible head holder designed to fit within special eight-channel intraoperative radiofrequency coils. Closed-magnet systems represent a larger percentage of iMRI systems that are currently being adopted worldwide.

15.3 Intracranial Tumor Surgery

The chief benefit of iMRI is in aiding with tumor resection (▶ Fig. 15.1). During surgery, the brain parenchyma becomes distorted due to the loss of cerebrospinal fluid, edema, and tumor resection. As surgery progresses, this brain shift can lead to inaccuracies with neuronavigation that is based on a preoperative scan. iMRI can assist surgical procedures by providing real-time updates of image-guided neuronavigation. Prior to the

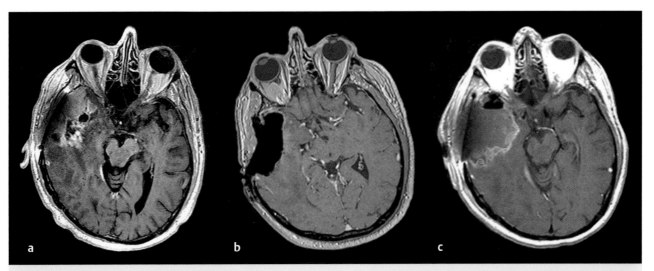

Fig. 15.1 Illustration of extent of resection (EOR) achieved with use of intraoperative magnetic resonance imaging scan in a high-grade glioma. (a) Preoperative contrast-enhanced T1 sequence showing right temporal lesion. (b) Intraoperative contrast-enhanced T1 sequence showing residual tumor medial border of resection cavity. (c) Postoperative contrast-enhanced T1 sequence illustrating gross total resection.

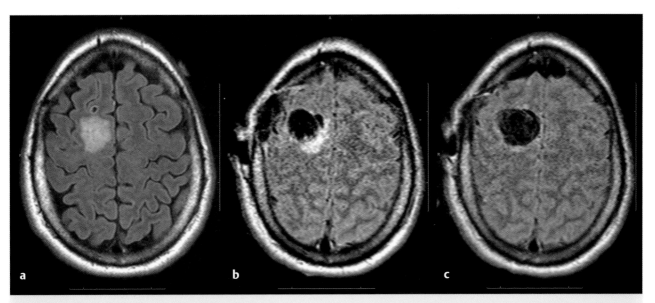

Fig. 15.2 Illustration of extent of resection (EOR) achieved with use of intraoperative magnetic resonance imaging scans in a low-grade glioma. (a) Preoperative T2 fluid-attenuated inversion recovery (FLAIR) sequence illustrating a right frontal lesion. (b) Intraoperative T2 FLAIR sequence illustrating residual T2 signal at posterior-medial border of resection cavity. (c) Second intraoperative T2 FLAIR sequence illustrating no residual T2 signal and gross total resection.

introduction of iMRI systems, a patient might have to return to the operating room in the case of inadequate resection. With iMRI a surgeon can access real-time imaging to assess the extent of tumor resection (EOTR) and carry out any necessary re-resection prior to concluding the operation, thus eliminating the risk of return to surgery for inadequate resections. With such a tool neurosurgeons are able to provide more complete resections and theoretically improve survival for patients with gliomas. The initial experience with iMRI showed no adverse events related to use, and most authors cited a perceived benefit in assisting with resection control.[17,22–28] Characteristically there was a great deal of heterogeneity in patient populations within these studies with a mixture of low-grade and malignant gliomas. In addition, not all tumors operated on were intended to undergo

gross total resection due to proximity to eloquent or critical structures.

15.3.1 Low-Grade Gliomas

Patients with low-grade gliomas represent a population that can potentially benefit greatly from surgery with iMRI (▶ Fig. 15.2). From a clinical standpoint, low-grade gliomas can have an initially indolent subclinical growth rate, but the normal pattern is for continuous growth and systematic progression to malignant transformation, in turn leading to neurologic disability and, ultimately, death.[29,30] From a treatment standpoint, there is a growing amount of evidence that EOTR can have a significant effect not only on the rate of tumor progression and overall

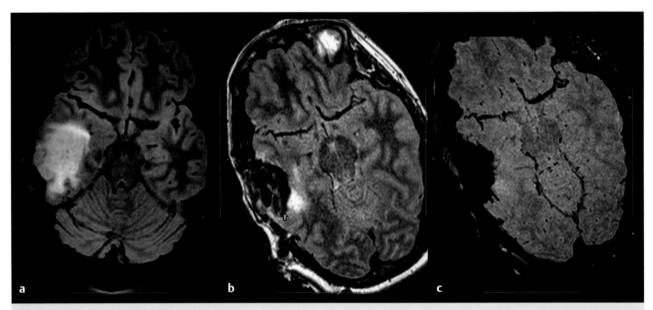

Fig. 15.3 Illustration of extent of resection (EOR) and use of intraoperative markers for resection control. (**a**) Preoperative T2 fluid-attenuated inversion recovery (FLAIR) sequence illustrating low-grade lesion in right temporal lobe. (**b**) Intraoperative T2 FLAIR sequence illustrating residual tumor and posterior-medial border of resection cavity. A flow void (arrow) at the posterior aspect is correlated with a vein seen grossly to help guide further resection of residual tumor. (**c**) Final intraoperative sequence illustrating no residual signal and gross total resection.

survival but also on the risk of anaplastic transformation.[31–38] Unfortunately, low-grade gliomas can present a unique surgical challenge because it can be difficult to distinguish tumor from brain parenchyma. When the iMRI was first introduced, the role of surgery in the treatment of low-grade gliomas was still somewhat controversial.

The Brigham and Women's Hospital group published a study describing the use of iMRI for the treatment of low-grade gliomas that illustrated a survival benefit.[39] The study was retrospective with no true control group. Surgical data were pooled and compared with survival data using national databases. Given the results, this study was the first to illustrate a benefit of surgical resection combined with the use of iMRI for patients with low-grade gliomas. Unfortunately, data on exact EOTR were not given; therefore, it is difficult to say what role the use of iMRI with surgical resection contributed to the observed survival benefit. Subsequent studies have tried to quantify the benefit of iMRI with volumetric studies evaluating EOTR. Senft et al published a study using a portable low-field scanner.[40] They found that, in low-grade glioma patients, iMRI resection control led to a 47.6% chance of further tumor. However, this was coupled with a 90.5% chance of meeting surgical goals compared to 100% in the high-grade glioma group. This difference was attributed to differences of low-field iMRI images compared to those of postoperative imaging obtained with high-field scanners. Hatiboglu et al published a prospective study that specifically evaluated the benefit in EOTR using iMRI.[41] This particular study used a closed magnet high-field system, where a scan would be conducted at the discretion of the surgeon. EOTR would be measured at the time of the first intraoperative scan and at the postoperative scan. They observed an increase of EOTR from 63 to 100%, 69 to 78%, and 57 to 71% for grades I, II, and III, respectively.

Despite a lack of class I evidence, it seems plausible that there is a potential clinical benefit with the regular use of iMRI in patients with low-grade gliomas. With an observed benefit in increasing EOTR with the use of iMRI in select studies coupled with an expanding body of literature supporting a correlation of EOTR and overall survival, it seems fairly evident that iMRI can, in the right hands, increase survival in low-grade glioma patients. Given its relatively lower incidence compared with high-grade gliomas, it seems unlikely that a randomized control study evaluating the use of iMRI—or surgery in general for low-grade gliomas—will ever come to fruition. Nevertheless, the evidence does suggest a tangible benefit with the use of iMRI in treating low-grade gliomas.

15.3.2 High-Grade Gliomas

Despite advancements in treatment modalities, the prognosis of surgically treated patients with high-grade gliomas remains poor.[42,43] The treatment paradigm is relatively simple: maximized surgical resection with preserved neurologic function followed by adjuvant therapy.[44,45,46] As in the case of low-grade gliomas, iMRI provides resection control through real-time updates to EOTR. Updated neuronavigation can also be obtained with iMRI using an intraoperative scan and recalibration before resuming a resection. In addition, intraoperative markers of distinct anatomical structures (i.e., blood vessels) can be identified by the neurosurgeon within a resection cavity and correlated radiographic images identified by a neuroradiologist on an intraoperative scan (▶ Fig. 15.3). This can provide useful orientation for increased resection control.

Kubben et al published a review examining the added benefit to iMRI for resection of high-grade gliomas and/or glioblastoma multiforme specifically.[47] Quantitative assessment on EOTR with the use of iMRI was one of the inclusion criteria for review. Twelve nonrandomized studies were identified with a total 439 patients. Gross total resection was one of the assessments for EOTR and was assessed in either qualitative or quantitative (through volumetric analysis) fashion (summarized in ▶ Table 15.1). Data on EOTR

Table 15.1 Study population and resection parameters of included studies

Study	N	Gross total resection		Intended	First iMRI	Last iMRI	Clinical performance	Complications	Survival
		Definition	Volumetry						
Knauth et al (1999)	41 HGG in 38 patients	NS	No	In 100%	37%	Not done (76% GTR on EPMRI)	NS	NS	NS
Wirtz et al (2000)	68 HGG including recurrences (62 GBM)	Removal of CE on iMRI, evaluated by neurosurgeon	No	NS	In 27% of HGG	Resection continued in 66% of HGG (no final iMRI result available)	NS in sub-population	NS in sub-population	Median 13.3 months for GTR vs. 9.2 months for STR (p = 0.0035)
Bohinski et al (2001)	30 HGG	Opinion of neuro-radiologist and neurosurgeon	No	NS in sub-population (in 30–40 gliomas)	Additional resection in 57% of HGG	NS	NS in sub-population	NS in sub-population	NS
Nimsky et al (2003)	32 GBM	Evaluation (by neurosurgeon?)	No	NS in sub-population	6/32 patients	7/32 patients	NS in sub-population	NS in sub-population	NS
Hirschberg et al (2005)	32 GBM[a]	Opinion of neurosurgeon and neuroradiologist	No	NS (seems to be 19/27 patients)	5/27 patients	NS	Improved 16%; unchanged 55%; deteriorated 29%	Two infections, three visual field defects	Mean 14.5 months vs. 12.1 months for matched control group without iMRI (p = 0.14)
Schneider et al (2005)	31 GBM	> 95% removal of CE (with necrosis) on T1Gd, measured by segmentation	Yes: sum of tumor area per slice × slice thickness (+ gap thickness)	NS	2/31 patients	11/31 patients	Deteriorated 13%	One rebleed, one edema, two new paresis	Median 537 days for GTR vs. 237 days for STR (p = 0.004)
Busse et al (2006)	24 GBM including recurrences	Consensus of neurosurgeon and neuroradiologist	No	NS	NS	Four GBM had total resection	NS in sub-population	NS in sub-population	NS
Muragaki et al (2006)	30 GBM	Removal of CE on T1Gd, measured by segmentation	Yes: sum of tumor area per slice × slice thickness	NS	NS	90% EOTR	NS in sub-population	NS in sub-population	NS
Nimsky et al (2006)	57 GBM	NS	No[b]	Not intended in (at least) 25/57 patients	Sixteen of 57 patients	23/57 patients	NS in sub-population	NS in sub-population	NS
Hatiboglu et al (2009)	27 GBM	> 95% EOTR (CE on T1Gd)	Yes: tumor area on vitrea by two neurosurgeons	NS	12 of 27 patients	24 of 27 patients	NS in sub-population	NS in sub-population	NS

Table 15.1 continued

Study	N	Gross total resection					Clinical performance	Complications	Survival
Lenaburg et al (2009)	35 GBM in 29 patients	Mathematical model	Yes: $4/3 \times \pi \times a \times b \times c$ (a, b, and c are diameters)	NS	NS (further resection in 72%)	27/35 cases had resection >95%	Deteriorated 1/35 cases	One respiratory failure (died); two wound infections leading to wound revision, one CSF leak	NS
Senft et al (2010)	41 GBM	No residual CE seen by neuroradiologist (masked to treatment group)	No	In 100%	NS	All 10 iMRI patients and 19/31 cNN patients (on EPMRI)	NS	NS	Median 74 weeks for GTR vs. 46 weeks for STR ($p < 0.001$); 88 weeks for iMRI vs. 68 weeks for cNN ($p = 0.07$)

Abbreviations: CE, contrast enhancement; cNN, conventional neuronavigation; CSF, cerebrospinal fluid; EOTR, extent of tumor resection; EPMRI, early postoperative MRI; GBM, glioblastoma multiforme; GTR, gross total resection; HGG, high-grade glioma; iMRI, intraoperative MRI; N, number of cases or patients; NS, not specified; STR, subtotal resection; T1Gd, T1-weighted MRI after gadolinium administration.

Note: If possible, only data on GBM were used (derived from text, tables, or figures). If not available, data for HGG were used.

[a]Originally 32 GBM were operated on for this study, but only 27 were described as having good image quality and were used for further analysis.

[b]In smaller study on volumetric assessment of glioma removal (excluded for overlapping data) the authors performed volumetry by applying manual segmentation on the VectorVision workstation, using coregistration of all imaging data sets.

Source: Modified with permission from Kubben PL, ter Meulen KJ, Schijns OEMG, ter Laak-Poort MP, van Overbeeke JJ, van Santbrink H. Intraoperative MRI-guided resection of glioblastoma multiforme: A systemic review. Lancet Oncol 2011;12:1062–1070.

during the first intraoperative scan were not provided in all studies. Where it was measured, EOTR was improved across all studies between the first and final iMRI scan. Four of the studies provided survival data, one of which had a matched control group without iMRI.[48] In this particular study, although not statistically significant to the level of 95% confidence ($p = 0.14$), survival was increased in the iMRI versus without-iMRI cohorts with a mean survival of 14.5 months and 12.1 months, respectively. In the study by Senft et al, two cohorts were examined, one with iMRI and another using conventional neuronavigation with gross total resection intended for all patients.[49] For all patients undergoing surgery (with or without iMRI) those with gross total resection had a median survival of 74 weeks versus 46 weeks for subtotal resections ($p < 0.001$). In addition, patients who had surgery with iMRI had a median survival of 88 weeks versus 68 weeks for those that had surgery without iMRI ($p = 0.07$). In the other two studies, comparisons were done between cohorts with gross total resection versus subtotal resection. Wirtz et al showed a statistically significant improved survival ($p = 0.0035$) with median survival of 13.3 months versus 9.2 months.[50] Schneider et al also showed improved survival with a median survival of 537 days versus 237 days ($p = 0.003$).[28] At the conclusion of this review, there was at best class 2 evidence to suggest a superiority of iMRI over conventional methods for surgery on high-grade gliomas.

One of the notable points of this review was made regarding attribution bias. With the poor prognosis of high-grade gliomas, in particular glioblastoma, neurosurgeons are careful to avoid additional deficits when resecting these lesions. With the availability of iMRI, a surgeon is given leave to take a more conservative approach with the expectation of an intraoperative scan to further guide a resection. Without iMRI, a surgeon may be compelled to be as aggressive as possible, with the expectation being to maximize a resection. This bias would serve to depress the EOTR during an initial scan and would falsely elevate the potential gain in EOTR when comparing a first iMRI scan versus the final postoperative scan. In addition, although EOTR can be a useful surrogate in assessing the usefulness of iMRI, the impact of iMRI on survival would be the most meaningful assessment of its value.

At the time of this writing, there is only one published randomized, controlled trial evaluating the effect of iMRI guidance on EOTR. Senft et al published a series of 24 glioma patients randomized to surgery with iMRI and 25 randomized to conventional surgery.[51] The tumor histology was predominantly World Health Organization (WHO) grade IV glioma (glioblastoma multiforme and gliosarcoma) with two grade III and one grade I gliomas. All patients included in the study were intended to have gross total resections. In the iMRI group 96% of patients achieved total tumor removal compared to 68% in the control group. Of the patients in the iMRI group, 33% underwent further resection after the iMRI scan. At 6 months, 67% of the iMRI group had stable disease, with only 36% in the conventional group ($p = 0.046$). Kaplan-Meier estimates of progression-free survival suggested a median of 226 days in the iMRI group and 154 days in the conventional group; however, this difference was not statistically significant. Nevertheless, class I evidence does exist showing that iMRI can have an impact in terms of maximizing EOTR, as well as improving survival. It will be interesting to see if future studies will further corroborate these findings.

15.3.3 Pituitary Tumors

Pituitary adenomas are preferentially approached transsphenoidally in the modern neurosurgical era.[52] Characterized by a generally indolent course, pituitary adenomas can represent a unique set of clinical challenges. In the case of nonfunctioning adenomas, indications for resection include neurologic deficit (most often in the form of visual field deficit with compression of the optic apparatus) or in the setting of documented growth. Functional adenomas can represent a unique clinical challenge with their endocrinological symptoms. Indeed, adrenocorticotropic hormone (ACTH)-secreting tumors causing Cushing disease can have severe health consequences with shortened survival compared to the general population.[53] From a surgical standpoint, extension of tumor superiorly into the suprasellar space or laterally into the cavernous sinus can offer technical challenges. With a transsphenoidal approach, visualization into the suprasellar space with an operative microscope is limited, and it can be difficult to assess whether there is residual tumor. Any residual tumor is typically treated with radiotherapy (in most cases stereotactic neurosurgery if there is sufficient space between residual tumor and the optic apparatus) or with reoperation, though both are associated with risks such as radiation side effects and cerebrospinal fluid (CSF) leakage, respectively.

Similar to its use in gliomas, iMRI can be a helpful adjunct for the surgical removal of pituitary tumors. In tumors that are surgically curable (i.e., tumors without a component of cavernous sinus invasion) complete resection can ensure a patient will not have to endure either radiotherapy or reoperation. There are several studies that have examined the use of iMRI.[21,24,54,55] Bohinski et al described their experience with 30 pituitary patients using a 0.3 T magnet.[21] One patient underwent a transsphenoidal approach initially, but on subsequent iMRI scan was found to have a significant hemorrhage extending into the third and lateral ventricles requiring emergent conversion into a standard craniotomy. Of the remaining 29 patients, 19 (66%) underwent further resection after the first intraoperative scan. Sixteen out of the 29 patients were scheduled to undergo gross total resection, whereas the remaining 13 were intended to undergo "optimal" subtotal resection, as deemed appropriate by the senior neurosurgeon. Out of the gross total resection group, 9 (56%) had residual tumor and underwent reexploration. In the subtotal resection group 10 (77%) required reexploration. The authors attribute this unusually high percentage of reexplorations to the learning curve associated with iMRI use, as well as limitations with the operating table, which in this particular configuration was fixed to the scanner and could not be maneuvered like a standard table. Schwartz et al published their experience with 15 patients who underwent endoscopically assisted transsphenoidal surgery with a 0.12 T magnet.[56] Three patients showed residual tumor on iMRI, which was identified using a scope with a 45-degree angle. Four patients had what appeared to be residual tumor, which on reexploration was found to be pooled blood or folds of arachnoid. The remaining eight had adequate resections based on the preoperative goals. Gerlach et al published a series in which 40 patients were operated using a 0.15 T scanner.[5] In this study only 7 (17.5%) patients required reexploration after intraoperative scan; however, an average increase of 77.4 minutes of anesthesia time and an average increase of 38.7 minutes of operative time were noted.

Nimsky et al published the results of 106 patients that had transsphenoidal surgery using a high-field 1.5 T scanner.[59] Eighty-five patients were intended to undergo complete removal, with 29 (34%) requiring reexploration, and of those, only 21 (72%) could undergo complete resection. The authors attributed an increase of total resection from 58 to 82% as a result of iMRI. In the remaining 21 patients where partial removal was intended, 8 (38%) underwent reexploration after intraoperative scan. The study also noted a lack of false-negative findings when comparing iMRI scans to later postoperative scans. To date, no class I evidence exists to suggest that iMRI in the setting of pituitary surgery has any tangible benefit. There is some class II evidence that suggests the use of iMRI can be helpful in achieving resection control. Whether or not the added cost of using an iMRI, as well as the increased amount of time under general anesthesia, translates to improved clinical outcome for pituitary tumors has yet to be determined.

15.3.4 Pediatric Tumors

The same advantages, whether real or theoretical, attributed to tumor surgery in adults with iMRI can also be applied to the pediatric population. For tumors of the pediatric population, there is a clear survival benefit to obtaining total tumor removal.[60] Therefore, any adjunct to maximize resection as well as eliminate the need for reoperation for residual tumor would be perceived as beneficial. Lesions of the pediatric population are characterized by an increased prevalence of cystic lesions, which by their nature can result in a significant amount of brain shift with drainage of the cyst fluid. iMRI can provide updated imaging to accommodate for any changes after partial cyst drainage and can also be used to verify the placement of catheters before conclusion of an operation.[61,62]

A number of studies have looked at the efficacy of low-field iMRI for pediatric tumors.[62-67] Nimsky et al described their experience using a 0.2 T magnet in 33 pediatric cases.[63] The indications for surgery were heterogeneous, including 9 cyst drainages, 6 resections for epilepsy, 6 pituitary lesions, and 12 brain tumors. The authors noted two tumor cases and three catheter placement cases where iMRI resulted in modification of surgical strategy. Samdani et al published a series of 20 pediatric patients undergoing surgery with a 0.12 T magnet.[65] The pathology findings were heterogeneous, with three cases of cortical dysplasia in addition to a mix of tumor histology. This study noted a learning curve in terms of additional anesthesia time required for iMRI scan, with a mean of 138 additional minutes for the first 10 cases versus 84 additional minutes for the last 10 cases. As far as added value provided by iMRI, they reported four cases where additional tumor was removed and one case of additional hippocampus removal. In addition, researchers noted confirmation of fenestration of cyst, confirmed cyst separation from ventricle, as well as one case where iMRI allowed for visualization of tumor adherence to the optic chiasm.

More recently there have been additional studies reporting the utility of high-field iMRI scanners for pediatric applications. Levy et al published a study of 105 procedures in 98 children over a 10-year period.[68] This series included five operations for spinal pathology. Of the remaining 100 cranial procedures, 55 were for tumor, 27 for epilepsy, 12 for vascular lesions, 3 for infection/inflammatory process, and 3 for CSF diversion or cyst drainage. The iMRI scanner in this case was used for three types of scans: a preoperative planning scan, an intradissection scan, and a quality-assurance scan. Intradissection scans were obtained in 80% (n = 84) of procedures with a mean time of 30 minutes required for the scan. Of the 55 cases for tumor, 49 underwent intradissection scans, and of these, 24 (49%) required additional resection. EOTR and impact on overall survival were not examined in this study. However, the authors did advocate the utility of iMRI by allowing the neurosurgeon to conduct an operation in a "stepwise manner." They argue that the availability of iMRI can allow for greater comfort in allowing for a temporary halt to the procedure to obtain updated imaging to further guide resection. Shah et al published a comparison of 42 iMRI-guided resections compared to 103 conventional resections without iMRI in the pediatric population.[69] The authors noted a significant increase in operative duration with a mean of 350 minutes for the iMRI group versus 243 minutes in the conventional group. In addition, length of hospitalization tended to be increased for the iMRI group at 8.2 days compared to 6.6 days for the conventional group. In 18 of the iMRI cases (42.9%), additional resection was required after intraoperative scanning. Both groups had similar rates of achieving surgical goals—79% versus 80% for iMRI and conventional resection, respectively. However, there was a 7.77% (n = 8) rate of reoperation within 2 weeks of the initial operation in the conventional group, with no cases of reoperation in the iMRI group. This difference was not found to be statistically significant. Despite this, the authors did advocate for the utility of iMRI in terms of overall cost savings, weighing costs of additional hospitalization, as well as for another surgical procedure versus the cost of an iMRI scan. However, the overall cost of installing the iMRI itself was not factored into this analysis. In addition, the authors also commented on the psychological benefit to the patient as well as parents, which they argue can be significant, especially in the pediatric population.

As with other applications for tumor surgery, iMRI does appear to be of some benefit in the pediatric population based on the literature. Unfortunately, class I evidence does not exist to support this. In addition, there is little outcome data in terms of overall survival for this particular subset of patients. Further study will be required to truly establish the efficacy and value of iMRI in pediatric patients.

15.4 Integration with Functional Imaging

The development of functional imaging modalities such as functional MRI (fMRI) with magnetoencephalography to identify areas of eloquent cortex as well as diffusion tensor MRI techniques (diffusion tensor imaging [DTI]) to visualize white matter fiber tracts have given rise to the concept of functional neuronavigation (▶ Fig. 15.4). The application and integration of fMRI with existing neuronavigational technology has been described in its utility to aid with tumor resection.[70,71,72,73] In particular, fMRI allows the neurosurgeon to plan an approach through a cortical entry point that is safe and removed from eloquent structures. With regard to application with iMRI, the information provided by fMRI to date has been integrated only

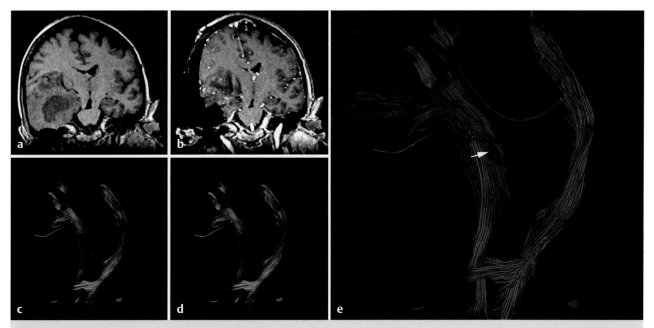

Fig. 15.4 Images of a 50-year-old woman with a right temporal World Health Organization grade IV glioblastoma. (**a**) Preoperative coronal T1-weighted magnetic resonance imaging scan (without contrast enhancement just after induction of anesthesia and head fixation). (**b**) In the corresponding intraoperative image, no contrast-enhancing tumor parts are visible. (**c,d**) Corresponding tractography of the pyramidal tracts. The superoinferior fiber orientation is color coded in blue; color coding of the anteroposterior direction is exchanged with the left/right direction because of the horizontal placement of the head for surgery during imaging. (**c**) Preoperative, (**d**) intraoperative, and (**e**) overlay of preoperative (blue) and intraoperative (gray) tractography of the pyramidal tracts depicting the inward shifting of the right pyramidal tract (white arrow). (Reprinted with permission from Nimsky C, Ganslandt O, Hastreiter P, et al. Preoperative and intraoperative diffusion tensor imaging-based fiber tracking in glioma surgery. Neurosurgery 2005;56:130–138.)

with preoperative neuronavigation planning.[72,73] The limitation here is that updated fMRI data cannot be provided during the middle of a resection in which a patient is under general anesthesia. DTI has also been described in its role to provide functional neuronavigation.[71,74,75,76] Integration of DTI with neuronavigation allows the neurosurgeon to avoid damaging white matter tracts that could result in significant morbidity to the patient. In addition, obtaining DTI with an intraoperative scan has also been examined.[77–81]

The first report of integrating DTI with iMRI was published by Mamata et al in 2001.[77] This study used a 0.5 T interventional scanner with three patient volunteers undergoing tumor resection. DTI was used to identify infarcts caused by surgery. In addition, white matter tracts were identifiable at the time of intraoperative scan and could therefore be avoided during surgery. This study showed the feasibility of obtaining DTI during an intraoperative scan with iMRI. With the feasibility of combining DTI with iMRI-guided surgery, other investigators sought to evaluate the utility of a wider-scale application of DTI tractography in patients undergoing surgery for tumor. Of particular interest were the degree and directionality of shift of white matter tracts during a tumor resection. Christopher Nimsky and his group at University Erlangen-Nuernberg reported on a series of 37 glioma patients who underwent both preoperative and intraoperative DTI fiber tracking using a 1.5 T magnet.[78,79] This study was primarily concerned with imaging of the pyramidal tracts. The authors noted a range of white matter tract movement of 8 mm of inward shift to 15 mm of outward shift. Of the 37 patients, 11 (29.7%) had inward shift, and 23 (62.2%) had outward shift, with 3 remaining patients with no remaining shift

during intraoperative scanning. The amount of white matter shift correlated statistically with the size of tumor ($r = 0.453$, $p < 0.01$), but the directionality of shift seemed unpredictable. Regarding added scan time, the authors reported that their standard protocol required 21 minutes, with the DTI measurement requiring another 5.5 minutes of scan time. The fiber tract computation and visualization also added another minute. The authors reported 1 of 37 patients who had a worsened preoperative motor deficit. However, the authors attributed this due to swelling as a result of venous insufficiency rather than with any inaccuracies of DTI tractography.

Similar to the Nimsky study, Romano et al also tried to study corticospinal tract shift during glioma surgery.[80] Using a 1.5 T magnet, the authors described 20 patients undergoing glioma surgery. They found a range of 9.7 mm of inward shift with 11 mm of outward shift. Outward shift was observed in 8 patients (40%), and inward shift was observed in 10 patients (50%), with the 2 remaining patients showing no shift. In their analysis, they found that the volume of peritumoral edema had a significant correlation with the amount of shift ($r = 0.691$, $p = 0.001$). In contrast with Nimsky et al's study, they found that shift magnitude had no correlation with tumor volume. The directionality of shift was also observed to be unpredictable in their study. In addition, the authors also acquired DTI data in 11 patients after opening the dura mater prior to tumor resection, with 7 patients displaying outward shift. In their analysis, they found a correlation between craniotomy size and shifting ($r = 0.69$, $p = 0.05$). No patients had worsening deficit with surgery, whereas, of the 18 patients who had preoperative deficits, 15 demonstrated neurologic improvement postoperatively.

DTI tractography with iMRI-guided surgery has also been applied to optic radiation. In a recent study, Sun et al performed preoperative, intraoperative, and postoperative tractography of the optic radiations in 44 patients with brain lesions.[81] Thirty-six of the 44 patients had gliomas. The authors were able to identify the optic radiations in all 44 patients in preoperative scans. This information was incorporated into their functional neuronavigation systems, and three-dimensional image data were incorporated into the operative microscope. This allowed the authors to create image contours to serve as a reminder of proximity to the optic radiations during the time of resection. No data on the extent of white matter shift were provided, but they did note the distance between the lesions with the optic tracts as identified on DTI tractography. Twenty-seven of the glioma patients were noted to have lesions within 5 mm of the optic radiation, of whom 12 had normal vision, and 15 had some form of visual field deficits. Postoperatively, the visual fields were improved in 4 patients, unchanged in 20, and worse in 3 patients. All nine patients who had lesion distances > 5 mm from the optic radiation had normal visual fields both pre- and postoperatively. In addition, the authors also provided data on EOTR and noted that 17 of the 36 glioma patients underwent reexploration after intraoperative scan. Total tumor removal was achieved in 9 of these 17 patients (52.9%), with partial tumor removal in the remainder to avoid damage to the optic radiation. The authors found a significant correlation between tumor distance to optic radiation with the amount of residual tumor after the first iMRI scan ($r = 0.38$, $p < 0.05$), but there was no significant correlation between tumor distance to optic radiation with the final extent of resection. The authors argued that, despite the proximity to the optic radiations, the information provided by updating DTI tractography during the iMRI scan facilitated more aggressive resections.

Functional neuroimaging has been successfully integrated into iMRI-guided surgery. DTI tractography has become an increasingly widespread and popular application to provide functional neuronavigation in the guidance of resection of intracranial lesions. It is likely that this trend will continue, and that there will be more reports of innovative applications of these modalities to assist with surgery of the nervous system.

15.5 Other iMRI Applications

iMRI-guided surgery has applications beyond that of tumor removal. Implementation with surgical treatment of epilepsy, deep brain stimulation (DBS), and some spine applications have also been described in the literature.[83] In addition, some novel sequences can also be applied to provide accurate image guidance for deep structures (▶ Fig. 15.5).

15.5.1 Epilepsy Surgery

Treatment of medically intractable temporal lobe epilepsy includes surgical resection of localized seizure foci in addition to specific structures. Greater surgical cure rates appear to be achieved when surgical resection is used to treat mesial temporal sclerosis or focal lesions.[83,84,85] Despite a reasonably high success rate, recurrences have been reported between 20 and 60%.[85,86,87] Whether or not the success of seizure control is directly related to the extent of resection in all cases is still

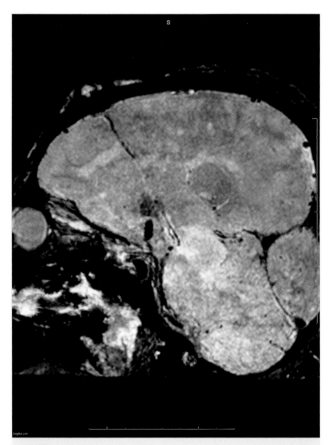

Fig. 15.5 Susceptibility-weighted imaging sequence imaging technique showing biopsy tract for brainstem glioma.

somewhat controversial. Some authors who advocate complete resection of the medial temporal structures, namely the amygdala and hippocampus, have evaluated the use of iMRI-guided epilepsy resections. The application of iMRI for epilepsy surgery has been described in some early reports.[16] Buchfelder et al examined the use of a 0.2 T iMRI in 58 cases of medically intractable epilepsy.[88] Notably, half of the cases were nonlesional, whereas the other half had lesions including cavernomas and neoplasms. They found that the intraoperative images were consistent with postoperative images obtained on high-field scanners, and that their iMRI scanner was able to provide images with enough resolution to assess the completeness of resection.

Schwartz et al published their experience with a 0.5 T scanner on five consecutive patients with medial temporal lobe epilepsy.[89] Intraoperative scans were obtained in all five patients after initial resection, and the authors found that in all five cases there was sufficient resection of the amygdala. However, they also found that all five patients had a small residual hippocampus, which was reexplored. Four of the five patients were seizure-free with no auras, whereas the fifth patient had a seizure after discontinuing antiepileptics. Mean follow-up was 8 months for this series. Kaibara et al examined the use of a 1.5 T iMRI system in 14 adult patients with epilepsy and mesial temporal lobe sclerosis identified on preoperative imaging.[90] In all 14 patients targeted resection of the amygdala and hippocampus, with a posterior margin of either the dorsal surface of the midbrain or the splenium of the corpus callosum, was intended.

Interdissection scans showed that in 7 of the 14 patients there was inadequate resection of either the amygdala or the hippocampus. This prompted reexploration with confirmation of an adequate resection prior to concluding the operation. Overall they found that 13 of 14 patients (93%) were seizure-free at last follow-up (mean follow-up of 17 months, minimum 12 months), and the remaining patient had unchanged seizure frequency. iMRI has been shown to be of utility for the surgical management of epilepsy, but the efficacy has not yet been shown in larger randomized series.

15.5.2 Deep Brain Stimulation

DBS has become a widespread application for the treatment of movement disorders. Success of DBS depends on the accuracy of lead placement.[91] Lead placement is traditionally dependent on preoperative imaging to identify the DBS target coupled with application of a stereotactic frame. This is refined with intraoperative microelectrode recording (MER) with the patient awake to help improve lead placement. iMRI applications of DBS placement have the potential to maintain high-fidelity accuracy while avoiding the complexities associated with MER. Starr and Larson have pioneered the application of DBS placement within an iMRI scanner.[92,93] The patient is placed supine under general anesthesia inside the bore of a 1.5 T iMRI scanner. Planning scans are obtained with the patient in the scanner, while the target and trajectory are identified. Trajectory guides with an alignment stem are affixed to the patient's scalp. The alignment stem is maneuvered into position manually until the stem is aligned with the target line using MR fluoroscopy. The stem is then locked into place. A ceramic stylet within a peel-away sheath is then advanced to the target. The tip of the ceramic stylet is confirmed with intraoperative scans, and is replaced with an MRI-compatible DBS electrode. Once lead placement is verified with a scan, the peel-away sheaths are removed and the leads are locked into place. In 29 patients, no intracerebral hemorrhages were reported, and 2 cases of infection required hardware removal. In assessing the accuracy of stereotaxy, the authors found a 29% improvement on their previously reported 3.2 mm mean difference between expected and actual tip locations.[94] However, one patient did have inadequate lead placement, which required subsequent revision. Newer systems have also been developed and tested by the same group of authors.[95] Therefore there is evidence to show the feasibility and accuracy of such iMRI-guided DBS platforms. A larger-scale comparison between more traditional methods of DBS placement compared with this near-real-time iMRI-guided DBS placement will be necessary to determine which method is superior.

References

[1] Apuzzo MLJ, Sabshin JK. Computed tomographic guidance stereotaxis in the management of intracranial mass lesions. Neurosurgery 1983; 12: 277–285

[2] Barnett GH, Kormos DW, Steiner CP, Weisenberger J. Intraoperative localization using an armless, frameless stereotactic wand. Technical note. J Neurosurg 1993; 78: 510–514

[3] Bucholz RD, Smith KR, Henderson J. Intraoperative localization using a three-dimensional optical digitizer. SPIE 1993;1894:312–322

[4] Galloway RL, Maciunas RJ. Stereotactic neurosurgery. Crit Rev Biomed Eng 1990; 18: 181–205

[5] Golfinos JG, Fitzpatrick BC, Smith LR, Spetzler RF. Clinical use of a frameless stereotactic arm: results of 325 cases. J Neurosurg 1995; 83: 197–205

[6] Guthrie BL, Adler JR, Jr. Computer-assisted preoperative planning, interactive surgery, and frameless stereotaxy. Clin Neurosurg 1992; 38: 112–131

[7] Kelly PJ, Kall BA, Goerss S, Earnest F. Present and future developments of stereotactic technology. Appl Neurophysiol 1985; 48: 1–6

[8] Maciunas RJ, Galloway RL, Jr, Fitzpatrick JM, Mandava VR, Edwards CA, Allen GS. A universal system for interactive image-directed neurosurgery. Stereotact Funct Neurosurg 1992; 58: 108–113

[9] Roberts DW, Strohbehn JW, Hatch JF, Murray W, Kettenberger H. A frameless stereotaxic integration of computerized tomographic imaging and the operating microscope. J Neurosurg 1986; 65: 545–549

[10] Watanabe E, Mayanagi Y, Kosugi Y, Manaka S, Takakura K. Open surgery assisted by the neuronavigator, a stereotactic, articulated, sensitive arm. Neurosurgery 1991; 28: 792–799, discussion 799–800

[11] Hammoud MA, Ligon BL, elSouki R, Shi WM, Schomer DF, Sawaya R. Use of intraoperative ultrasound for localizing tumors and determining the extent of resection: a comparative study with magnetic resonance imaging. J Neurosurg 1996; 84: 737–741

[12] Lunsford LD. A dedicated CT system for the stereotactic operating room. Appl Neurophysiol 1982; 45: 374–378

[13] Lunsford LD, Martinez AJ. Stereotactic exploration of the brain in the era of computed tomography. Surg Neurol 1984; 22: 222–230

[14] Lunsford LD, Parrish R, Albright L. Intraoperative imaging with a therapeutic computed tomographic scanner. Neurosurgery 1984; 15: 559–561

[15] Shalit MN, Israeli Y, Matz S, Cohen ML. Intra-operative computerized axial tomography. Surg Neurol 1979; 11: 382–384

[16] Black PM, Moriarty T, Alexander E, III et al. Development and implementation of intraoperative magnetic resonance imaging and its neurosurgical applications. Neurosurgery 1997; 41: 831–842, discussion 842–845

[17] Black PM, Alexander E, III, Martin C et al. Craniotomy for tumor treatment in an intraoperative magnetic resonance imaging unit. Neurosurgery 1999; 45: 423–431, discussion 431–433

[18] Lewin JS. Interventional MR imaging: concepts, systems, and applications in neuroradiology. AJNR Am J Neuroradiol 1999; 20: 735–748

[19] Mislow JMK, Golby AJ, Black PM. Origins of intraoperative MRI. Neurosurg Clin N Am 2009; 20: 137–146

[20] Hadani M, Spiegelman R, Feldman Z, Berkenstadt H, Ram Z. Novel, compact, intraoperative magnetic resonance imaging-guided system for conventional neurosurgical operating rooms. Neurosurgery 2001; 48: 799–807, discussion 807–809

[21] Bohinski RJ, Warnick RE, Gaskill-Shipley MF et al. Intraoperative magnetic resonance imaging to determine the extent of resection of pituitary macroadenomas during transsphenoidal microsurgery. Neurosurgery 2001; 49: 1133–1143, discussion 1143–1144

[22] Knauth M, Wirtz CR, Tronnier VM, Aras N, Kunze S, Sartor K. Intraoperative MR imaging increases the extent of tumor resection in patients with high-grade gliomas. AJNR Am J Neuroradiol 1999; 20: 1642–1646

[23] Nimsky C, Fujita A, Ganslandt O, Von Keller B, Fahlbusch R. Volumetric assessment of glioma removal by intraoperative high-field magnetic resonance imaging. Neurosurgery 2004; 55: 358–370, discussion 370–371

[24] Nimsky C, Ganslandt O, Tomandl B, Buchfelder M, Fahlbusch R. Low-field magnetic resonance imaging for intraoperative use in neurosurgery: a 5-year experience. Eur Radiol 2002; 12: 2690–2703

[25] Nimsky C, Ganslandt O, Von Keller B, Romstöck J, Fahlbusch R. Intraoperative high-field-strength MR imaging: implementation and experience in 200 patients. Radiology 2004; 233: 67–78

[26] Ntoukas V, Krishnan R, Seifert V. The new generation polestar n20 for conventional neurosurgical operating rooms: a preliminary report. Neurosurgery 2008; 62 Suppl 1: 82–89, discussion 89–90

[27] Schneider JP, Schulz T, Schmidt F et al. Gross-total surgery of supratentorial low-grade gliomas under intraoperative MR guidance. AJNR Am J Neuroradiol 2001; 22: 89–98

[28] Schneider JP, Trantakis C, Rubach M et al. Intraoperative MRI to guide the resection of primary supratentorial glioblastoma multiforme—a quantitative radiological analysis. Neuroradiology 2005; 47: 489–500

[29] Duffau H. Surgery of low-grade gliomas: towards a 'functional neurooncology'. Curr Opin Oncol 2009; 21: 543–549

[30] Soffietti R, Baumert BG, Bello L et al. European Federation of Neurological Societies. Guidelines on management of low-grade gliomas: report of an EFNS-EANO Task Force. Eur J Neurol 2010; 17: 1124–1133

[31] Keles GE, Lamborn KR, Berger MS. Low-grade hemispheric gliomas in adults: a critical review of extent of resection as a factor influencing outcome. J Neurosurg 2001; 95: 735–745

[32] McGirt MJ, Chaichana KL, Attenello FJ et al. Extent of surgical resection is independently associated with survival in patients with hemispheric infiltrating low-grade gliomas. Neurosurgery 2008; 63: 700–707, author reply 707–708

[33] McGirt MJ, Chaichana KL, Gathinji M et al. Independent association of extent of resection with survival in patients with malignant brain astrocytoma. J Neurosurg 2009; 110: 156–162

[34] Sanai N, Berger MS. Glioma extent of resection and its impact on patient outcome. Neurosurgery 2008; 62: 753–764, discussion 264–266

[35] Sanai N, Berger MS. Operative techniques for gliomas and the value of extent of resection. Neurotherapeutics 2009; 6: 478–486

[36] Sanai N, Chang S, Berger MS. Low-grade gliomas in adults. J Neurosurg 2011; 115: 948–965

[37] Sanai N, Polley MY, Berger MS. Insular glioma resection: assessment of patient morbidity, survival, and tumor progression. J Neurosurg 2010; 112: 1–9

[38] Smith JS, Chang EF, Lamborn KR et al. Role of extent of resection in the long-term outcome of low-grade hemispheric gliomas. J Clin Oncol 2008; 26: 1338–1345

[39] Claus EB, Horlacher A, Hsu L et al. Survival rates in patients with low-grade glioma after intraoperative magnetic resonance image guidance. Cancer 2005; 103: 1227–1233

[40] Senft C, Seifert V, Hermann E, Franz K, Gasser T. Usefulness of intraoperative ultra low-field magnetic resonance imaging in glioma surgery. Neurosurgery 2008; 63 Suppl 2: 257–266, discussion 266–267

[41] Hatiboglu MA, Weinberg JS, Suki D et al. Impact of intraoperative high-field magnetic resonance imaging guidance on glioma surgery: a prospective volumetric analysis. Neurosurgery 2009; 64: 1073–1081, discussion 1081

[42] Kowalczuk A, Macdonald RL, Amidei C et al. Quantitative imaging study of extent of surgical resection and prognosis of malignant astrocytomas. Neurosurgery 1997; 41: 1028–1036, discussion 1036–1038

[43] Kreth FW, Berlis A, Spiropoulou V et al. The role of tumor resection in the treatment of glioblastoma multiforme in adults. Cancer 1999; 86: 2117–2123

[44] Lacroix M, Abi-Said D, Fourney DR et al. A multivariate analysis of 416 patients with glioblastoma multiforme: prognosis, extent of resection, and survival. J Neurosurg 2001; 95: 190–198

[45] Laws ER, Shaffrey ME, Morris A, Anderson FA, Jr. Surgical management of intracranial gliomas—does radical resection improve outcome? Acta Neurochir Suppl (Wien) 2003; 85: 47–53

[46] Nicolato A, Gerosa MA, Fina P, Iuzzolino P, Giorgiutti F, Bricolo A. Prognostic factors in low-grade supratentorial astrocytomas: a uni-multivariate statistical analysis in 76 surgically treated adult patients. Surg Neurol 1995; 44: 208–221, discussion 221–223

[47] Kubben PL, ter Meulen KJ, Schijns OEMG, ter Laak-Poort MP, van Overbeeke JJ, van Santbrink H. Intraoperative MRI-guided resection of glioblastoma multiforme: a systematic review. Lancet Oncol 2011; 12: 1062–1070

[48] Hirschberg H, Samset E, Hol PK, Tillung T, Lote K. Impact of intraoperative MRI on the surgical results for high-grade gliomas. Minim Invasive Neurosurg 2005; 48: 77–84

[49] Senft C, Franz K, Blasel S et al. Influence of iMRI-guidance on the extent of resection and survival of patients with glioblastoma multiforme. Technol Cancer Res Treat 2010; 9: 339–346

[50] Wirtz CR, Knauth M, Staubert A et al. Clinical evaluation and follow-up results for intraoperative magnetic resonance imaging in neurosurgery. Neurosurgery 2000; 46: 1112–1120, discussion 1120–1122

[51] Senft C, Bink A, Franz K, Vatter H, Gasser T, Seifert V. Intraoperative MRI guidance and extent of resection in glioma surgery: a randomised, controlled trial. Lancet Oncol 2011; 12: 997–1003

[52] Wilson CB. A decade of pituitary microsurgery. The Herbert Olivecrona lecture. J Neurosurg 1984; 61: 814–833

[53] Stewart PM, Krone NP. The adrenal cortex. In: Melmed S, Polonsky KS, Larson MD, Kronenberg H.M. eds. Williams Textbook of Endocrinology. 12th ed. Philadelphia, PA: Saunders; 2011:479–544

[54] Pergolizzi RS, Jr, Nabavi A, Schwartz RB et al. Intra-operative MR guidance during trans-sphenoidal pituitary resection: preliminary results. J Magn Reson Imaging 2001; 13: 136–141

[55] Schulder M, Salas S, Brimacombe M et al. Cranial surgery with an expanded compact intraoperative magnetic resonance imager. Technical note. J Neurosurg 2006; 104: 611–617

[56] Schwartz TH, Stieg PE, Anand VK. Endoscopic transsphenoidal pituitary surgery with intraoperative magnetic resonance imaging. Neurosurgery 2006; 58 Suppl: ONS44–ONS51, discussion ONS44–ONS51

[57] Gerlach R, du Mesnil de Rochemont R, Gasser T et al. Feasibility of Polestar N20, an ultra-low-field intraoperative magnetic resonance imaging system in resection control of pituitary macroadenomas: lessons learned from the first 40 cases. Neurosurgery 2008; 63: 272–284, discussion 284–285

[58] Fahlbusch R, Thapar K. New developments in pituitary surgical techniques. Best Pract Res Clin Endocrinol Metab 1999; 13: 471–484

[59] Nimsky C, von Keller B, Ganslandt O, Fahlbusch R. Intraoperative high-field magnetic resonance imaging in transsphenoidal surgery of hormonally inactive pituitary macroadenomas. Neurosurgery 2006; 59: 105–114, discussion 105–114

[60] Finlay JL, Wisoff JH. The impact of extent of resection in the management of malignant gliomas of childhood. Childs Nerv Syst 1999; 15: 786–788

[61] Lancon JA, Killough KR, Dhillon G, Parent AD. Interventional magnetic resonance imaging guided aspiration and biopsy of a cystic midbrain tumor. Pediatr Neurosurg 1999; 30: 151–156

[62] Vitaz TW, Hushek S, Shields CB, Moriarty T. Changes in cyst volume following intraoperative MRI-guided Ommaya reservoir placement for cystic craniopharyngioma. Pediatr Neurosurg 2001; 35: 230–234

[63] Nimsky C, Ganslandt O, Gralla J, Buchfelder M, Fahlbusch R. Intraoperative low-field magnetic resonance imaging in pediatric neurosurgery. Pediatr Neurosurg 2003; 38: 83–89

[64] Roth J, Beni Adani L, Biyani N, Constantini S. Intraoperative portable 0.12-tesla MRI in pediatric neurosurgery. Pediatr Neurosurg 2006; 42: 74–80

[65] Samdani AF, Schulder M, Catrambone JE, Carmel PW. Use of a compact intraoperative low-field magnetic imager in pediatric neurosurgery. Childs Nerv Syst 2005; 21: 108–113, discussion 114

[66] Vitaz TW, Hushek SG, Shields CB, Moriarty TM. Interventional MRI-guided frameless stereotaxy in pediatric patients. Stereotact Funct Neurosurg 2002; 79: 182–190

[67] Vitaz TW, Hushek S, Shields CB, Moriarty T. Intraoperative MRI for pediatric tumor management. Acta Neurochir Suppl (Wien) 2003; 85: 73–78

[68] Levy R, Cox RG, Hader WJ, Myles T, Sutherland GR, Hamilton MG. Application of intraoperative high-field magnetic resonance imaging in pediatric neurosurgery. J Neurosurg Pediatr 2009; 4: 467–474

[69] Shah MN, Leonard JR, Inder G et al. Intraoperative magnetic resonance imaging to reduce the rate of early reoperation for lesion resection in pediatric neurosurgery. J Neurosurg Pediatr 2012; 9: 259–264

[70] Ganslandt O, Fahlbusch R, Nimsky C et al. Functional neuronavigation with magnetoencephalography: outcome in 50 patients with lesions around the motor cortex. J Neurosurg 1999; 91: 73–79

[71] Guye M, Parker GJ, Symms M et al. Combined functional MRI and tractography to demonstrate the connectivity of the human primary motor cortex in vivo. Neuroimage 2003; 19: 1349–1360

[72] Kober H, Nimsky C, Möller M, Hastreiter P, Fahlbusch R, Ganslandt O. Correlation of sensorimotor activation with functional magnetic resonance imaging and magnetoencephalography in presurgical functional imaging: a spatial analysis. Neuroimage 2001; 14: 1214–1228

[73] Nimsky C, Ganslandt O, Kober H et al. Integration of functional magnetic resonance imaging supported by magnetoencephalography in functional neuronavigation. Neurosurgery 1999; 44: 1249–1255, discussion 1255–1256

[74] Clark CA, Barrick TR, Murphy MM, Bell BA. White matter fiber tracking in patients with space-occupying lesions of the brain: a new technique for neurosurgical planning? Neuroimage 2003; 20: 1601–1608

[75] Hendler T, Pianka P, Sigal M et al. Delineating gray and white matter involvement in brain lesions: three-dimensional alignment of functional magnetic resonance and diffusion-tensor imaging. J Neurosurg 2003; 99: 1018–1027

[76] Yamada K, Kizu O, Mori S et al. Brain fiber tracking with clinically feasible diffusion-tensor MR imaging: initial experience. Radiology 2003; 227: 295–301

[77] Mamata Y, Mamata H, Nabavi A et al. Intraoperative diffusion imaging on a 0.5 Tesla interventional scanner. J Magn Reson Imaging 2001; 13: 115–119

[78] Nimsky C, Ganslandt O, Hastreiter P et al. Intraoperative diffusion-tensor MR imaging: shifting of white matter tracts during neurosurgical procedures—initial experience. Radiology 2005; 234: 218–225

[79] Nimsky C, Ganslandt O, Hastreiter P et al. Preoperative and intraoperative diffusion tensor imaging-based fiber tracking in glioma surgery. Neurosurgery 2005; 56: 130–137, discussion 138

[80] Romano A, D'Andrea G, Calabria LF et al. Pre- and intraoperative tractographic evaluation of corticospinal tract shift. Neurosurgery 2011; 69: 696–704, discussion 704–705

[81] Sun GC, Chen XL, Zhao Y et al. Intraoperative high-field magnetic resonance imaging combined with fiber tract neuronavigation-guided resection of cerebral lesions involving optic radiation. Neurosurgery 2011; 69: 1070–1084, discussion 1084

[82] Woodard EJ, Leon SP, Moriarty TM, et al: Initial experience with intraoperative magnetic resonance imaging in spine surgery. Spine 2001;26:410–417

[83] Berkovic SF, McIntosh AM, Kalnins RM et al. Preoperative MRI predicts outcome of temporal lobectomy: an actuarial analysis. Neurology 1995; 45: 1358–1363

[84] Spencer DD, Spencer SS, Mattson RH, Williamson PD, Novelly RA. Access to the posterior medial temporal lobe structures in the surgical treatment of temporal lobe epilepsy. Neurosurgery 1984; 15: 667–671

[85] Wyler AR, Hermann BP, Richey ET. Results of reoperation for failed epilepsy surgery. J Neurosurg 1989; 71: 815–819

[86] Awad IA, Nayel MH, Lüders H. Second operation after the failure of previous resection for epilepsy. Neurosurgery 1991; 28: 510–518

[87] Wiebe S, Blume WT, Girvin JP, Eliasziw M Effectiveness and Efficiency of Surgery for Temporal Lobe Epilepsy Study Group. A randomized, controlled trial of surgery for temporal-lobe epilepsy. N Engl J Med 2001; 345: 311–318

[88] Buchfelder M, Fahlbusch R, Ganslandt O, Stefan H, Nimsky C. Use of intraoperative magnetic resonance imaging in tailored temporal lobe surgeries for epilepsy. Epilepsia 2002; 43: 864–873

[89] Schwartz TH, Marks D, Pak J et al. Standardization of amygdalohippocampectomy with intraoperative magnetic resonance imaging: preliminary experience. Epilepsia 2002; 43: 430–436

[90] Kaibara T, Myles ST, Lee MA, Sutherland GR. Optimizing epilepsy surgery with intraoperative MR imaging. Epilepsia 2002; 43: 425–429

[91] Papavassiliou E, Rau G, Heath S et al. Thalamic deep brain stimulation for essential tremor: relation of lead location to outcome. Neurosurgery 2008; 62 Suppl 2: 884–894

[92] Martin AJ, Larson PS, Ostrem JL et al. Placement of deep brain stimulator electrodes using real-time high-field interventional magnetic resonance imaging. Magn Reson Med 2005; 54: 1107–1114

[93] Starr PA, Martin AJ, Ostrem JL, Talke P, Levesque N, Larson PS. Subthalamic nucleus deep brain stimulator placement using high-field interventional magnetic resonance imaging and a skull-mounted aiming device: technique and application accuracy. J Neurosurg 2010; 112: 479–490

[94] Starr PA, Christine CW, Theodosopoulos PV et al. Implantation of deep brain stimulators into the subthalamic nucleus: technical approach and magnetic resonance imaging-verified lead locations. J Neurosurg 2002; 97: 370–387

[95] Larson PS, Starr PA, Bates G, Tansey L, Richardson RM, Martin AJ. An optimized system for interventional magnetic resonance imaging-guided stereotactic surgery: preliminary evaluation of targeting accuracy. Neurosurgery 2012; 70 Suppl Operative: 95–103, discussion 103

16 On the Horizon: Ultra-High-Field MR

Steffen Sammet and Alexander Radbruch

16.1 Introduction

Ultra-high-field (UHF) magnetic resonance imaging (MRI) appeared on the horizon in the late 1980s when the first 4 T systems were installed in the United States at the University of Alabama, Birmingham; at the National Institutes of Health, Bethesda, Maryland; and at the Center for Magnetic Resonance Research of the University of Minnesota, Minneapolis.[1] These early systems had multiple engineering challenges, and many technological developments were necessary before diagnostic quality MRI scans could be obtained.[2] For more than a decade these high-field systems were mainly used in research, but there was always interest in exploiting the gain in signal-to-noise ratio (SNR) from UHF MRI for clinical applications. In 1998 the first human 8 T MRI system was installed at The Ohio State University, Columbus, which was then followed by a 7 T system at the University of Minnesota.[3] These two UHF systems were still investigational devices, built in part from in-house components. The 7 T system's 90-cm bore size was superior to the 8 T magnet's 80-cm bore size in terms of patient comfort and gradient performance.[4] The same bore-size advantage existed for 3 T systems compared to 4 T systems, and therefore the subsequent commercial MRI systems were built at 3 T and 7 T.[5] The current era of UHF MRI began when three leading manufacturers of clinical MR systems, Siemens Healthcare, Philips Healthcare, and General Electric Healthcare, introduced their first commercial 7 T systems. The commercial availability of 7 T from these established vendors led to a new momentum for UHF MRI. More than 50 7 T MRI systems have been installed and are operational worldwide today. The development of self-shielded 7 T magnets has significantly reduced the costs of siting UHF MRI systems in hospital environments and will enable 7 T MRI to eventually integrate into clinical workflows. The first results have demonstrated the advantages of UHF, especially in neuroradiological applications, including increased SNR,[6] improved sensitivity for functional brain imaging,[7] and increased spectral resolution for magnetic resonance spectroscopy (MRS).[8]

16.2 Challenges of Ultra-High-Field MRI

Promising results of the first 7 T MRI studies, however, elucidated some of the new challenges associated with UHF MRI technology. At higher field strengths variations of the static magnetic field, B_0, degrade image quality, especially in systems with larger bore sizes.[9] Especially fast gradient sequences are sensitive to the central field nonuniformities due to accumulation of phase errors during the scan. For example, the ultrafast echoplanar imaging (EPI) MRI pulse sequence uses long readout and data sampling durations resulting in enhanced distortion artifacts at UHF.[10] EPI is an essential sequence for functional magnetic resonance imaging (fMRI) and diffusion-weighted imaging (DWI). These imaging techniques are widely used in assessing brain function; therefore, solutions to B_0

nonuniformity at UHF were critically needed for neuroimaging applications. Technology was developed that improved B_0 field inhomogeneities by at least an order of magnitude through the introduction of additional subsidiary windings known as active shims.[11,12]

At UHF not only the static magnetic field B_0 shows variations but also the radiofrequency (RF) field B_1.[13] The Larmor frequency of protons

$$\omega_o = \gamma \cdot B_0$$

is 300 MHz at 7 T, and the wavelength in tissue is thus shortened to around 14 cm. As a consequence, alternating B_1 RF fields show considerable variations across the field of view and lead to variations in SNR and contrast across the image.[14] Therefore, considerable resources were invested in the development of RF coils to improve both sensitivity and homogeneity. A novel technique called B_1-shimming, or RF-shimming, has demonstrated promising results and might become the method of choice to improve the homogeneity of the RF field at UHF. Another promising solution to B_1-inhomogeneities at UHF is the concept of traveling wave MRI. Traveling wave MRI radically changes the design of the RF technology. The bore of the magnet is used as a wave guide coupled to an antenna that is positioned at the end of the bore or as a small dipole close to the patient within the bore of the magnet. The bore of the magnet acts like a high-pass filter for traveling waves. For a typical 60 cm bore size of a 7 T magnet the cutoff frequency for the high-pass filter is very close to 298 MHz, corresponding to the hydrogen Larmor frequency at 7 T. The high dielectric constant of the human body diffracts the energy of the RF field at the surface of the body, and consequently the energy flows into the body. The entire bore of the magnet acts essentially as a very long RF coil.[15]

The higher static magnetic field B_0 at UHF creates a longer magnetization vector in tissue. The increased magnitude of the magnetization vector requires more energy deposition of the RF field B_1 and leads subsequently to an increased specific absorption rate (SAR) and additional patient safety concerns at UHF.[16,17] An increased static magnetic field B_0 also leads to an increase of the spin-lattice relaxation time T_1 and to a decrease of the spin-spin relaxation time T_2 caused by spin diffusion and exchange. These relaxation time changes lead to modified contrasts at UHF and need to be considered in sequence design and parameter selection.[18]

Inside the MRI bore there are three gradient coils (G_x, G_y, G_z) that vary the static magnetic field B_0 depending on the position. The gradient coils are built with wound wires or etched copper plates on fiberglass and are embedded in epoxy resin.[19] Switching currents in the gradients coils are used for spatial excitation and encoding of the spins. The gradients in MRI scanners are defined by the gradient strength, the gradient rise time, and the region of uniformity.[20] Lorentz forces on the current-carrying wires within the high static magnetic field B_0 of the main magnet cause vibrations at audible frequencies. The acoustic noises from the gradient coils can potentially damage the patient's hearing unless precautions are taken, such as earplugs or noise-reducing headphones. Therefore, multiple methods have been considered to reduce the acoustic noise and vibrations generated by the gradient coils, especially at UHG strengths, for example, by placing the gradients on rubber supports or vacuum-sealed gradient coil assemblies mounted directly on the floor so that they are mechanically decoupled from the magnet.[21] At UHF strengths fast gradient echo sequences are frequently used to profit from the high static field strength. These sequences require quick gradient rise times and rapidly switching gradients, which can induce noticeable vibration artifacts in the images. The electric fields generated by the gradients can also cause peripheral nerve stimulations and tingling sensations in patients.[22,23,24]

Safety studies on the first 8 T MRI system in Columbus, Ohio, led the U.S. Food and Drug Administration (FDA) to classify MRI up to 8 T as a nonsignificant risk.[25,26] This does not apply to patients with metallic implants. During an MRI examination, a metallic implant may interact with the static field B_0, RF field B_1, or gradient fields, and lead to translational or rotational motion, heating, device malfunction, or a combination of these effects.[27] These effects have been studied for many clinically relevant implants at 1.5 T and 3 T, resulting in metallic implants with FDA-approved labeling for MRI procedures that are acceptable if specific conditions are met. At field strengths above 3 T only a few systematic MRI safety assessments of metallic implants have been performed; therefore, patients with metallic implants are excluded from participating in UHF MRI studies in most institutions at the moment.[28] Therefore, new UHF MRI testing procedures for implants need to be designed and implemented. Despite all challenges, several human MRI systems with even higher field strengths, such as 9.4 T, 11.7 T, and even 14 T are either in planning or already operational.[29,30]

16.3 Potential of Ultra-High-Field MRI

16.3.1 Higher Signal-to-Noise Ratio

The impetus for UHF MRI is primarily the improvement in SNR afforded by higher main magnetic field strengths. SNR increases approximately linearly with the magnetic field strength.[14,31]

An increased SNR in MRI can be used to do the follows:

- Achieve higher spatial resolution (i.e., smaller voxel sizes)
- Shorten the often long measurement times in clinical MRI
- Open possibilities for MRI and MRS for nuclei that are less abundant than the hydrogen nucleus (e.g., ^{13}C, ^{17}O, ^{19}F, ^{23}Na, ^{31}P, ^{35}Cl, ^{39}K) to provide important physiological information about pathological changes or drug distribution noninvasively[32,33]
- Improve the detection of low-concentration metabolites in proton magnetic resonance spectroscopy[34]

These important advantages of a higher SNR offer great potential for improved neuro-oncological MRI. Smaller voxel sizes may lead to improved detection of small cancerous lesions and metastases. Faster scan times shorten imaging sequences and protocols, thus reducing motion artifacts from restless patients.[35]

The high SNR of UHF MRI can also be exploited to compensate for inherent SNR losses of parallel imaging techniques (e.g.,

sensitivity encoding [SENSE], simultaneous acquisition of spatial harmonics [SMASH], partially parallel imaging with localized sensitivities [PILS[, generalized autocalibrating partially parallel acquisitions [GRAPPA]). These parallel imaging techniques are widely used to accelerate MRI acquisition by using phased-array coils that increase imaging speed without the need to have faster gradient switching.[36]

16.3.2 Enhanced-Contrast Mechanisms

UHF MRI offers advantages to enhance contrast mechanisms in neuro-oncology in several MR imaging techniques.

Susceptibility- or T_2*-Weighted MRI

Susceptibility increases linearly with field strength B_0. Magnetic susceptibility is a dimensionless quantity and describes how a bulk material is magnetized when exposed to an external field. Magnetic susceptibility also describes the distortion of a magnetic field caused by the spatial variations of magnetic susceptibility in biological tissue.[37] Magnetic susceptibility is directly related to T_2* relaxation time. Functional and physiological brain processes, as well as pathological alterations that change blood oxygenation in the brain, can be better assessed by T_2* contrast imaging at UHF. Deoxygenated blood in the brain vasculature functions as an endogenous contrast agent and has been shown to better display tumor microvasculature with UHF MRI.[38,39]

Blood Oxygenation Level Dependent

Oxygenation sensitive imaging techniques, such as blood oxygenation level dependent (BOLD), profit as well from increased susceptibility contrast at UHF.[40] The oxygen-transporting protein hemoglobin changes from the diamagnetic oxyhemoglobin to the paramagnetic deoxyhemoglobin when it unloads oxygen in tissue. Deoxyhemoglobin can therefore serve as an intrinsic paramagnetic contrast agent. The oxygen consumption of activated brain areas increases and leads to a vasodilatation and consequently to an increased blood flow and blood volume. The increased arterial blood flow is not matched by the local oxygen consumption; therefore, an excess of oxygen is present in the draining veins, and an increased concentration of the diamagnetic oxyhemoglobin is found. Under brain activation the T_2* decay due to signal dephasing is therefore reduced in the vicinity of the vein, which leads to an increased signal. In functional MRI (fMRI) the enhanced signal changes can be used to better map activated brain areas due to the increase in image contrast.[41] fMRI can be used to localize functional brain areas and spare brain structures with essential function during therapy.[42] BOLD contrast can also be used to measure oxygen extraction fraction with the quantitative BOLD (qBOLD) technique.[43]

Contrast-Enhanced MR Angiography

UHF contrast-enhanced MR angiography (MRA) provides the possibility of higher-resolution images with improved differentiation between tissue and enhancing vessels. UHF MRA also shows an increased sensitivity for subtle alterations of the blood–brain barrier with minimal contrast uptake. Tumor recurrence can potentially be detected at an earlier time point, allowing for an earlier adaption of the therapy. The increased sensitivity to contrast enhancement as well as the high-spatial resolution of UHF MRI may also improve the detection of small metastases[44] and better differentiate these lesions from normal brain structures. Higher resolution also improves the detection of metastases in the vicinity of other enhancing structures, such as meninges, falx, and veins. An increased conspicuity of these lesions can influence treatment when solitary metastasis or multiple metastases are questioned. Higher field strengths may also be used to better visualize the arterial vasculature in tumors, which might provide additional information about neoangiogenic vessels.[45]

Perfusion MRI

Perfusion MRI describes techniques that use endogenous or exogenous tracers to evaluate the perfusion of blood in the cerebral capillaries. In neuro-oncological imaging, perfusion MRI is used to differentiate active tumor areas from surrounding healthy tissue and from necrotic tumor areas. Perfusion MRI can be used for tumor staging and evaluation of tumor response because it can visualize neoangiogenesis in tumors, especially at UHF.[46]

The perfusion technique dynamic contrast enhanced (DCE) MRI uses contrast agents to shorten the relaxation times T_1 and T_2 to create a contrast change during the passage of a contrast agent bolus. T_1-weighted techniques show a signal increase with contrast agent concentration, whereas T_2- or T_2^*-weighted techniques show a signal decrease. Contrast changes in the T_1-weighted technique DCE MRI provide transfer constants, such as k_{trans} (volume transfer constant between blood plasma and extravascular extracellular space [EES]), k_{ep} (rate constant between plasma and EES), and V_e (volume of the EES per unit volume of tissue), and help to assess tumor angiogenesis.[47] The first in vivo DCE MRI studies showed the potential of this perfusion technique at UHF.[48]

Contrast changes in T_2^*-weighted perfusion imaging are proportional to the concentration of contrast agent and therefore directly related to the relative cerebral blood volume (rCBV). Hemodynamic maps including mean transit time (MTT), time to peak (TTP), time of arrival, negative integral, and index can also be calculated in T_2^*-weighted perfusion imaging. At higher field strengths, lower contrast agent concentrations can be used to create the same T_2^*, contrast due to enhanced susceptibility contrast at UHF.[49]

The perfusion technique arterial spin labeling (ASL) uses blood as an endogenous tracer. In ASL the longitudinal magnetization of arterial blood proximal to the tissue of interest is changed (tagged), and then monitored during the passage to the tissue of interest. ASL at UHF strengths profits from an increased SNR as well as longer T_1 values of the blood. Increasing T_1 values of blood at higher field strengths contribute to a long-lasting ASL contrast to better delineate the passage of the arterial bolus through the capillaries. Nevertheless, UHF B_1-inhomogeneities can lead to a decreased efficiency of the inversion of the arterial bolus. These limitations can be partly compensated with adiabatic inversion pulses, but these pulses come with the expense of increased specific absorption rate (SAR).[50]

Diffusion MRI

DWI and diffusion tensor imaging (DTI) are techniques for studying the diffusion of water molecules and the integrity of white matter noninvasively in the human brain in vivo.[51] Diffusion MRI benefits from the inherent sensitivity benefit at UHF due to a related boost in SNR. DWI and DTI use single-shot EPI (sshEPI) due to its speed and its robustness to motion artifacts. At UHF MRI sshEPI shows severe distortions related to B_0 inhomogeneities and image blurring from a fast T_2^* decay.[52] Parallel imaging techniques can improve image quality of DWI and DTI at UHF strengths by shortening the echo train length, thus mitigating susceptibility-induced distortion and T_2^*-related blurring.[53]

MRS

MRS measures the concentration of chemical compounds (metabolites) in the human brain noninvasively. MRS is used in neuro-oncology to assess pathological processes by evaluation of concentration changes of related metabolites.[54] For example, an increased ratio of choline to creatine (Cho:Cr), a reduced ratio of N-acetylaspartate to creatine (NAA:Cr), an increased ratio of myoinositol to creatine (MI:Cr), and the presence of lipids or lactate are useful diagnostic measurements to differentiate benign from malignant tumors. MRS has also shown clinical potential in grading tumors. Metabolic maps have the ability to evaluate peritumoral regions and differentiate regions of recurrent tumor from radiation necrosis. The low sensitivity and specificity of the MRS is a limiting factor at lower field strengths. The sensitivity of MRS is limited by low metabolite concentrations, which also restrict the spatial resolution of multivoxel spectroscopic imaging techniques. MRS at high field strengths profits from a higher SNR as well as increased spectral resolution. A higher spectral resolution aids in differentiating compounds with small chemical shift differences and a higher SNR helps to detect metabolites with low concentrations.[55] Higher magnetic field strengths can also improve the detection of low-abundance nuclei such as ^{13}C, ^{17}O, ^{19}F, ^{23}Na, ^{31}P, ^{35}Cl, and ^{39}K.[34]

Time-of-Flight MRA

Time-of-flight MRA (TOF-MRA) is improved at higher static magnetic field strengths by increased intravascular signals as well as longer T_1 relaxation times of static tissues.[56] Longer T_1 values lead to significantly better background signal suppression and thus better vessel-to-background conspicuity.[57] Due to the increased resolution and sensitivity for flow at UHF it is possible to better assess tumor vessels directly and possibly quantify the extent of neovascularization.[58]

Phase Contrast MRA

Phase contrast MRA measures phase differences between flowing blood and surrounding stationary tissue to encode blood velocity. The most common method to encode velocity is the application of a bipolar gradient between the excitation pulse and the readout. This bipolar gradient of a given intensity and time will dephase moving spins in proportion to their velocity. The encoding gradient can be adjusted to encode flows within a

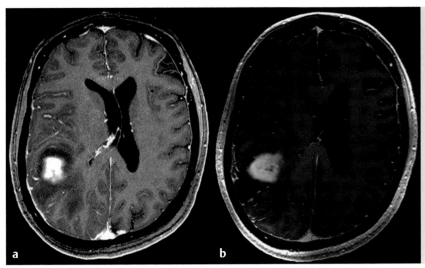

Fig. 16.1 Right temporal glioblastoma on contrast-enhanced T1-weighted images. Images at 3 T in (**a**) (repetition time [TR] 1.7 ms, echo time [TE] 4.64 ms, pixel spacing 0.5 × 0.5 mm) and at 7 T in (**b**) (TR 2.8 ms, TE 3.0 ms, pixel spacing 0.286 × 0.286 mm). Infiltration of the tumor delineates better on the 7 T images in (**b**).

certain velocity range or various velocity encoding (venc) values. The surrounding stationary tissue has identical signal in both acquisitions and will be subtracted so that only blood vessels are depicted and can be clearly visualized and identified. The increase of SNR at UHF enables the acquisition of smaller voxel sizes that result in better identification of vessel contours and subsequently better delineation of pathological processes.[59]

16.4 Application of UHF MRI in Brain Tumors

The introduction of UHF MRI within neuro-oncological imaging has the potential to improve the two most urgent challenges within brain tumor imaging: evaluation of differential diagnosis and therapy response assessment. The increased field strength allows an improved visualization of structures within the tumor on MRI sequences that are used on a routine basis, such as T2 or susceptibility-weighted imaging (SWI). Moreover, the increased frequency dispersion from the higher field results in an enhanced spectral resolution, or chemical shift, that can be exploited within MRS to quantify metabolite peaks that overlap at lower field strengths.[60] Finally, the increased field strength facilitates the use of techniques that are not applied in a clinical setting at lower field strengths, such as sodium imaging[61] or chemical exchange saturated transfer imaging.[62,63] With these new techniques new insights on tumor pathophysiology can potentially be obtained.[64,65] In the following, routine sequences as well as advanced imaging techniques and their potential value for the improvement of brain tumor imaging are discussed. Because 7 T is not approved for routine application in most countries, the majority of the presented results are still preliminary and not proven within large patient collectives.

16.4.1 T1-Weighted Imaging

Contrast-enhanced T1-weighted images still play an important role for imaging of high-grade glioma within daily clinical decision making. According to the recently introduced Radiology Assessment in Neuro-Oncology (RANO) criteria, progressive

disease of high-grade glioma is defined by at least a 25% increase in the sum of the products of perpendicular diameters of the enhancing lesion or appearance of any new lesion.[66] Even though the contrast in T1-weighted images at UHF-MRI is inherently reduced due to shorter relaxation times[60,67] a good contrast can still be obtained at UHF-MRI (▶ Fig. 16.1).

16.4.2 T2-Weighted Imaging

Assessment of T2-weighted images is particularly important in tumors that do not present any contrast enhancement. Even in enhancing high-grade gliomas the assessment of T2-weighted images has gained importance since RANO criteria acknowledged for the first time the so-called T2-progress. According to these criteria, a significant T2-signal increase qualifies for progressive disease even if there is no increase of contrast-enhancing tumor portions on T1-weighted images.[66,68] A major limitation of this approach is that T2-signal increase is often nonspecific, and infiltrative tumor progression cannot be differentiated reliably from other causes of T2-signal increase, such as a change in steroid dosing or radiation effects.[69] Therefore, RANO criteria recommend evaluating any imaging pattern on T2-weighted images that suggests infiltrating tumor, including mass effect (e.g., thickening of the corpus callosum or infiltration of the cortical ribbon).[66]

Due to the increased spatial resolution UHF-MRI displays more details of the tumor substructure, such as small vessels or microbleeds (▶ Fig. 16.2 and ▶ Fig. 16.3). The superior delineation of the internal tumor structure on T2-weighted images can potentially be used to assess T2 progress more accurately, even though this is not yet proven.

16.4.3 Susceptibility-Weighted Imaging

The basis of the assessment of brain tumors on SWI are low signal intensity structures—so-called intratumoral susceptibility signals (ITSS)—that usually cannot be visualized on conventional MRI. Park et al defined ITSS as low signal intensity and a fine linear or dotlike structure, with or without conglomeration, seen within the tumor.[70] Qualitative and quantitative efforts

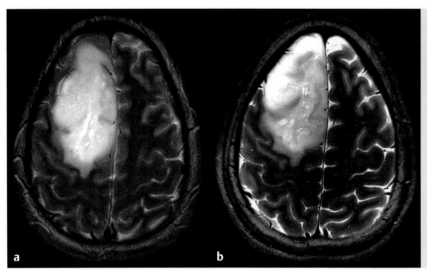

Fig. 16.2 Low-grade glioma in the right frontal lobe. Images at 3 T in (**a**) (repetition time [TR] 12 ms, echo time [TE] 57 ms, pixel spacing 0.286 × 0.286 mm) and at 7 T in (**b**) (TR 5.1 ms, TE 86 ms, pixel spacing 0.599 × 0.599 mm). Substructures within the tumor delineate better on the 7 T images.

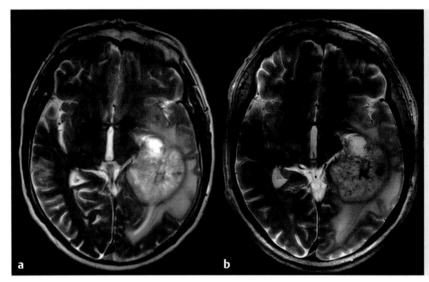

Fig. 16.3 Glioblastoma in the left temporal lobe. Image at 3 T in (**a**) (repetition time [TR] 12 ms, echo time [TE] 57 ms, pixel spacing 0.286 × 0.286 mm) and at 7 T in (**b**) (TR 5.1 ms, TE 86 ms, pixel spacing 0.599 × 0.599 mm). Both examinations took place on the same day. Substructures within the tumor delineate better on the 7 T image.

have been made to characterize ITSS and exploit their appearance for differential diagnosis of brain tumors (▶ Fig. 16.4).[71,72] Pathophysiological correlates of the ITSS are mostly microbleeds, vessels, or calcifications.[73] At lower field strengths the differentiation of ITSS in vessels or microbleeds is often impossible, whereas the increased sensitivity to susceptibility contrast at UHF-MRI enables the differentiation between microbleeds and vessels in some cases. Interestingly, Moenninghoff et al described the presence of a tortuous microvasculature that was not apparent at 1.5 T and corresponded to histological staining for abnormal vascularity on histology.[74] Finally, quantitative susceptibility mapping (QSM), an advanced postprocessing technique of the phase signal, benefits from the increased field strength at UHF-MRI and enables a clear differentiation between a paramagnetic origin of ITSS, such as deoxyhemoglobin, methemoglobin, hemosiderin, and ferritin, or a diamagnetic origin, such as calcifications.[73,75,76]

16.4.4 Time-of-Flight Angiography

Currently TOF angiography is the most commonly used non-contrast-enhanced MRA.[77] Although TOF angiography at 3 T is known as a reliable method for the evaluation of patients with cerebrovascular disease and for the noninvasive detection of intracranial aneurysms,[78,79] it is rarely used in tumor imaging protocols within clinical praxis. This is because tumor vessels usually cannot be visualized at 3 T and additional TOF angiography only provides information about a potential displacement of the main cerebral arteries due to tumor growth.

Generally, high-grade gliomas are characterized by vascular proliferation of tumor vessels, which differentiates them from other brain tumors, such as low-grade gliomas.[80] Hence direct visualization of tumor vessels could potentially contribute to the differential diagnosis of glioblastoma. Furthermore, the increasing use of antiangiogenic agents such as bevacizumab in

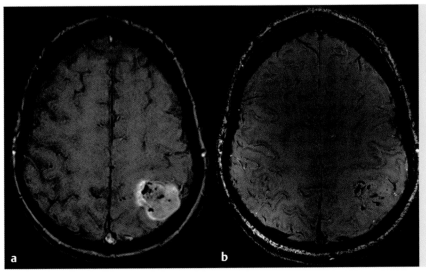

Fig. 16.4 Glioblastoma in the left parietal lobe. Contrast-enhanced susceptibility-weighted image at 3 T in (**a**) and susceptibility-weighted image at 7 T in (**b**). Intratumoral susceptibility signals (ITSS) display with higher resolution on the 7 T image.

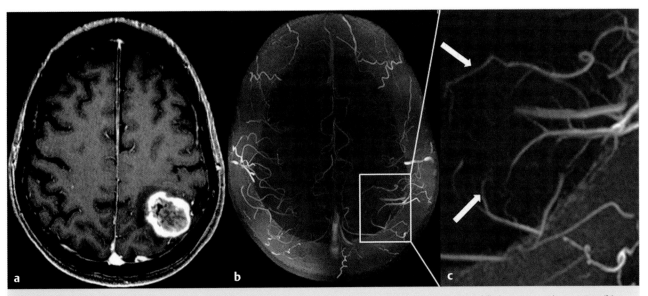

Fig. 16.5 Glioblastoma in the left parietal lobe. Contrast-enhanced T1-weighted image at 3 T in (**a**) and time-of-flight angiography at 7 T in (**b**) (enlarged in **c**). Tumor vessels display within the glioblastoma (**c**) (white arrows).

the treatment of glioblastoma highlights the potential of the visualization of tumor vessels for response assessment.

TOF angiography at UHF-MRI potentially visualizes the tumor vessels of high-grade gliomas directly (▶ Fig. 16.5) and hence opens the possibility for direct monitoring of antiangiogenic therapies.

16.4.5 Chemical Exchange Saturated Transfer Imaging

Finally, UHF-MRI enables the use of imaging techniques that provide metabolic information with high resolution. Namely chemical exchange saturation transfer (CEST) imaging benefits from the increased field strength at UHF-MRI. CEST MRI is a noninvasive MRI technique that is sensitive to the tissue-specific concentration of endogenous mobile proteins and peptides, respectively.[62,81] Multiple metabolites within brain

tumors have exchangeable protons and thus become endogenous agents with distinct chemical shifts. These differences make CEST a technology with the potential for frequency selective molecular imaging.[81] The first results have already demonstrated the possibility to identify and differentiate grades of glioma with CEST imaging.[82,83,84,85]

Signal contrast related to mobile proteins results from saturation of their exchanging protons by selective RF irradiation. Protons in a saturated state transfer to the free bulk water yielding a reduction of local z-magnetization of water protons. This leads to a signal accumulation in the water pool, which allows an indirect MRI of mobile proteins. At low saturation powers (e.g., 0.6–0.8 T) CEST signal at –2 to –5 ppm should be predominantly mediated by nuclear Overhauser enhancement (NOE) effects.[63,86,87] Initial examinations of high-grade gliomas at 7 T[87] found that NOE-mediated CEST effects significantly drop in tumor tissue. However, pH differences play a potential role

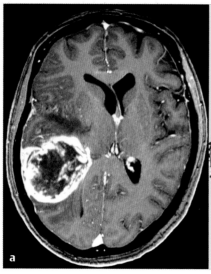 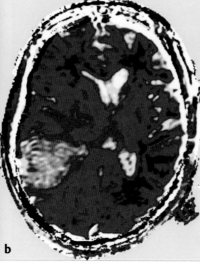

Fig. 16.6 Glioblastoma in the right temporal lobe. Contrast-enhanced T1-weighted images at 3 T in (**a**). In (**b**) chemical exchange saturated effects at 3.5 ppm are visualized. The enhancement can clearly be differentiated from the necrosis on the chemical exchange saturation transfer (CEST) image, without the use of contrast agent. It is assumed that the contrast at 3.5 ppm is mainly generated by the nuclear Overhauser enhancement effect.

within the CEST effect,[88] and future studies should highlight the pathophysiological origin of areas presenting different CEST signals within brain tumors (▸ Fig. 16.6).

References

[1] Bomsdorf H, Helzel T, Kunz D, Röschmann P, Tschendel O, Wieland J. Spectroscopy and imaging with a 4 tesla whole-body MR system. NMR Biomed 1988; 1: 151–158

[2] Hoult DI, Lee D. Shimming a superconducting nuclearmagnetic resonance imaging magnet with steel. Rev Sci Instrum 1985; 56: 131–135

[3] Robitaille P-ML, Warner R, Jagadeesh J et al. Design and assembly of an 8 tesla whole-body MR scanner. J Comput Assist Tomogr 1999; 23: 808–820

[4] Warner R, Pittard S, Feenan PJ, Goldi F, Abduljalil AM, Robitaille PML. Design and manufacture of the world's first whole body MRI magnet operating at a field strength above 7.0 Tesla: initial findings. Proc Int Soc Magn Reson Med 1998:254

[5] Robitaille PML, Abduljalil AM, Kangarlu A et al. Human magnetic resonance imaging at 8 T. NMR Biomed 1998; 11: 263–265

[6] Hoult DI, Richards RE. The signal-to-noise ratio of the nuclear magnetic resonance experiment. J Magn Reson 1976; 24: 71–83

[7] Yacoub E, Shmuel A, Pfeuffer J et al. Imaging brain function in humans at 7 Tesla. Magn Reson Med 2001; 45: 588–594

[8] Mekle R, Mlynárik V, Gambarota G, Hergt M, Krueger G, Gruetter R. MR spectroscopy of the human brain with enhanced signal intensity at ultrashort echo times on a clinical platform at 3 T and 7 T. Magn Reson Med 2009; 61: 1279–1285

[9] Asner FM. High-Field Superconducting Magnets. Oxford, England: Oxford University Press; 1999

[10] Stehling MK, Turner R, Mansfield P. Echo-planar imaging: magnetic resonance imaging in a fraction of a second. Science 1991; 254: 43–50

[11] de Graaf RA, Brown PB, McIntyre S, Rothman DL, Nixon TW. Dynamic shim updating (DSU) for multislice signal acquisition. Magn Reson Med 2003; 49: 409–416

[12] Roopchansingh V, Jesmanowicz A, Hyde JS. Magnetic field homogeneity improvement in the lower frontal lobe by combined resistive and passive shims with a user-defined mask. Proc Int Soc Magn Reson Med 2004;11:1650

[13] Roe , mer PB, Edelstein WA, Hayes CE, Souza SP, Mueller OM. The NMR phased array. Magn Reson Med 1990; 16: 192–225

[14] Vaughan JT, Garwood M, Collins CM et al. 7 T vs. 4T: RF power, homogeneity, and signal-to-noise comparison in head images. Magn Reson Med 2001; 46: 24–30

[15] Brunner DO, Paška J, Froehlich J, Pruessmann KP. Traveling-wave RF shimming and parallel MRI. Magn Reson Med 2011; 66: 290–300

[16] Bottomley PA, Edelstein WA. Power deposition in whole-body NMR imaging. Med Phys 1981; 8: 510–512

[17] Collins CM, Smith MB. Signal-to-noise ratio and absorbed power as functions of main magnetic field strength, and definition of "90 degrees " RF pulse for the head in the birdcage coil. Magn Reson Med 2001; 45: 684–691

[18] Bottomley PA, Foster TH, Argersinger RE, Pfeifer LM. A review of normal tissue hydrogen NMR relaxation times and relaxation mechanisms from 1–100 MHz: dependence on tissue type, NMR frequency, temperature, species, excision, and age. Med Phys 1984; 11: 425–448

[19] Turner R. Gradient coil design: a review of methods. Magn Reson Imaging 1993; 11: 903–920

[20] Chapman BLW. Gradients: the heart of the MRI machine. Curr Med Imag Rev 2006; 2: 131–138

[21] Chapman BLW, Mansfield P. Quiet gradient coils: Active acoustically and magnetically screened distribuited transverse gradient designs. Meas Sci Technol 1995; 6: 349–354

[22] Reilly JP. Peripheral nerve stimulation by induced electric currents: exposure to time-varying magnetic fields. Med Biol Eng Comput 1989; 27: 101–110

[23] Schmitt F, Stehling MK, Turner R. Physiological side effects of fast gradient switching. In: Echo-Planar Imaging. New York, NY: Springer; 1998:201–252

[24] Glover PM. Interaction of MRI field gradients with the human body. Phys Med Biol 2009; 54: R99–R115

[25] Kangarlu A, Burgess RE, Zhu H et al. Cognitive, cardiac, and physiological safety studies in ultra high field magnetic resonance imaging. Magn Reson Imaging 1999; 17: 1407–1416

[26] Chakeres DW, Bornstein R, Kangarlu A. Randomized comparison of cognitive function in humans at 0 and 8 Tesla. J Magn Reson Imaging 2003; 18: 342–345

[27] Schenck JF. Safety of strong, static magnetic fields. J Magn Reson Imaging 2000; 12: 2–19

[28] Schenck JF. Physical interactions of static magnetic fields with living tissues. Prog Biophys Mol Biol 2005; 87: 185–204

[29] Vedrine P, Aubert G, Beaudet F et al. The whole body 11.7 T MRI magnet for Iseult/INUMAC project. IEEE Trans Appl Supercond 2008; 18: 868–873

[30] Schild T, Abdel Maksoud W, Aubert G et al. The Iseult/INUMAC whole body 11.7 T MRI magnet R&D program. IEEE Trans Appl Supercond 2010; 20: 702–705

[31] Hoult DI, Phil D. Sensitivity and power deposition in a high-field imaging experiment. J Magn Reson Imaging 2000; 12: 46–67

[32] Twieg DB, Hetherington HP, Ponder SL, den Hollander J, Pohost GM. Spatial resolution in 31 P metabolite imaging of the human brain at 4.1 T. J Magn Reson B 1994; 104: 153–158

[33] Chu WJ, Hetherington HP, Kuzniecky RI et al. Is the intracellular pH different from normal in the epileptic focus of patients with temporal lobe epilepsy? A 31 P NMR study. Neurology 1996; 47: 756–760

[34] Pan JW, Mason GF, Vaughan JT, Chu WJ, Zhang Y, Hetherington HP. 13C editing of glutamate in human brain using J-refocused coherence transfer spectroscopy at 4.1 T. Magn Reson Med 1997; 37: 355–358

[35] Yuh WT, Christoforidis GA, Koch RM et al. Clinical magnetic resonance imaging of brain tumors at ultrahigh field: a state-of-the-art review. Top Magn Reson Imaging 2006; 17: 53–61

[36] Pruessmann KP, Weiger M, Scheidegger MB, Boesiger P. SENSE: sensitivity encoding for fast MRI. Magn Reson Med 1999; 42: 952–962

[37] Abduljalil AM, Robitaille P-ML. Macroscopic susceptibility in ultra high field MRI. J Comput Assist Tomogr 1999; 23: 832–841

[38] Christoforidis GA, Bourekas EC, Baujan M et al. High resolution MRI of the deep brain vascular anatomy at 8 Tesla: susceptibility-based enhancement of the venous structures. J Comput Assist Tomogr 1999; 23: 857–866

[39] Christoforidis GA, Kangarlu A, Abduljalil AM et al. Susceptibility-based imaging of glioblastoma microvascularity at 8 T: correlation of MR imaging and postmortem pathology. AJNR Am J Neuroradiol 2004; 25: 756–760

[40] Duong TQ, Yacoub E, Adriany G et al. High-resolution, spin-echo BOLD, and CBF fMRI at 4 and 7 T. Magn Reson Med 2002; 48: 589–593

[41] Lee S-P, Silva AC, Ugurbil K, Kim SG. Diffusion-weighted spin-echo fMRI at 9.4 T: microvascular/tissue contribution to BOLD signal changes. Magn Reson Med 1999; 42: 919–928

[42] Olman CA, Ugurbil K, Schrater P, Kersten D. BOLD fMRI and psychophysical measurements of contrast response to broadband images. Vision Res 2004; 44: 669–683

[43] Yacoub E, Van De Moortele PF, Shmuel A, Uğurbil K. Signal and noise characteristics of Hahn SE and GE BOLD fMRI at 7 T in humans. Neuroimage 2005; 24: 738–750

[44] Mönninghoff C, Maderwald S, Theysohn JM et al. Imaging of brain metastases of bronchial carcinomas with 7 T MRI - initial results. Rofo 2010; 182: 764–772

[45] Yuh WTC, Christoforidis GA, Mayr NA et al. Ultrahigh field clinical MR imaging: challenge and excitement. US Radiology 2011; 3: 16–22

[46] Prabhakaran V, Nair VA, Austin BP et al. Current status and future perspectives of magnetic resonance high-field imaging: a summary. Neuroimaging Clin N Am 2012; 22: 373–397, xii

[47] Larsson HB, Courivaud F, Rostrup E, Hansen AE. Measurement of brain perfusion, blood volume, and blood-brain barrier permeability, using dynamic contrast-enhanced T(1)-weighted MRI at 3 tesla. Magn Reson Med 2009; 62: 1270–1281

[48] Liang J, Sammet S, Yang X, Jia G, Takayama Y, Knopp MV. Intraindividual in vivo comparison of gadolinium contrast agents for pharmacokinetic analysis using dynamic contrast enhanced magnetic resonance imaging. Invest Radiol 2010; 45: 233–244

[49] Zwanenburg JJ, Versluis MJ, Luijten PR, Petridou N. Fast high resolution whole brain T2* weighted imaging using echo planar imaging at 7 T. Neuroimage 2011; 56: 1902–1907

[50] Wells JA, Siow B, Lythgoe MF, Thomas DL. The importance of RF bandwidth for effective tagging in pulsed arterial spin labeling MRI at 9.4 T. NMR Biomed 2012; 25: 1139–1143

[51] Basser PJ, Mattiello J, LeBihan D. MR diffusion tensor spectroscopy and imaging. Biophys J 1994; 66: 259–267

[52] van Gelderen P, de Vleeschouwer MHM, DesPres D, Pekar J, van Zijl PCM, Moonen CTW. Water diffusion and acute stroke. Magn Reson Med 1994; 31: 154–163

[53] Le Bihan D. Looking into the functional architecture of the brain with diffusion MRI. Nat Rev Neurosci 2003; 4: 469–480

[54] Hetherington HP, Mason GF, Pan JW et al. Evaluation of cerebral gray and white matter metabolite differences by spectroscopic imaging at 4.1 T. Magn Reson Med 1994; 32: 565–571

[55] Pan JW, Mason GF, Pohost GM, Hetherington HP. Spectroscopic imaging of human brain glutamate by water-suppressed J-refocused coherence transfer at 4.1 T. Magn Reson Med 1996; 36: 7–12

[56] von Morze C, Xu D, Purcell DD et al. Intracranial time-of-flight MR angiography at 7 T with comparison to 3 T. J Magn Reson Imaging 2007; 26: 900–904

[57] von Morze C, Purcell DD, Banerjee S et al. High-resolution intracranial MRA at 7 T using autocalibrating parallel imaging: initial experience in vascular disease patients. Magn Reson Imaging 2008; 26: 1329–1333

[58] Heverhagen JT, Bourekas E, Sammet S, Knopp MV, Schmalbrock P. Time-of-flight magnetic resonance angiography at 7 Tesla. Invest Radiol 2008; 43: 568–573

[59] Stamm AC, Wright CL, Knopp MV, Schmalbrock P, Heverhagen JT. Phase contrast and time-of-flight magnetic resonance angiography of the intracerebral arteries at 1.5, 3 and 7 T. Magn Reson Imaging 201 3; 31: 545–549

[60] Lupo JM, Li Y, Hess CP, Nelson SJ. Advances in ultra-high field MRI for the clinical management of patients with brain tumors. Curr Opin Neurol 2011; 24: 605–615

[61] Nagel AM, Laun FB, Weber MA, Matthies C, Semmler W, Schad LR. Sodium MRI using a density-adapted 3D radial acquisition technique. Magn Reson Med 2009; 62: 1565–1573

[62] Zaiss M, Bachert P. Chemical exchange saturation transfer (CEST) and MR Z-spectroscopy in vivo: a review of theoretical approaches and methods. Phys Med Biol 2013; 58: R221–R269

[63] Zaiss M, Kunz P, Goerke S, Radbruch A, Bachert P. MR imaging of protein folding in vitro employing nuclear-Overhauser-mediated saturation transfer. NMR Biomed 2013; 26: 1815–1822

[64] Jones CK, Schlosser MJ, van Zijl PC, Pomper MG, Golay X, Zhou J. Amide proton transfer imaging of human brain tumors at 3 T. Magn Reson Med 2006; 56: 585–592

[65] Nagel AM, Bock M, Hartmann C et al. The potential of relaxation-weighted sodium magnetic resonance imaging as demonstrated on brain tumors. Invest Radiol 2011; 46: 539–547

[66] Wen PY, Macdonald DR, Reardon DA et al. Updated response assessment criteria for high-grade gliomas: response assessment in neuro-oncology working group. J Clin Oncol 2010; 28: 1963–1972

[67] Ladd ME. High-field-strength magnetic resonance: potential and limits. Top Magn Reson Imaging 2007; 18: 139–152

[68] Radbruch A, Lutz K, Wiestler B et al. Relevance of T2 signal changes in the assessment of progression of glioblastoma according to the Response Assessment in Neurooncology criteria. Neuro-oncol 2012; 14: 222–229

[69] Lutz K, Wiestler B, Graf M et al. Infiltrative patterns of glioblastoma: identification of tumor progress using apparent diffusion coefficient histograms. J Magn Reson Imaging 201 4; 39: 1096–1103

[70] Park MJ, Kim HS, Jahng GH, Ryu CW, Park SM, Kim SY. Semiquantitative assessment of intratumoral susceptibility signals using non-contrast-enhanced high-field high-resolution susceptibility-weighted imaging in patients with gliomas: comparison with MR perfusion imaging. AJNR Am J Neuroradiol 2009; 30: 1402–1408

[71] Radbruch A, Wiestler B, Kramp L et al. Differentiation of glioblastoma and primary CNS lymphomas using susceptibility weighted imaging. Eur J Radiol 2013; 82: 552–556

[72] Radbruch A, Graf M, Kramp L et al. Differentiation of brain metastases by percentagewise quantification of intratumoral-susceptibility-signals at 3Tesla. Eur J Radiol 2012; 81: 4064–4068

[73] Deistung A, Schweser F, Wiestler B et al. Quantitative susceptibility mapping differentiates between blood depositions and calcifications in patients with glioblastoma. PLoS ONE 2013; 8: e57924

[74] Moenninghoff C, Maderwald S, Theysohn JM et al. Imaging of adult astrocytic brain tumours with 7 T MRI: preliminary results. Eur Radiol 2010; 20: 704–713

[75] Schweser F, Deistung A, Lehr BW, Reichenbach JR. Differentiation between diamagnetic and paramagnetic cerebral lesions based on magnetic susceptibility mapping. Med Phys 2010; 37: 5165–5178

[76] Schweser F, Deistung A, Lehr BW, Reichenbach JR. Quantitative imaging of intrinsic magnetic tissue properties using MRI signal phase: an approach to in vivo brain iron metabolism? Neuroimage 2011; 54: 2789–2807

[77] Miyazaki M, Lee VS. Nonenhanced MR angiography. Radiology 2008; 248: 20–43

[78] Urbach H, Dorenbeck U, von Falkenhausen M et al. Three-dimensional time-of-flight MR angiography at 3 T compared to digital subtraction angiography in the follow-up of ruptured and coiled intracranial aneurysms: a prospective study. Neuroradiology 2008; 50: 383–389

[79] Willinek WA, Born M, Simon B et al. Time-of-flight MR angiography: comparison of 3.0-T imaging and 1.5-T imaging—initial experience. Radiology 2003; 229: 913–920

[80] Wen PY, Kesari S. Malignant gliomas in adults. N Engl J Med 2008; 359: 492–507

[81] Liu G, Song X, Chan KW, McMahon MT. Nuts and bolts of chemical exchange saturation transfer MRI. NMR Biomed 2013; 26: 810–828

[82] Zhou J, Tryggestad E, Wen Z et al. Differentiation between glioma and radiation necrosis using molecular magnetic resonance imaging of endogenous proteins and peptides. Nat Med 2011; 17: 130–134

[83] Wen Z, Hu S, Huang F et al. MR imaging of high-grade brain tumors using endogenous protein and peptide-based contrast. Neuroimage 2010; 51: 616–622

[84] Jia G, Abaza R, Williams JD et al. Amide proton transfer MR imaging of prostate cancer: a preliminary study. J Magn Reson Imaging 2011; 33: 647–654

[85] Rivlin M et al. Molecular imaging of tumors and metastases using chemical exchange saturation transfer (CEST) MRI Scientific Reports 2013; 3: 3045

[86] Zhou J, Hong X, Zhao X, Gao JH, Yuan J. APT-weighted and NOE-weighted image contrasts in glioma with different RF saturation powers based on magnetization transfer ratio asymmetry analyses. Magn Reson Med 2013; 70: 320–327

[87] Jones CK, Huang A, Xu J et al. Nuclear Overhauser enhancement (NOE) imaging in the human brain at 7 T. Neuroimage 2013; 77: 114–124

[88] Jin T, Wang P, Zong X, Kim SG. Magnetic resonance imaging of the Amine-Proton EXchange (APEX) dependent contrast. Neuroimage 2012; 59: 1218–1227

17 On the Horizon: Tumor Genomics

Rivka R. Colen, Faisal Tai, and Pascal O. Zinn

17.1 Introduction

Imaging genomics is an emerging field that links specific imaging characteristics (also termed radiophenotypes or phenotypes) to the underlying genomic composition of tissues or tumors, such as glioblastoma multiforme (GBM) (▶ Fig. 17.1).[1,2] Imaging features, specifically those shown on magnetic resonance imaging (MRI), have been shown to correlate with the underlying histopathological composition of tumors.[3,4,5,6,7,8] Specifically, imaging features have been shown to correlate with DNA/RNA-based and protein-based whole-genome data.[1,2,9,10,11,12,13,14] Conventional imaging features such as tumor location and border, signal intensity, and contrast enhancement as well as the advanced techniques of magnetic resonance perfusion (MRP) and diffusion-weighted imaging (DWI) are used in imaging genomics.[1,10,11,15,16,17,18,19,20] Several significant associations have been established for a variety of cancers, including liver cancer,[21] non–small cell lung cancer,[22] and glial cell tumors.[9,10,11,12,16]

This chapter reviews the field to date with a focus on brain tumors. The growth in this field is largely due to advances in genomic sequencing technology from which large amounts of genomic data have been acquired after having been derived through surgical biopsies. First, the Human Genome Project, the largest collaborative biological project to date, introduced sequencing efforts to map the human genome. The advent of microarray technology enabled the analysis of thousands of genomics events simultaneously. More recently, the high demand for low-cost sequencing has driven the development of next-generation sequencing technology that enables high-throughput sequencing and processing of thousands to millions of sequences simultaneously. Such technological tools are enabling researchers in the field of imaging genomics to make large strides and advancements in this field.

17.2 Genomics in Glioma

17.2.1 Genomic Markers in Glioblastoma Multiforme

Genetics and *genomics* have different meanings; whereas genetics is the study of heredity and looks at the functioning and composition of single genes, genomics is the study of genes and looks at their combined network functions and their influence on growth and development. Genomics addresses all genes and their interrelationships, including large gene and signaling networks. Outside stimuli and the surrounding tumor microenvironment can cause changes in gene expression, microRNA (miRNA) levels, promoter methylation, and cellular phenotype, which is a collective phenomenon termed epigenetics. Epigenetic modifications provide cellular diversity and tumor heterogeneity,[23,24,25,26] and markers of these modifications can have diagnostic or prognostic value. *O6-methylguanine-DNA methyl transferase (MGMT)* promoter methylation and *isocitrate dehydrogenase 1 (IDH1)* mutation status have shown promise as prognostic and predictive genomic biomarkers.[27,28] Confirmed by multiple clinical trials, epigenetic-mediated gene silencing through *MGMT* promoter methylation is one of the most important prognostic factors for progression-free and overall survival and is an important predictive genomic biomarker for treatment response to alkylating agents such as temozolomide[27,29,30]; consequently, the MGMT assay has become one of the most requested molecular assays in clinical neuro-oncology.[31] Similarly, *IDH1* mutations, the most common mutation in secondary GBMs (seen in 50–88% of secondary GBMs), can differentiate primary from secondary GBMs and indicate a better prognosis in patients whose tumor harbors this mutation.[31,32] The diagnostic and prognostic value of *IDH1* mutation status is likely to result in revisions to the current World Health Organization (WHO) classification scheme for GBM.[31]

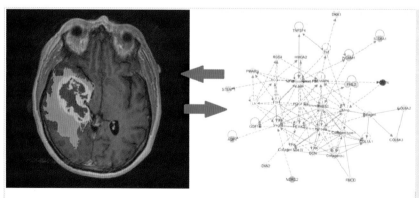

Fig. 17.1 Imaging genomic mapping in glioblastoma multiforme (GBM). Imaging, specifically magnetic resonance imaging, can be correlated with the underlying genomic composition of the tumors, as demonstrated here using the Ingenuity Pathway Analysis network, which demonstrates the molecular networks associated with imaging phenotypes, specifically an invasion/edema phenotype in a GBM patient. (Used with the permission of Zinn PO, Mahajan B, Sathyan P, et al. Radiogenomic mapping of edema/cellular invasion MRI-phenotypes in glioblastoma multiforme. PLoS ONE 2011;6(10):e25451.)

Important underlying cancer-related genetics are miRNAs, small, noncoding RNA molecules that function as negative gene regulators and potent silencers of gene expression via transcriptional and posttranslational modification on target genes.[33] A single miRNA may regulate more than 100 messenger RNAs (mRNAs) and, as such, miRNAs are crucial regulators of cell proliferation and differentiation and significant players in the maintenance of glioma stem cells.[34] The most commonly upregulated and comprehensively studied miRNA in GBM is miRNA-21, a major oncogenic miRNA that targets tumor suppressor pathways in GBM and is involved in glioma invasion, apoptosis, and migration.[35,36]

17.2.2 Genomic Classification of GBM

Initial studies identified two clinically, defined subtypes and, more recently, molecular-genetic defined subtypes of GBM: primary and secondary.[37,38] These subtypes are typically seen in patients of different ages and have distinct genomic profiles with differential gene transcription patterns.[39,40] Primary GBMs, also termed de novo, are defined as tumors that present without a prior history or histopathological evidence of a lower-grade astrocytoma. Secondary GBMs are defined as those that arose by malignant transformation of a lower-grade astrocytoma.[37,41] Approximately 95% of GBMs are primary GBMs; these are typically seen in older patients (age > 50 years),[37] and are genomically characterized by a higher incidence of *epidermal growth factor receptor (EGFR)* gene amplifications/mutations and a low incidence of *tumor protein 53 (TP53)* mutations.[42] Secondary GBM accounts for only 5% of all GBMs; these are found predominantly in younger patients (age < 50 years),[32,37] and are genomically characterized by frequent *TP53* mutations and infrequently by *EGFR* amplification/mutations.[42] Recent studies found *IDH1* and *IDH1* mutation status to be the most accurate predictors of secondary GBM, because patients whose tumors harbored the *IDH1* mutation have longer overall survival (31 vs. 15 months)[28,32,43] and better response to temozolomide.[44]

The development of The Cancer Genome Atlas (TCGA) advanced the understanding of the genomic basis of cancer. A national network of research and technology teams, the TCGA began in 2006 to characterize more than 20 tumor types and has generated a comprehensive, large-scale, multidimensional analysis of the cancer genome. The first cancer studied out of this work was GBM.[38] The resultant genomic characterization of GBM provides insight into differential genomic profiles and molecular heterogeneity in a single tumor (intratumoral heterogeneity) and among different individuals with the "same" histologically defined tumor (interindividual heterogeneity).[39,40] This heterogeneity is now well recognized and has led to the recognition of the individuality of genomic signatures, which has since affected drug development and drug target discovery strategies.

Leveraging the comprehensive genomic, clinical, and survival data afforded by TCGA, Verhaak et al[40] classified GBMs into four molecular subtypes by using integrated multidimensional genomic data and genomic aberrations to establish patterns of somatic mutations and DNA copy numbers. The classical subtype harbored the genomic aberrations most common to GBM; these tumors demonstrate *EGFR* and chromosome 7

amplifications and *cyclin-dependent kinase inhibitor 2A (CDKN2A)* locus and chromosome 10 deletions. The mesenchymal subtype showed a high frequency of neurofibromin 1 (NF1) mutations/deletions and high expression levels of *chitinase-3-like protein 1 (CHI3L1)* and *MET* proto-oncogene. The proneural subtype had characteristics similar to secondary GBM, such as occurrence in younger patients, *platelet-derived growth factor receptor alpha (PDGFRA)*, and *IDH1 and TP53 mutations*. The neural subtype was strongly associated with neural, oligodendrocytic, and astrocytic gene signatures. Likewise, Phillips et al[45] divided high-grade glioma into three subtypes: proneural, proliferative, and mesenchymal; these subtypes demonstrated significant prognostic value independent of the WHO tumor grade and/or the presence of necrosis. Phillips et al also found that *PDGFRA* amplification correlated with higher-grade glioma. Molecular analysis of low-grade glioma (LGG) is under way, and we anticipate that the data will provide similar molecular subclassification of LGGs.

17.3 Imaging Genomics in Glioblastoma and Other Gliomas

Of the gliomas, GBM has been the one most studied in great detail and its molecular networks and subtypes based on MRI have been reported.[1] Initially conducted studies correlating radiophenotypical features to genomic data of brain tumors involved associations of imaging to single genetic characteristics such as the codeletion of *1p* and *19q*,[46] *TP53* overexpression,[47] *EGFR* amplification,[9] and *MGMT* promoter methylation in gliomas.[48] These have been followed by studies that identify hundreds and thousands of genes that correlate to a particular imaging phenotype.[11,16] In recent years, a small number of studies that apply advanced MRI techniques of MRP, DWI, and MR spectroscopy (MRS) have been published.[10]

17.3.1 Imaging Genomics in GBM

Qualitative Imaging Genomic Correlative Analyses

Most of the early research in imaging genomics correlated genotypes to qualitative conventional MRI tumor characteristics (phenotypes or radiophenotypes), such as contrast enhancement and tumor border integrity.[9,49] Diehn et al[9] found that *EGFR* overexpression was associated with a high ratio of contrast enhancement to necrosis within the same tumor. Aghi et al[49] demonstrated that *EGFR*-overexpressing (primary) GBMs, compared with *TP53*-mutated (secondary) GBMs and GBMs without *TP53* mutations or *EGFR* overexpression, had a higher ratio of T2-bright volume to enclosed T1-enhancing volume, possibly due to angiogenesis and edema caused by high levels of *vascular endothelial growth factor (VEGF)*. Aghi et al[49] also found that *EGFR*-overexpressing GBMs had lower T2 border sharpness coefficients than tumors that did not overexpress *EGFR*, resulting in fuzzy borders that suggested a high degree of tumor invasion; *EGFR* amplification has also been found to be correlated with resistance to radiation therapy,[50] and Schlegel et al[51] reported that older patients with GBM whose tumors did not have *TP53* mutations had an increase in overall survival

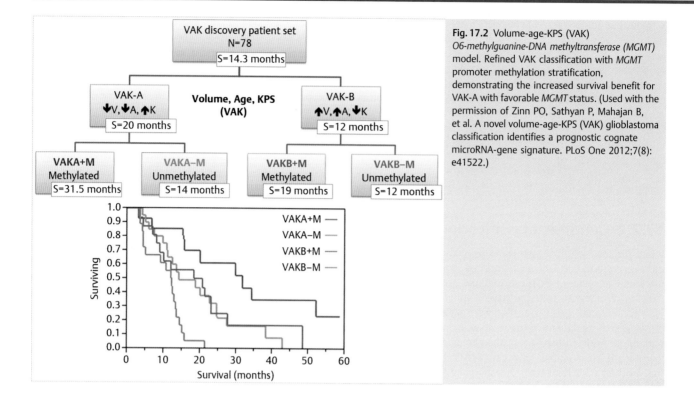

Fig. 17.2 Volume-age-KPS (VAK) *O6-methylguanine-DNA methyltransferase (MGMT)* model. Refined VAK classification with *MGMT* promoter methylation stratification, demonstrating the increased survival benefit for VAK-A with favorable *MGMT* status. (Used with the permission of Zinn PO, Sathyan P, Mahajan B, et al. A novel volume-age-KPS (VAK) glioblastoma classification identifies a prognostic cognate microRNA-gene signature. PLoS One 2012;7(8): e41522.)

compared with patients whose tumors had *TP53* mutations. Mut et al[47] looked exclusively at imaging characteristics related to *TP53* expression in GBM and found that tumors with low *TP53* expression (<50% as shown by immunohistochemical staining) demonstrated heterogeneous enhancement and ill-defined borders on postcontrast T1-weighted images, whereas those with higher *TP53* expression demonstrated well-defined borders and ring enhancement pattern on postcontrast T1-weighted images; the latter also had more favorable prognoses and longer overall survival times. Mut et al[47] found no relationship between *TP53* expression and location and number of lesions, size of the enhancing lesion and perilesional edema, mass effect, and tumor necrosis. However, our group recently demonstrated, via transcription factor analysis, that *TP53* was associated with high necrosis volumes in male patients with GBM.[52] Relatedly, *IDH1* mutation is most commonly seen in GBMs located in the frontal lobe.[53] However, some studies have found no significant correlation between genotype and tumor location.[54,55,56]

MGMT promoter methylation status has also been shown to correlate with imaging features; Drabycz et al[57] found that ring enhancement was significantly associated with unmethylated *MGMT* promoter status,[57] and another study found that ill-defined borders were more common in the *MGMT* promoter methylated tumors.[58] Eoli et al[48] found that unmethylated *MGMT* promoter status in GBM was associated with *17p* and *TP53* mutations, and that these tumors are predominantly ring enhancing with necrosis, and were usually located in the temporal lobe. By contrast, GBMs with methylated *MGMT* promoter status demonstrated more homogeneous enhancement, were found mostly in the frontal lobe, and were associated with prolonged overall survival. Methylated *MGMT* promoter status and *TP53* expression were also correlated with survival differences in the *volume-age-KPS* (VAK) classification system proposed by

Zinn et al,[15] in which tumors were categorized based on the total volume of tumor on preoperative MRI, the patient's age, and the patient's Karnofsky performance scale score (▶ Fig. 17.2). Low T1-enhancing tumor volume (<30,000 mm³ or <40 mm in diameter) was significantly associated with *TP53* activation (▶ Fig. 17.3).

Diehn et al[9] found that the expression of genes implicated in hypoxia and angiogenesis was associated with contrast enhancement; and the expression of genes involved in proliferation and cell cycle was associated with mass effect. Pope et al[11] found the overexpression of *interleukin-8* and *VEGF* to be associated with complete enhancement rather than incomplete enhancement in GBMs. Using GBM samples obtained by image-guided stereotactic biopsies, Van Meter et al[14] revealed differences between the expression of 623 genes between samples obtained from the enhancing core and those obtained from the periphery of tumors. The genes associated with the enhancing tumor core included *VEGF, platelet derived growth factor (PDGF), matrix metalloproteinase 1 (MMP-1)*, and genes involved in signaling pathways displaying characteristics favoring tumor aggression, cell migration, angiogenesis, cell adhesion, tumor proliferation, cell–cell communication, and cell motility. Genes associated with the enhancing periphery of the tumor were involved in central nervous system development and cell expansion such as *EGFR* and the *v-akt murine thymoma viral oncogene homologue 1 (ATK-1)* mRNA.

Quantitative Imaging Genomic Analysis

The first comprehensive large-scale quantitative imaging genomic analysis was performed by our group[16] and demonstrated the ability of MRI to predict the underlying genomic composition of GBM (▶ Fig. 17.4).[16] In this study, using GBM patient data from TCGA, we found that a high peritumoral MRI

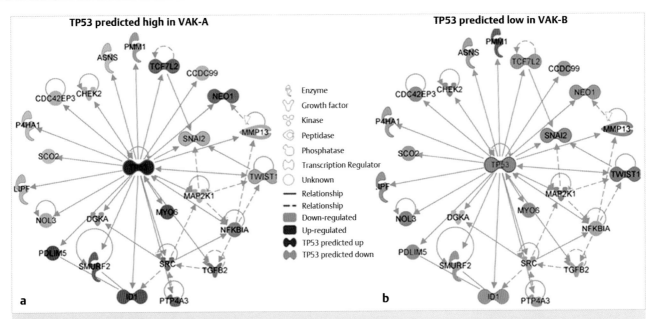

Fig. 17.3 *Volume-age-KPS (VAK)* molecular characterization. *TP53* activation and inhibition across VAK-A and VAK-B patient classes together with molecular regulatory networks of differentially regulated genes. (Used with the permission of Zinn PO, Sathyan P, Mahajan B, et al. A novel volume-age-KPS (VAK) glioblastoma classification identifies a prognostic cognate microRNA-gene signature. PLoS One 2012;7(8):e41522.)

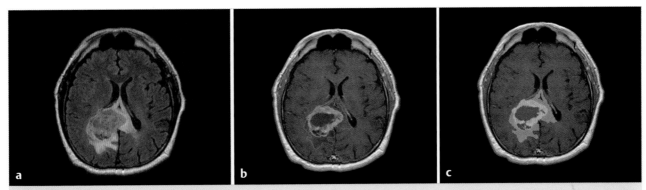

Fig. 17.4 Quantitative volumetric brain tumor imaging mapping. A 55-year-old man with a right temporal glioblastoma multiforme (GBM). (a) Axial fluid-attenuated inversion recovery (FLAIR) image demonstrates segmentation (in blue) of the region of FLAIR hyperintensity corresponding to the area of edema/tumor infiltration. Notice the segmented enhancement (yellow) and necrosis (orange) that has been segmented on the T1-weighted imaging (T1WI) postcontrast. (b) The segmented edema/tumor infiltration (blue), enhancement (yellow), and necrosis (orange) are seen overlaid on a base postcontrast T1WI. (c) Axial postcontrast enhanced T1WI demonstrates the segmentation of the enhancement (yellow) and necrosis (orange).

fluid-attenuated inversion recovery (FLAIR) volume was linked to 53 genes associated with cancer, cellular migration/invasion, cell morphology, and cell signaling. High peritumoral FLAIR volume was also associated with high expression of *periostin (POSTN)*, a gene known to be involved in tumor invasion in other cancers.[1] *POSTN* and its corresponding miR-219 were associated with the mesenchymal subtype compared to the proneural subtype, and, further, were significantly correlated with overall survival and time to disease progression (▶ Fig. 17.5).[16,40] *CXCR4*, a chemokine related to cell proliferation and migration, has also been linked to areas of increased intensity and peritumoral signal abnormality on T2-weighted images.[59,60] The first imaging genomic validation (in vitro and in vivo) study, also performed by Zinn et al,[16] confirmed that high FLAIR signal intensity volume was associated with high *POSTN* levels and the degree of cellular invasion in orthotopic xenograft models.

More recently, Naeini et al[18] found associations between the GBM subtypes and tumor volumetry on MRI. They found that the volume of contrast enhancement, the volume of central necrosis, the combined volume of contrast enhancement and central necrosis, and the ratio of T2/ FLAIR to contrast enhancement and necrosis differed significantly between the mesenchymal and nonmesenchymal subtypes. Naeini et al also found that the volume ratio of T2 hyperintensity to contrast enhancement and central necrosis was significantly lower in the mesenchymal subtype than in the nonmesenchymal GBM subtypes and was a significant predictor of survival.[18] Gutman et al[12] also found associations between MRI features and GBM subtypes (▶ Table 17.1). In this study, the proneural subtype demonstrated significantly lower contrast enhancement in tumor volume, whereas the mesenchymal subtype demonstrated a lower non-contrast-enhancing tumor component. On T2/FLAIR

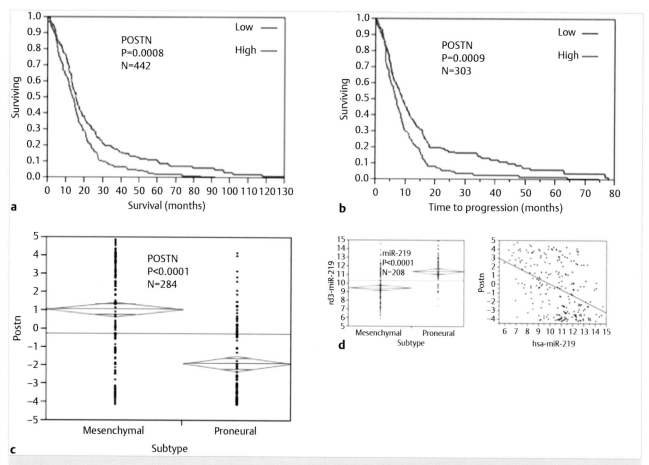

Fig. 17.5 Kaplan-Meier curves for *periostin*. (**a**) Overall survival and (**b**) progression-free survival. (**c**) *Periostin* expression levels across the two main glioblastoma multiforme (GBM) subtypes: mesenchymal and proneural. (**d**) Expression levels of miR-219 across the mesenchymal and proneural subtypes and in addition the inverse correlation ($R^2 = 0.204$) with periostin. (Used with the permission of Zinn PO, Mahajan B, Sathyan P, et al. Radiogenomic mapping of edema/cellular invasion MRI-phenotypes in glioblastoma multiforme. PLoS ONE 2011;6(10):e25451.)

images, GBMs with *EGFR* mutations were significantly larger, and GBMs with *TP53* mutations were smaller than their respective wild-type GBMs; a weak association was also found between *CDKN2A* deletion and necrosis.[12]

Advanced MRI Genomics

Advanced MRI sequences, such as MRP, MRS, and DWI, have been shown to correlate with the underlying genomic composition of tumors. Barajas et al[61] found that GBMs with high relative cerebral blood volume (rCBV) values were associated with elevated expression levels of *VEGF* and genes responsible for tumor aggressiveness, hypoxia, and mitosis; apparent diffusion coefficient (ADC) values in GBM were inversely correlated with genes involved in tumor aggressiveness, hypoxia, and mitosis.[61] Moon et al[58] found that tumors with methylated *MGMT* promoter status had higher ADC values, possibly due to heterogeneity or lower cellularity, and lower fractional anisotropy (FA) values than did tumors with unmethylated *MGMT* promoter status.

More recently, Jain et al[10] showed that rCBV measurements provided important prognostic information independent of the

molecular subclasses as defined by Verhaak et al,[40] and that further strengthened the GBM subclassifications (▶ Fig. 17.6). Furthermore, patients with higher rCBV showed worse prognoses and lower overall 2-year survival rates than did patients with lower rCBV. Jain et al[62] had previously demonstrated a correlation between rCBV and expression levels of genes involved in angiogenesis.

Recently MRS has been shown to be a potential predictor of *IDH1* and *IDH2* mutation status by detecting 2-hydroxyglutarate (2-HG), an oncometabolite produced when *IDH* genes are mutated.[17,63,64] Patients whose gliomas harbor *IDH1* and *IDH2* mutations are known to have better outcomes than patients whose tumors do not have these mutations. Choi et al[64] successfully detected 2-HG levels noninvasively using MRS in patients with gliomas, and Andronesi et al[63] had similar findings when studying 2-HG levels in tumors containing *IDH1* and *IDH2* mutations using high-resolution magic angle spinning (HR-MAS) MRS. These studies supported the use of MRS as a possible medium to further study genetic associations that might ultimately enable clinicians to diagnose patients noninvasively.

Table 17.1 Associations between imaging features and Verhaak subtypes based on original categoric ranges of VASARI feature set

No. of tumors present of each subtype (out of 70) according to percentage of total abnormal tissue				
Neuroimaging feature and subtype	0–5%	6–33%	34–67%	68–95%	p-value
Edema					
Classic	3 (4.35)	4 (5.8)	9(13.04)	0	0.09
Mesenchymal	4 (5.8)	8 (11.59)	11 (15.94)	2 (2.9)	
Neural	2 (2.9)	9. (13.04)	3 (4.35)	0	
Proneural	7 (10.14)	3 (4.35)	4 (5.8)	0	
Total	16 (23.2)	24 (34.8)	27 (39.1)	2 (2.9)	
Contrast-enhanced tumor					
Classic	0	13 (18.57)	3 (4.29)	0	0.02
Mesenchymal	1 (1.43)	19 (27.14)	5 (7.14)	0	
Neural	0	13 (18.57)	2 (2.86)	0	
Proneural	5 (7.14)	6 (8.57)	2 (2.86)	1 (1.43)	
Total	6 (8.6)	51 (72.9)	12 (17.1)	1 (1.4)	
Necrotic					
Classic	1 (1.43)	13 (18.57)	2 (2.86)		0.16
Mesenchymal	7 (10)	13 (18.57)	5 (7.14)		
Neural	3 (4.29)	8 (11.43)	4 (5.71)		
Proneural	5 (7.14)	4 (5.71)	5 (7.14)		
Total	16 (22.9)	38 (54.3)	16 (22.9)		
Nonenhanced tumor					
Classic	10 (14.29)	4 (5.71)	2 (2.86)	0	<0.01
Mesenchymal	20 (28.57)	4 (5.71)	0	1 (1.43)	
Neural	4 (5.71)	6 (8.57)	4 (5.71)	1 (1.43)	
Proneural	4 (5.71)	4 (5.71)	3 (4.29)	3 (4.29)	
Total	38 (54.3)	18 (25.7)	9 (12.9)	5 (7.1)	

Note: Numbers in parentheses are percentages. p-values were obtained with the Fisher exact test.
Source: Used with the permission of Gutman DA, Cooper LAD, Hwang SN, et al. MR imaging predictors of molecular profile and survival: multi-institutional study of the TCGA glioblastoma data set. Radiology 2013;267:560–569.

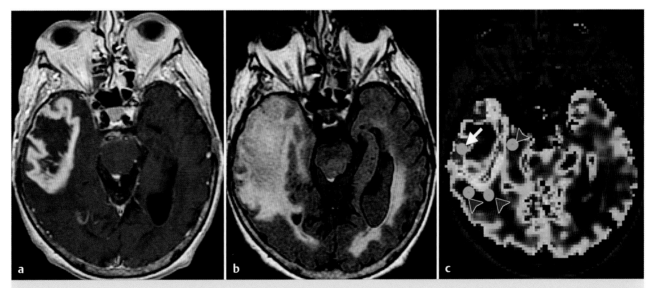

Fig. 17.6 Perfusion imaging strengthens the molecular subclassification of glioblastoma multiforme (GBM). Patient with right temporal GBM, axial (**a**) contrast-enhanced T1-weighted, (**b**) fluid-attenuated inversion recovery images, and (**c**) cerebral blood volume parametric maps at the same axial level. (Used with permission from Jain R, Poisson L, Narang J, et al. Genomic mapping and survival prediction in glioblastoma: molecular subclassification strengthened by hemodynamic imaging biomarkers. Radiology 2013;267:212–220.)

17.4 Imaging Genomics in Oligodendroglioma

Zlatescu et al,[46] in a study that helped form the concept of imaging genomics by linking genomic changes to tumor location, found that the loss of *1p* and *19q* chromosomes was more commonly associated with bilateral than with unilateral oligodendrogliomas. Zlatescu et al also showed that this mutation was not usually seen in tumors located in temporal lobe, insula, and diencephalon; Mueller et al[65] demonstrated that temporal lobe tumors are related to *TP53* mutations. Another study[66] found that oligodendrogliomas with intact *1p* were most likely to be in the temporal lobe location, whereas those with *1p* deletions were more likely to be in the frontal lobe; tumors with *1p* deletions have increased chemosensitivity, prolonging the patient's survival.[67]

Megyesi et al[68] found that oligodendrogliomas with *1p* deletions had indistinct borders on T1-weighted images, mixed signal intensities on T1- and T2-weighted images, paramagnetic susceptibility changes, and calcification; those with intact *1p* had sharper borders, uniform intensity, no changes in paramagnetic effects on susceptibility, and no calcification; *19q* deletion was not found to be strongly associated with the imaging features seen in the tumors with *1p* deletion. MR image texture can also be interpreted based on spatial frequency using Stockwell-transform (S-transform) analysis, which was previously used to study histopathology in multiple sclerosis[69]; homogeneous smooth images appear as strong low frequencies and heterogeneous regions appear as strong high frequencies. Brown et al,[70] in a study using postcontrast T1- and T2-weighted images, concluded that oligodendrogliomas with *1p/19q* deletions could be distinguished from those with intact alleles by using S-transform analysis in intermediate frequencies.

Advanced imaging genomic correlations in oligodendroglioma have also been studied. Jenkinson et al[71] were among the first to link rCBV to *1p/19q* status; they found that rCBV was much higher in oligodendrogliomas with *1p/19q* deletion than tumors with intact *1p/19q* alleles. Subsequent studies confirmed the link between high rCBV and the loss of *1p/19q*.[72] In a study by Kapoor et al,[73] the correlation between high rCBV and the loss of *1p/19q* held true only for low-grade oligodendrogliomas; Law et al[74] found that high rCBV correlated with *1p* but not *19q* deletion. Emblem et al,[75] using histogram analysis, revealed that rCBV distribution in low-grade oligodendrogliomas was more heterogeneous in tumors with a *1p/19q* loss than in tumors with intact *1p/19q* alleles.

Positron-emission tomography (PET) radiotracer uptake characteristics have also been found to correlate with genomic tumor compositions. In a study of oligodendrogliomas using single-photon emission computed tomography (SPECT), Walker et al[76] found that low-grade oligodendrogliomas with *1p/19q* deletions had high ^{201}Tl and ^{18}F-fluorodeoxyglucose (FDG) uptake that was independent of contrast enhancement. Stockhammer et al[77] observed similar findings that *1p/19q* loss in grade II oligodendrogliomas was associated with high glucose uptake on FDG-PET.

17.5 Imaging Proteomics

The correlation of imaging with proteomics has been described by Hobbs et al,[13] who, using MRI-guided tissue biopsies, found that the biopsied regions of contrast enhancement and non-contrast enhancement in the same person had different protein expression profiles. Furthermore, although some similarity in protein expression was seen between the non-contrast-enhanced regions of different individuals, the protein expression in the contrast-enhanced regions was unique to each individual.

17.6 Conclusion

In recent years, studies from several institutions and authors have begun to correlate image findings with genomic data and, in the process, there have been numerous articles and research projects giving birth to an entirely new field of "imaging genomics."[1,9,10,15] It has arisen from continuous progress in imaging technologies, the discovery of new genetic data, and the improvement of gene-sequencing technologies. Many imaging genomic studies discuss qualitative and quantitative parameters based on imaging, predominantly MRI phenotypes, and correlate these characteristics to the underlying genomic composition of brain tumors. Initially, single genetic associations involving the loss of *1p/19q*, overexpression of *TP53*, *EGFR* amplification, and *MGMT* methylation were studied in gliomas[9,46,47,48]; these were followed by linking imaging features such as contrast enhancement and signal intensity on T1- and T2-weighted images to hundreds of genes.[11,13,14,16,18,78] However, it was not until 2011 that the first comprehensive analysis relating MRI-volumetrics to large-scale genetic and mRNA expression profiles in GBM was published,[29] establishing imaging genomics as a field on the frontier of noninvasive diagnosis, especially in cancer, and drug development. Furthermore, the first in vitro and in vivo validation of imaging genomics has also been done.[16]

Imaging genomics has prognostic value as well as far-reaching implications for the prevention, early treatment, and monitoring of brain tumors. The possibility of noninvasively diagnosing the genotype of tumors allows for better treatment and an improved outlook for patients. Imaging patterns and biomarkers can be linked to genomic data, forming the basis for noninvasive diagnosis, targeted therapy, targeted biopsies, and the potential elimination of repeat biopsies or resections. Therapy can also be easily adapted based on this genomic information that was obtained noninvasively.

17.7 Acknowledgments

The authors would like to thank Ginu Thomas, MD, for critically reviewing the manuscript.

References

[1] Zinn PO, Colen RR. Imaging genomic mapping in glioblastoma. Neurosurgery 2013; 60 Suppl 1: 126–130

[2] Jaffe CC. Imaging and genomics: is there a synergy? Radiology 2012; 264: 329–331

[3] Kelly PJ, Daumas-Duport C, Kispert DB, Kall BA, Scheithauer BW, Illig JJ. Imaging-based stereotaxic serial biopsies in untreated intracranial glial neoplasms. J Neurosurg 1987; 66: 865–874

[4] Pavlisa G, Rados M, Pavlisa G, Pavic L, Potocki K, Mayer D. The differences of water diffusion between brain tissue infiltrated by tumor and peritumoral vasogenic edema. Clin Imaging 2009; 33: 96–101

[5] Al-Okaili RN, Krejza J, Wang S, Woo JH, Melhem ER. Advanced MR imaging techniques in the diagnosis of intraaxial brain tumors in adults. Radiographics 2006; 26 Suppl 1: S173–S189

[6] Law M, Yang S, Babb JS et al. Comparison of cerebral blood volume and vascular permeability from dynamic susceptibility contrast-enhanced perfusion MR imaging with glioma grade. AJNR Am J Neuroradiol 2004; 25: 746–755

[7] Le Bihan D, Turner R, Douek P, Patronas N. Diffusion MR imaging: clinical applications. AJR Am J Roentgenol 1992; 159: 591–599

[8] Cho YD, Choi GH, Lee SP, Kim JK. (1)H-MRS metabolic patterns for distinguishing between meningiomas and other brain tumors. Magn Reson Imaging 2003; 21: 663–672

[9] Diehn M, Nardini C, Wang DS et al. Identification of noninvasive imaging surrogates for brain tumor gene-expression modules. Proc Natl Acad Sci U S A 2008; 105: 5213–5218

[10] Jain R, Poisson L, Narang J et al. Genomic mapping and survival prediction in glioblastoma: molecular subclassification strengthened by hemodynamic imaging biomarkers. Radiology 2013; 267: 212–220

[11] Pope WB, Chen JH, Dong J et al. Relationship between gene expression and enhancement in glioblastoma multiforme: exploratory DNA microarray analysis. Radiology 2008; 249: 268–277

[12] Gutman DA, Cooper LA, Hwang SN et al. MR imaging predictors of molecular profile and survival: multi-institutional study of the TCGA glioblastoma data set. Radiology 2013; 267: 560–569

[13] Hobbs SK, Shi G, Homer R, Harsh G, Atlas SW, Bednarski MD. Magnetic resonance image-guided proteomics of human glioblastoma multiforme. J Magn Reson Imaging 2003; 18: 530–536

[14] Van Meter T, Dumur C, Hafez N, Garrett C, Fillmore H, Broaddus WC. Microarray analysis of MRI-defined tissue samples in glioblastoma reveals differences in regional expression of therapeutic targets. Diagn Mol Pathol 2006; 15: 195–205

[15] Zinn PO, Sathyan P, Mahajan B et al. A novel volume-age-KPS (VAK) glioblastoma classification identifies a prognostic cognate microRNA-gene signature. PLoS ONE 2012; 7: e41522

[16] Zinn PO, Mahajan B, Sathyan P et al. Radiogenomic mapping of edema/cellular invasion MRI-phenotypes in glioblastoma multiforme. PLoS One 2011;6: e25451

[17] Pope WB, Prins RM, Albert Thomas M et al. Non-invasive detection of 2-hydroxyglutarate and other metabolites in IDH1 mutant glioma patients using magnetic resonance spectroscopy. J Neurooncol 2012; 107: 197–205

[18] Naeini KM, Pope WB, Cloughesy TF et al. Identifying the mesenchymal molecular subtype of glioblastoma using quantitative volumetric analysis of anatomic magnetic resonance images. Neuro-oncol 2013; 15: 626–634

[19] Ellingson BM, Lai A, Harris RJ et al. Probabilistic radiographic atlas of glioblastoma phenotypes. AJNR Am J Neuroradiol 2013; 34: 533–540

[20] Pope WB, Mirsadraei L, Lai A et al. Differential gene expression in glioblastoma defined by ADC histogram analysis: relationship to extracellular matrix molecules and survival. AJNR Am J Neuroradiol 2012; 33: 1059–1064

[21] Rutman AM, Kuo MD. Radiogenomics: creating a link between molecular diagnostics and diagnostic imaging. Eur J Radiol 2009; 70: 232–241

[22] Gevaert O, Xu J, Hoang CD et al. Non-small cell lung cancer: identifying prognostic imaging biomarkers by leveraging public gene expression microarray data—methods and preliminary results. Radiology 2012; 264: 387–396

[23] Burger JA, Kipps TJ. CXCR4: a key receptor in the crosstalk between tumor cells and their microenvironment. Blood 2006; 107: 1761–1767

[24] Heddleston JM, Hitomi M, Venere M et al. Glioma stem cell maintenance: the role of the microenvironment. Curr Pharm Des 2011; 17: 2386–2401

[25] Heddleston JM, Li Z, McLendon RE, Hjelmeland AB, Rich JN. The hypoxic microenvironment maintains glioblastoma stem cells and promotes reprogramming towards a cancer stem cell phenotype. Cell Cycle 2009; 8: 3274–3284

[26] Lathia JD, Heddleston JM, Venere M, Rich JN. Deadly teamwork: neural cancer stem cells and the tumor microenvironment. Cell Stem Cell 2011; 8: 482–485

[27] Hegi ME, Diserens AC, Gorlia T et al. MGMT gene silencing and benefit from temozolomide in glioblastoma. N Engl J Med 2005; 352: 997–1003

[28] Yan H, Parsons DW, Jin G et al. IDH1 and IDH2 mutations in gliomas. N Engl J Med 2009; 360: 765–773

[29] Hegi ME, Liu L, Herman JG et al. Correlation of O6-methylguanine methyltransferase (MGMT) promoter methylation with clinical outcomes in glioblastoma and clinical strategies to modulate MGMT activity. J Clin Oncol 2008; 26: 4189–4199

[30] Esteller M, Toyota M, Sanchez-Cespedes M et al. Inactivation of the DNA repair gene O6-methylguanine-DNA methyltransferase by promoter hypermethylation is associated with G to A mutations in K-ras in colorectal tumorigenesis. Cancer Res 2000; 60: 2368–2371

[31] von Deimling A, Korshunov A, Hartmann C. The next generation of glioma biomarkers: MGMT methylation, BRAF fusions and IDH1 mutations. Brain Pathol 2011; 21: 74–87

[32] Parsons DW, Jones S, Zhang X et al. An integrated genomic analysis of human glioblastoma multiforme. Science 2008; 321: 1807–1812

[33] Stahlhut Espinosa CE, Slack FJ. The role of microRNAs in cancer. Yale J Biol Med 2006; 79: 131–140

[34] Cheng L, Bao S, Rich JN. Potential therapeutic implications of cancer stem cells in glioblastoma. Biochem Pharmacol 2010; 80: 654–665

[35] Papagiannakopoulos T, Shapiro A, Kosik KS. MicroRNA-21 targets a network of key tumor-suppressive pathways in glioblastoma cells. Cancer Res 2008; 68: 8164–8172

[36] Gabriely G, Wurdinger T, Kesari S et al. MicroRNA 21 promotes glioma invasion by targeting matrix metalloproteinase regulators. Mol Cell Biol 2008; 28: 5369–5380

[37] Ohgaki H, Dessen P, Jourde B et al. Genetic pathways to glioblastoma: a population-based study. Cancer Res 2004; 64: 6892–6899

[38] Cancer Genome Atlas Research Network. Comprehensive genomic characterization defines human glioblastoma genes and core pathways. Nature 2008; 455: 1061–1068

[39] Phillips HS, Kharbanda S, Chen R et al. Molecular subclasses of high-grade glioma predict prognosis, delineate a pattern of disease progression, and resemble stages in neurogenesis. Cancer Cell 2006; 9: 157–173

[40] Verhaak RG, Hoadley KA, Purdom E et al. Cancer Genome Atlas Research Network. Integrated genomic analysis identifies clinically relevant subtypes of glioblastoma characterized by abnormalities in PDGFRA, IDH1, EGFR, and NF1. Cancer Cell 2010; 17: 98–110

[41] Kleihues P, Ohgaki H. Primary and secondary glioblastomas: from concept to clinical diagnosis. Neuro-oncol 1999; 1: 44–51

[42] Robertson T, Koszyca B, Gonzales M. Overview and recent advances in neuropathology. Part 1: Central nervous system tumours. Pathology 2011; 43: 88–92

[43] Nobusawa S, Watanabe T, Kleihues P, Ohgaki H. IDH1 mutations as molecular signature and predictive factor of secondary glioblastomas. Clin Cancer Res 2009; 15: 6002–6007

[44] SongTao Q, Lei Y, Si G et al. IDH mutations predict longer survival and response to temozolomide in secondary glioblastoma. Cancer Sci 2012; 103: 269–273

[45] Phillips JJ, Aranda D, Ellison DW et al. PDGFRA amplification is common in pediatric and adult high-grade astrocytomas and identifies a poor prognostic group in IDH1 mutant glioblastoma. Brain Pathol 2013; 23: 565–573

[46] Zlatescu MC, TehraniYazdi A, Sasaki H et al. Tumor location and growth pattern correlate with genetic signature in oligodendroglial neoplasms. Cancer Res 2001; 61: 6713–6715

[47] Mut M, Turba UC, Botella AC, Baskurt E, Lopes MB, Shaffrey ME. Neuroimaging characteristics in subgroup of GBMs with p53 overexpression. J Neuroimaging 2007; 17: 168–174

[48] Eoli M, Menghi F, Bruzzone MG et al. Methylation of O6-methylguanine DNA methyltransferase and loss of heterozygosity on 19q and/or 17p are overlapping features of secondary glioblastomas with prolonged survival. Clin Cancer Res 2007; 13: 2606–2613

[49] Aghi M, Gaviani P, Henson JW, Batchelor TT, Louis DN, Barker FG, II. Magnetic resonance imaging characteristics predict epidermal growth factor receptor amplification status in glioblastoma. Clin Cancer Res 2005; 11: 8600–8605

[50] Barker FGI, II, Simmons ML, Chang SM et al. EGFR overexpression and radiation response in glioblastoma multiforme. Int J Radiat Oncol Biol Phys 2001; 51: 410–418

[51] Schlegel J, Merdes A, Stumm G et al. Amplification of the epidermal-growth-factor-receptor gene correlates with different growth behaviour in human glioblastoma. Int J Cancer 1994; 56: 72–77

[52] Colen RR, Wang J, Gutman DA, Singh S, Zinn PO. Imaging genomic mapping reveals gender-specific oncogenic associations of cell death in glioblastoma. Radiology 2014 [in Press]

[53] Carrillo JA, Lai A, Nghiemphu PL et al. Relationship between tumor enhancement, edema, IDH1 mutational status, MGMT promoter methylation, and survival in glioblastoma. AJNR Am J Neuroradiol 2012; 33: 1349–1355

[54] Walker C, du Plessis DG, Joyce KA et al. Molecular pathology and clinical characteristics of oligodendroglial neoplasms. Ann Neurol 2005; 57: 855–865

[55] van den Bent MJ, Looijenga LH, Langenberg K et al. Chromosomal anomalies in oligodendroglial tumors are correlated with clinical features. Cancer 2003; 97: 1276–1284

[56] Felsberg J, Erkwoh A, Sabel MC et al. Oligodendroglial tumors: refinement of candidate regions on chromosome arm 1p and correlation of 1p/19q status with survival. Brain Pathol 2004; 14: 121–130

[57] Drabycz S, Roldán G, de Robles P et al. An analysis of image texture, tumor location, and MGMT promoter methylation in glioblastoma using magnetic resonance imaging. Neuroimage 2010; 49: 1398–1405

[58] Moon WJ, Choi JW, Roh HG, Lim SD, Koh YC. Imaging parameters of high grade gliomas in relation to the MGMT promoter methylation status: the CT, diffusion tensor imaging, and perfusion MR imaging. Neuroradiology 2012; 54: 555–563

[59] Stevenson CB, Ehtesham M, McMillan KM et al. CXCR4 expression is elevated in glioblastoma multiforme and correlates with an increase in intensity and extent of peritumoral T2-weighted magnetic resonance imaging signal abnormalities. Neurosurgery 2008; 63: 560–569, discussion 569–570

[60] McMillan KM, Ehtesham M, Stevenson CB, Edgeworth ML, Thompson RC, Price RR. T2 detection of tumor invasion within segmented components of glioblastoma multiforme. J Magn Reson Imaging 2009; 29: 251–257

[61] Barajas RF, Jr, Hodgson JG, Chang JS et al. Glioblastoma multiforme regional genetic and cellular expression patterns: influence on anatomic and physiologic MR imaging. Radiology 2010; 254: 564–576

[62] Jain R, Narang J, Gutierrez J et al. Correlation of immunohistologic and perfusion vascular parameters with MR contrast enhancement using image-guided biopsy specimens in gliomas. Acad Radiol 2011; 18: 955–962

[63] Andronesi OC, Kim GS, Gerstner E et al. Detection of 2-hydroxyglutarate in IDH-mutated glioma patients by in vivo spectral-editing and 2D correlation magnetic resonance spectroscopy. Sci Transl Med 2012; 4: 116ra4

[64] Choi C, Ganji SK, DeBerardinis RJ et al. 2-hydroxyglutarate detection by magnetic resonance spectroscopy in IDH-mutated patients with gliomas. Nat Med 2012; 18: 624–629

[65] Mueller W, Hartmann C, Hoffmann A et al. Genetic signature of oligoastrocytomas correlates with tumor location and denotes distinct molecular subsets. Am J Pathol 2002; 161: 313–319

[66] Laigle-Donadey F, Martin-Duverneuil N, Lejeune J et al. Correlations between molecular profile and radiologic pattern in oligodendroglial tumors. Neurology 2004; 63: 2360–2362

[67] Eoli M, Bissola L, Bruzzone MG et al. Reclassification of oligoastrocytomas by loss of heterozygosity studies. Int J Cancer 2006; 119: 84–90

[68] Megyesi JF, Kachur E, Lee DH et al. Imaging correlates of molecular signatures in oligodendrogliomas. Clin Cancer Res 2004; 10: 4303–4306

[69] Zhang Y, Wells J, Buist R, Peeling J, Yong VW, Mitchell JR. A novel MRI texture analysis of demyelination and inflammation in relapsing-remitting experimental allergic encephalomyelitis. Med Image Comput Comput Assist Interv 2006; 9: 760–767

[70] Brown R, Zlatescu M, Sijben A et al. The use of magnetic resonance imaging to noninvasively detect genetic signatures in oligodendroglioma. Clin Cancer Res 2008; 14: 2357–2362

[71] Jenkinson MD, Smith TS, Joyce KA et al. Cerebral blood volume, genotype and chemosensitivity in oligodendroglial tumours. Neuroradiology 2006; 48: 703–713

[72] Whitmore RG, Krejza J, Kapoor GS et al. Prediction of oligodendroglial tumor subtype and grade using perfusion weighted magnetic resonance imaging. J Neurosurg 2007; 107: 600–609

[73] Kapoor GS, Gocke TA, Chawla S et al. Magnetic resonance perfusion-weighted imaging defines angiogenic subtypes of oligodendroglioma according to 1p19q and EGFR status. J Neurooncol 2009; 92: 373–386

[74] Law M, Brodsky JE, Babb J et al. High cerebral blood volume in human gliomas predicts deletion of chromosome 1p: Preliminary results of molecular studies in gliomas with elevated perfusion. J Magn Reson Imaging 2007; 25: 1113–1119

[75] Emblem KE, Scheie D, Due-Tonnessen P et al. Histogram analysis of MR imaging-derived cerebral blood volume maps: combined glioma grading and identification of low-grade oligodendroglial subtypes. AJNR Am J Neuroradiol 2008; 29: 1664–1670

[76] Walker C, du Plessis DG, Fildes D et al. Correlation of molecular genetics with molecular and morphological imaging in gliomas with an oligodendroglial component. Clin Cancer Res 2004; 10: 7182–7191

[77] Stockhammer F, Thomale UW, Plotkin M, Hartmann C, Von Deimling A. Association between fluorine-18-labeled fluorodeoxyglucose uptake and 1p and 19q loss of heterozygosity in World Health Organization Grade II gliomas. J Neurosurg 2007; 106: 633–637

[78] Guccione S, Yang YS, Shi G, Lee DY, Li KC, Bednarski MD. Functional genomics guided with MR imaging: mouse tumor model study. Radiology 2003; 228: 560–568

18 On the Horizon: Going Beyond Conventional MR Contrast Agents

Josep Puig and Wilson B. Chwang

18.1 Why We Need More Than What Is Available

In patients with brain tumors, contrast-enhanced magnetic resonance imaging (MRI) with gadolinium (Gd)-based agents is essential for characterization of disease extent, planning surgical resection, delineating appropriate radiosurgical target volumes, and following patients for disease recurrence.[1,2] Effective management of patients with brain tumors depends on accurate detection and delineation of lesions. Enhancement of intra-axial brain tumors using Gd chelates is based primarily on disruption of the blood–brain barrier and/or abnormal vascularity, which allows the agent to accumulate within the lesion.[3] Contrast enhancement thus improves the demarcation of pathological tissue from normal brain.

Several factors affect the degree of signal enhancement of a lesion from Gd chelates, including magnetic resonance (MR) field strength, sequence parameters, and individual properties of the contrast agent itself, as well as the dose and concentration of the agent. The ideal MR contrast agent would perfectly delineate the margins of the tumor, thus showing its size and extent and clarifying its relationships with other structures; moreover, it would enable tumor enhancement to be distinguished from treatment-related enhancement. The ideal MR contrast agent would also make it possible to obtain reliable information on tumor grade based on assessment of the microvasculature with functional techniques. However, the intrinsic infiltrative nature of some brain tumors, particularly glioblastomas, makes it a real challenge to reliably delineate their margins and extent.[4]

Chelate-bound Gd ions (Gd^{3+}) were first used for MRI purposes in the early 1980s, and many Gd-chelate contrast agents for MR brain imaging are now commercially available.[5,6] Contrast agents are used in approximately one third of all MRI scans of the central nervous system.[7] Gd-based agents can be classified based on molarity and protein-binding capacity. The most widely used contrast agents are gadopentetate dimeglumine (Gd-DTPA), gadoteridol (Gd-HP-DO3A), gadoterate (Gd-DOTA), gadodiamide (Gd-DTPA-BMA), gadoversetamide (Gd-DTPA-BMEA), and gadobenate dimeglumine (Gd-BOPTA). These are water soluble, extracellular, non-tissue-specific compounds that do not bind to proteins (except Gd-BOPTA, which has transient weak protein-binding properties).[5] These extravascular contrast agents are all supplied at a standardized concentration of 0.5 mmol/mL. Although their molecular structures differ, these small-molecular-weight compounds have similar pharmacokinetic profiles and physicochemical properties that result in their quick diffusion from the blood into the extracellular space for both normal and pathological tissues and transient accumulation in areas with an abnormal blood–brain barrier, leading to faster T1 relaxation times and demonstrable contrast enhancement.[8]

Extravascular contrast agents have similar T1 relaxivities (4.3–5 L/mmol/s) and are routinely given at a standard dose of 0.1 mmol/kg body weight. Numerous studies have shown that the enhancement characteristics of these non-protein-binding contrast agents are virtually indistinguishable at this dose.[9–17] Another extravascular contrast agent, gadobutrol (Gd-BT-DO3A-butriol), is a double-concentrated, nonionic macrocyclic Gd chelate with potential advantages for clinical imaging.[18,19] The low osmolality and viscosity of gadobutrol make it possible to double the concentration of Gd chelate.[20] Recent studies have shown that the higher relaxivity of gadobutrol in comparison with other non-protein-binding Gd-based agents can improve enhancement in different ways, increasing in vivo T1 shortening per injected volume at the standard dose.[21,22,23,24]

On the other hand, the protein-binding properties of a Gd-based contrast agent can also affect brain tumor contrast enhancement substantially. As the protein-bound fraction of contrast agent increases, the time that the contrast material remains inside blood vessels also increases. This increased intravascular availability improves tumor enhancement. Previous studies have demonstrated that even the weak protein-binding properties of gadobenate dimeglumine provide better tumor enhancement, resulting in superior lesion depiction and delineation, compared to non-protein-binding agents such as gadopentetate dimeglumine or gadoterate dimeglumine.[8–12]

To overcome the limitations of extravascular contrast agents, including rapid clearance from the blood pool and consequent suboptimal reduction of T1 relaxation times in blood, new, intravascular contrast agents have been designed for MRI (▶ Table 18.1).[25] Examples include Gd-based molecules with significantly stronger protein binding and various macromolecular contrast agents (MMCAs), including superparamagnetic iron oxide nanoparticles. Experimental studies and early clinical trials have shown the benefits of intravascular contrast agents, including increased sensitivity and diagnostic accuracy.

Gadofosveset trisodium (MS-325, Ablavar, Lantheus Medical Imaging, North Bilerica, MA), an intravascular contrast agent, forms reversible noncovalent bonds with albumin. It has relatively low relaxivity in its unbound state, but unbound gadofosveset accounts for only about 15% of the compound in human blood; the remaining 85% is bound to albumin (▶ Fig. 18.1).[26] This slows the tumbling rate of the complex, resulting in a four- to fivefold increase in blood relaxivity at 1.5 T in comparison with extracellular Gd-based agents.[27] In addition, like MMCA, gadofosveset has a long terminal half-life and remains confined to the vascular pool. Furthermore, there is a high concentration of albumin in the interstitial space of gliomas, and it is reasonable to expect that gadofosveset will bind to this albumin in addition to the albumin in blood, leading to greater lesion enhancement.[28] Recently, improved enhancement with gadofosveset trisodium in comparison with extravascular agents has been demonstrated in a variety of human brain tumors.[29,30]

Detailed characterization of the tumor vasculature provides a better understanding of the complex mechanisms associated with tumor growth and is especially important in monitoring therapy. In this direction, experimental and some early clinical

Table 18.1 Conventional versus newer magnetic resonance contrast agents for brain tumor imaging

	Conventional MR contrast agents	Newer MR contrast agents
Examples	• Gadopentetate dimeglumine (Gd-DTPA) • Gadoteridol (Gd-HP-DO3A) • Gadoterate (Gd-DOTA) • Gadodiamide (DTPA-BMA) • Gadobutrol (Gd-BT-DO3A-butriol) • Gadobenate dimeglumine (Gd-BOPTA)	• Blood pool contrast agents • Albumin–(Gd-DTPA) • Dextran–(Gd-DTPA) • Liposomal-Gd contrast agents • Iron oxide nanoparticles (USPIO)
Paramagnetic agent	Gd	Gd, iron[a]
Molecular weight (kDa)	< 1	> 10–30
Distribution	Interstitial, extravascular	Intravascular, intracellular[b]
Plasma half-life (hours)	1.5	> 14
Excretion	Renal	Renal/MPS[c]
Mechanism of enhancement	Equal distribution throughout extracellular space with abnormal blood–brain barrier; nonbinding to serum proteins[d]; untargeted agents	Intravascular and extravascular enhancement; capable of binding to serum proteins; targeted agents
Dosage (mmol/kg body weight)	0.1–0.3	0.03[e]
T1 relaxativity (R1; mmol/s)	< 5	> 19
MR perfusion imaging	First-pass imaging	First-pass imaging, steady-state imaging
Advantages	Determination of disease extent; planning surgical resection; delineation of radiosurgical volumes	Greater tumor enhancement; persistent high intravascular enhancement; better delineation of microvessels; long window scan imaging; lower dosage; convection-enhanced delivery of drugs using liposomes
Drawbacks	Vascular half-life relatively short; enhancement only a few minutes after administration	Most remain in preclinical stage

[a]Iron oxide nanoparticles and some liposomes.
[b]Ultrasmall superparamagnetic iron oxide (USPIO) particles.
[c]Iron oxide nanoparticles accumulate into the mononuclear phagocytic system (MPS).
[d]Transient weak protein-binding properties for gadobenate dimeglumine.
[e]Gadofosveset trisodium.

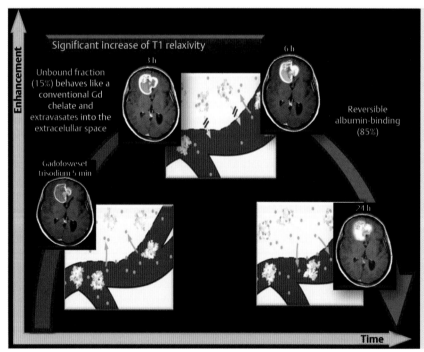

Fig. 18.1 Mechanism of tissue enhancement for the intravascular contrast agent gadofosveset.

studies have shown the potential of MMCAs for characterizing tumor angiogenesis by dynamic contrast-enhanced MRI based on the ability to assess microvessel permeability and fractional plasma volume. Although most MMCAs are still under development, these contrast media will potentially enable qualitative and quantitative, physiologically based imaging evaluation of tumor microvessels and the response to angiogenesis inhibitors. Although many are not yet approved for clinical use, they do show promise for brain tumor imaging applications.

This chapter reviews several groups of the newest MR contrast agents for brain tumor imaging. We discuss the advantages and limitations of each group, using examples from our experience and from the literature, with the understanding that newer contrast agents are needed to overcome the current limitations and improve our diagnostic capabilities.

18.2 Blood Pool Agents

Gd-based agents can be classified based on molarity and protein-binding capacity. The typical extravascular contrast agents have similar pharmacokinetic and physicochemical profiles that result in their transient accumulation in areas with an abnormal blood–brain barrier. Extravascular contrast agents have similar T1 relaxivities (4.3–5 L/mmol/s) and are given at a standard dose of 0.1 mmol/kg of body weight. They exhibit rapid clearance from the blood pool, which results in unsatisfactory reduction of T1 relaxation times in blood. To overcome this problem, new protein-binding Gd compounds have been designed for use as intravascular blood pool agents.

Although not currently approved for brain tumor imaging in the United States, gadofosveset is the first blood pool agent approved for clinical use with MR angiography in the European Union, Canada, and the United States. Gadofosveset binds strongly but reversibly to albumin in plasma, leading to higher relaxivity (4 or 5 times higher) and better vascular retention, resulting in longer intravascular half-life (~16 h vs. ~90 min). The diagnostic accuracy of gadofosveset-enhanced MRI for evaluating vascular stenoses and aneurysms of abdominal vessels in patients with aortoiliac occlusive disease is similar to that of conventional angiography.[31] A recent report showed that gadofosveset MR angiography is also useful in the follow-up of intracranial aneurysms.[32]

The usefulness of gadofosveset trisodium in imaging glioblastomas has recently been evaluated. Puig et al[30] demonstrated advantages for gadofosveset over gadobutrol, an extravascular contrast agent, for imaging histologically proven glioblastoma in a clinical setting. Interestingly, in the subjective analysis, readers rated images obtained 6 hours after gadofosveset administration more useful for diagnosis, and this impression was confirmed by the increases in quantitative enhancement parameters (▶ Fig. 18.2). The greater enhancement seen 6 hours after gadofosveset injection may be attributable to greater accumulation in the interstitial fluid of tumors due to the so-called trapping effect of contrast molecules: after unbound gadofosveset molecules pass through the impaired blood–brain barrier, they bind with albumin within the tumor, resulting in strongly reduced backflow rates and increased relaxivity. These findings are in line with previous preclinical studies performed using rat brain glioma models, which concluded that the

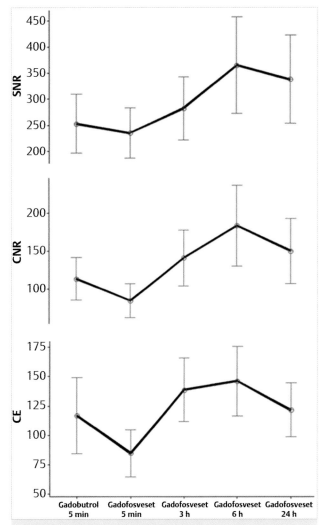

Fig. 18.2 Comparison of quantitative enhancement characteristics between gadobutrol and gadofosveset trisodium. Error bars reflect the standard deviations at each time point. SNR, signal-to-noise ratio; CNR, contrast-to-noise ratio; CE, contrast enhancement. (Used with permission from Puig J, Blasco G, Essig M, et al. Albumin-binding MR blood pool contrast agent improves diagnostic performance in human brain tumour: comparison of two contrast agents for glioblastoma. Eur Radiol 2013;23(4):1093–1101.)

pharmacodynamic effect of protein binding increases the relaxivity of the contrast agent, thereby increasing the MR signal. Adzamli et al[33] found two- to threefold stronger enhancement with albumin-binding agents (including gadofosveset) compared to the nonbinding extravascular contrast agent gadoversetamide, on a per mole basis. Furthermore, Wintersperger et al[34] demonstrated that the protein-binding capacity of experimental gadolinium chelates (bound fraction of ~50–90%) increased contrast-to-noise ratio and contrast enhancement in rat brain glioma in comparison with the non-protein-binding agent gadopentetate dimeglumine and the weak protein-binding agent gadobenate dimeglumine. This is important because gadobenate dimeglumine has been extensively evaluated in brain tumors, and significantly greater lesion-to-brain contrast has been demonstrated in multiple clinical trials and in experimental models in comparison with other extravascular agents.[7,35,36,37]

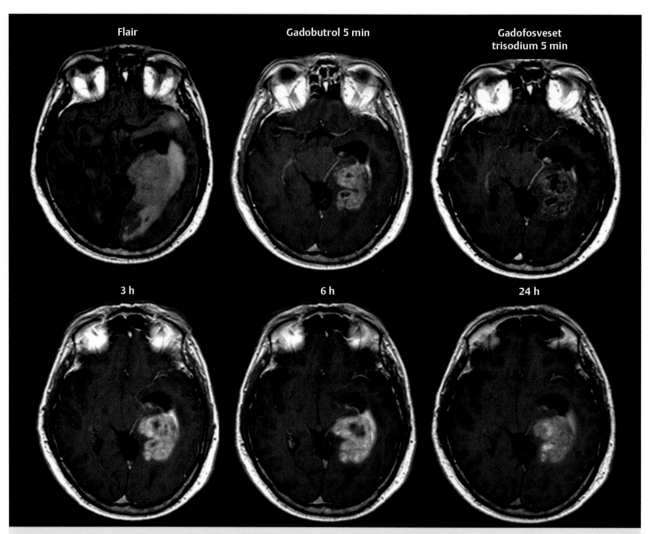

Fig. 18.3 Blood pool contrast agents may improve tumor delineation. A 63-year-old man with histologically confirmed glioblastoma. Axial fluid-attenuated inversion recovery (FLAIR) and T1-weighted magnetic resonance images obtained after intravenous administration of gadobutrol and gadofosveset trisodium show a large tumor in the left occipital and temporal lobes. Images obtained 3 and 6 hours after administration of the blood pool contrast agent gadofosveset show greater enhancement and depict the extent of disease more clearly. The overall enhancing tumor volume is larger with gadofosveset trisodium. Progressive enhancement inside the rim, usually in a patchy pattern, could reflect the presence of islands of surviving tumor cells within regions undergoing macroscopic necrosis.

The more pronounced and prolonged enhancement achieved with gadofosveset trisodium that results in improved diagnostic end points can be attributed to the markedly greater T1 relaxivity of this agent at 1.5 T (19 ± 1 L/mmol/s compared with 4.7 ± 0.2 L/mmol/s for gadobutrol).[18,33] The relaxivity of gadofosveset is dramatically increased when the complex is bound to protein because transient interactions of the contrast-effective moiety of gadofosveset with albumin decrease the tumbling rate of the molecule (called the receptor-induced magnetization enhancement effect) and increase its persistence in blood.[27] Extravascular Gd-based agents have a blood half-life of 90 minutes; they diffuse rapidly into the tumor, so enhancement peaks within the first few minutes after they are administered.[5] By contrast, the intravascular contrast agent gadofosveset has a blood half-life of approximately 16 hours, and peak enhancement is not achieved until several hours after administration.[26] Immediately after injection, the unbound fraction of gadofosveset molecules (about 15%) passes through the blood–brain barrier and also causes the glomerular filtration rate to increase. However, after a few circulation cycles, the remaining molecules of gadofosveset are homogeneously distributed throughout the vascular blood in the albumin-bound state (about 85%) (see ▶ Fig. 18.1).[38]

Serum proteins like albumin can extravasate from blood into tumors as a consequence of the breakdown of the blood–brain barrier (through openings in the endothelial junction or by pinocytosis) and increased vascular permeability.[28,39] Previous studies have shown that the bound fraction of gadofosveset has significantly stronger relaxation effects than the unbound fraction as a result of the larger size and resultant longer rotational correlation time of the molecule.[27,33,38,40] Six hours after gadofosveset administration has been proposed as the optimal time for scanning to evaluate glioblastoma in humans (▶ Fig. 18.3, ▶ Fig. 18.4, ▶ Fig. 18.5, and ▶ Fig. 18.6).

A contrast agent for MRI of brain tumors should provide high T1 contrast. Contrast enhancement of brain tumors is based on

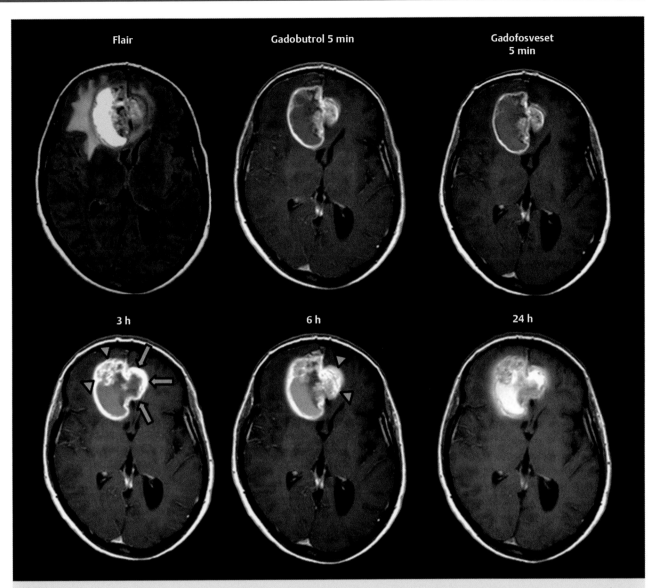

Fig. 18.4 Large enhancing bifrontal tumor. The delineation and enhancement of the lesion are markedly better and more homogeneous with gadofosveset (arrows). Note in particular the better delineation of a hypervascular component of the lesion (arrowheads). FLAIR, fluid-attenuated inversion recovery. (Used with permission from Puig J, Blasco G, Essig M, et al. Albumin-binding MR blood pool contrast agent improves diagnostic performance in human brain tumour: comparison of two contrast agents for glioblastoma. Eur Radiol 2013;23(4):1093–1101.)

complex pathophysiological changes in the tumor and the adjacent brain tissue, primarily due to disruption of the blood–brain barrier and increased capillary permeability.[3] Two types of brain tumor enhancement are important. Extravascular enhancement occurs when the contrast agent permeates through the vessel wall and accumulates in the perivascular interstitial fluid. Intravascular enhancement occurs when blood flow or volume increases due to the tumor's increased or pathological vascularity; contrast material in blood results in enhancement proportional to increases in blood flow or volume, reflecting the vascular component or angiogenesis of the tumor. The increase in tissue relaxivities brought about by gadofosveset's binding to intravascular and extravasated serum albumin, together with its longer half-life, results in greater enhancement in tissues with increased microvascularization or extravasation, making brain tumors more conspicuous on

T1-weighted images and enabling better delineation of their extension (see ▶ Fig. 18.4, ▶ Fig. 18.5, and ▶ Fig. 18.6). Gliomas usually extend beyond the areas demarcated on T2-weighted or conventional Gd-based contrast-enhanced T1-weighted MRI, so improved delineation of the borders and extension of gliomas can be useful for planning surgical resection and/or radiation therapy and might contribute to a more accurate understanding of brain tumors.[41,42]

One aspect of tumor physiology that may represent tumor aggressiveness is vascular leakage. Vascular leakage reflects the spread of increased vascularity, the rupture of the blood–brain barrier, or both; it arises from both focal areas with severe vascular abnormalities and regions with mild vascular abnormalities in which leakage often extends into the unenhanced abnormal region (peritumoral edema).[43] Peritumoral edema, which is unenhanced on T1-weighted images after the

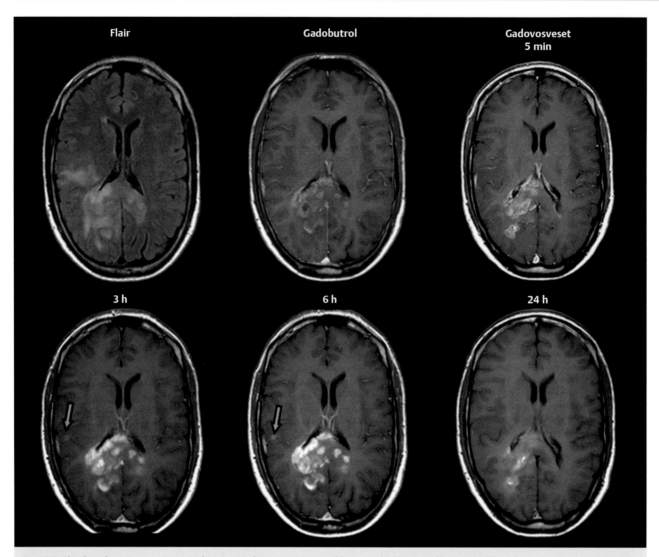

Fig. 18.5 Blood pool contrast agents may detect more lesions. A 43-year-old man with a large glioblastoma. Although the lesion was visible with gadobutrol, in images acquired 3 and 6 hours after gadofosveset administration, markedly improved definition of lesion margins enables the extension of the tumor into the splenium in the adjacent occipital lobe to be better defined. An additional nodule was seen in the right parietal area (arrows). FLAIR, fluid-attenuated inversion recovery. (Used with permission from Puig J, Blasco G, Essig M, et al. Albumin-binding MR blood pool contrast agent improves diagnostic performance in human brain tumour: comparison of two contrast agents for glioblastoma. Eur Radiol 2013;23(4):1093–1101.)

administration of classical contrast agents, has been described as an area of infiltration surrounding the tumor in which tumor cells coexist with tumor-secreted vascular permeability factors.[44] A high degree of vascular permeability indicates an abnormality of the blood–brain barrier and presumably reflects a larger size pore or disruption of the endothelial junctions.[45] Thus the magnitude of the opening in the blood–brain barrier seems to be a surrogate marker for tumor aggressiveness. Recently, Cao et al[43,46] determined the volume of vascular leakage from the transfer constant of the extravascular contrast agent Gd-DTPA from plasma to tissue in dynamic contrast-enhanced imaging; they found that vascular leakage volume predicted survival better than the fluid-attenuated inversion recovery (FLAIR) and post-Gd T1 tumor volumes, suggesting that vascular leakage could be a surrogate marker for the aggressiveness of high-grade gliomas. In Puig et al's[30] study, enhancement had dispersed into the area of peritumoral edema

24 hours after gadofosveset trisodium injection in slightly more than half of the glioblastomas.

This peritumoral enhancement could be explained by the presence of albumin in the peritumoral edema, which is supported by the finding of albumin concentrations as high as 19.2 mg/mL in peritumoral edema in cat brains after xeno-transplantation of cell clones from primary rat tumors.[47] Recently, Pronin et al[48] described the dispersion of Gd-DTPA enhancement into the area of peritumoral edema in the time interval between 5 minutes and 6 hours after injection in an 11-patient cohort study, with the highest average increase in volume of contrast observed at 6 hours. On the other hand, an increase in the volume of enhancement over time has also been demonstrated in animal models of glioblastomas, although this increase might not depend on the infiltrative and edematous patterns or might not be closely related with peritumoral edema.[49] Given that the extent of vascular leakage estimated by

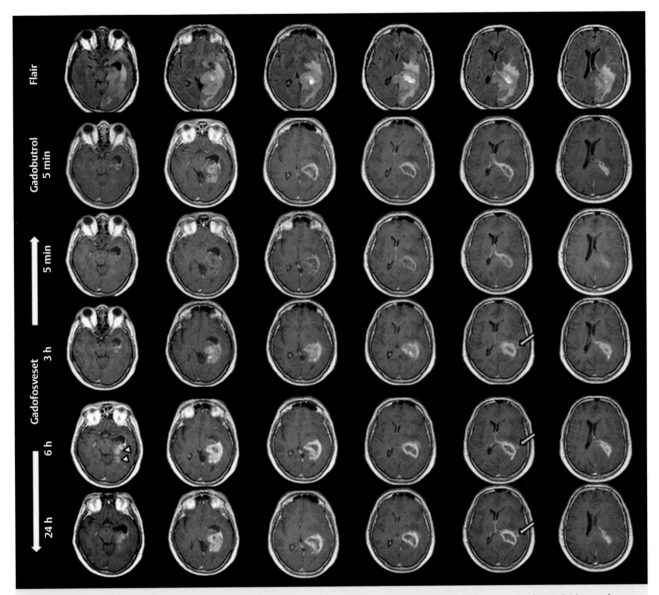

Fig. 18.6 A 63-year-old man with histologically confirmed glioblastoma in the left occipital and temporal lobes. Images obtained 6 hours after gadofosveset administration show greater enhancement and depict the extent of disease more clearly (arrowheads). The overall enhancing tumor volume is larger with gadofosveset. A small additional lesion is clearly demonstrated in the late post-gadofosveset scans (arrows). FLAIR, fluid-attenuated inversion recovery. (Used with permission from Puig J, Blasco G, Essig M, et al. Albumin-binding MR blood pool contrast agent improves diagnostic performance in human brain tumour: comparison of two contrast agents for glioblastoma. Eur Radiol 2013;23(4):1093–1101.)

the transfer constant of Gd-DTPA might help predict tumor aggressiveness and survival in patients with high-grade glioma,[43] further research should address whether dispersion of gadofosveset over time from the initial site of enhancement to the periphery on T1-weighted imaging is useful for predicting survival.

Moreover, in the overwhelming majority of tumors with a central necrotic and/or cystic cavity, enhancement was observed in the cavity 24 hours after gadofosveset administration.[30] This finding, which has also been reported after gadopentetate dimeglumine and gadobenate dimeglumine administration in experimental brain tumors,[7,50] reflects the delayed wash-in and delayed washout of the contrast agent from the poorly vascularized necrotic area.[51,52] The leakage of

intracellular proteins into the extracellular space after lysis of necrotic cells could also contribute to these phenomena.

Another advantage associated with the high relaxivity of gadofosveset is the possibility of reducing the dose of Gd (by a factor of 4) in terms of number of Gd ions administered, compared to conventional Gd chelates. This is important because whether nephrogenic systemic fibrosis develops depends not only on the stability of the Gd-based agents applied but also on the cumulative Gd dose administered.[53] Although gadobutrol is considered a relatively safe agent because its macrocyclic structures favor higher kinetic stability than linear chelates,[22,54,55] gadofosveset at a dose of 0.03 mmol/kg body weight yielded better enhancement than the gadobutrol at a dose of 0.1 mmol/kg body weight; thus gadofosveset represents a lower risk of nephrogenic systemic fibrosis without compromising image quality.

The experience to date suggests that the use of gadofosveset trisodium might have important clinical implications, particularly in intraoperative imaging for the real-time assessment of tumor resection. Generally, the first step in the multimodal treatment of glioma patients is surgery aiming to resect as much of the tumor as possible without inducing disabling neurologic deficits. Gross total resection in which no contrast-enhancing tumor remains after resection is associated with extended overall survival and progression-free survival in low-grade and high-grade gliomas (> 7 month increase in median survival), although no class 1 supporting evidence is available.[56–60] The accurate intraoperative assessment of tumor margins can be difficult for neurosurgeons; moreover, the functional relevance of brain tissue precludes widening resections to include a safety margin.

To optimize the extent of resection, intraoperative imaging methods, including computed tomography (CT), ultrasonography, 5-aminolevulinic acid, and MRI have been established in operating rooms, enabling surgeons to better see the extent of lesions and serving as immediate resection control. Of these intraoperative imaging methods, high-field intraoperative MRI scanners provide the highest resolution for detecting contrast-enhancing tissue tumor remnants and are considered essential in the surgical management of glioblastomas.[58] Intraoperative MRI could influence the course of surgery by enabling additional resection in 10 to 70% of cases, and it could increase the number of gross total resections to nearly 100%.[58,60] The greater enhancement provided by gadofosveset, at least in the first 6 hours after a single dose, might enable greater volumes of tumor to be resected, thus increasing the percentage of patients in whom the maximum amount of tumor can be safely resected. However, the dispersion of gadofosveset at 24 hours follow-up is also a potential source of errors: a long delay in scanning after contrast injection might lead to overestimation of the volume of enhancing tumor and misinterpretation of the extent of the zone of enhancement, resulting in the resection of initially nonenhancing white matter.

Blood pool contrast agents such as gadofosveset are likely to play a central role in the evaluation of tumor angiogenesis. Angiogenesis is vital to tumor growth. When a tumor exceeds a diameter of 1 to 2 mm, diffusion from the surrounding vasculature alone is no longer sufficient to provide nutrients to the outer cells of the tumor; the tumor induces the growth of new vessels to supply nutrients and possibly to remove biological end products secreted by rapidly dividing cancer cells. Blood pool contrast agents result in both intravascular enhancement, related to blood flow, and interstitial enhancement, related to vessel permeability. The persistent strong intravascular enhancement of gadofosveset allows for the acquisition of high-resolution images in the steady state, enabling better delineation of vessel pathology, abnormal vascular beds, and increased vascularity associated with fast-growing tumors (▶ Fig. 18.7). There is an urgent clinical need for accurate, noninvasive imaging biomarkers to quantify tumor angiogenesis and to monitor the response to treatment. Furthermore, if blood pool contrast agents are validated as surrogate markers for treatment outcome, they will be very useful in the development of new tumor angiogenesis inhibitors. Thus the ability of MR

techniques using blood pool contrast agents to reveal changes in tumor microvascularity is likely to accelerate the development, testing, and monitoring of new antiangiogenic drugs.

Overall, the future of blood pool contrast imaging is promising. However, although it seems reasonable to expect that the greater diagnostic information available on gadofosveset-enhanced images would help improve the efficacy of therapeutic procedures, particularly with regard to better definition of the target volumes at radiosurgery, a more comprehensive understanding of the precise extent to which greater diagnostic information contributes to improved patient management would be required to prove this point conclusively. Future studies are necessary to fully explore the true clinical potential of gadofosveset as well as its advantages over the currently established Gd-based agents for contrast-enhanced MRI in the diagnosis and follow-up of brain tumors.

18.3 Macromolecular Contrast Agents

MMCAs for MRI have been defined as paramagnetic or superparamagnetic compounds with molecular weights higher than 10 or 30 kDa.[61,62,63] There are many types of MMCA, such as albumin–(Gd-DTPA) complexes, gadofosveset (already described), dextran–(Gd-DTPA) complexes, liposomes, and iron oxide nanoparticles. These contrast agents remain largely within the intravascular space of normal tissues, but they can extravasate from damaged or otherwise hyperpermeable microvessels and accumulate in the interstitial space.[64,65,66] The hyperpermeability of tumor microvessels to macromolecular solutes has been demonstrated in many tumor types.[67] Preclinical studies have shown the utility of MMCAs for the detection and measurement of this characteristic macromolecular leakiness of malignant tumors.[68]

Dynamic contrast-enhanced MRI using MMCAs enables assessment of the tumor vasculature based on the differential distribution of the contrast agent within normal and pathological tissues. Quantitative assays of both morphologic and functional properties can provide useful diagnostic insight into tissue angiogenesis. MRI enhanced with MMCAs has been used experimentally for the characterization of tumor microvessels in a wide range of malignant tumor types. Kinetic analysis of dynamic contrast-enhanced MR data can be used to estimate microvascular permeability and tumor blood volume (▶ Fig. 18.8). By measuring these functional tumor properties, an accurate, noninvasive, and quantitative description of the tumor microcirculation can be acquired, improving the specificity of imaging examinations for diagnosis, treatment, and in vivo monitoring of antitumor therapy.

18.3.1 Albumin–(Gd-DTPA) Complexes

Albumin–(Gd-DTPA) complexes consist of a human protein backbone with multiple (typically 30–35) covalently bound Gd chelates; these water-soluble MMCAs have molecular weights of about 90 kDa.[61,64] The ability of dynamic MRI enhanced with albumin–(Gd-DTPA)$_{30}$ to quantitatively define the characteristics of tumor microvessels, including transendothelial permeability and fractional plasma volume, has been shown in several

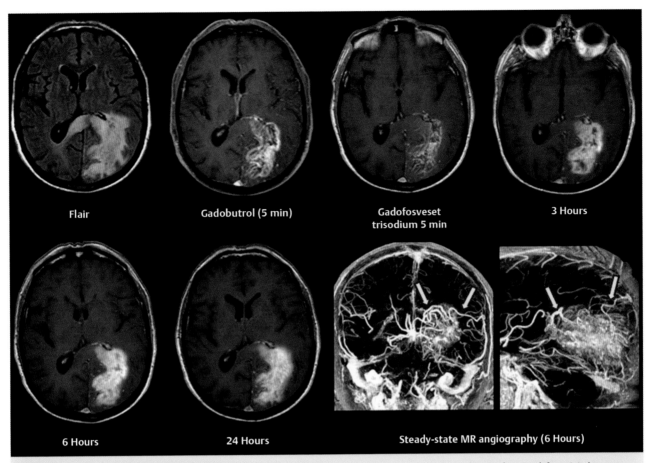

Fig. 18.7 Blood pool contrast agents detect tumor angiogenesis. Glioblastoma multiforme presenting as a large enhancing left occipital tumor. Although the lesion is clearly visible with gadobutrol, the markedly improved definition of margins 6 hours after gadofosveset administration shows the extension of tumor into the splenium better. Thanks to the long intravascular half-life of gadofosveset, we were able to obtain a high-resolution contrast-enhanced magnetic resonance angiogram that allowed us to identify some of the neovessels. FLAIR, fluid-attenuated inversion recovery.

experimental cancer models, including breast, prostate, and ovarian adenocarcinomas.[61,69] Albumin–(Gd-DTPA)$_{30}$-enhanced MRI can also potentially be used to monitor the effect of antiangiogenic therapy exemplified by anti–vascular endothelial growth factor (VEGF) antibody (Avastin, Genetech, South San Francisco, CA). Tumor microvascular permeability of human breast tumors and human ovarian carcinoma decrease significantly after anti-VEGF antibody administration.[70,71] However, the clinical use of albumin-(Gd-DTPA) complexes has not been approved due to their potential immunogenic properties and prolonged partial retention in the body (about 17% at 2 weeks).[72] MRI enhanced with albumin-(Gd-DTPA) complexes with a low dose of Gd (0.03 mmol) yields a relatively low contrast-to-noise ratio in tumors, and relatively long scan times (30–45 min) are typically used due to the progressive extravasation of albumin-(Gd-DTPA) complexes.[61]

18.3.2 Dextran–(Gd-DTPA) Complexes

Dextran–(Gd-DTPA) complexes are linear polysaccharides composed of a polymer of glucose molecules. Gd-DTPA moieties can be covalently attached to each dextran molecule via an easily hydrolysable bond.[73] Wang et al[74] first evaluated dextran–(Gd-DTPA) as an MMCA. By complexing 15 Gd-DTPA chelates to each

dextran molecule, they created a compound with a molecular weight of approximately 75 kDa that remained in the intravascular space for at least 1 h after injection and enhanced the liver, spleen, kidneys, and myocardium. Dextran is broken down more rapidly than albumin and has a shorter biological half-life (43 min). The distribution and subsequent elimination of dextran–(Gd-DTPA) complexes are dependent on their molecular weight and charge.[75] Dextran–(Gd-DTPA) complexes have been investigated for MR angiography,[76,77] imaging acute myocardial infarction,[78] and cardiac perfusion studies.[79] Sirlin et al[80] compared dextran–(Gd-DTPA) with low molecular weight contrast agents in rabbits with VX2 thigh tumors. However, dextrans of higher molecular weights have been associated with an increased incidence of anaphylactic reactions and are considered unsuitable for clinical use.[75]

18.3.3 Liposomal-Gd Contrast Agents

Liposomes are artificial spherical vesicles composed of a lipid bilayer that serves to separate its internal aqueous core from the external medium. The usefulness of liposomal-Gd contrast agents has been demonstrated in animal models. The Gd chelates can be encapsulated within the interior core of the liposome (core-encapsulated Gd liposomes), conjugated on the

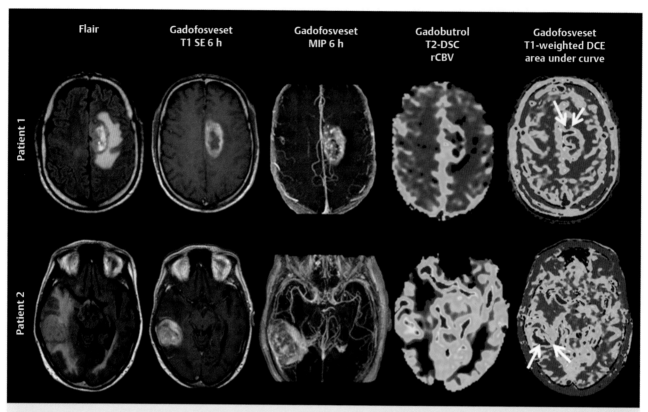

Fig. 18.8 Blood–brain barrier breakdown evaluated by blood pool contrast agents in pretreatment glioblastomas. T2*-weighted dynamic susceptibility contrast imaging using an extracellular agent shows focal increase in cerebral blood volume (CBV) values in the enhancing rim in Patient 1 and inside the lesion in Patient 2. T1-weighted dynamic contrast-enhanced permeability maps show markedly increased permeability within the lesion (arrows), consistent with severe blood–brain barrier damage. Both cases show the underestimation of relative CBV (rCBV) in the setting of severe blood–brain barrier breakdown. DCE, dynamic contrast enhanced; DSC, dynamic susceptibility contrast. MIP, maximum intensity projection; SE, spin-echo.

internal and external surfaces of the liposome bilayer (surface-conjugated Gd liposomes), or incorporated using both approaches (core-encapsulated, surface-conjugated Gd liposomes).[81] The micellar structures have a surface coating of polyethylene glycol that provides long blood circulation half-life. For MR angiography applications, long-circulating liposomal formulations provide uniform signal intensity and stable enhancement over an extended period of imaging.[82] In comparison to conventional extravascular contrast agents, liposomes provide a unique nanoparticle platform because they confer specific properties with respect to target specificity, pharmacokinetics, therapy monitoring, and signal amplification in contrast agents.[81] In preclinical studies, liposomal contrast agents for MRI have shown promising results for MR angiography of the neurovasculature[83] as well as for real-time monitoring of drug infusion to brain tumors.[84]

The T1 relaxivity of liposomal-Gd contrast agents is determined by interactions between the Gd atoms and the bulk water molecules. The core encapsulation of Gd chelates results in lower T1 relaxivities compared with conventional contrast agents as a result of slow transport of water molecules across the lipid bilayer.[85] Ghaghada et al[86] showed that a liposomal-Gd contrast agent that remained within vessels longer enabled good visualization of microvessels in the spines of mice,

whereas extravascular contrast agents demonstrated rapid extravasation from normal vessels into the surrounding extravascular space. Additionally, higher T1 relaxivities achieved using surface-conjugated Gd liposomes has enabled ultra-high-resolution imaging of the circle of Willis and perforating vessels.

The blood–brain barrier poses a significant challenge for delivery of drug macromolecules into the brain. Convection-enhanced delivery (CED) circumvents the blood–brain barrier through direct intracerebral infusion using a hydrostatic pressure gradient to transfer therapeutic compounds. In preclinical studies, liposomes have been used for CED of drugs, expanding the CED-based approach to the treatment of brain tumors.[87] In addition, liposomes could be delivered systemically to monitor the efficacy of neoadjuvant therapies for brain tumors. Liposomal contrast agents' property of remaining in the circulation for long periods could be exploited to measure nanoparticle-based transvascular permeability in brain tumors as well as fractional blood volume during antiangiogenic therapy.[88]

Given the encouraging results from preclinical studies, clinical trials in humans should be forthcoming. MMCA applications in brain tumor imaging might become an adjuvant modality for diagnosing and targeting tumors as well as for monitoring the response to therapy.

Table 18.2 Available superparamagnetic iron oxide nanoparticles used as magnetic resonance contrast agents

Name	Developer	Coating Agent	Size (nm)[a]	Clinical dose (μmol Fe/kg)	Relaxivity (mM[-1] sec[-1])[b]
Ferumoxides AMI-25 Feridex/Endorem	Guerbet AMAG Pharmaceuticals, Inc., Waltham, MA	Dextran T10	120–180 (SPIO)	30	$r_1 = 10.1$ $r_2 = 120$
Ferucarbotran SH U 555 A Resovist	Bayer Schering Pharma AG, Whippany, NJ	Carboxydextran	60 (SPIO)	8–12	$r_1 = 9.7$ $r_2 = 189$
Ferumoxtran-10 AMI-227 Combidex/Sinerem	Guerbet AMAG Pharmaceuticals, Inc.	Dextran T10, T1	15–30 (USPIO)	45	$r_1 = 9.9$ $r_2 = 65$
Ferumoxytol Code 7228	AMAG Pharmaceuticals, Inc.	Polyglucose sorbitol carboxymethyl ether	30 (USPIO)	18–74	$r_1 = 15$ $r_2 = 89$
SH U 555 C Supravist	Bayer Schering Pharma AG	Carboxydextran	21 (USPIO)	40	$r_1 = 10.7$ $r_2 = 38$
Feruglose NC-100150 Clariscan	GE Healthcare, Kentwood, MI	Pegylated starch	20 (USPIO)	36	na
VSOP-C184	Ferropharm, Teltow, Germany	Citrate	7 (VSPIO)	15–75	$r_1 = 14$ $r_2 = 33.4$
Gadoteridol (ProHance)	Bracco Diagnostics, Inc., Monroe Township, NJ	NA	1 (GBCA)	100 (μmol (Gd)/kg)	$r_1 = 4$ $r_2 = 6$

Abbreviations: GBCA, gadolinium-based contrast agent; na, not available; SPIO, superparamagnetic iron oxide particles; USPIO, ultrasmall superparamagnetic iron oxide particles; VSPIO, very small superparamagnetic iron oxide particles.
Source: Table taken from Weinstein JS, Varallyay CG, Dosa E, et al. Superparamagnetic iron oxide nanoparticles: diagnostic magnetic resonance imaging and potential therapeutic applications in neurooncology and central nervous system inflammatory pathologies, a review. J Cereb Blood Flow Metab 2010;30(1):15–35. With permission from Nature Publishing Group.
[a]Hydrodynamic diameter, laser light scattering.
[b]Relaxometric properties (mM[-1] sec[-1]) at 1.5 T, 37°C, water or in plasma; per mM Gd, or Fe.

18.4 Iron Oxide Nanoparticles

Superparamagnetic iron oxide nanoparticles have been used as MR contrast agents for over 20 years, and there has been much recent interest in their use for brain tumor imaging. Measuring from 20 to 180 nm, these particles are significantly larger than most Gd-based agents, which are on the order of 1 nm. Based on their size, they can be classified into standard superparamagnetic iron oxide particles (SPIO), ultrasmall superparamagnetic iron oxide (USPIO) particles, and very small superparamagnetic iron oxide particles (VSPIO). Their very long half-life and high relaxivities make these particles particularly attractive for use as MR contrast agents.[89] Many different types of iron oxide nanoparticles are being used for clinical and experimental imaging applications (▶ Table 18.2). Most belong to the ultrasmall category (10–50 nm), so they are commonly referred to as simply USPIOs.

USPIOs are composed of an iron oxide core, either magnetite (Fe_3O_4) or maghemite (γFe_2O_3), surrounded by a hydrophilic monomer or polymer coating, which determines their circulation time and uptake within the tissues.[90] Various surface modifications have also been introduced for the purpose of targeting specific cell types, such as chlorotoxin for targeting glioma cells in animal models[91] or various monoclonal antibodies. Different formulations influence the surface charge of the molecule as well as the overall size. Because of their relatively large size, USPIOs remain in the circulation for longer than most traditional Gd-based contrast agents, particularly at earlier time points after injection, and they can be used as both blood pool agents and intracellular imaging agents.[92,93] They are taken up by Kupffer cells in the liver, monocytes, macrophages, and by glial cells and dendritic cells in the brain, and applications for both liver imaging and brain imaging have been developed.

The primary USPIOs used for neuroimaging applications are ferumoxytol and ferumoxtran-10. Ferumoxtran-10 belongs to the first generation of iron oxide nanoparticles; because it must be given as a slow intravenous infusion to limit toxicity, it cannot be used for MR angiography or dynamic studies that require a rapid bolus. However, enhancement of brain tumors with ferumoxtran-10 peaks 24 hours after injection and slowly declines in the following days. Ferumoxtran-10 significantly improves the delineation of brain tumors compared to standard Gd agents, allowing for better visualization of tumor margins due to its lower diffusion and increased uptake by the tumor cells.[94] Thus, like other blood pool contrast agents, it has the potential to improve the accuracy of surgical resection and reduce the rate of residual tumor following surgery. Hunt et al[95] showed that a single preoperative dose of ferumoxtran-10 can provide a stable imaging marker of brain tumors during intraoperative MRI, avoiding the problem of artifactual enhancement of non-tumor tissue due to disruption of the blood–brain barrier during surgery that is common with conventional Gd contrast agents (▶ Fig. 18.9).

On the other hand, ferumoxytol is the first USPIO nanoparticle that can be used as an intravenous bolus injection without any significant toxicity.[96] Ferumoxytol has also been studied in comparison to Gd-based agents for brain tumor imaging; it has the advantages of high relaxivities and little extravasation into the interstitial space, although it does eventually begin to leak through the blood–brain barrier. Enhancement of brain tumors with ferumoxytol also peaks approximately 24 hours after injection, and enhancement continues to be present even 72 hours after injection.[92] The half-life of ferumoxytol is approximately 14 hours. Clearance of ferumoxytol from the central nervous system has not been well studied,

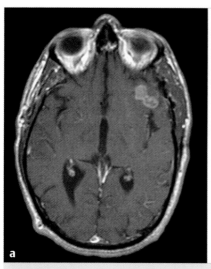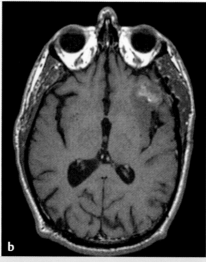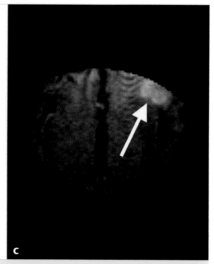

Fig. 18.9 A 41-year-old patient with anaplastic oligodendroglioma. Preoperative gadolinium-enhanced (**a**) and ferumoxtran-10-enhanced (**b**) images and intraoperative ferumoxtran-10-enhanced image (**c**) show the utility of ultrasmall superparamagnetic iron oxide particles in intraoperative magnetic resonance imaging. Arrow points to the area of the tumor enhancement. (Used with permission from Hunt MA, Bagó AG, Neuwelt EA. Single-dose contrast agent for intraoperative MR imaging of intrinsic brain tumors by using ferumoxtran-10. AJNR Am J Neuroradiol 2005;26(5):1084–1088.)

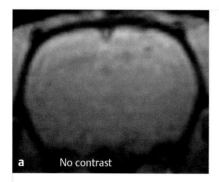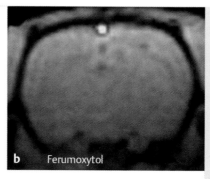

No contrast   Ferumoxytol

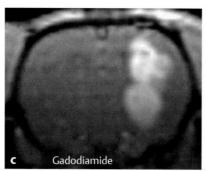

Gadodiamide

Fig. 18.10 Comparison of (**a**) nonenhanced, (**b**) ferumoxytol-enhanced, and (**c**) gadodiamide-enhanced images of rat brain glioma. Sixty seconds following injection of contrast agent, there is no enhancement seen with ferumoxytol, which acts as a blood pool agent, as opposed to gadodiamide, which extravasates rapidly. (Used with permission from Varallyay CG, Muldoon LL, Gahramanov S, et al. Dynamic MRI using iron oxide nanoparticles to assess early vascular effects of antiangiogenic versus corticosteroid treatment in a glioma model. J Cereb Blood Flow Metab 2009;29(4):853–860.)

so the long-term consequences of ferumoxytol accumulation in the brain are unknown. However, renal clearance has not been observed, so ferumoxytol is advantageous for patients with chronic renal failure who are unable to receive Gd-based agents.

The utility of USPIOs for brain tumor imaging has been shown in dynamic susceptibility-weighted contrast MRI. This imaging technique enables the generation of maps to characterize tumor vasculature in terms of cerebral blood volume (CBV), cerebral blood flow, and mean transit time. In a tumor model using human U87 MG glioma cells, ferumoxytol was found to estimate CBV more accurately than gadodiamide, which extravasates more readily and underestimates the true CBV of the tumor (▶ Fig. 18.10 and ▶ Fig. 18.11).[97] USPIOs also promise to play an important role in evaluating the response to antiangiogenic treatment. In murine models, ferumoxtran-10 was better at detecting glioma compared to a Gd-based agent following treatment with vandetanib,[98] and feruglose was useful in measuring fractional blood volume in prolactinomas following treatment with the antiangiogenic agent ZD6126.[99] Results

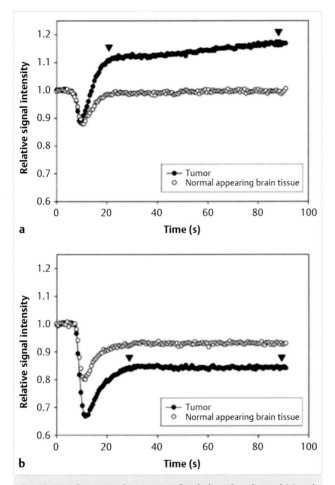

Fig. 18.11 Relative signal intensities of gadodiamide-enhanced (**a**) and ferumoxytol-enhanced (**b**) tumors over time. Gadodiamide results in increased signal intensity compared to normal brain, due to extravasation of the contrast agent, whereas ferumoxytol remains in the intravascular compartment and reaches a plateau over time. (Used with permission from Varallyay CG, Muldoon LL, Gahramanov S, et al. Dynamic MRI using iron oxide nanoparticles to assess early vascular effects of antiangiogenic versus corticosteroid treatment in a glioma model. J Cereb Blood Flow Metab 2009;29(4):853–860.)

18.5 Conclusion

In the management of patients with brain tumors, imaging needs to characterize the disease and determine its extent to enable accurate planning of treatment and to evaluate the response to treatment. Contrast-enhanced MRI is an essential tool for brain imaging; however, advances in the development of contrast agents are needed to maximize the potential utility of the technique and to further our understanding of the pathophysiology of brain tumors.

References

[1] Albert FK, Forsting M, Sartor K, Adams HP, Kunze S. Early postoperative magnetic resonance imaging after resection of malignant glioma: objective evaluation of residual tumor and its influence on regrowth and prognosis. Neurosurgery 1994; 34: 45–60, discussion 60–61

[2] Kondziolka D, Patel A, Lunsford LD, Kassam A, Flickinger JC. Stereotactic radiosurgery plus whole brain radiotherapy versus radiotherapy alone for patients with multiple brain metastases. Int J Radiat Oncol Biol Phys 1999; 45: 427–434

[3] Smirniotopoulos JG, Murphy FM, Rushing EJ, Rees JH, Schroeder JW. Patterns of contrast enhancement in the brain and meninges. Radiographics 2007; 27: 525–551

[4] Jensen TR, Schmainda KM. Computer-aided detection of brain tumor invasion using multiparametric MRI. J Magn Reson Imaging 2009; 30: 481–489

[5] Essig M, Weber MA, von Tengg-Kobligk H, Knopp MV, Yuh WT, Giesel FL. Contrast-enhanced magnetic resonance imaging of central nervous system tumors: agents, mechanisms, and applications. Top Magn Reson Imaging 2006; 17: 89–106

[6] Giesel FL, Mehndiratta A, Essig M. High-relaxivity contrast-enhanced magnetic resonance neuroimaging: a review. Eur Radiol 2010; 20: 2461–2474

[7] Cavagna FM, Maggioni F, Castelli PM et al. Gadolinium chelates with weak binding to serum proteins. A new class of high-efficiency, general purpose contrast agents for magnetic resonance imaging. Invest Radiol 1997; 32: 780–796

[8] Colosimo C, Manfredi R, Tartaglione T. Contrast enhancement issues in the MR evaluation of the central nervous system. Eur Radiol 1997; 7 Suppl 5: 231–237

[9] Grossman RI, Rubin DL, Hunter G et al. Magnetic resonance imaging in patients with central nervous system pathology: a comparison of OptiMARK (Gd-DTPA-BMEA) and Magnevist (Gd-DTPA). Invest Radiol 2000; 35: 412–419

[10] Oudkerk M, Sijens PE, Van Beek EJ, Kuijpers TJ. Safety and efficacy of dotarem (Gd-DOTA) versus magnevist (Gd-DTPA) in magnetic resonance imaging of the central nervous system. Invest Radiol 1995; 30: 75–78

[11] Yuh WTC, Fisher DJ, Engelken JD et al. MR evaluation of CNS tumors: dose comparison study with gadopentetate dimeglumine and gadoteridol. Radiology 1991; 180: 485–491

[12] Colosimo C, Knopp MV, Barreau X et al. A comparison of Gd-BOPTA and Gd-DOTA for contrast-enhanced MRI of intracranial tumours. Neuroradiology 2004; 46: 655–665

[13] Myhr G, Rinck PA, Børseth A. Gadodiamide injection and gadopentetate dimeglumine. A double-blind study in MR imaging of the CNS. Acta Radiol 1992; 33: 405–409

[14] Balériaux D, Matos C, De Greef D. Gadodiamide injection as a contrast medium for MRI of the central nervous system: a comparison with gadolinium-DOTA. Neuroradiology 1993; 35: 490–494

[15] Valk J, Algra PR, Hazenberg CJ, Slooff WB, Svaland MG. A double-blind, comparative study of gadodiamide injection and gadopentetate dimeglumine in MRI of the central nervous system. Neuroradiology 1993; 35: 173–177

[16] Brugières P, Gaston A, Degryse HR et al. Randomised double blind trial of the safety and efficacy of two gadolinium complexes (Gd-DTPA and Gd-DOTA). Neuroradiology 1994; 36: 27–30

[17] Akeson P, Jonsson E, Haugen I, Holtås S. Contrast-enhanced MRI of the central nervous system: comparison between gadodiamide injection and gadolinium-DTPA. Neuroradiology 1995; 37: 229–233

[18] Tombach B, Heindel W. Value of 1.0- M gadolinium chelates: review of preclinical and clinical data on gadobutrol. Eur Radiol 2002; 12: 1550–1556

correlating CBV and long-term survival are mixed, possibly due to imprecision in measuring CBV[100,101]; USPIOs may make it possible to calculate CBV more accurately and thus to better distinguish true tumor progression from pseudoprogression and to better predict survival.

In addition to tumor imaging, USPIOs' ability to show blood barrier disruption might also be useful in other conditions such as inflammation, stroke, epilepsy, and trauma.[102,103,104,105] Moreover, like other blood pool contrast agents such as gadofosveset, USPIOs can be used to visualize arterial stenoses.[106] However, one drawback to using USPIOs is these particles cannot be distinguished from endogenous iron in the setting of acute hemorrhage. Overall, however, USPIOs promise to have at least a complementary role to traditional Gd-based contrast agents. Not only have USPIOs surpassed Gd-based agents with regard to tumor detection and characterization in preclinical studies but, unlike Gd-based agents, they are not eliminated through the kidneys so they can be used in patients with renal failure.

[19] Le Duc G, Corde S, Charvet AM et al. In vivo measurement of gadolinium concentration in a rat glioma model by monochromatic quantitative computed tomography: comparison between gadopentetate dimeglumine and gadobutrol. Invest Radiol 2004; 39: 385–393

[20] Cheng KT. Gadobutrol. 2006 Molecular Imaging and Contrast Agent Database (National Center for Biotechnology Information [US] Web site). 2004–2010. http://www.ncbi.nlm.nih.gov/books/NBK23589. Accessed January 24, 2012

[21] Giesel FL, Mehndiratta A, Risse F et al. Intraindividual comparison between gadopentetate dimeglumine and gadobutrol for magnetic resonance perfusion in normal brain and intracranial tumors at 3 Tesla. Acta Radiol 2009; 50: 521–530

[22] Attenberger UI, Runge VM, Jackson CB et al. Comparative evaluation of lesion enhancement using 1 M gadobutrol vs. 2 conventional gadolinium chelates, all at a dose of 0.1 mmol/kg, in a rat brain tumor model at 3T. Invest Radiol 2009; 44: 251–256

[23] Rohrer M, Bauer H, Mintorovitch J, Requardt M, Weinmann HJ. Comparison of magnetic properties of MRI contrast media solutions at different magnetic field strengths. Invest Radiol 2005; 40: 715–724

[24] Morelli JN, Runge VM, Vu L, Loynachan AT, Attenberger UI. Evaluation of gadodiamide versus gadobutrol for contrast-enhanced MR imaging in a rat brain glioma model at 1.5 and 3 T. Invest Radiol 2010; 45: 810–818

[25] Mohs AM, Lu ZR. Gadolinium(III)-based blood-pool contrast agents for magnetic resonance imaging: status and clinical potential. Expert Opin Drug Deliv 2007; 4: 149–164

[26] Farooki A, Narra V, Brown J. Gadofosveset (EPIX/Schering). Curr Opin Investig Drugs 2004; 5: 967–976

[27] Caravan P. Protein-targeted gadolinium-based magnetic resonance imaging (MRI) contrast agents: design and mechanism of action. Acc Chem Res 2009; 42: 851–862

[28] Seitz RJ, Wechsler W. Immunohistochemical demonstration of serum proteins in human cerebral gliomas. Acta Neuropathol 1987; 73: 145–152

[29] Essig M, Rohrer M, Giesel F et al. Human brain tumor imaging with a protein-binding MR contrast agent: initial experience. Eur Radiol 2010; 20: 218–226

[30] Puig J, Blasco G, Essig M et al. Albumin-binding MR blood pool contrast agent improves diagnostic performance in human brain tumour: comparison of two contrast agents for glioblastoma. Eur Radiol 2013; 23: 1093–1101

[31] Goyen M, Edelman M, Perreault P et al. MR angiography of aortoiliac occlusive disease: a phase III study of the safety and effectiveness of the blood-pool contrast agent MS-325. Radiology 2005; 236: 825–833

[32] Kau T, Gasser J, Celedin S et al. MR angiographic follow-up of intracranial aneurysms treated with detachable coils: evaluation of a blood-pool contrast medium. AJNR Am J Neuroradiol 2009; 30: 1524–1530

[33] Adzamli K, Yablonskiy DA, Chicoine MR et al. Albumin-binding MR blood pool agents as MRI contrast agents in an intracranial mouse glioma model. Magn Reson Med 2003; 49: 586–590

[34] Wintersperger BJ, Runge VM, Tweedle MF, Jackson CB, Reiser MF. Brain tumor enhancement in magnetic resonance imaging: dependency on the level of protein binding of applied contrast agents. Invest Radiol 2009; 44: 89–94

[35] Knopp MV, Runge VM, Essig M et al. Primary and secondary brain tumors at MR imaging: bicentric intraindividual crossover comparison of gadobenate dimeglumine and gadopentetate dimeglumine. Radiology 2004; 230: 55–64

[36] Colosimo C, Demaerel P, Tortori-Donati P et al. Comparison of gadobenate dimeglumine (Gd-BOPTA) with gadopentetate dimeglumine (Gd-DTPA) for enhanced MR imaging of brain and spine tumours in children. Pediatr Radiol 2005; 35: 501–510

[37] Kuhn MJ, Picozzi P, Maldjian JA et al. Evaluation of intraaxial enhancing brain tumors on magnetic resonance imaging: intraindividual crossover comparison of gadobenate dimeglumine and gadopentetate dimeglumine for visualization and assessment, and implications for surgical intervention. J Neurosurg 2007; 106: 557–566

[38] Lauffer RB, Parmelee DJ, Dunham SU et al. MS-325: albumin-targeted contrast agent for MR angiography. Radiology 1998; 207: 529–538

[39] Hossmann KA, Hürter T, Oschlies U. The effect of dexamethasone on serum protein extravasation and edema development in experimental brain tumors of cat. Acta Neuropathol 1983; 60: 223–231

[40] Caravan P, Cloutier NJ, Greenfield MT et al. The interaction of MS-325 with human serum albumin and its effect on proton relaxation rates. J Am Chem Soc 2002; 124: 3152–3162

[41] Johnson PC, Hunt SJ, Drayer BP. Human cerebral gliomas: correlation of postmortem MR imaging and neuropathologic findings. Radiology 1989; 170: 211–217

[42] Giese A, Westphal M. Treatment of malignant glioma: a problem beyond the margins of resection. J Cancer Res Clin Oncol 2001; 127: 217–225

[43] Cao Y, Nagesh V, Hamstra D et al. The extent and severity of vascular leakage as evidence of tumor aggressiveness in high-grade gliomas. Cancer Res 2006; 66: 8912–8917

[44] Halperin EC, Bentel G, Heinz ER, Burger PC. Radiation therapy treatment planning in supratentorial glioblastoma multiforme: an analysis based on post mortem topographic anatomy with CT correlations. Int J Radiat Oncol Biol Phys 1989; 17: 1347–1350

[45] Kelly PJ, Daumas-Duport C, Scheithauer BW, Kall BA, Kispert DB. Stereotactic histologic correlations of computed tomography- and magnetic resonance imaging-defined abnormalities in patients with glial neoplasms. Mayo Clin Proc 1987; 62: 450–459

[46] Nagesh V, Chenevert TL, Tsien CI et al. Quantitative characterization of hemodynamic properties and vasculature dysfunction of high-grade gliomas. NMR Biomed 2007; 20: 566–577

[47] Hossmann KA. Hemodynamic and metabolic disturbances in experimental peritumoral edema. In: Johansson BB, Owman C, Widner H, eds. Pathophysiology of the Blood–Brain Barrier. New York, NY: Elsevier Science; 1990:369–380

[48] Pronin IN, McManus KA, Holodny AI, Peck KK, Kornienko VN. Quantification of dispersion of Gd-DTPA from the initial area of enhancement into the peritumoral zone of edema in brain tumors. J Neurooncol 2009; 94: 399–408

[49] Farace P, Tambalo S, Fiorini S et al. Early versus late GD-DTPA MRI enhancement in experimental glioblastomas. J Magn Reson Imaging 2011; 33: 550–556

[50] Els T, Bockhorst K, Hoehn-Berlage M. NMR contrast enhancement of brain tumours: Comparison of the blood brain barrier tracer GdDTPA and tumour-selective contrast agent MnTPPS. MAGMA 1993; 1: 126–133

[51] Baxter LT, Jain RK. Transport of fluid and macromolecules in tumors. II. Role of heterogeneous perfusion and lymphatics. Microvasc Res 1990; 40: 246–263

[52] Goldacre RJ, Sylven B. On the access of blood-borne dyes to various tumour regions. Br J Cancer 1962; 16: 306–322

[53] Fries P, Runge VM, Bücker A et al. Brain tumor enhancement in magnetic resonance imaging at 3 tesla: intraindividual comparison of two high relaxivity macromolecular contrast media with a standard extracellular gd-chelate in a rat brain tumor model. Invest Radiol 2009; 44: 200–206

[54] Hahn G, Sorge I, Gruhn B et al. Pharmacokinetics and safety of gadobutrol-enhanced magnetic resonance imaging in pediatric patients. Invest Radiol 2009; 44: 776–783

[55] Hammerstingl R, Adam G, Ayuso JR et al. Comparison of 1.0 M gadobutrol and 0.5 M gadopentetate dimeglumine-enhanced magnetic resonance imaging in five hundred seventy-two patients with known or suspected liver lesions: results of a multicenter, double-blind, interindividual, randomized clinical phase-III trial. Invest Radiol 2009; 44: 168–176

[56] Lacroix M, Abi-Said D, Fourney DR et al. A multivariate analysis of 416 patients with glioblastoma multiforme: prognosis, extent of resection, and survival. J Neurosurg 2001; 95: 190–198

[57] Sanai N, Berger MS. Glioma extent of resection and its impact on patient outcome. Neurosurgery 2008; 62: 753–764, discussion 264–266

[58] Kuhnt D, Becker A, Ganslandt O, Bauer M, Buchfelder M, Nimsky C. Correlation of the extent of tumor volume resection and patient survival in surgery of glioblastoma multiforme with high-field intraoperative MRI guidance. Neuro-oncol 2011; 13: 1339–1348

[59] Senft C, Bink A, Franz K, Vatter H, Gasser T, Seifert V. Intraoperative MRI guidance and extent of resection in glioma surgery: a randomised, controlled trial. Lancet Oncol 2011; 12: 997–1003

[60] Senft C, Franz K, Blasel S et al. Influence of iMRI-guidance on the extent of resection and survival of patients with glioblastoma multiforme. Technol Cancer Res Treat 2010; 9: 339–346

[61] Preda A, van Vliet M, Krestin GP, Brasch RC, van Dijke CF. Magnetic resonance macromolecular agents for monitoring tumor microvessels and angiogenesis inhibition. Invest Radiol 2006; 41: 325–331

[62] Daldrup-Link HE, Brasch RC. Macromolecular contrast agents for MR mammography: current status. Eur Radiol 2003; 13: 354–365

[63] Padhani AR. MRI for assessing antivascular cancer treatments. Br J Radiol 2003; 76: S60–S80

[64] Brasch RC. New directions in the development of MR imaging contrast media. Radiology 1992; 183: 1–11

[65] Demsar F, Roberts TP, Schwickert HC et al. A MRI spatial mapping technique for microvascular permeability and tissue blood volume based on macromolecular contrast agent distribution. Magn Reson Med 1997; 37: 236–242

[66] Shames DM, Kuwatsuru R, Vexler V, Mühler A, Brasch RC. Measurement of capillary permeability to macromolecules by dynamic magnetic resonance

imaging: a quantitative noninvasive technique. Magn Reson Med 1993; 29: 616–622

[67] Jain RK. Barriers to drug delivery in solid tumors. Sci Am 1994; 271: 58–65

[68] Brasch R, Turetschek K. MRI characterization of tumors and grading angiogenesis using macromolecular contrast media: status report. Eur J Radiol 2000; 34: 148–155

[69] Su MY, Mühler A, Lao X, Nalcioglu O. Tumor characterization with dynamic contrast-enhanced MRI using MR contrast agents of various molecular weights. Magn Reson Med 1998; 39: 259–269

[70] Pham CD, Roberts TP, van Bruggen N et al. Magnetic resonance imaging detects suppression of tumor vascular permeability after administration of antibody to vascular endothelial growth factor. Cancer Invest 1998; 16: 225–230

[71] Turetschek K, Preda A, Novikov V et al. Tumor microvascular changes in antiangiogenic treatment: assessment by magnetic resonance contrast media of different molecular weights. J Magn Reson Imaging 2004; 20: 138–144

[72] White D, Wang S-C, Aicher K, et al. Albumin-(Gd-DTPA)15–20: whole body clearance, and organ distribution of gadolinium. In: Proceedings of the Society of Magnetic Resonance in Medicine, 8th Annual Meeting; Amsterdam; August 12–18,1989;807

[73] Barrett T, Kobayashi H, Brechbiel M, Choyke PL. Macromolecular MRI contrast agents for imaging tumor angiogenesis. Eur J Radiol 2006; 60: 353–366

[74] Wang SC, Wikström MG, White DL et al. Evaluation of Gd-DTPA-labeled dextran as an intravascular MR contrast agent: imaging characteristics in normal rat tissues. Radiology 1990; 175: 483–488

[75] Mehvar R. Dextrans for targeted and sustained delivery of therapeutic and imaging agents. J Control Release 2000; 69: 1–25

[76] Kroft LJ, Doornbos J, Benderbous S, de Roos A. Equilibrium phase MR angiography of the aortic arch and abdominal vasculature with the blood pool contrast agent CMD-A2-Gd-DOTA in pigs. J Magn Reson Imaging 1999; 9: 777–785

[77] Loubeyre P, Canet E, Zhao S, Benderbous S, Amiel M, Revel D. Carboxymethyl-dextran-gadolinium-DTPA as a blood-pool contrast agent for magnetic resonance angiography. Experimental study in rabbits. Invest Radiol 1996; 31: 288–293

[78] Wikström M, Martinussen HJ, Wikström G et al. MR imaging of acute myocardial infarction in pigs using Gd-DTPA-labeled dextran. Acta Radiol 1992; 33: 301–308

[79] Casali C, Janier M, Canet E et al. Evaluation of Gd-DOTA-labeled dextran polymer as an intravascular MR contrast agent for myocardial perfusion. Acad Radiol 1998; 5 Suppl 1: S214–S218

[80] Sirlin CB, Vera DR, Corbeil JA, Caballero MB, Buxton RB, Mattrey RF. Gadolinium-DTPA-dextran: a macromolecular MR blood pool contrast agent. Acad Radiol 2004; 11: 1361–1369

[81] Ghaghada KB, Colen RR, Hawley CR, Patel N, Mukundan S, Jr. Liposomal contrast agents in brain tumor imaging. Neuroimaging Clin N Am 2010; 20: 367–378

[82] Ayyagari AL, Zhang X, Ghaghada KB, Annapragada A, Hu X, Bellamkonda RV. Long-circulating liposomal contrast agents for magnetic resonance imaging. Magn Reson Med 2006; 55: 1023–1029

[83] Howles GP, Ghaghada KB, Qi Y, Mukundan S, Jr, Johnson GA. High-resolution magnetic resonance angiography in the mouse using a nanoparticle blood-pool contrast agent. Magn Reson Med 2009; 62: 1447–1456

[84] Krauze MT, Forsayeth J, Park JW, Bankiewicz KS. Real-time imaging and quantification of brain delivery of liposomes. Pharm Res 2006; 23: 2493–2504

[85] Ghaghada K, Hawley C, Kawaji K, Annapragada A, Mukundan S, Jr. T1 relaxivity of core-encapsulated gadolinium liposomal contrast agents—effect of liposome size and internal gadolinium concentration. Acad Radiol 2008; 15: 1259–1263

[86] Ghaghada KB, Bockhorst KH, Mukundan S, Jr, Annapragada AV, Narayana PA. High-resolution vascular imaging of the rat spine using liposomal blood pool MR agent. AJNR Am J Neuroradiol 2007; 28: 48–53

[87] Mehta AI, Choi BD, Ajay D et al. Convection enhanced delivery of macromolecules for brain tumors. Curr Drug Discov Technol 2012; 9: 305–310

[88] Persigehl T, Bieker R, Matuszewski L et al. Antiangiogenic tumor treatment: early noninvasive monitoring with USPIO-enhanced MR imaging in mice. Radiology 2007; 244: 449–456

[89] Weinstein JS, Varallyay CG, Dosa E et al. Superparamagnetic iron oxide nanoparticles: diagnostic magnetic resonance imaging and potential therapeutic applications in neurooncology and central nervous system inflammatory pathologies, a review. J Cereb Blood Flow Metab 2010; 30: 15–35

[90] Thorek DL, Chen AK, Czupryna J, Tsourkas A. Superparamagnetic iron oxide nanoparticle probes for molecular imaging. Ann Biomed Eng 2006; 34: 23–38

[91] Lyons SA, O'Neal J, Sontheimer H. Chlorotoxin, a scorpion-derived peptide, specifically binds to gliomas and tumors of neuroectodermal origin. Glia 2002; 39: 162–173

[92] Neuwelt EA, Várallyay CG, Manninger S et al. The potential of ferumoxytol nanoparticle magnetic resonance imaging, perfusion, and angiography in central nervous system malignancy: a pilot study. Neurosurgery 2007; 60: 601–611, discussion 611–612

[93] Metz S, Bonaterra G, Rudelius M, Settles M, Rummeny EJ, Daldrup-Link HE. Capacity of human monocytes to phagocytose approved iron oxide MR contrast agents in vitro. Eur Radiol 2004; 14: 1851–1858

[94] Enochs WS, Harsh G, Hochberg F, Weissleder R. Improved delineation of human brain tumors on MR images using a long-circulating, superparamagnetic iron oxide agent. J Magn Reson Imaging 1999; 9: 228–232

[95] Hunt MA, Bagó AG, Neuwelt EA. Single-dose contrast agent for intraoperative MR imaging of intrinsic brain tumors by using ferumoxtran-10. AJNR Am J Neuroradiol 2005; 26: 1084–1088

[96] Neuwelt EA, Hamilton BE, Varallyay CG et al. Ultrasmall superparamagnetic iron oxides (USPIOs): a future alternative magnetic resonance (MR) contrast agent for patients at risk for nephrogenic systemic fibrosis (NSF)? Kidney Int 2009; 75: 465–474

[97] Varallyay CG, Muldoon LL, Gahramanov S et al. Dynamic MRI using iron oxide nanoparticles to assess early vascular effects of antiangiogenic versus corticosteroid treatment in a glioma model. J Cereb Blood Flow Metab 2009; 29: 853–860

[98] Claes A, Gambarota G, Hamans B et al. Magnetic resonance imaging-based detection of glial brain tumors in mice after antiangiogenic treatment. Int J Cancer 2008; 122: 1981–1986

[99] Robinson SP, Howe FA, Griffiths JR, Ryan AJ, Waterton JC. Susceptibility contrast magnetic resonance imaging determination of fractional tumor blood volume: a noninvasive imaging biomarker of response to the vascular disrupting agent ZD6126. Int J Radiat Oncol Biol Phys 2007; 69: 872–879

[100] Lev MH, Ozsunar Y, Henson JW et al. Glial tumor grading and outcome prediction using dynamic spin-echo MR susceptibility mapping compared with conventional contrast-enhanced MR: confounding effect of elevated rCBV of oligodendrogliomas [corrected]. AJNR Am J Neuroradiol 2004; 25: 214–221

[101] Oh J, Henry RG, Pirzkall A et al. Survival analysis in patients with glioblastoma multiforme: predictive value of choline-to-N-acetylaspartate index, apparent diffusion coefficient, and relative cerebral blood volume. J Magn Reson Imaging 2004; 19: 546–554

[102] Muldoon LL, Varallyay P, Kraemer DF et al. Trafficking of superparamagnetic iron oxide particles (Combidex) from brain to lymph nodes in the rat. Neuropathol Appl Neurobiol 2004; 30: 70–79

[103] Rausch M, Sauter A, Fröhlich J, Neubacher U, Radü EW, Rudin M. Dynamic patterns of USPIO enhancement can be observed in macrophages after ischemic brain damage. Magn Reson Med 2001; 46: 1018–1022

[104] Akhtari M, Bragin A, Cohen M et al. Functionalized magnetonanoparticles for MRI diagnosis and localization in epilepsy. Epilepsia 2008; 49: 1419–1430

[105] Hoehn M, Wiedermann D, Justicia C et al. Cell tracking using magnetic resonance imaging. J Physiol 2007; 584: 25–30

[106] Tang TY, Howarth SP, Miller SR et al. Correlation of carotid atheromatous plaque inflammation using USPIO-enhanced MR imaging with degree of luminal stenosis. Stroke 2008; 39: 2144–2147

[107] Corot C, Robert P, Idee JM, Port M. Recent advances in iron oxide nanocrystal technology for medical imaging. Adv Drug Deliv Rev 2006;58:1471–1504

19 On the Horizon: Molecular Imaging

Sanath Kumar, Meser M. Ali, and Ali S. Arbab

19.1 Introduction

The majority of brain tumors are metastatic and half of them are from lung cancers. The most common primary brain tumors are gliomas, meningiomas, pituitary adenomas, and nerve sheath tumors. Gliomas make up more than 50% of all primary brain tumors and are ased on the cellular types, genetic makeup, and aggressiveness; gliomas are divided into different classification and grades. Among them glioblastoma multiforme (GBM) is considered a more aggressive and devastating tumor, which is hypervascular, heterogeneous, highly infiltrative in nature. The current treatments, including surgical resection, radiotherapy, and chemotherapy, do not increase the post treatment survival to an acceptable level. Although the overall incidence of GBM is much lower compared to that of other cancers, such as breast, cervical, and lung, its poor prognosis makes GBM one of the most challenging cancers for the scientific community. Clinicians and basic scientists are seeking the cause of treatment failure and recurrence of GBM. Mechanisms of resistance are being studied at genetic and molecular levels. However, to understand the changes at molecular and genetic levels requires in vivo techniques that can predict the changes that may cause resistance to the applied treatments. The current in vivo imaging modalities that are being extensively used in the clinical setting are not deciphering the problem that may arise at the initial stages of resistance/tolerance to treatment. Current U.S. Food and Drug Administration (FDA)-approved imaging modalities and techniques cannot predict the effect or failure of applied treatments until it is too late. Investigators, including us, are trying to determine the targets to predict the development of resistance and tolerance to applied treatments which can be detected by in vivo imaging. The targets could be molecular markers, receptors, protein–protein interactions, events of neovascularization, epigenetic of neovascularization or drug resistance, accumulation of progenitor and immunogenic cells, cancer stem cells, and so on. FDA-approved or preclinical imaging modalities can be used to understand the mechanisms of resistance and recurrence and of early prediction of treatment failure. To understand the molecular mechanisms in GBM recurrence, molecular imaging techniques are gaining popularity in both clinical and preclinical studies. For successful implementation of molecular imaging techniques, involvement of chemists is essential to make contrast agents for different imaging modalities and to make agents that target receptor/ligands. This chapter discusses the current development and use of different molecular contrast agents as well as the use of cells as imaging probes.

19.2 What Is Molecular Imaging?

The broad definition of molecular imaging should include both in vivo and in vitro imaging techniques to understand the molecular mechanisms or processes of intra- and extracellular functions (e.g., signaling, protein–protein interaction, gene and protein expression, receptor–ligands interaction, cellular metabolism, etc.), mechanisms of tissue damage, oxygen or pH status of any tissues, development of tumor, interaction of tumor with surrounding tissues, mechanisms of neovascularization, and the interaction of endothelial cells with tumor cells and others. Unlike traditional imaging techniques, molecular imaging uses probes or biomarkers to target specific pathways or mechanisms for the area of interests. Many in vitro and in vivo imaging modalities have been developed for molecular imaging. FDA-approved clinically relevant imaging modalities such as magnetic resonance imaging (MRI), single photon emission computed tomography (SPECT), positron-emission tomography (PET), and even optical imaging are being used as imaging modalities for understanding the molecular events in cancer and in other diseases.

19.3 Why Molecular Imaging for Glioma?

Traditionally GBMs (or high-grade gliomas) are treated with surgery, radiotherapy, and adjuvant chemotherapy. At present, neither the surgeon and nor the radiation oncologist relies on the molecular mechanisms or genetic aberration in primary or recurrent GBM. However, in regard to chemotherapy and adjuvant therapy, medical oncologists are focusing more on the possible molecular characteristics of GBM or the presence of any genetic aberration to counter the primary or recurrent GBM by adjusting possible appropriate adjuvant therapy.[1,2,3,4] At present, in the clinical setting, these changes are determined from a biopsy or explanted tumor samples. Newer blood tests to find out relevant micro-RNA or released cytokines/growth factors are far from clinical use. Therefore molecular imaging could allow oncologists to change treatment strategies, when necessary, based on imaging findings in respect to resistance to applied treatments and/or development of newer genetic aberration in the recurrent GBM. All clinically approved imaging modalities, such as MRI, SPECT, and PET, are being used to determine the characteristics of tumor tissues/cells, as well as different molecular mechanisms involved in the primary and recurrent GBM. However, when the question of understanding the basic molecular mechanisms arises, both SPECT and PET have advantages over MRI. There are many clinically approved radiopharmaceuticals available to determine the early recurrence of GBM by nuclear medicine techniques, such as SPECT or PET, by exploiting the enhanced use of amino acids (e.g., tyrosine, methionine) by tumors, use of glucose by tumors, DNA repair and multiplication, protein–protein interaction, expression of different receptors on tumor cells, and its associated vascularity. Different clinical and preclinical imaging modalities and probes can be used to understand the strength of molecular imaging and its future use in patient management.

19.4 MRI for Molecular Imaging of Primary and Recurrent Glioma

MRI is a very versatile imaging modality. Understanding tissue characteristics by using different image sequences itself can be regarded as molecular imaging. For example, creating T1 and T2 relaxation maps can determine the endogenous magnetic properties of tissues, which can be used to differentiate between normal and abnormal structures in the brain. Diffusion-weighted imaging (DWI) can differentiate high-grade from low-grade and treated from nontreated tumor by determining water movement.[5,6,7] Clinically applicable sequences as well as sequences under development can be used in clinical and preclinical settings to understand the molecular mechanism involved in primary GBM, along with the effects of treatment and the changes in molecules in recurrent glioma with or without the administration of specific molecular probes. A detailed description and usage of various clinically relevant sequences are not the scope of this chapter; Chapters 4, 5, 6, and 7 earlier in the book describe different sequences and techniques. This chapter provides a brief description of the sequences not discussed elsewhere in the book.

19.4.1 MRI in the Clinical Setting

Proton Density

Proton density (spin density)-weighted images are produced by selecting the scan parameters to minimize the effects of T1 and T2 relaxation, resulting in an image dependent primarily on the proton per unit volume of tissue being imaged. Proton density contrast gives a quantitative summary of the number of protons per unit tissue. The higher the number of protons in a given tissue, the greater the transverse component of magnetization, and the brighter the signal on the proton density contrast image. Conversely the lower the number of protons in a given tissue, the lower the transverse magnetization and the darker the signal on the proton density image. Proton density images are useful for distinguishing tumor and edema from adjacent cerebrospinal fluid (CSF), which may appear similar to high-signal areas on heavily T2-weighted images. Proton density MRI has been used to study treatment response in GBM patients following adjuvant antiangiogenic treatment.[8] The amount of signal change was predictive of long-term progression free survival and overall survival in GBM patients after bevacizumab treatment.[8]

Electrolytes (Na +)

Sodium MRI (^{23}Na MRI) is increasingly becoming an attractive potential marker for predicting therapeutic response after anticancer treatment. The high rate of mitotic activity in the tumors is preceded by the sustained depolarization of the cell membrane.[9] This leads to an increase in intracellular sodium concentration inside the tumor cell lines, including glial cells.[10,11,12] Changes in the total sodium concentration are known to be a good indicator of oncological treatment effect, including cell lysis.[13] This increase in total sodium concentration is readily measurable using ultrashort echo time sodium MRI. Unlike many other imaging modalities, the change in sodium concentration is limited by blood–brain barrier (BBB) changes. It has been evaluated to assess treatment response of GBM tumors in patients.[13] This technique seems to provide valuable information on tumor progression and response, especially when combined with a PET scan.[13]

Peptides

MR spectroscopic and proteomic studies have shown that human brain tumors have a greater macromolecular protein concentration, compared to the normal brain, and the concentration increases with tumor grade.[14] Amide protein transfer (APT) imaging is a novel MRI technique based on amide proton signals from endogenous cellular proteins and peptides. One of the biggest advantages of APT MRI is that it does not require administration of an exogenous contrast agent. APT imaging has been used in preclinical models to reliably distinguish between brain tumor recurrence and radiation necrosis.[15] It has been used for imaging patients with brain tumors, and APT contrast has shown to be superior when compared to conventional MRI in distinguishing tumor tissue from peritumoral edema.[16] Clinical studies have also revealed the potential use of APT imaging in noninvasive diagnosis of the tumor grade.[17] Another potential clinical utility of APT imaging is the noninvasive identification of heterogeneity in high-grade brain tumors.[18] This could potentially be useful in the planning of a surgical resection and radiation therapy of heterogeneous tumors like GBM.

USPIO-Based Contrast

Magnetic nanoparticles have the potential to be used as contrast agents in MRI because they possess unique magnetic properties, along with the ability to function at the cellular level of biological interactions. Intravenous administration of ferumoxtran, an ultra-small paramagnetic iron oxide particle, has been shown to produce enhancement that is comparable to that of gadolinium in malignant brain tumors.[19] Neuwelt et al compared the ferumoxtran imaging with gadolinium enhancement in a series of seven patients.[20] They observed that the ferumoxtran-enhancing lesions could be well detected even with a low Tesla magnet (0.15 T). Ferumoxtran was also able to detect areas of tumors that did not enhance with gadolinium. The ferumoxtran signal was detectable 2 to 5 days after administration.[20] The mechanism for additional and persistent MR signal change of iron oxide particles is due to the long plasma half-life and intracellular trapping by reactive cells (astrocytes, macrophages), rather than tumor cells in and around the tumor. Thus magnetic nanoparticles seem to be an attractive contrast agent to be used during intraoperative resection and postoperative follow up in patients with malignant brain tumors. Unfortunately ferumoxtran did not receive full FDA approval. However, another iron-oxide based nanoparticle "ferumoxytol" has been approved for clinical use in patients with end stage renal failure.[21] Dr. Neuwelt's group at the Oregon Health and Science University is recruiting patients to use ferumoxytol to assess the early response in patients with GBM by way of MRI. Studies from this group have shown that cerebral blood volume measurements using dynamic perfusion MRI with ferumoxytol USPIO, is promising for more accurate detection of therapeutic responses to antiangiogenic therapy.[22]

19.4.2 Preclinical Setting

Metabolites

MR spectroscopic imaging has already been established for clinical use to determine different metabolites in GBM before and after treatments. Hyperpolarized ^{13}C MR metabolic imaging is gaining momentum to determine metabolic status in tumors. Hyperpolarized ^{13}C MR metabolic imaging can be used to determine different metabolites, including pyruvate, acetate, succinate, fumarate, choline, and fructose in glioma and other tumors.[23–28] A disadvantage of hyperpolarized ^{13}C MR technique is that a special setup (hardware) is needed, and the full benefit of this technique in the clinical setting has yet to be finalized.

Gene Expression

Detection of the expression of an endogenous gene in a glioma has yet to be detected by MRI. However, to understand the kinetics of tumor growth, investigators have transduced glioma cells with genes that can accumulate administered contrast agents or iron.[29,30,31] Weissleder et al first showed that engineered transferrin receptor-transduced tumor cells can accumulate iron, which makes the implanted cell easy to observe under in vivo MRI.[32] Investigators also used the ferritin gene for uptake of endogenous iron by the transduced cells so that it could be detected by in vivo MRI. A cell with a reporter gene is used to determine tumor invasion and migration kinetics before and after treatment; however, the technique has not produced a practical solution for the study of tumor kinetics. There are many obstacles with this approach: (1) 100% of the cells should be transduced and should remain transduced following multiple divisions, (2) the expression of a reporter gene or genes of interest that are sufficient enough to cause detectable MR signals (e.g., accumulation of iron by ferritin), and (3) a transduced gene should not alter the function of the cells. Investigations with iron-labeled stem cells showed slower migration[33]; therefore, iron accumulation in glioma cells may alter the migratory and invasive capacity of implanted glioma.

CEST and PARACEST MRI

During the last decade, MRI contrast agents have been developed that can be selectively detected through chemical exchange saturation transfer (CEST).[11] These contrast agents contain protons that undergo chemical exchange with protons of surrounding water molecules, such as protons in amine or amide groups in the covalent structure of the agent, or protons in water molecules that are noncovalently bound to the contrast agent.[34,35] The narrow band of radiofrequencies that are applied at the chemical shift of the exchangeable proton of the CEST agent can selectively saturate the MR signal of the proton, causing the MR signal to be eliminated. Subsequent chemical exchange of the saturated proton on the CEST agent with a proton on a water molecule transfers the saturation to the water, which reduces the total detectable MR signal of water. This approach was first demonstrated by Balaban et al using low molecular weight diamagnetic molecules containing exchangeable -OH or -NH groups.[11] They showed that the MR contrast can be turned on/off by applying a saturating irradiation pulse, and since chemical exchange between such groups and bulk water is pH dependent, such systems can potentially be used to image tissue pH. Although some diamagnetic CEST (DIACEST) agents have chemical shifts as large as 6.33 ppm, most DIACEST agents have chemical shifts of 1 to 4 ppm, which limits the design of CEST agents to slowly exchanging amide, amine,

imine, guanidinium, indole, pyrimidine, imidazole, and alcoholic chemical groups.[36] Paramagnetic CEST (PARACEST) agents contain lanthanide ions that increase the chemical shifts of amide, amine, and alcoholic groups of up to about ± 50 ppm, which allows PARACEST agents to be designed with chemical groups that have much faster chemical exchange rates.[34,37] In addition, PARACEST agents can be designed to noncovalently bind to a water molecule with sufficient strength, so that the water molecule exchanges with surrounding water at a rate that is slow enough to generate a CEST effect.[35] The proximity to the lanthanide ion can cause the bound water to resonate at CEST-detectable chemical shifts as large as 580 ppm, which further expands the chemical design of CEST agents.[38] Therefore, a wide variety of CEST agents can be designed with many types of labile protons at different chemical shifts, which may be selectively detected during the same MRI study.

Endogenous CEST for Glioma Detection

Glioma cells have been labeled with iron oxide of various types to sufficiently alter T2 without overt loss of biological function.[39,40,41] However, these contrast effects tend to fade with time because of cell leakage or cell division. Gilad and coworkers reported an alternative approach to overcome these problems by transfecting glioma cells to produce a lysine-rich protein (LRP) that can then be detected by CEST imaging.[42] Amide protons from LRP have a chemical shift of 3.76 ppm. Selective saturation within this chemical shift range initiate to generate a CEST effect.[43] Genetically transfected glioma cells, implanted into a mouse brain, were easily differentiated from control cells by CEST imaging by applying a selective presaturation pulse at the resonant frequency of the LRP amide resonance (▶ Fig. 19.1). The images show CEST contrast only in the region where the engineered cells had been implanted, demonstrating that unique CEST activation systems such as this may be useful for cell tracking. Because the LRP is produced by the genetic machinery of the cell, its concentration should, in principle, be maintained even after many cell divisions. Furthermore, different cells could be encoded to produce different markers for CEST that require different activation frequencies. This would allow two, or more, types of cells to be tracked simultaneously by applying an appropriate frequency-selective presaturation pulse to follow the cells of interest. This example demonstrates one of the main advantages of CEST imaging—CEST contrast can be turned on selectively by simply adding a presaturation pulse to an imaging sequence. The apparent negative image contrast generated by CEST activation is not a drawback in this case because a control CEST image that uses a different activation frequency (typically at an equal frequency offset on the opposite side of the water frequency) must be gathered so that the difference image can be displayed as a positive image, a negative image, or a colorized image.[44] This makes it difficult to selectively activate the CEST agent in tissues where the bulk water signal can be rather broad. Nevertheless, Gilad et al have shown that CEST can be amplified by using exogenous macromolecules with large numbers of exchanging sites or endogenous proteins or peptides.[42] This technique can be translated to clinical use if sufficient knowledge is available to manipulate and use different proteins (that has CEST effect) in the tumors before and after treatments.

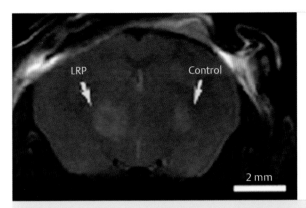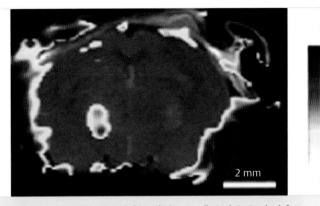

Fig. 19.1 An image of a mouse brain implanted with glioma cells expressing lysine-rich protein (LRP) (left) and glioma cells (right). On the left is an anatomical image, on the right a colorized difference image of the areas that exhibit chemical exchange saturation transfer (CEST) has been overlaid on the anatomical image. The LRP gives rise to a significant change in water signal intensity, allowing the genetically modified cells to be easily identified and tracked by CEST imaging. The area of CEST intensity around the skull is thought to be due to field inhomogeneities. (Images are reproduced with permission from Gilad AA, McMahon MT, Walczak P, et al. Artificial reporter gene providing MRI contrast based on proton exchange. Nat Biotechnol 2007;25(2):217–219.)

PARACEST Agent

PARACEST-based MRI contrast agents have advantages relative to T1- or T2-relaxivity MRI contrast agents. For many years, a major criticism of PARACEST MRI methods has been the apparent inability to apply PARACEST agents to in vivo animal models, which would appear to obviate clinical translation of these methods. Therefore, it is essential to develop in vivo studies using novel PARACEST imaging probes.

To improve in vivo detection sensitivity, PARACEST agents have been conjugated to nanocarriers such as dendrimers, linear polymers, and other high molecular weight macromolecules such as adenovirus particles.[45,46,47] For example, Eu-DOTA-Gly$_4$ PARACEST agents have been conjugated to a G5PAMAM dendrimer via the 1-ethyl-3-(3-dimethylamino-propyl) carbodiimide hydrochloride/N-hydroxysuccinimidyl (EDC/NHS) coupling method. Matrix-assisted laser desorpted ionization (MALDI) mass spectrometry analysis of the DOTA-Gly-conjugated G5PAMAM dendrimer indicated that a range of 34 to 51 ligands were covalently attached to the surface of a G5-PAMAM dendrimer, with a weighted average of approximately 41 ligands per dendrimer.[48] Eu-G5-DL680 showed a CEST peak at +55 ppm, which demonstrated that the presence of the fluorescent agent (DL680) on Eu-G5-DL680 did not affect the agent's ability to generate CEST.[49] It has been reported that 1.62 and 1.43 mM Eu-DOTA-Gly and Yb-DOTA-Gly are required to achieve a 3% CEST effect in solution, which may limit in vivo application.[50] The solution study showed that 45 µM G5-Eu is required to generate 3% of the CEST effect. Therefore, coupling 41 PARACEST agents to the dendrimer resulted in a 36-fold improvement in sensitivity (on a per dendrimer basis), which shows that the CEST effect almost exactly scaled with the concentration of the agent on the dendrimer.[48]

Detection of Glioma with PARACEST Agent

An anatomical magnetic resonance (MR) image showed the location of the U87 glioma (▶ Fig. 19.2a). The CEST MR image

contrast before and after the administration of the PARACEST agents was used to determine the dynamic change in % CEST during the study (▶ Fig. 19.2b). Based on image noise, a CEST effect of 5.2% or higher had a 95% probability that the CEST effect was real. The MR images prior to injection showed no significant CEST effect, but this significance threshold was exceeded immediately after injection of the agent. A strong CEST effect was first visualized at the tumor rim at 2.8 minutes after the injection, which can be attributed to the hypervascular rim typically observed in malignant glioma tumors.[51] The CEST effect persisted during the remainder of the MRI study, which was attributed to the enhanced permeability and retention (EPR) effect that is typically observed with nano-sized agents in glioma tumors.[49] For comparison, the contralateral brain tissue did not show a statistically significant CEST effect throughout the MRI scan session. The temporal results shown in ▶ Fig. 19.3 c demonstrate variability in the baseline measurement prior to the injection, which was attributed to pulse imperfections. This variability was greater after injection of the agent, which was attributed to motion artifacts (despite the use of a stereotactic holder) and pulse imperfections. This "noise" in ▶ Fig. 19.2c has been observed in similar in vivo CEST MRI studies.[48,50,52,53] This result indicated that CEST MRI could detect the presence of the dual modality contrast agent in the glioma, which detected the glioma with excellent specificity relative to normal brain tissue. This experimental approach required the acquisition of CEST MR images at only one saturation frequency, which simplified the acquisition method relative to approaches that require multiple saturation frequencies. This approach also accounted for static effects that influence the contrast of an MR image with selective saturation, including endogenous magnetization transfer, direct saturation of water, and B$_0$ and B$_1$ magnetic field inhomogeneities. However, the use of one saturation frequency cannot account for other dynamic changes caused by the agent. For example, macrocyclic Eu(III) chelates have recently been shown to have a significant T2ex (exchange of spin) rate that can cause dynamic darkening of the image.[54] Although Eu(III) chelates have very low T1 relaxivities, the high ratio of Eu(III)

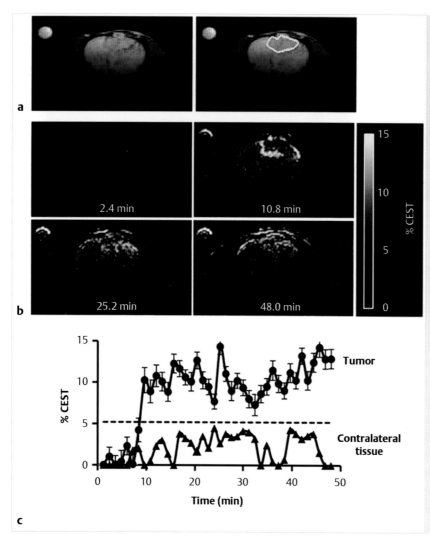

Fig. 19.2 In vivo chemical exchange saturation transfer (CEST) magnetic resonance imaging (MRI). (a) The left panel shows an anatomical image that identifies the location of the tumor prior to administration of the agent. The right panel highlights the location of the tumor. (b) Parametric CEST maps detected the agent in the U87 tumor but not in the contralateral tissue. The maps are labeled with the time point relative to injection. (c) The temporal change in CEST shows rapid accumulation and persistence of the agent in the U87 tumor. CEST was greater than the 95% probability threshold in the U87 tumor but was less than the probability threshold for the contralateral tissue.

chelates per dendrimer may compensate for low T1 relaxivity and may possibly cause a change in image contrast. Yet the statistically significant and dynamic changes in image contrast after injection still ensure that the MRI method detected the agent.

Macroscopic fluorescence imaging validated that the CEST MRI results were generated by accumulation of the dual-modality contrast agent in the glioma.[49] In vivo fluorescence imaging showed accumulation of the contrast agent in the brain (▶ Fig. 19.3a). The comparison of ex vivo fluorescence imaging (▶ Fig. 19.3b) and the anatomical MR image (▶ Fig. 19.3b) further confirmed that the accumulation occurred in the glioma site (▶ Fig. 19.3c). The ex vivo study may have also been accomplished by detecting the fluorescence from Eu(III) in the chelate. However, Eu(III) chelates typically have weak fluorescence, so that the in vivo study would have been difficult to accomplish based on Eu(III) fluorescence.[55] Therefore, we elected to use the Dylight 680 fluorophore (Thermo Fisher Scientific, Inc., Rockford, IL) for the in vivo and ex vivo studies for consistency.[49]

19.5 Nuclear Medicine for Molecular Imaging of Primary and Recurrent Glioma

Nuclear medicine techniques have advantages over other in vivo imaging modalities in respect to matured radiochemistry techniques, availability of the wide range of clinically usable radioisotopes, availability of ligand chemistry to target the wide range of useful receptors in tumor cells or cells associated with neovasculatures, and cellular metabolisms. Other advantages of nuclear medicine would be the possibility of treatment using established ligand-receptor reaction by tagging it with Beta-emitters of usable radioisotopes. The list of useful radiopharmaceuticals for targeting primary or recurrent glioma and its associated neovascularization can be found in the Molecular Imaging and Contrast Agent Database (MICAD) developed by the National Institutes of Health (NIH) (http://www.ncbi.nlm.nih.gov/books/NBK22999/). Despite being strongly developed, radiochemistry, available useful radiopharmaceuticals, and

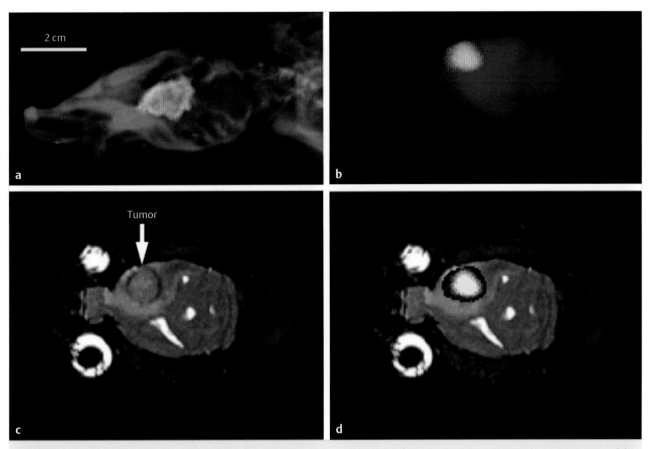

Fig. 19.3 Macroscopic fluorescence imaging. (**a**) The in vivo fluorescent image of the rat head overlayed on an X-ray image shows the presence of the agent in the U87 tumor in the brain. (**b**) The ex vivo fluorescence image of whole brain also detected the agent in the brain (fluorescent image was overlayed on X-ray image of the whole brain). (**c**) The coronal magnetic resonance (MR) image shows the location of the U87 tumor. (**d**) The ex vivo fluorescence image was also overlayed on the MR image to show that the agent was located in the U87 glioma. The anatomy of the brain was correlated between MRI and X-ray images.

nuclear medicine techniques are not being fully used in the detection of primary and recurrent GBM. The reason behind the suboptimal use might be due to the lack of anatomical demarcation on nuclear medicine images alone, the cost of radiopharmaceuticals and associated instruments, and tighter regulation for using radioisotopes.

19.5.1 SPECT Imaging

Single photon emission computed tomography (SPECT) using thallium 201 (^{201}Tl), [99]mTc-tetrofosmin, [99]mTc-sestamibi, and ^{123}I-iodo-a-methyl tyrosine (IMT) radiotracers has been used to evaluate the proliferation and treatment response of gliomas.[56] Studies have shown a linear correlation between tracer uptake during SPECT and tumor proliferation and aggressiveness.[57] SPECT has also been shown to reliably differentiate between tumor recurrence and radiation necrosis.[58] [201]Tl was one of the first tracers studied; it has the advantage of a relative absence of tracer uptake in normal brain parenchyma, providing a better contrast between tumor and normal brain tissue.[59] Uptake of ^{201}Tl depends on the cell membrane potential and Na+-K+-ATPase activity. It is thought that malignant cells and metabolically active cells will have more cell membrane potential and Na+-K+-ATPase activity compared to dying or nonmetaboli-

cally active cells.[60,61,62] Therefore, ^{201}Tl can distinguish the recurrent tumor from radiation necrosis.[63,64] Similarly, uptake of Tc-99-terofosmin or Tc-99m-MIBI depends on the mitochondrial potential of cells and involves the Na+-K+-ATPase, Na+/H+ antiport, and Na+-K+-Cl− cotransport system.[60,62] Malignant cells as well as myocardial cells are shown to have more mitochondria compared to surrounding normal cells. Tc-99m-MIBI is also helpful in understanding the chemotherapy resistance and presence of p-glycoprotein in malignant cells.[65,66,67] These three agents (^{201}Tl, Tc-99m-MIBI, and Tc-99m-tetrofosmin) predict the cell membrane potential, ion transport system, and molecular mechanisms of drug resistance by malignant cells.

Amino acid analogue 3-[^{123}I]iodo-alpha-methyl-L-tyrosine (IMT) has been used in the clinical setting to diagnose recurrent glioma using SPECT studies.[68,69,70] Mechanisms of uptake of IMT have been determined and compared with those of 3H-methyl-L-methionine (3H-MET) in glioma cells.[71] 3H-MET showed involvement of the Na+-dependent L amino acid transport system, whereas IMT uptake was independent of Na+ but involved the "L" amino acid transport system. Neither agent involved the "A" amino acid transport system. The investigators concluded that, due to similarity in the tracer uptake mechanism, IMT SPECT and (11)C-MET positron-emission tomography (PET) could be used for the diagnostic evaluation of glioma with similar clinical relevance.

Unlike the PET scan, functional metabolic imaging with SPECT is less expensive and is widely available. Hence, SPECT imaging is a cost-effective, noninvasive imaging modality that could be used to aid in the diagnosis and evaluation of treatment response of gliomas.

19.5.2 PET imaging

In contrast to imaging modalities like MRI or computed tomographic (CT) scans, which provide anatomical information, PET scans are unique because they provide metabolic information about the tumors.[72] Most tumors are characterized by an increase in glucose uptake and glycolysis.[73] Clinical PET scan studies are performed using a glucose-based probe, [18F] fluoro-deoxyglucose ([18F]FDG). [18F]FDG is transported into the cancer cells by glucose transporters (GLUT1 and GLUT3), and, like glucose, it is phosphorylated via hexokinase to form [18F] FDG-6-phosphate. However, in contrast to glucose-6-phosphate, [18F] FDG-6-phosphate undergoes slow metabolism and is effectively trapped in the tumor cell.[74] Because glucose is the obligatory energy substrate in the normal brain, increased [18F] FDG uptake by the surrounding normal brain during PET scan of brain tumors is unavoidable. However, [18F] FDG-PET has been shown to be useful in identifying high-grade gliomas because they exhibit higher glucose uptake than the normal brain.[75] Delbeke et al reported that the diagnosis of high-grade gliomas could be made with high sensitivity and specificity when the ratio of tumor to white matter exceeds 1.5, and the ratio of tumor to gray matter exceeds 0.6.[76]

Unfortunately, [18F] FDG-PET has been shown to have poor predictive value for diagnosing low-grade gliomas, postoperative residual tumor, and recurrent tumor.[77,78,79] This is due to the fact that these clinical entities exhibit similar or lower FDG uptake compared to the surrounding normal brain.[80] Also, false-negative and false-positive FDG uptake values are seen in Alzheimer disease and during the posttreatment period, respectively. Efforts have been made to improve the diagnostic accuracy of [18F] FDG-PET in low-grade tumors, residual disease after resection, and recurrent tumors. Coregistration of PET images with MR images, and delayed imaging have been shown to improve the contrast between normal brain gray matter from residual or recurrent tumors.[81,82]

Amino acid–based probes, [11C] MET, [18F] FET, and [18F] FDOPA, have also been used in clinical PET imaging. These probes have low cerebral uptake, resulting in improved detection of low-grade lesions. Unlike MRI, [11C] MET uptake by tumors is not dependent on the disruption of the BBB.[83] Increased uptake of methionine by cancer cells results from an increased transport by L-amino acid transporters, secondary to enhanced protein synthesis, increased need for polyamines, and a high rate of transmethylation and transsulfuration reactions.[84] Clinical studies using [11C] MET-PET have shown it to be useful in differentiating clinical entities, including high-grade gliomas, low-grade gliomas, and residual and recurrent tumors.[85,86] Amino acids labeled with 18F, such as O-(2-[18F] fluoroethyl)-L-tyrosine (FET), are presently under investigation for clinical purposes. This artificial amino acid is not incorporated into proteins, but it exhibits high uptake in tumor cells because of increased transport via the amino acid transport systems L and B[0, +].[87] [18F] FET-PET has been shown to reliably distinguish between tumor recurrence and benign lesions.[88] The [18F] fluorinated L-DOPA analogue, [18F] FDOPA, has been shown to be more sensitive and specific than [18F] FDG-PET for evaluating recurrent low-grade tumors and for distinguishing tumor recurrence from radiation necrosis.[89] In mammalian cells, L-DOPA is synthesized from the amino acid L-tyrosine by the enzyme tyrosine hydroxylase. L-DOPA is a precursor of the neurotransmitters dopamine, norepinephrine, and epinephrine. L-DOPA is taken up by the brain through the BBB mediated by large neutral amino acid transporters.

Treatment response is usually monitored by anatomical changes on CT or MRI scans, which usually takes months or years to develop. The ability to measure cell proliferation in a tumor could be potentially used to monitor treatment response after treatment, well before any anatomical changes are evident. Different radiopharmaceuticals have been developed to determine the proliferative status of tumor cells in both in vitro and in vivo settings. L-[1-(11)C]tyrosine (TYR) PET reagent has been developed to measure the protein synthesis rate in brain tumors.[90] The investigators used the PET reagent in 20 patients and compared it with proliferative markers (Ki-67) in biopsy samples. It is concluded that the protein synthesis rate and proliferation are an independent process and are not suitable for determination of tumor cell proliferation in vivo.[90] [18F]fluoro-deoxyadenosine and [18F]fluoroethyluracil have also been developed to use as PET agents to determine tumor proliferation.[91] However, these agents are not being used in the clinical setting. [18F]5-fluoro-2-deoxyuridine (FdUrd) was used to determine tumor cell proliferation in both preclinical and clinical settings and then compared with FDG-PET.[92,93] The investigators concluded that FDG-PET is better than FdUrd-PET.[93] [18F] 3'-deoxy-3'-fluorothymidine (FLT)-based PET scan has been used in vivo to monitor tumor proliferation following treatment.[94,95,96] Currently FLT is said to be a better-suited PET agent for determining tumor cell proliferation.

19.6 Cells as Imaging Probes for Glioma

19.6.1 Targeting Neovasculatures Using Stem Cells

GBM is a highly vascular and therapy-resistant central nervous system neoplasm. The formation of blood vessels occurs by two mechanisms: vasculogenesis and angiogenesis. Vasculogenesis is the process where blood vessels are formed de novo by in situ differentiation of the primitive progenitors (i.e., angioblasts) into mature endothelial cells, and this was thought to take place only during embryonic development.[97] In contrast, angiogenesis occurs during both embryonic development and postnatal life and is defined as a process that gives rise to new blood vessels by the proliferation and migration of preexisting differentiated endothelial cells.[98,99] It was generally considered that blood vessel formation during postnatal life was restricted to angiogenesis only, and for decades, tumor vascularization was thought to be the exclusive result of the sprouting of new vessels from preexisting ones. However, recent studies demonstrated the existence of additional angiogenic and vasculogenic mechanisms associated with tumor growth, such as intussusceptive angiogenesis, vessel cooption, vasculogenic mimicry, lymphangiogenesis, and the recruitment of endothelial progenitor cells (EPCs).[100–105]

Current evidence from recent publications indicates the involvement of both angiogenesis and vasculogenesis processes for glioma growth (tumor growth).[101,102,105] Tumor angiogenesis is supported by endothelial cells originating from sprouting and cooption of neighboring preexisting vessels.[106,107,108] It may also be supported by the mobilization and functional incorporation of bone marrow–derived EPCs as shown previously in xenografted lymphoma, lung cancer, and other tumors.[109–113] With emerging new insights into vasculogenesis, investigators are looking into possible mechanisms of how bone marrow-derived progenitor cells (BMPCs) or EPCs, migrate and incorporate into tumor neovascularization.[103] One of the mechanisms that has been pointed out is the involvement of the stromal cell derived factor (SDF)-1-chemokine receptor type 4 (CXCR4) axis.[114,115,116] SDF-1α is a chemokine that is expressed in tumor cells and released in the circulation following hypoxia in the tumor (with the upregulation of HIF-1α).[117,118,119] In an experiment, Heissig et al[120] determined the mechanisms of releasing hematopoietic stem cells (HSCs) and EPCs from bone marrow. Under steady-state conditions, quiescent c-Kit + HSCs or EPCs reside in a niche in close contact with stromal cells. Membrane-bound cytokines, such as membrane-bound Kit ligand (mKitL), not only convey survival signals but also support the adhesion of stem cells to the stroma. Increased chemokine/cytokine, such as SDF-1α and vascular endothelial growth factor (VEGF), induce upregulation of MMP-9, resulting in the release of soluble Kit ligand (sKitL). sKitL confers signals that transfer c-Kit + HSCs or EPCs from a quiescent to a proliferative state, and enhances mobility of VEGFR2 + EPCs and LinαSca-1 + c-Kit + repopulating cells, translocating them into a vascular-enriched niche, favoring differentiation and mobilization to the peripheral circulation. SDF-1α is a strong chemoattractant for CXCR4 positive cells.

In vivo determination of the involvement of host BMPCs or EPCs in the formation of neovascularization in tumors is challenging. To be detected by in vivo imaging modalities, the host bone marrow cells should carry a reporter, such as a fluorescent protein, or genes that can be targeted later (e.g., luciferase or sodium iodide symporter or specific promoter mediated activation of gene). However, this reporter should be present in BMPCs but not in other cell types. In the making of a transgenic animal model, having such conditional gene expression would be difficult, but with chimeric animal models, bone marrow cells of recipient animals should be replaced with bone marrow cells from animals expressing different reporters, such as green fluorescent protein-positive (GFP +) bone marrow cells.[102,121,122] Recently, a chimeric animal model has been developed in our laboratory to determine the involvement of BMPC in the tumor neovascularization in a glioma. Sublethally irradiated athymic mice received bone marrow cells from GFP + transgenic mice.[123] GFP + bone marrow cells were transplanted in athymic mice 24 hours following sublethal irradiation. The tumors were implanted after 28 days when the flow cytometric analysis showed more than 70% engraftment of the GFP + cells. Migration and accumulation of transplanted bone marrow cells in the implanted gliomas were determined by optical imaging (Kodak, Carestream multispectral system, Carestream Health, Inc.,

Rochester, NY), along with proper excitation and emission profiles. Optical imaging showed a gradual increase in GFP intensity in the tumors, and multiple GFP + cells lining the blood vessels and other infrastructures of the tumors were observed under a fluorescent microscope (▶ Fig. 19.4).

On the other hand exogenously administered EPC can be used to determine the neovascularization in a glioma. Because of the slower active neovascularization in radiation necrosis, differentiation between recurrent GBM and radiation necrosis can be done using EPC as imaging probes. We have used different imaging modalities to detect the implanted glioma in animal models using EPCs.[124,125] EPCs can be labeled with iron oxides and nanoparticles. The accumulation of these magnetically labeled cells can be detected at the sites of the implanted gliomas by MRI (▶ Fig. 19.5). EPCs can also be labeled with In-111-oxine, which is an FDA agent. In-111-oxine-labeled cells are being routinely used in clinics to determine hidden infection or T cell reactivity. We have used In-111-labeled cord blood EPC to determine the neovascularization in implanted gliomas. SPECT images showed early migration and accumulation of In-111-labeled EPCs to the sites of the gliomas (see ▶ Fig. 19.5). In-111-labeled EPCs can be used to differentiate recurrent GMB from radiation necrosis based on active neovascularization in the tumor but not in radiation necrosis.

Exogenously labeled EPCs are being used, and transduced EPCs can also be used to detect implanted gliomas, based on active neovascularization. The transduced EPCs can be used both for tracking and for gene delivery/therapy vehicles. Recently we have used lentiviral vectors carrying human sodium iodide symporter genes to transduce cord blood EPCs. The human sodium iodide symporter (hNIS) is an intrinsic transmembrane glycoprotein that mediates the transport of iodide into thyroid follicular cells.[126,127] This transport system also transports Tc-99 m pertechnetate (Tc-99m) that can be imaged by a gamma camera.[128,129] Visualization and quantification of Tc-99 m activity at the site of interest (following administration of transduced cells) would provide the evidence of homing, viability, and expression of the exogenous hNIS gene in transduced cells. The in vivo use of genetically modified EPCs requires that the duration and level of expression of the encoded transgene need to be monitored. Ideally, the monitoring system should also be able to monitor cell homing and viability and demonstrate the persistence of site-specific gene expression in vivo. Expression of hNIS with resultant Tc-99 m uptake can conveniently be imaged with SPECT or a gamma camera that can determine hNIS expression in vivo, which will indicate the effectiveness of the EPC to carry the gene of interest to the tumor site. Collected EPCs were cultured and transduced to carry hNIS. Cellular viability, differential capacity, and Tc-99 m uptake were determined. Five to ten million EPCs were intravenously administered and Tc-99-SPECT images were acquired on day 8 to determine the accumulation of EPCs and expression of transgenes (increased activity of Tc-99m) in the tumors. Transduced EPCs were also magnetically labeled, and the accumulation of cells was confirmed by MRI and histochemistry (▶ Fig. 19.6). SPECT analysis showed increased activity of Tc-99 m in the tumors that received transduced EPCs, indicative of the expression of a transgene (hNIS). The activity of Tc-99 m in the tumors was also dependent on the number of administered transduced EPCs. MRI showed the accumulation

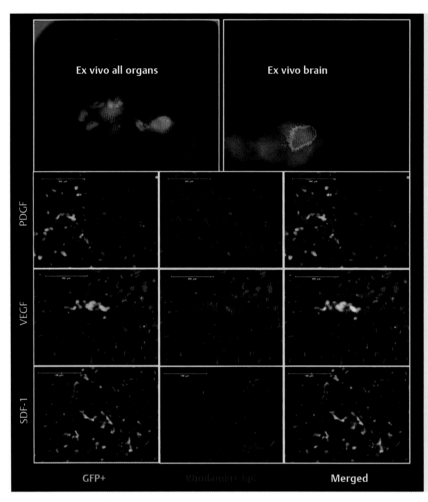

Fig. 19.4 Migration and accumulation of bone marrow–derived progenitor cells (BMPCs) in glioma. Involvement of green fluorescent protein-positive (GFP +) bone marrow cells was determined in a chimeric mouse model of human glioma. Optical images show increased GFP + signal intensity at the site of implanted glioma. Immunohistochemistry (IHC) images show expression of platelet derived growth factor (PDGF), vascular endothelial growth factor (VEGF), and stromal cell derived factor (SDF)-1α (red in middle column) at the vicinity of GFP + cells (green in left column) in the glioma.

of magnetically labeled EPCs. Immunohistochemical analysis showed iron and hNIS positive and human CD31 and von Willebrand factor (vWF) positive cells in the tumors.[130]

19.6.2 Targeting Tumor Antigens Using Cytotoxic T-Cell (CTL)

Tumor immunology has long been a focus of cell-based vaccine therapy research, and dendritic, as well as T cells, are considered to be the best candidates for developing such therapies. Dendritic cell (DC)-based vaccination therapy against recurrent glioma uses the patient's own DCs that are pulsed ex vivo with the derived glioma cell-lysate or apoptotic glioma cells and is currently being used in clinical trials.[131,132,133,134] Investigators have identified specific glioma-associated antigens (GAAs), which are being used to pulse DCs.[135,136,137] There are more than 10 active clinical trials sponsored by the National Cancer Institute (NCI) targeting primary as well as recurrent glioma that use primed DC–based vaccination (www.cancer.gov/clinicaltrials). Apoptotic tumor cells, tumor cell lysate, and GAA (peptides) are being used to prime the DCs in these clinical trials. It was shown that autologous administration of these tumor cell lysate-pulsed DCs initiated immunogenic activity against glioma cells, delaying tumor recurrence, and/or decreasing the recurrence rate.[133,134,138,139] Animal studies also showed an increased number of CTLs compared to the control or prevaccination levels in experimental glioma, which used cell-lysate-pulsed DC therapy, indicating in vivo sensitization of T cells to gliomas, presumably due to the administered primed DCs.[140,141,142] Studies describing the accumulation of DCs and CTLs at the site of tumors indicated the initiation of a tumor-based immune reaction.[143,144] In addition, in vivo effectiveness of CTLs that were sensitized in vitro by DCs was demonstrated in a rat glioma model, as reported by Merchant et al.[145] Animal experiments performed by our group also demonstrated initiation of cellular immunity in syngeneic Fisher rats.[146] In these experiments, we used magnetically labeled sensitized splenocytes (sensitized T cells) to detect the tumor by cellular MRI. We have also been able to make glioma-specific CTLs ex vivo by using glioma cell lysate-pulsed DCs, and we used them to differentiate implanted human glioma from radiation necrosis in a rat model by way of cellular MRI.[147]

The method of priming DCs using tumor-associated antigens (TAAs) is more specific than priming with whole tumor cell lysate. Investigators have identified tumor-specific antigens (peptides), and these antigens can be used to pulse DCs to initiate antigen-specific CTLs when administered into the hosts.

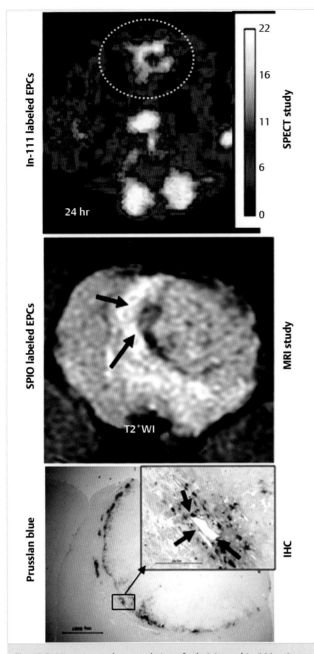

Fig. 19.5 Migration and accumulation of administered In-111-oxine and superparamagnetic iron oxide particles (SPIO) labeled endothelial progenitor cells (EPCs) in tumor. Five million In-111-labeled EPCs followed by 5 million magnetically labeled EPCs were administered in the same rat. Single photon emission computed tomographic (SPECT) images were obtained on days 0, 1, and 3. SPECT images of the tumor obtained at 24 h showed increased activity at the site of tumor indicating accumulation of In-111-labeled EPCs. Magnetic resonance imaging (MRI) was obtained by a clinical 3 T system on day 7 following the last SPECT. Note the low signal intensity areas on T2*-weighted imaging (black arrows) indicating accumulation of iron-positive cells, which is proved by 3,3'-diaminobenzidine (DAB)-enhanced Prussian blue staining. Inset shows the iron-positive cells lining the blood vessels.

Zhang et al have profiled the antigens in 20 different types of human glioma cell lines and concluded that all the cells exhibited multiple TAAs, which can be used to prime DCs to initiate CTLs.[137] The authors identified a few important antigens, such as melanoma-2 (Aim-2), B-cyclin, EphA2, GP100, h1, 6-N-acetylglucosaminyltransferaseV (GnT-V), IL13Ra2, Her2/neu, hTert, Mage, Mart-1, Sart-1, and survivin. Based on their results, Dr. Okada's group (at University of Pittsburgh Medical Center [UPMC]) and other investigators have identified three important antigens (EphA2, IL13Ra2, survivin) for priming DCs, and used them as vaccines for glioma treatment.[148,149] NCI-sponsored clinical trials are under way to make GAA-pulsed DCs for vaccination use in patients with recurrent glioma. In these proposals, the investigators prime the autologous DCs with specific peptides by simple incubation during the conversion of adherent peripheral blood mononuclear cells to mature DCs.

Lymphocytes have been in use for decades to detect different disease conditions, such as xenografted tumors in rodents, renal allograft, autoimmune thyroid disease, and metastatic melanoma.[150,151,152,153] Autologous lymphocytes have been labeled with radioactive isotopes, and accumulation at specific sites has been detected by nuclear medicine imaging.[154,155] Autologous lymphocyte labeling with radioactive isotopes, such as In-111-oxine, along with administration into patients, are FDA-approved procedures for diagnostic purposes. Chin et al has reported the use of tumor-infiltrating lymphocytes, collected from resected tumor specimens, and expanded ex vivo using recombinant interleukin (IL)-2 as imaging probes by labeling with In-111-oxine.[156] However, the authors did not notice any accumulation of In-111 labeled lymphocytes at the sites of metastasis. Lymphocytes have also been labeled with iron oxides to track the migration by MRI; however, there has been no report of making tumor-specific CTLs ex vivo for the detection of tumors by in vivo imaging. Previously, our group has reported making sensitized splenocytes (CTLs) in vivo in syngeneic Fisher-344 rats by implanting 9 L gliosarcoma cells. These CTLs were collected from the spleen and used as an imaging probe to detect the implanted tumor in another set of rats carrying the 9 L glioma in the brain.[146] The in vivo experiment produced CTLs that showed specificity by accumulating in and around the implanted tumors, whereas splenocytes collected from control rats did not show significant accumulation in the implanted tumors. The CTLs (sensitized splenocytes) were also able to differentiate implanted tumor from radiation necrosis because there was no accumulation at the sites of radiation injury (necrosis). Based on the results of sensitized splenocytes, we have started making CTLs in an ex vivo setting to sensitize T cells against implanted U-251 gliomas, using glioma cell lysate-pulsed DCs. We have created a cytotoxic T cell ex vivo using collected cord blood CD14 + and CD2/3 + cells,[147] and also used glioma cell lysate to prime the DCs. These cytotoxic T cells were used as imaging probes by labeling them with iron oxide nanoparticles or In-111-oxine. We have used these labeled cytotoxic T cells to detect implanted glioma in animal models (▶ Fig. 19.7).

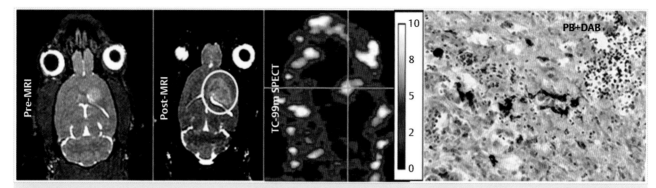

Fig. 19.6 Migration and accumulation of transgenic superparamagnetic iron oxide particles (SPIO)-labeled endothelial progenitor cells (EPCs) in tumor. Ten million transgenic human sodium iodide symporter (hNIS) carrying EPCs (half of them were labeled with SPIO) were intravenously (IV) administered in a glioma-bearing rat. Magnetic resonance imaging (MRI) and Tc-99 m single photon emission computed tomography (SPECT) were performed on day 7 and 8, respectively. Note the low signal intensity areas on magnetic resonance imaging (MRI) in tumor following IV administration of SPIO-labeled EPCs (Post-MRI, circle). SPECT images show increased accumulation of Tc-99 m in the tumor. DAB-enhanced Prussian blue staining shows the presence of iron-positive cells.

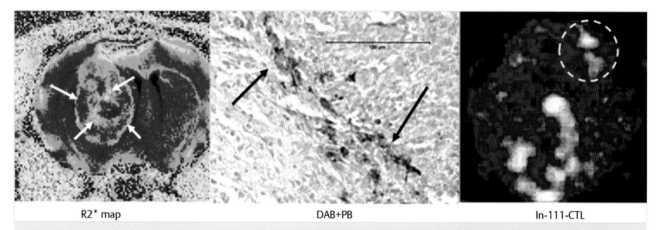

Fig. 19.7 Magnetic resonance imaging (MRI) and single photon emission computed tomographic (SPECT) images to detect an implanted glioma using cytotoxic T cells (CTLs). Magnetically labeled CTLs were intravenously (IV) administered and T2*-weighted imaging (T2*WI) was acquired. R2* map created from the T2*WI showed accumulation of CTLs in the tumor both at the periphery and in the center (white arrows). DAB-enhanced Prussian blue (PB) stain showed iron-positive cells (black arrows). In-111-Oxine-labeled CTL also showed accumulation in the tumors (24 h after IV injection, white circle).

19.7 Optical Imaging for Molecular Imaging of Primary and Recurrent Glioma

19.7.1 Clinical Setting

Optical imaging techniques including bioluminescence and fluorescence imaging are emerging as powerful tools in the molecular imaging of glioma. Bioluminescence refers to light produced by the enzymatic reaction of a luciferase enzyme with its substrate. In fluorescence imaging, an external light of appropriate wavelength is used to excite a target fluorescent molecule, followed almost immediately by the release of a longer-wavelength, and lower-energy light for imaging. Targets for fluorescence imaging may be endogenous molecules (e.g., collagen or hemoglobin), fluorescent proteins (green fluorescent protein and related molecules), or optical contrast agents with fluorescent molecules. Optical imaging has largely been used in preclinical glioma models to evaluate the margin status and the extent of surgical resection.[157] In an experimental rodent model, using intravenous fluorescein and topical acriflavine dyes, intraoperative confocal microscopy was able to detect histological features and tumor infiltration in glioblastomas.[158] However, intraoperative confocal microscopy using optical imaging techniques can be used to provide high-resolution real-time images of tissues in vivo. This technology has been adapted by neurosurgeons in the form of a handheld rigid probe, that displays images in real time on an attached external monitor at magnifications of up to × 1,000. The technology is also being used in patients to verify the margin status following surgical resection of a variety of brain tumors.[159,160,161]

19.7.2 Preclinical Setting

Optical imaging is becoming a strong option as a modality for preclinical glioma research and treatment. The availability of a wide range of fluorescent and bioluminescent probes enables investigators to identify the site of interest without the interference of background activity before and after treatments. Moreover, the excitation and emission profiles of near infrared fluorescent probes allow investigators to pinpoint the site of interaction in the tumor microenvironment. Optical imaging is being used as an alternate method to determine the tumor burden following treatment. Tumor volume interpolated from bioluminescent imaging (BLI) in implanted glioma showed a significant correlation with the tumor volume measured by MRI.[162] The same investigators also used near-infrared dye tagged deoxyglucose to determine the uptake in intracranial gliomas.[162] This is a development that can easily be translated to clinics, where patients can be injected with this probe, tagged with 2-deoxyglucose (like the FDG-PET agent), 24 hours before the surgery. The surgeons can determine the margin of the tumor using a near-infrared fluorescent imaging device. Zhao et al[163] have used near-infrared dye tagged human monoclonal antibody against phosphatidylserine (PS) to determine the effect on a glioma before and after irradiation. PS is strictly located in the inner leaflet of the plasma membrane bilayer in most normal cell types, including the vascular endothelium. Loss of PS asymmetry occurs during apoptosis and necrosis, resulting in the exposure of PS on the external surface of the cells. Investigators have also exploited endogenous fluorescent properties of glioma cells to detect the tumor by optical imaging. Glioma tumors provide significant endogenous fluorescence from protoporphyrin IX (PpIX) and this is enhanced with aminolevulinic acid (ALA). Kepshire et al[164] showed the advantage of fluorescent tomographic imaging when interfaced with microCT, to detect implanted glioma. Optical imaging is an emerging technique and is beyond the scope of this chapter. Readers are referred to recent reviews for further information.[165,166,167,168,]

19.8 Conclusion and Future Directions

It is proven beyond doubt that the molecular imaging techniques have unique advantage over traditional imaging methods in the diagnosis, treatment, and follow-up of glioma. Some of the advantages include (1) noninvasive imaging of tumor microenvironment before and after treatment, allowing optimization of therapies; (2) assess treatment response well before changes are apparent on traditional imaging like CT or MRI; (3) investigate changes at cellular level of biological interactions in real-time; and (4) accurately delineate tumor for enhanced drug delivery. Currently, there are many challenges to routine implementation of molecular imaging such as poor resolution and the prohibitive cost of designing novel contrast agents to be used in clinical trials. However, the future of molecular imaging in glioma appears to be promising. As we move toward personalized treatment approach based on genomic profile of individual patient, molecular imaging has the potential to play an important role in glioma management. In the meantime, every effort should be made to improve the design and development of imaging agents and techniques for clinical use.

References

[1] Liu X, Shi Y, Maag DX et al. Iniparib nonselectively modifies cysteine-containing proteins in tumor cells and is not a bona fide PARP inhibitor. Clin Cancer Res 2012; 18: 510–523

[2] Wick W, Weller M, Weiler M, Batchelor T, Yung AW, Platten M. Pathway inhibition: emerging molecular targets for treating glioblastoma. Neuro-oncol 2011; 13: 566–579

[3] Sasine JP, Savaraj N, Feun LG. Topoisomerase I inhibitors in the treatment of primary CNS malignancies: an update on recent trends. Anticancer Agents Med Chem 201 0; 10: 683–696

[4] Carrillo JA, Lai A, Nghiemphu PL et al. Relationship between tumor enhancement, edema, IDH1 mutational status, MGMT promoter methylation, and survival in glioblastoma. AJNR Am J Neuroradiol 2012; 33: 1349–1355

[5] Tien RD, Felsberg GJ, Friedman H, Brown M, MacFall J. MR imaging of high-grade cerebral gliomas: value of diffusion-weighted echoplanar pulse sequences. AJR Am J Roentgenol 1994; 162: 671–677

[6] Van Cauter S, Veraart J, Sijbers J et al. Gliomas: diffusion kurtosis MR imaging in grading. Radiology 2012; 263: 492–501

[7] Hein PA, Eskey CJ, Dunn JF, Hug EB. Diffusion-weighted imaging in the follow-up of treated high-grade gliomas: tumor recurrence versus radiation injury. AJNR Am J Neuroradiol 2004; 25: 201–209

[8] Ellingson BM, Cloughesy TF, Lai A et al. Quantification of edema reduction using differential quantitative T2 (DQT2) relaxometry mapping in recurrent glioblastoma treated with bevacizumab. J Neurooncol 2012; 106: 111–119

[9] Cone CD, Jr. The role of the surface electrical transmembrane potential in normal and malignant mitogenesis. Ann N Y Acad Sci 1974; 238: 420–435

[10] Nagy I, Lustyik G, Lukács G, Nagy V, Balázs G. Correlation of malignancy with the intracellular Na + :K + ratio in human thyroid tumors. Cancer Res 1983; 43: 5395–5402

[11] Ward KM, Aletras AH, Balaban RS. A new class of contrast agents for MRI based on proton chemical exchange dependent saturation transfer (CEST). J Magn Reson 2000; 143: 79–87

[12] Ignelzi RJ. An analysis of the nuclear sodium content of human normal glia as well as tumors of glial and nonglial origin. Neurol Res 1983; 5: 79–84

[13] Laymon CM, Oborski MJ, Lee VK et al. Combined imaging biomarkers for therapy evaluation in glioblastoma multiforme: correlating sodium MRI and F-18 FLT PET on a voxel-wise basis. Magn Reson Imaging 2012; 30: 1268–1278

[14] Howe FA, Barton SJ, Cudlip SA et al. Metabolic profiles of human brain tumors using quantitative in vivo 1 H magnetic resonance spectroscopy. Magn Reson Med 2003; 49: 223–232

[15] Zhou J, Tryggestad E, Wen Z et al. Differentiation between glioma and radiation necrosis using molecular magnetic resonance imaging of endogenous proteins and peptides. Nat Med 2011; 17: 130–134

[16] Jones CK, Schlosser MJ, van Zijl PC, Pomper MG, Golay X, Zhou J. Amide proton transfer imaging of human brain tumors at 3 T. Magn Reson Med 2006; 56: 585–592

[17] Zhou J, Blakeley JO, Hua J et al. Practical data acquisition method for human brain tumor amide proton transfer (APT) imaging. Magn Reson Med 2008; 60: 842–849

[18] Wen Z, Hu S, Huang F et al. MR imaging of high-grade brain tumors using endogenous protein and peptide-based contrast. Neuroimage 2010; 51: 616–622

[19] Varallyay P, Nesbit G, Muldoon LL et al. Comparison of two superparamagnetic viral-sized iron oxide particles ferumoxides and ferumoxtran-10 with a gadolinium chelate in imaging intracranial tumors. AJNR Am J Neuroradiol 2002; 23: 510–519

[20] Neuwelt EA, Várallyay P, Bagó AG, Muldoon LL, Nesbit G, Nixon R. Imaging of iron oxide nanoparticles by MR and light microscopy in patients with malignant brain tumours. Neuropathol Appl Neurobiol 2004; 30: 456–471

[21] Landry R, Jacobs PM, Davis R, Shenouda M, Bolton WK. Pharmacokinetic study of ferumoxytol: a new iron replacement therapy in normal subjects and hemodialysis patients. Am J Nephrol 2005; 25: 400–410

[22] Varallyay CG, Muldoon LL, Gahramanov S et al. Dynamic MRI using iron oxide nanoparticles to assess early vascular effects of antiangiogenic versus corticosteroid treatment in a glioma model. J Cereb Blood Flow Metab 2009; 29: 853–860

[23] Wiesinger F, Weidl E, Menzel MI et al. IDEAL spiral CSI for dynamic metabolic MR imaging of hyperpolarized [1–13C]pyruvate. Magn Reson Med 2012; 68: 8–16

[24] Chaumeil MM, Ozawa T, Park I et al. Hyperpolarized 13C MR spectroscopic imaging can be used to monitor Everolimus treatment in vivo in an orthotopic rodent model of glioblastoma. Neuroimage 2012; 59: 193–201

[25] Sasao A, Hirai T, Iriguchi N et al. 13C MR imaging of methionine-rich gliomas at 4.7T: a pilot study. Magn Reson Med Sci 2011; 10: 139–142

[26] Park I, Bok R, Ozawa T et al. Detection of early response to temozolomide treatment in brain tumors using hyperpolarized 13C MR metabolic imaging. J Magn Reson Imaging 2011; 33: 1284–1290

[27] Park I, Larson PE, Zierhut ML et al. Hyperpolarized 13C magnetic resonance metabolic imaging: application to brain tumors. Neuro-oncol 2010; 12: 133–144

[28] Day SE, Kettunen MI, Cherukuri MK et al. Detecting response of rat C6 glioma tumors to radiotherapy using hyperpolarized [1- 13C]pyruvate and 13C magnetic resonance spectroscopic imaging. Magn Reson Med 2011; 65: 557–563

[29] Cohen B, Dafni H, Meir G, Harmelin A, Neeman M. Ferritin as an endogenous MRI reporter for noninvasive imaging of gene expression in C6 glioma tumors. Neoplasia 2005; 7: 109–117

[30] Ono K, Fuma K, Tabata K, Sawada M. Ferritin reporter used for gene expression imaging by magnetic resonance. Biochem Biophys Res Commun 2009; 388: 589–594

[31] Wang J, Xie J, Zhou X et al. Ferritin enhances SPIO tracking of C6 rat glioma cells by MRI. Mol Imaging Biol 2011; 13: 87–93

[32] Weissleder R, Moore A, Mahmood U et al. In vivo magnetic resonance imaging of transgene expression. Nat Med 2000; 6: 351–355

[33] Janic B, Iskander AS, Rad AM, Soltanian-Zadeh H, Arbab AS. Effects of ferumoxides-protamine sulfate labeling on immunomodulatory characteristics of macrophage-like THP-1 cells. PLoS ONE 2008; 3: e2499

[34] Zhang S, Michaudet L, Burgess S, Sherry AD. The amide protons of an ytterbium(III) dota tetraamide complex act as efficient antennae for transfer of magnetization to bulk water. Angew Chem Int Ed Engl 2002; 41: 1919–1921

[35] Zhang S, Winter P, Wu K, Sherry AD. A novel europium(III)-based MRI contrast agent. J Am Chem Soc 2001; 123: 1517–1518

[36] Liu G, Li Y, Pagel MD. Design and characterization of a new irreversible responsive PARACEST MRI contrast agent that detects nitric oxide. Magn Reson Med 2007; 58: 1249–1256

[37] Woods M, Woessner DE, Zhao P et al. Europium(III) macrocyclic complexes with alcohol pendant groups as chemical exchange saturation transfer agents. J Am Chem Soc 2006; 128: 10155–10162

[38] Terreno E, Castelli DD, Cravotto G, Milone L, Aime S. Ln(III)-DOTAMGly complexes: a versatile series to assess the determinants of the efficacy of paramagnetic chemical exchange saturation transfer agents for magnetic resonance imaging applications. Invest Radiol 2004; 39: 235–243

[39] Bernas LM, Foster PJ, Rutt BK. Magnetic resonance imaging of in vitro glioma cell invasion. J Neurosurg. 2007;106(2):306–313

[40] Zhang F, Xie J, Liu G, He Y, Lu G, Chen X. In vivo MRI tracking of cell invasion and migration in a rat glioma model. Mol Imaging Biol. 2011;13(4):695–701

[41] Mamani JB, Malheiros JM, Cardoso EF, Tannús A, Silveira PH, Gamarra LF. In vivo magnetic resonance imaging tracking of C6 glioma cells labeled with superparamagnetic iron oxide nanoparticles. Einstein (Sao Paulo). 2012;10(2):164–170

[42] Gilad AA, McMahon MT, Walczak P et al. Artificial reporter gene providing MRI contrast based on proton exchange. Nat Biotechnol 2007; 25: 217–219

[43] Goffeney N, Bulte JW, Duyn J, Bryant LH, Jr, van Zijl PC. Sensitive NMR detection of cationic-polymer-based gene delivery systems using saturation transfer via proton exchange. J Am Chem Soc 2001; 123: 8628–8629

[44] Sherry AD, Woods M. Chemical exchange saturation transfer contrast agents for magnetic resonance imaging. Annu Rev Biomed Eng 2008; 10: 391–411

[45] Pikkemaat JA, Wegh RT, Lamerichs R et al. Dendritic PARACEST contrast agents for magnetic resonance imaging. Contrast Media Mol Imaging 2007; 2: 229–239

[46] Wu Y, Zhou Y, Ouari O et al. Polymeric PARACEST agents for enhancing MRI contrast sensitivity. J Am Chem Soc 2008; 130: 13854–13855

[47] Vasalatiy O, Gerard RD, Zhao P, Sun X, Sherry AD. Labeling of adenovirus particles with PARACEST agents. Bioconjug Chem 2008; 19: 598–606

[48] Ali MM, Yoo B, Pagel MD. Tracking the relative in vivo pharmacokinetics of nanoparticles with PARACEST MRI. Mol Pharm 2009; 6: 1409–1416

[49] Ali MM, Bhuiyan MP, Janic B et al. A nano-sized PARACEST-fluorescence imaging contrast agent facilitates and validates in vivo CEST MRI detection of glioma. Nanomedicine (Lond) 2012; 7: 1827–1837

[50] Ali MM, Liu G, Shah T, Flask CA, Pagel MD. Using two chemical exchange saturation transfer magnetic resonance imaging contrast agents for molecular imaging studies. Acc Chem Res 2009; 42: 915–924

[51] Tovi M. MR imaging in cerebral gliomas analysis of tumour tissue components. Acta Radiol Suppl 1993; 384: 1–24

[52] Sheth VR, Liu G, Li Y, Pagel MD. Improved pH measurements with a single PARACEST MRI contrast agent. Contrast Media Mol Imaging 2012; 7: 26–34

[53] Sheth VR, Li Y, Chen LQ, Howison CM, Flask CA, Pagel MD. Measuring in vivo tumor pHe with CEST-FISP MRI. Magn Reson Med 2012; 67: 760–768

[54] Soesbe TC, Togao O, Takahashi M, Sherry AD. SWIFT-CEST: a new MRI method to overcome T_2 shortening caused by PARACEST contrast agents. Magn Reson Med 2012; 68: 816–821

[55] Josan JS, De Silva CR, Yoo B et al. Fluorescent and lanthanide labeling for ligand screens, assays, and imaging. Methods Mol Biol 2011; 716: 89–126

[56] Alexiou GA, Fotopoulos AD, Tsiouris S, Voulgaris S, Kyritsis AP. 99mTc-tetrofosmin SPECT for the evaluation of cerebral lesions. Eur J Nucl Med Mol Imaging 2010; 37: 2403–2404

[57] Alexiou GA, Tsiouris S, Goussia A et al. Evaluation of glioma proliferation by 99mTc-Tetrofosmin. Neuro-oncol 2008; 10: 104–105

[58] Alexiou GA, Fotopoulos AD, Papadopoulos A, Kyritsis AP, Polyzoidis KS, Tsiouris S. Evaluation of brain tumor recurrence by (99m)Tc-tetrofosmin SPECT: a prospective pilot study. Ann Nucl Med 2007; 21: 293–298

[59] Oriuchi N, Tamura M, Shibazaki T et al. Clinical evaluation of thallium-201 SPECT in supratentorial gliomas: relationship to histologic grade, prognosis and proliferative activities. J Nucl Med 1993; 34: 2085–2089

[60] Arbab AS, Koizumi K, Toyama K, Araki T. Uptake of technetium-99m-tetrofosmin, technetium-99m-MIBI and thallium-201 in tumor cell lines. J Nucl Med 1996; 37: 1551–1556

[61] Arbab AS, Koizumi K, Toyama K, Arai T, Araki T. Ion transport systems in the uptake of 99Tcm-tetrofosmin, 99Tcm-MIBI and 201Tl in a tumour cell line. Nucl Med Commun 1997; 18: 235–240

[62] Arbab AS, Koizumi K, Toyama K, Arai T, Araki T. Technetium-99m-tetrofosmin, technetium-99m-MIBI and thallium-201 uptake in rat myocardial cells. J Nucl Med 1998; 39: 266–271

[63] Slizofski WJ, Krishna L, Katsetos CD et al. Thallium imaging for brain tumors with results measured by a semiquantitative index and correlated with histopathology. Cancer 1994; 74: 3190–3197

[64] Tomura N, Izumi J, Anbai A et al. Thallium-201 SPECT in the evaluation of early effects on brain tumors treated with stereotactic irradiation. Clin Nucl Med 2005; 30: 83–86

[65] Andrews DW, Das R, Kim S, Zhang J, Curtis M. Technetium-MIBI as a glioma imaging agent for the assessment of multi-drug resistance. Neurosurgery 1997; 40: 1323–1332, discussion 1333–1334

[66] Vergote J, Moretti JL, de Vries EG, Garnier-Suillerot A. Comparison of the kinetics of active efflux of 99mTc-MIBI in cells with P-glycoprotein-mediated and multidrug-resistance protein-associated multidrug-resistance phenotypes. Eur J Biochem 1998; 252: 140–146

[67] Sun SS, Hsieh JF, Tsai SC, Ho YJ, Lee JK, Kao CH. Expression of mediated P-glycoprotein multidrug resistance related to Tc-99m MIBI scintimammography results. Cancer Lett 2000; 153: 95–100

[68] Kuwert T, Woesler B, Morgenroth C et al. Diagnosis of recurrent glioma with SPECT and iodine-123-alpha-methyl tyrosine. J Nucl Med 1998; 39: 23–27

[69] Riemann B, Kopka K, Stögbauer F et al. Kinetic parameters of 3-[(123)I]iodo-L-alpha-methyl tyrosine ([(123)I]IMT) transport in human GOS3 glioma cells. Nucl Med Biol 2001; 28: 217–222

[70] Samnick S, Bader JB, Hellwig D et al. Clinical value of iodine-123-alpha-methyl-L-tyrosine single-photon emission tomography in the differential diagnosis of recurrent brain tumor in patients pretreated for glioma at follow-up. J Clin Oncol 2002; 20: 396–404

[71] Langen KJ, Mühlensiepen H, Holschbach M, Hautzel H, Jansen P, Coenen HH. Transport mechanisms of 3-[123I]iodo-alpha-methyl-L-tyrosine in a human glioma cell line: comparison with [3H]methyl]-L-methionine. J Nucl Med 2000; 41: 1250–1255

[72] Basu S, Alavi A. Molecular imaging (PET) of brain tumors. Neuroimaging Clin N Am 2009; 19: 625–646

[73] Warburg O. On the origin of cancer cells. Science 1956; 123: 309–314

[74] Spence AM, Muzi M, Graham MM et al. Glucose metabolism in human malignant gliomas measured quantitatively with PET, 1-[C-11]glucose and FDG: analysis of the FDG lumped constant. J Nucl Med 1998; 39: 440–448

[75] Di Chiro G. Positron emission tomography using [18F] fluorodeoxyglucose in brain tumors. A powerful diagnostic and prognostic tool. Invest Radiol 1987; 22: 360–371

[76] Delbeke D, Meyerowitz C, Lapidus RL et al. Optimal cutoff levels of F-18 fluorodeoxyglucose uptake in the differentiation of low-grade from high-grade brain tumors with PET. Radiology 1995; 195: 47–52

[77] Olivero WC, Dulebohn SC, Lister JR. The use of PET in evaluating patients with primary brain tumours: is it useful? J Neurol Neurosurg Psychiatry 1995; 58: 250–252

[78] Ricci PE, Karis JP, Heiserman JE, Fram EK, Bice AN, Drayer BP. Differentiating recurrent tumor from radiation necrosis: time for re-evaluation of positron emission tomography? AJNR Am J Neuroradiol 1998; 19: 407–413

[79] Kawai N, Kagawa M, Miyake K et al. [Use of 11F-fluorothymidine positron emission tomography in brain tumor] No Shinkei Geka 2009; 37: 657–664

[80] Chao ST, Suh JH, Raja S, Lee SY, Barnett G. The sensitivity and specificity of FDG PET in distinguishing recurrent brain tumor from radionecrosis in patients treated with stereotactic radiosurgery. Int J Cancer 2001; 96: 191–197

[81] Wang SX, Boethius J, Ericson K. FDG-PET on irradiated brain tumor: ten years' summary. Acta Radiol 2006; 47: 85–90

[82] Spence AM, Muzi M, Mankoff DA et al. 18F-FDG PET of gliomas at delayed intervals: improved distinction between tumor and normal gray matter. J Nucl Med 2004; 45: 1653–1659

[83] Roelcke U, Radü EW, von Ammon K, Hausmann O, Maguire RP, Leenders KL. Alteration of blood-brain barrier in human brain tumors: comparison of [18F]fluorodeoxyglucose, [11C]methionine and rubidium-82 using PET. J Neurol Sci 1995; 132: 20–27

[84] Leskinen-Kallio S, Någren K, Lehikoinen P, Ruotsalainen U, Joensuu H. Uptake of 11C-methionine in breast cancer studied by PET. An association with the size of S-phase fraction. Br J Cancer 1991; 64: 1121–1124

[85] Herholz K, Hölzer T, Bauer B et al. 11C-methionine PET for differential diagnosis of low-grade gliomas. Neurology 1998; 50: 1316–1322

[86] Sonoda Y, Kumabe T, Takahashi T, Shirane R, Yoshimoto T. Clinical usefulness of 11C-MET PET and 201Tl SPECT for differentiation of recurrent glioma from radiation necrosis. Neurol Med Chir (Tokyo) 1998; 38: 342–347, discussion 347–348

[87] Wester HJ, Herz M, Weber W et al. Synthesis and radiopharmacology of O-(2-[18F]fluoroethyl)-L-tyrosine for tumor imaging. J Nucl Med 1999; 40: 205–212

[88] Pöpperl G, Götz C, Rachinger W, Gildehaus FJ, Tonn JC, Tatsch K. Value of O-(2-[18F]fluoroethyl)- L-tyrosine PET for the diagnosis of recurrent glioma. Eur J Nucl Med Mol Imaging 2004; 31: 1464–1470

[89] Chen W, Silverman DH, Delaloye S et al. 18F-FDOPA PET imaging of brain tumors: comparison study with 18F-FDG PET and evaluation of diagnostic accuracy. J Nucl Med 2006; 47: 904–911

[90] de Wolde H, Pruim J, Mastik MF, Koudstaal J, Molenaar WM. Proliferative activity in human brain tumors: comparison of histopathology and L-[1-(11)C]tyrosine PET. J Nucl Med 1997; 38: 1369–1374

[91] Kim CG, Yang DJ, Kim EE et al. Assessment of tumor cell proliferation using [18F]fluorodeoxyadenosine and[18F]fluoroethyluracil. J Pharm Sci 1996; 85: 339–344

[92] Carnochan P, Brooks R. Radiolabelled 5-iodo-2-deoxyuridine: a promising alternative to [18F]-2-fluoro-2-deoxy-D-glucose for PET studies of early response to anticancer treatment. Nucl Med Biol 1999; 26: 667–672

[93] Buchmann I, Vogg AT, Glatting G et al. [18F]5-fluoro-2-deoxyuridine-PET for imaging of malignant tumors and for measuring tissue proliferation. Cancer Biother Radiopharm 2003; 18: 327–337

[94] Eckel F, Herrmann K, Schmidt S et al. Imaging of proliferation in hepatocellular carcinoma with the in vivo marker 18F-fluorothymidine. J Nucl Med 2009; 50: 1441–1447

[95] Buck AK, Herrmann K, Shen C, Dechow T, Schwaiger M, Wester HJ. Molecular imaging of proliferation in vivo: positron emission tomography with [18F]fluorothymidine. Methods 2009; 48: 205–215

[96] Barwick T, Bencherif B, Mountz JM, Avril N. Molecular PET and PET/CT imaging of tumour cell proliferation using F-18 fluoro-L-thymidine: a comprehensive evaluation. Nucl Med Commun 2009; 30: 908–917

[97] Risau W, Flamme I. Vasculogenesis. Annu Rev Cell Dev Biol 1995; 11: 73–91

[98] Folkman J, Shing Y. Angiogenesis. J Biol Chem 1992; 267: 10931–10934

[99] Folkman J. Seminars in Medicine of the Beth Israel Hospital, Boston. Clinical applications of research on angiogenesis. N Engl J Med 1995; 333: 1757–1763

[100] Hillen F, Griffioen AW. Tumour vascularization: sprouting angiogenesis and beyond. Cancer Metastasis Rev 2007; 26: 489–502

[101] Döme B, Hendrix MJC, Paku S, Tóvári J, Tímár J. Alternative vascularization mechanisms in cancer: Pathology and therapeutic implications. Am J Pathol 2007; 170: 1–15

[102] Yu L, Su B, Hollomon M, Deng Y, Facchinetti V, Kleinerman ES. Vasculogenesis driven by bone marrow-derived cells is essential for growth of Ewing's sarcomas. Cancer Res 2010; 70: 1334–1343

[103] Patenaude A, Parker J, Karsan A. Involvement of endothelial progenitor cells in tumor vascularization. Microvasc Res 2010; 79: 217–223

[104] El Hallani S, Boisselier B, Peglion F et al. A new alternative mechanism in glioblastoma vascularization: tubular vasculogenic mimicry. Brain 2010; 133: 973–982

[105] Folkins C, Shaked Y, Man S et al. Glioma tumor stem-like cells promote tumor angiogenesis and vasculogenesis via vascular endothelial growth factor and stromal-derived factor 1. Cancer Res 2009; 69: 7243–7251

[106] Zhang ZG, Zhang L, Jiang Q, Chopp M. Bone marrow-derived endothelial progenitor cells participate in cerebral neovascularization after focal cerebral ischemia in the adult mouse. Circ Res 2002; 90: 284–288

[107] Tomanek RJ, Schatteman GC. Angiogenesis: new insights and therapeutic potential. Anat Rec 2000; 261: 126–135

[108] Hotfilder M, Nowak-Göttl U, Wolff JE. Tumorangiogenesis: a network of cytokines. Klin Padiatr 1997; 209: 265–270

[109] Asahara T, Murohara T, Sullivan A et al. Isolation of putative progenitor endothelial cells for angiogenesis. Science 1997; 275: 964–967

[110] Reyes M, Dudek A, Jahagirdar B, Koodie L, Marker PH, Verfaillie CM. Origin of endothelial progenitors in human postnatal bone marrow. J Clin Invest 2002; 109: 337–346

[111] Rafii S, Lyden D, Benezra R, Hattori K, Heissig B. Vascular and haematopoietic stem cells: novel targets for anti-angiogenesis therapy? Nat Rev Cancer 2002; 2: 826–835

[112] Lyden D, Hattori K, Dias S et al. Impaired recruitment of bone-marrow-derived endothelial and hematopoietic precursor cells blocks tumor angiogenesis and growth. Nat Med 2001; 7: 1194–1201

[113] Jiang Y, Jahagirdar BN, Reinhardt RL et al. Pluripotency of mesenchymal stem cells derived from adult marrow. Nature 2002; 418: 41–49

[114] Shichinohe H, Kuroda S, Yano S, Hida K, Iwasaki Y. Role of SDF-1/CXCR4 system in survival and migration of bone marrow stromal cells after transplantation into mice cerebral infarct. Brain Res 2007; 1183: 138–147

[115] Jin DK, Shido K, Kopp HG et al. Cytokine-mediated deployment of SDF-1 induces revascularization through recruitment of CXCR4 + hemangiocytes. Nat Med 2006; 12: 557–567

[116] Petit I, Jin D, Rafii S. The SDF-1-CXCR4 signaling pathway: a molecular hub modulating neo-angiogenesis. Trends Immunol 2007; 28: 299–307

[117] Ceradini DJ, Kulkarni AR, Callaghan MJ et al. Progenitor cell trafficking is regulated by hypoxic gradients through HIF-1 induction of SDF-1. Nat Med 2004; 10: 858–864

[118] Arbab AS, Janic B, Knight RA et al. Detection of migration of locally implanted AC133 + stem cells by cellular magnetic resonance imaging with histological findings. FASEB J 2008; 22: 3234–3246

[119] Moore MA, Hattori K, Heissig B et al. Mobilization of endothelial and hematopoietic stem and progenitor cells by adenovector-mediated elevation of serum levels of SDF-1, VEGF, and angiopoietin-1. Ann N Y Acad Sci 2001; 938: 36–45, discussion 45–47

[120] Heissig B, Hattori K, Dias S et al. Recruitment of stem and progenitor cells from the bone marrow niche requires MMP-9 mediated release of kit-ligand. Cell 2002; 109: 625–637

[121] Sheikh AY, Lin SA, Cao F et al. Molecular imaging of bone marrow mononuclear cell homing and engraftment in ischemic myocardium. Stem Cells 2007; 25: 2677–2684

[122] Sengupta N, Caballero S, Mames RN, Butler JM, Scott EW, Grant MB. The role of adult bone marrow-derived stem cells in choroidal neovascularization. Invest Ophthalmol Vis Sci 2003; 44: 4908–4913

[123] Schaefer BC, Schaefer ML, Kappler JW, Marrack P, Kedl RM. Observation of antigen-dependent CD8 + T-cell/ dendritic cell interactions in vivo. Cell Immunol 2001; 214: 110–122

[124] Varma NR, Janic B, Iskander AS et al. Endothelial progenitor cells (EPCs) as gene carrier system for rat model of human glioma. PLoS ONE 2012; 7: e30310

[125] Janic B, Jafari-Khouzani K, Babajani-Feremi A et al. MRI tracking of FePro labeled fresh and cryopreserved long term in vitro expanded human cord blood AC133 + endothelial progenitor cells in rat glioma. PLoS ONE 2012; 7: e37577

[126] Dai G, Levy O, Carrasco N. Cloning and characterization of the thyroid iodide transporter. Nature 1996; 379: 458–460

[127] Smanik PA, Liu Q, Furminger TL et al. Cloning of the human sodium iodide symporter. Biochem Biophys Res Commun 1996; 226: 339–345

[128] Barton KN, Xia X, Yan H et al. A quantitative method for measuring gene expression magnitude and volume delivered by gene therapy vectors. Mol Ther 2004; 9: 625–631

[129] Chen L, Altman A, Mier W, Lu H, Zhu R, Haberkorn U. 99mTc-pertechnetate uptake in hepatoma cells due to tissue-specific human sodium iodide symporter gene expression. Nucl Med Biol 200 2; 2006: 575–580

[130] Janic B, Arbab AS. Cord blood endothelial progenitor cells as therapeutic and imaging probes. Imaging Med 2012; 4: 477–490

[131] Van Gool S, Maes W, Ardon H, Verschuere T, Van Cauter S, De Vleeschouwer S. Dendritic cell therapy of high-grade gliomas. Brain Pathol 2009; 19: 694–712

[132] Yamanaka R. Dendritic-cell- and peptide-based vaccination strategies for glioma. Neurosurg Rev 2009; 32: 265–273, discussion 273

[133] Yamanaka R, Abe T, Yajima N et al. Vaccination of recurrent glioma patients with tumour lysate-pulsed dendritic cells elicits immune responses: results of a clinical phase I/II trial. Br J Cancer 2003; 89: 1172–1179

[134] Yamanaka R, Yajima N, Abe T et al. Dendritic cell-based glioma immunotherapy (review).(review) Int J Oncol 2003; 23: 5–15

[135] Saka M, Amano T, Kajiwara K et al. Vaccine therapy with dendritic cells transfected with Il13ra2 mRNA for glioma in mice. J Neurosurg 20 10; 113: 270–279

[136] Hatano M, Eguchi J, Tatsumi T et al. EphA2 as a glioma-associated antigen: a novel target for glioma vaccines. Neoplasia 2005; 7: 717–722

[137] Zhang JG, Eguchi J, Kruse CA et al. Antigenic profiling of glioma cells to generate allogeneic vaccines or dendritic cell-based therapeutics. Clin Cancer Res 2007; 13: 566–575

[138] Ni HT, Spellman SR, Jean WC, Hall WA, Low WC. Immunization with dendritic cells pulsed with tumor extract increases survival of mice bearing intracranial gliomas. J Neurooncol 2001; 51: 1–9

[139] Yang L, Ng KY, Lillehei KO. Cell-mediated immunotherapy: a new approach to the treatment of malignant glioma. Cancer Contr 2003; 10: 138–147

[140] Yu JS, Wheeler CJ, Zeltzer PM et al. Vaccination of malignant glioma patients with peptide-pulsed dendritic cells elicits systemic cytotoxicity and intracranial T-cell infiltration. Cancer Res 2001; 61: 842–847

[141] Yu JS, Liu G, Ying H, Yong WH, Black KL, Wheeler CJ. Vaccination with tumor lysate-pulsed dendritic cells elicits antigen-specific, cytotoxic T-cells in patients with malignant glioma. Cancer Res 2004; 64: 4973–4979

[142] Fields RC, Shimizu K, Mulé JJ. Murine dendritic cells pulsed with whole tumor lysates mediate potent antitumor immune responses in vitro and in vivo. Proc Natl Acad Sci U S A 1998; 95: 9482–9487

[143] Smithers M, O'Connell K, MacFadyen S et al. Clinical response after intradermal immature dendritic cell vaccination in metastatic melanoma is associated with immune response to particulate antigen. Cancer Immunol Immunother 20 13; 2003: 41–52

[144] Dembic Z, Schenck K, Bogen B. Dendritic cells purified from myeloma are primed with tumor-specific antigen (idiotype) and activate CD4 + T cells. Proc Natl Acad Sci U S A 2000; 97: 2697–2702

[145] Merchant RE, Baldwin NG, Rice CD, Bear HD. Adoptive immunotherapy of malignant glioma using tumor-sensitized T lymphocytes. Neurol Res 1997; 19: 145–152

[146] Arbab AS, Rad AM, Iskander AS et al. Magnetically-labeled sensitized splenocytes to identify glioma by MRI: a preliminary study. Magn Reson Med 2007; 58: 519–526

[147] Arbab AS, Janic B, Jafari-Khouzani K et al. Differentiation of glioma and radiation injury in rats using in vitro produce magnetically labeled cytotoxic T-cells and MRI. PLoS ONE 2010; 5: e9365

[148] Okano F, Storkus WJ, Chambers WH, Pollack IF, Okada H. Identification of a novel HLA-A*0201-restricted, cytotoxic T lymphocyte epitope in a human glioma-associated antigen, interleukin 13 receptor alpha2 chain. Clin Cancer Res 2002; 8: 2851–2855

[149] Hatano M, Kuwashima N, Tatsumi T et al. Vaccination with EphA2-derived T cell-epitopes promotes immunity against both EphA2-expressing and EphA2-negative tumors. J Transl Med 2004; 2: 40

[150] Pontes JE, Frost P, Pokorny M, Smith J. Gamma camera imaging of renal allografts using 111-InOx labelled autologous lymphocytes. Invest Urol 1980; 17: 451–453

[151] Clark DC, Morton ME, Dettman GL. Localization of 99mTc-labeled immune splenocytes at tumor site and detection by gamma camera imaging. Invest Radiol 1978; 13: 121–126

[152] Pozzilli P, Pozzilli C, Pantano P, Negri M, Andreani D, Cudworth AG. Tracking of indium-111-oxine labelled lymphocytes in autoimmune thyroid disease. Clin Endocrinol (Oxf) 1983; 19: 111–116

[153] Fisher B, Packard BS, Read EJ et al. Tumor localization of adoptively transferred indium-111 labeled tumor infiltrating lymphocytes in patients with metastatic melanoma. J Clin Oncol 1989; 7: 250–261

[154] Milgram R, Goodwin DA. Human scanning with In-111 oxine labeled autologous lymphocytes. Clin Nucl Med 1985; 10: 30–34

[155] Grimfors G, Schnell PO, Holm G et al. Tumour imaging of indium-111 oxine-labelled autologous lymphocytes as a staging method in Hodgkin's disease. Eur J Haematol 1989; 42: 276–283

[156] Chin Y, Janssens J, Bleus J, Zhang J, Raus J. In vivo distribution of radio-labeled tumor infiltrating lymphocytes in cancer patients. In Vivo 1993; 7: 27–30

[157] Haglund MM, Hochman DW, Spence AM, Berger MS. Enhanced optical imaging of rat gliomas and tumor margins. Neurosurgery 1994; 35: 930–940, discussion 940–941

[158] Sankar T, Delaney PM, Ryan RW et al. Miniaturized handheld confocal microscopy for neurosurgery: results in an experimental glioblastoma model. Neurosurgery 2010; 66: 410–417, discussion 417–418

[159] Eschbacher J, Martirosyan NL, Nakaji P et al. In vivo intraoperative confocal microscopy for real-time histopathological imaging of brain tumors. J Neurosurg 2012; 116: 854–860

[160] Sanai N, Snyder LA, Honea NJ et al. Intraoperative confocal microscopy in the visualization of 5-aminolevulinic acid fluorescence in low-grade gliomas. J Neurosurg 2011; 115: 740–748

[161] Sanai N, Eschbacher J, Hattendorf G et al. Intraoperative confocal microscopy for brain tumors: a feasibility analysis in humans. Neurosurgery 2011; 68 Suppl Operative: 282–290, discussion 290

[162] Zhou H, Luby-Phelps K, Mickey BE, Habib AA, Mason RP, Zhao D. Dynamic near-infrared optical imaging of 2-deoxyglucose uptake by intracranial glioma of athymic mice. PLoS ONE 2009; 4: e8051

[163] Zhao D, Stafford JH, Zhou H, Thorpe PE. Near-infrared Optical Imaging of Exposed Phosphatidylserine in a Mouse Glioma Model. Transl Oncol 2011; 4: 355–364

[164] Kepshire DS, Gibbs-Strauss SL, O'Hara JA et al. Imaging of glioma tumor with endogenous fluorescence tomography [published correction available in J Biomed Opt. 2009 May-Jun;14(3):039802. Gibbs-Strauss, Summer L corrected to Gibbs-Struass, Summer L]. J Biomed Opt 2009; 14: 030501

[165] Wen PY, Kesari S. Malignant gliomas in adults. N Engl J Med. 2008;359:492–507

[166] James ML, Gambhir SS. A molecular imaging primer: modalities, imaging agents, and applications. Physiol Rev. 2012;92:897–965

[167] Luker GD, Luker KE. Optical imaging: current applications and future directions. J Nucl Med. 2008;49:1–4

[168] Ntziachristos V, Yoo JS, van Dam GM. Current concepts and future perspectives on surgical optical imaging in cancer. J Biomed Opt. 2010;15:066024